Poisoning

The home is loaded with poisons: Cosmetics, Detergents, Bleaches, Cleaning Solutions, Glue, Lye, Paint, Turpentine, Kerosene, Gasoline and other petroleum products, Alcohol, Aspirin and other medications, and on and on.

1. Small children are most often the victims of accidental poisoning. If a child has swallowed or is suspected to have swallowed any substance that might be poisonous, assume the worst—TAKE ACTION.

2. Call your Poison Control Center. If none is in your area, call your emergency medical rescue squad. Bring suspected item and container with you.

3. What you can do if the victim is unconscious:

   A. Make sure patient is breathing. If not, tilt head back and perform mouth to mouth breathing. Do not give anything by mouth. Do not attempt to stimulate person. **Call Emergency Rescue Squad immediately.**

4. If the victim is vomiting:

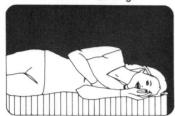

   A. Roll him or her over onto **the left side** so that the person will not choke on what is brought up.

5. Be prepared. Determine and verify your Poison Control Center and Fire Department Rescue Squad Numbers and keep them on your telephone.

Drug Overdose

A drug overdose is a poisoning. Alcohol is as much a poison as stimulants, tranquilizers, narcotics, hallucinogens or inhalants. Don't take drunkenness lightly.   Too much alcohol can kill.

1. Call for emergency help at once.

2. Check the victim's breathing and pulse. If breathing has stopped or is very weak give Rescue Breathing. Caution: Reviving victims of alcohol poisoning can be violent. Be careful! They can harm themselves and others.

3. While waiting for help:

   A. Watch breathing.
   B. Cover the person with a blanket for warmth.
   C. **Do not** throw water on the victim's face.
   D. **Do not** give **liquor** or a stimulant.

Remember: alcohol in combination with certain other drugs **can be deadly!**

Burns

1. Minor burns caused by fire, covering only a small area of the body:

   A. Can be treated with **cold running water** or an **ice pack** applied for 20 to 30 minutes to relieve swelling and pain.
   B. Do not use grease of any kind. Cold running water is the best first aid.

2. Serious burns:

   A. Require prompt professional care. **Call for help immediately.**
   B. Wrap the victim in a **clean, wet sheet** or towel moistened at room temperature.
   C. **Burn victims need fluid.** Give the victim **all the water he or she desires.**
   D. **Do not attempt to clean the burns** or remove clothing or other particles attached to the burnt area.
   E. Keep the victim lying down, calm and reassured.

3. Eye burns:

   A. Should be **flushed with large amounts of water.** Then cover the eye with a damp, clean towel and **get emergency medical care** as soon as possible.

4. Electrical burns:

   A. Are difficult to detect. A person who has received a severe electrical shock may have badly burned underlying tissue, though the surface skin shows little evidence.
   B. **Get the victim prompt medical attention.** Unattended electrical burns can lead to serious complications.

5. Chemical burns:

   A. Should be washed with **plenty of cool, running water.** Get the victim into **a cool shower,** if possible.
   B. After 10 minutes, wrap him or her in a wet, clean sheet and **get emergency medical attention without delay.**

THE NEW ILLUSTRATED
MEDICAL AID
ENCYCLOPEDIA

First Aid and Emergencies

Medical Contributors

James A. Brussel, M.D.
Assistant Commissioner
Department of Mental Hygiene
State of New York

J. Moore Campbell, M.D.
Clinical Professor of Surgery
School of Medicine
University of Oklahoma

Everett N. Cobb, D.D.S.
Assistant Professor of Operative Dentistry
School of Dentistry
Georgetown University

E.V. Cowdry, Ph.D.
Professor Emeritus of Anatomy
School of Medicine
Washington University

Loren T. DeWind, M.D.
Assistant Clinical Professor of Medicine
School of Medicine
University of Southern California
and California College of Medicine

Mauricio J. Dulfano, M.D.
Assistant Professor of Medicine
School of Medicine
Tufts University

Thomas W. Farmer, M.D.
Head, Division of Neurology
School of Medicine
The University of North Carolina

Roald N. Grant, M.D.
Director of Professional Education
American Cancer Society

Leonard D. Grayson, M.D.
Clinical Assistant, Allergy Clinic
Medical School
Washington University

Robert A. Hansen, M.D.
Medical Director
Travelers Insurance Company, Los Angeles

Wade B. Irwin Sr., D.D.S.
Assistant Professor of Operative Dentistry
School of Dentistry
Georgetown University

Naomi M. Kanof, M.D.
Chairman, Editorial Board
The Journal of Investigative Dermatology

Jules Kaplan, M.D.
Instructor, Department of Otolaryngology
Medical School
Northwestern University

Mitchell Kory, Ph.D.
Senior Scientist
The Lilly Research Laboratories

Frank W. Newell, M.D.
Professor of Ophthalmology
Eye Research Laboratories
The University of Chicago

Art. H. Panayis, M.D.
Assistant Chief
Department of Obstetrics-Gynecology
Baltimore City Hospitals

Ira A. Roschelle, M.D.
Chief Resident Orthopedic Surgeon
Hospital for Joint Diseases, New York

Isadore Rossman, M.D.
Chief of Professional Services
Home Care Department
Montefiore Hospital, New York

Goodrich C. Schauffler, M.D.
Associate Clinical Professor of
Gynecology and Obstetrics, Medical School
University of Oregon

Lendon H. Smith, M.D.
Assistant Clinical Professor of Pediatrics
Medical School
University of Oregon

Frederick C. Thorne, M.D., Ph.D.
Editor, *Journal of Clinical Psychology*

James L. Troupin, M.D.
Director of Professional Education
The American Public Health Association

S.O. Waife, M.D.
Assistant Director, Medical Research Division
The Lilly Research Laboratories

Editor

Leroy E. Burney, M.D.
Vice President of Health Sciences
Temple University
Formerly Surgeon General
of the United States

Editorial Assistant

Genon Hickerson Neblett

Updating Editors

Alice C. Ewing

John A. Fribley

Teri K. Mitchell

ROYAL PUBLISHERS, INC.
NASHVILLE, TENNESSEE 37214

Published in Nashville, Tennessee, by Thomas Nelson, Inc., Publishers and distributed in Canada by Lawson Falle, Ltd., Cambridge, Ontario.

A compilation of material from earlier editions:
    ©1978 Royal Publishers, Inc.
    ©1965, 1972 Stravon Publishers, Inc.

Library of Congress Cataloging-in-Publication Data

The New illustrated medical aid encyclopedia.

    Includes index.
    1. Medicine, Popular--Dictionaries. I. Brussel,
James Arnold, 1905-   . II. Burney, Leroy E.
(Leroy Edgar), 1906-   . III. Title: Medical aid
encyclopedia.
RC81.A2N438 1988   610'.3'21   88-4630
ISBN 0-8407-3007-1

Manufactured in the United States of America

2 3 4 5 6 7 8 9 10 - 97 96 95 94 93 92 91 90 89 88

Preface

L IKE MOST PEOPLE IN our country, you and your family are today more health-conscious than ever before. At the same time, dramatic progress has been made, and continues to be made, in developing new lifesaving and life-giving medical techniques. Every day doctors learn more about the human body, its chemistry, its physical reactions, and its interrelation with the mind.

This encyclopedia attempts to coordinate this new knowledge and relate it to your own interest in good health, in ways that will help you and your family obtain the fullest possible benefits from the major advances of modern medicine. The distinguished physicians and scientists who have written this book present what they consider to be the essential, up-to-date facts on the symptoms, diagnosis, prevention, and treatment of the diseases and disabilities we are likely to encounter today. They tell the facts simply, in language the layman can readily grasp.

As a better informed family—and using this book for ready reference—you will know when to seek medical advice, and will be better able to understand and follow such advice as well as whatever treatment your physician prescribes. Please keep in mind, however, that this is *not* an encyclopedia of home remedies, nor does it replace the need for professional medical care. Importantly, it does outline for you the steps to be taken should an emergency arise, telling you exactly what to do and what not to do until the doctor comes. There are also suggestions on how to care for members of your family at home.

Many changes have occurred in our society within our lifetime which affect the patterns of illness and disability and make it more essential than ever before for you to be well informed. Our population continues to increase—every year adds two to three million more. The two age groups with the greatest proportional gains are the very young and the aging. More than all others, these two groups require medical care. In addition, their health problems are fairly unique: congenital defects, immunization, and infant nutrition are important problems in the very young; cancer, chronic diseases, and mental health are most prevalent among the aging.

The number of reported cases of venereal disease, sexually transmitted diseases, has soared during the past decade. The numbers continue to rise each month in cases of AIDS, genital herpes, and others. Doctors and research teams have discovered several related complications including pelvic inflammatory disease (PID), recurring infections, and sterility. What can be cured? How does one contract these diseases and how may they be avoided? These and other questions are answered in the special section, Sexually Transmitted Diseases.

Our population is highly mobile—about thirty-five million change residence each year. This increases the family's problems in connection with establishing a relationship with a family doctor or with specialists. On the other hand—and this is an indication of our increased health consciousness—where thirty years ago the average person saw a doctor two or three times a year at best, today the annual average has risen to five visits and even more, especially in the cities. As the cost of medical care continues to rise, more people are turning to nonprescription medications. The FDA has increased the number and variety available to the public without a doctor's prescription. With the help of your pharmacist, you can treat minor symptoms of colds and flus, cuts, burns, and many others. Helpful information appears in the special section covering over-the-counter medications.

In 1930 almost half of all patient visits were made in homes—today only one visit in ten is a home call by the physician. Care has been moved from the home to the hospital or other health care institution. This is as it should be, since hospitals are equipped with staffs possessing a broad range of skills; with laboratories to perform the ever-increasing number of tests to aid your own doctor in making a correct diagnosis and instituting proper treatment; with X-ray and other expensive and complex resources, all of which are essential to modern diagnosis and treatment.

Again, many surgical operations are being performed which only ten or fifteen years ago were considered impossible. For example, entire lungs are removed, various types of heart defects are repaired, segments of blood vessels are replaced by synthetic substitutes, and corneas are transplanted from one eye to another to restore sight. Patients are being helped by new heart drugs, improved anesthesia, bone graft banks and blood vessel banks, artificial heart, lung, and kidney machines, and many other miraculous lifesaving devices.

These and many other new developments are discussed in our book, making it possible for you to have an intelligent opinion about the progress of modern medicine as you read about it in magazines and the daily press. For instance, programs, such as community-wide polio immunization and fluoridation of the water supply, demand broad support for success; but such support is not possible without a well-informed public.

Moreover, encouraging and gratifying as our medical advances may be, their great promise is not yet being fulfilled for the simple reason that not enough of us are making the fullest possible use of this ever-increasing body of scientific knowledge. Only the well-informed can effectively apply such knowledge, preventing disease before it ever begins, and if it does, preventing irreparable damage by early diagnosis and treatment. To give only one example—it is all-important for every woman to know at what age—and how often—she should begin to avail herself of that effective early-screening technique for detection of cancer of the cervix, the life-saving cell cytology test.

It cannot be emphasized too often that keeping you and your family healthy requires you to be well informed, to accept personal responsibility for initiative and action in this area. The important diseases which strike today are no longer those susceptible to mass prevention and treatment, as was the case a generation ago. In the first part of this century, for instance, the major causes of illness and death in children were the diarrheas and dysenteries and such contagious diseases as diphtheria, whooping cough, and measles. The first two groups have been effectively controlled and all but eradicated by means of safe water supply, improved disposal of human waste, pasteurization of milk, refrigeration, and the availability of canned baby foods. Typhoid has almost disappeared except for an occasional minor outbreak, not so much as a result of what each individual does for himself but of what the community has done for all of us by developing a safe, chlorinated water supply, replacing pit privies with sewage systems, and enacting milk and food ordinances to ensure sanitary standards and quality.

Where once whole communities were incapacitated due to malaria, today state, regional, and local government mosquito-eradication programs have so changed the picture that it is now rare to have a case of malaria reported in any of our Southern states. Mass immunization with improved vaccines against diptheria, whooping cough, poliomyelitis and, most recently, measles have largely controlled these diseases on a mass basis.

All of this serves to underscore that the average increased life expectancy at birth to seventy years, as well as the lowered mortality rates, are due in the main to our rising educational and economic levels, improved environment, and the development of preventive biologics. Yet the fact remains that the average life expectancy at the age of fifty has increased by only three or four years since 1900. This only emphasizes that the prevention and treatment of heart disease, cancer, arthritis, diabetes, mental illness, and the other chronic diseases do not respond to mass therapy, and hence require vigilance and initiative on your part in recognizing early symptoms and seeking prompt medical advice and care.

This encyclopedia can be of invaluable help to you in meeting this individual responsibility more intelligently, for it makes accurate information on symptoms, as well as sound advice on when to seek diagnosis and treatment, readily available. Descriptions of diseases and disabling illnesses are followed by the specialists' suggestions as to accepted forms of treatment. It is also explained how and to what extent symptoms may vary in individual cases, and that therapy must therefore be related to individual needs.

The highly qualified authors have presented their best opinions on the diagnosis and treatment of a broad spectrum of diseases and health problems. But since, as we have just mentioned, individual treatment of a specific disease may vary to some extent, you will be wise to follow your own physician's advice carefully, inasmuch as he is the one diagnosing and treating you—or someone in your family—as an individual.

How to use this health care guide

THE MEDICAL AID ENCYCLOPEDIA FOR THE HOME is the first of five sections and consists of a series of alphabetically arranged medical entries; the second covers first aid and emergencies; the third explains the use of nonprescription medicines; the fourth covers sexually transmitted diseases; the fifth consists of patients' questions and doctors' answers; the last describes various public agencies that, under certain conditions, can be of great help to the family. In addition to the six sections, there are hundreds of illustrations, including eighty pages of full-color plates. These eighty pages are designed as ten 8-page color inserts. Each insert may be considered either as descriptive of some part of the main text, or as a complete unit in itself. To help the reader quickly find what he is looking for there is a comprehensive index at the end of the book. An Emergency Survival Guide is printed on the endsheet.

The section containing the medical entries describes most of today's common diseases, giving symptoms and treatment (if known), and because of the alphabetical arrangement it is a simple matter to turn to the right page to find the sought-for-entry.

The First Aid and Emergencies section contains a general discussion followed by an alphabetically arranged description of the most common first aid and emergency situations and methods of coping with them.

The Over-the-Counter Medications section gives general information on nonprescription drugs, including FDA standards, labeling, food and drug interactions. You will learn how to choose and make the most of your local pharmacist. In addition there is a comprehensive section on the most common pain reliever, aspirin, with a helpful dosage schedule for children.

The Sexually Transmitted Diseases section explains the symptoms and possible complications of the most prevalent infections. This section includes a detailed chart outlining signs, symptoms, and special considerations. The material should answer some of your questions and lead you to sources for further information.

The Question and Answer section contains typical questions put to doctors by their patients and the doctors' answers. The questions and answers are arranged in groups, thus questions of a cardiac nature are grouped together, just as questions of a psychological nature are grouped together, etc.

The Helpful Public Agencies section describes the services of a wide range of public and semipublic organizations that aid the family with information or direct help in dealing with the problems of communicable diseases, prenatal and infant care, school health services, medical and hospital care, etc.

The reader should refer to the comprehensive index in order to find entries or discussions that at first glance do not appear in the book. Frequently, an entry is listed by its medical name, but the index will also list it by its common (popular) name. Occasionally (where no separate entry for a disease can be found), a discussion of the particular disease or condition is included in a general discussion covering an entire group of diseases, but the index will contain a reference to this specific condition or ailment and, of course, the page number where it is mentioned will be given.

Contents

Color Inserts

Anatomical and Medical illustrations by
Leonard D. Dank

Illustrations by
George Geygan
Tom Armstrong
Ellen Zink

MEDICAL AID ENCYCLOPEDIA

FOR THE HOME

Medical Encyclopedia

ABDOMINAL PAIN Pain in the abdominal region is a symptom of many diseases which may either be of no consequence at all or extremely serious. Pain may arise from structures within the abdomen, or it may be referred from an extra-abdominal site.

Common abdominal disorders which cause pain include: appendicitis, gastroenteritis, peptic ulcer, colitis, hernias, intestinal obstructions, tumors, regional ileitis, diverticulitis, and colic. Many genito-urinary disorders, such as kidney stones, urinary-tract infections, tumors, pregnancy and its complications, inflammation of the pelvis, menstrual cramps, and ovarian cysts can cause abdominal pain. Diseases of associated organs (gallbladder, liver, pancreas, and peritoneum) are other sources.

Conditions that arise in other locations but may cause abdominal pain include: pneumonia, heart disease, neuritis, disorders of the blood, blood clots, systemic infections, spinal arthritis, and poisons such as lead and arsenic.

Symptoms. The description of the pain is most important in helping the physician in determining the cause. Such characteristics as onset, location, severity, and the methods that the patient uses to obtain relief are important. Certain types of pain are more or less characteristic of a specific condition. Thus, pain which occurs after eating a fatty meal and which tends to radiate under the right shoulder blade is often seen in cholecystitis. Peptic ulcer pain often occurs one or two hours after eating and is sharply localized in the upper mid-abdomen. Acute intestinal obstruction will often cause increasingly severe colicky pain with relief between spasms. Flank pain which is associated with bloody urine and which radiates into the genitalia or inner thigh is commonly seen with kidney stones. Tubal (ectopic) pregnancy can cause severe abdominal pain, and a history of a missed period with sudden shock and vaginal bleeding should alert one to this possibility. A coronary thrombosis may cause abdominal pain. Shingles (herpes zoster), which is a virus infection of the nerve root, can cause severe burning abdominal pain which is difficult to differentiate from other conditions until the characteristic blisters appear.

ABORTION An abortion occurs when a pregnancy is terminated before the unborn child has developed enough to survive outside the womb. An aborted pregnancy may be the result of a physical or psychological disorder (and may be termed a miscarriage). Also, an abortion may be deliberately induced by a physician because of complications that threaten the well-being of the woman, or because the woman chooses not to complete her pregnancy.

A baby born before the fifth month of pregnancy rarely survives. At this stage the baby weighs about a pound and, although a few babies of this weight have lived, babies usually must be carried for at least six and a half to seven months before the infant's organs are developed enough to allow normal physical and mental development. Babies delivered before the fifth month are therefore called abortions or miscarriages. Babies born between the fifth and seventh months are called immature, and their chances of survival are very poor. Those born between the seventh and ninth months are called premature, weighing less than five and one half pounds; with modern pediatric care most of them do very well. Finally, full-term babies are those born during the last month of pregnancy; they usually weigh over five and one half pounds.

Approximately 10 percent of all pregnancies end as miscarriages; many of these could be prevented with proper and specialized obstetrical care.

Common causes of miscarriages are abnormalities of the sperm or of the egg (ovum), resulting in abnormal conception. Such abnormalities usually cannot be treated and produce early miscarriages. There may be inefficiently functioning glands in the mother, such as the thyroid and the ovaries; such abnormalities can usually be detected and treated. Deformities of the womb (uterus)—tumors, congenital malformations, or inability of the mouth of the womb to hold the fetus (incompetent cervix)—may cause miscarriages. Nutritional and other chronic disorders, including emotional stress, may also precipitate a miscarriage.

Symptoms. Most miscarriages start with moderate vaginal bleeding, which is usually followed by lower abdominal pains (cramps), passage of clots of blood, and eventually the passage of the fetus and afterbirth. However, "spotting" or slight bleeding during early pregnancy is not necessarily a sign of foredoomed miscarriage; if such a condition occurs a physician should be consulted.

If the whole fetus and afterbirth are delivered, the miscarriage is termed complete. If, however, only parts of them are expelled, the miscarriage is incomplete. Occasionally the fetus dies in the womb and remains there for days or weeks before it is delivered.

Treatment. The treatment of an impending or completed miscarriage should always be undertaken by a qualified physician. The pregnant woman should always seek advice at the first evidence of bleeding or of lower-abdominal pains. In consultation with the patient, a decision will be made whether the pregnancy can continue, or whether the patient's best interests require an abortion.

Medical techniques currently used to induce abortion include vacuum aspiration, where the uterus lining including the embryo is removed by suction, and dilation and curettage, where the cervix is dilated and the womb lining plus the embryo is then scraped out. Abortion may also be induced by the injection of a saline solution into the amniotic sac.

A 1973 Supreme Court ruling established the legality of abortion "on request," and within the first trimester of a pregnancy the decision to abort is solely between the woman and her physician. After this period, states may limit or even prohibit abortions, excepting those that safeguard the woman's health or life.

For religious, moral, and other reasons, however, many women oppose abortion. If only because of the emotional trauma an abortion may cause, women should be aware of all of their options, including giving the child for adoption or foster care and keeping the child to rear themselves.

ABRASION   Abrasion is the abnormal wearing-away of the surface of a tooth, usually due to some mechanical cause. This may occur on any exposed surface of the tooth, including a portion of the root, if it is not protected by the covering of the gingiva. Abnormal wearing-away of teeth should be distinguished from that which is normal (attrition).

When abrasion results from faulty brushing, the abraded region is usually located on the area of the necks of the teeth which face the lips or cheeks, and the area is wedge-shaped. It is interesting to note that abrasion due to overzealous brushing, or to the use of excessively abrasive cleaning agents, will be more severe on the left side of the arch for right handed "brushers" and on the right side for left handed ones.

Abrasion may also be caused by other factors:

1. Toothpick, dental floss, and dental tape—the indiscriminate use of any of these may result in abrasion of the surfaces between the teeth at their neck.
2. The repeated biting of thread; opening of bobby pins; holding of tacks, nails, needles, or a pipe in the teeth may result in an abraded area on the biting edge, which is notched.
3. The habitual use of chewing tobacco, betel nuts, or the accidental ingestion of abrasive agents such as sand (sand-blasters) or other dust will result in the abrasion of the biting surfaces of the crowns.

Abrasion which results in a thinning or loss of the protective enamel may result in exposure of the more sensitive underlying dentin, resulting in pain which may require treatment by the dentist.

ABSCESS   This term describes a localized collection of pus within the tissues which is surrounded by a "limiting" membrane. The symptoms of an abscess may be swelling, redness, pain, and heat. Two important types are: periapical abscess—one occurring at the apical (apex) region of a tooth due to the death of the pulp tissue (see ROOT-CANAL TREATMENT); and periodontal abscess—one occurring in the tissues immediately surrounding the tooth, such as gingiva, bone, or the periodontal membrane. An abscess which breaks through its limiting membrane, burrowing through the surrounding bone to the external soft tissue, may result in a gum boil. As the contents accumulate, increased pressure will cause rupture of tissue and drainage of the pus into the oral cavity.

ABSCESS, PERITONSILLAR   If infection of the palatine tonsils breaks through the surrounding tissues, an abscess—a localized collection of pus—can occur.

Symptoms. The patient has great difficulty in swallowing and there is a bad odor to the breath. There is also difficulty in opening the mouth because of inflammation of the jaw muscles.

Treatment. The abscess should be cut into (incised) and drained by the physician. Rapid relief of pain usually occurs when the pressure is relieved.

ABSCESS, RETROPHARYNGEAL   An abscess-formation behind the pharyngeal wall and in front of the neck bones or vertebrae (visible in infants and very young children) may be secondary to an infection of the pharynx.

Symptoms. There is difficulty in breathing and sore throat associated with fever.

Treatment. The abscess must be drained in such a way that the infected material is not sucked into the lungs. Antibiotics are used after the drainage.

ABSORPTION   Absorption as used in a biologic sense, is the transport of materials across a barrier and incorporation into the tissue itself. Food and water, from one end of the alimentary canal to the other, may still be considered to be "outside" the body. Not until the substances cross the thin cellular lining of the stomach and intestines, and are picked up by the circulating blood and lymph, do the products of digestion become part of the body, that is, become "absorbed."

Little except alcohol is absorbed in the stomach. The basic components of food (protein, fat, and carbohydrate) must be sufficiently digested, broken down into smaller basic molecular units, before they can be absorbed. Digestion is carried out through the action of enzymes, chiefly in the first foot or so of the small intestine (duodenum). Absorption of foodstuff, however, takes place largely in the latter part of the small intestine (jejunum and ileum).

Water is absorbed, excreted back into the digestive canal, and reabsorbed, in a continuous dynamic state of flux. Most of the water, including the liquid portion of the gastrointestinal juices, is finally absorbed in the large intestine. When motility is increased, there is insufficient time for water reabsorption; the bowel contents are then liquid (diarrhea). Prolonged activity of reabsorptive mechanisms leads to the dry stool of constipation.

Absorption involves complex physical factors, such as the size and concentration of the molecules; water-salt concentration; surface tension; and active transport by the cells, which do chemical work and use energy in the process of transferring molecules across cell membranes.

Proteins and carbohydrates are broken down into their component parts: amino acids and simple sugars, respectively. These are then absorbed directly in the blood capillaries in the intestinal walls and carried by the circulating blood to the liver where they undergo many chemical changes.

Fat is split into fatty acids and glycerol in the intestine. These, in a complex way, are absorbed by tiny lymphatic vessels (lacteals) which eventually collect into larger vessels that empty into the veins.

The absorption of drugs, vitamins, and minerals is also based on passive diffusion or active transport mechanisms, many of which are still poorly understood.

ACCOMMODATION   The crystalline lens of the eye is changed in shape by the action of the ciliary muscle so that objects are clearly focused on the back of the eye. Thus the normal individual is able to see objects clearly both at near and far distances. With increasing age the lens loses its elasticity, and after the age of forty to forty-five, glasses are necessary for clear vision at near distance.

ACHLORHYDRIA   This term refers to the complete absence of acid-production by the stomach. It has been estimated that this condition is present in between 10 and 20 per cent of all individuals over the age of fifty and is therefore usually not associated with any particular disease or symptom. The importance of the condition lies in the fact that several serious disorders may be associated with absence of acid: pernicious anemia, gastric polyps, cancer of the stomach, and (sometimes) certain vitamin deficiency diseases. Less commonly, it may accompany certain chronic diseases such as nephritis, diabetes, chronic alcoholism, chronic cholecystitis, and colitis.

Symptoms. Few if any symptoms can be specifically ascribed to achlorhydria. Complete digestion of proteins and fats will still occur due to pancreatic and intestinal enzymes. Rarely, some cases of diarrhea may be associated with achlorhydria and respond to administration of dilute hydrochloric acid by mouth. Achlorhydria may be produced by X-irradiation of the stomach, a treatment sometimes resorted to for chronic peptic ulcer.

Treatment. Usually little or no treatment is required, but it is desirable to have reasonably frequent medical check-ups because of the possibility of the existence of certain conditions which are occasionally associated with it. The diet should be balanced and easily digestible.

ACIDOSIS   The body has a superb mechanism for maintaining the proper acidity-alkalinity of its tissues. This delicate and sensitive system involves: (1) buffering substances in the blood; (2) sensing areas in the central nervous system; and (3) careful control of carbon dioxide-oxygen transfer in the lungs.

A state of excess acidity not compensated for by bodily means is known as acidosis. (In reality, the term is used when there is depletion of alkali.) This condition occurs in connection with several disorders, among them, uncontrolled diabetes, kidney disease, and severe diarrhea.

The body normally produces an excess quantity of acidic substances. Most are neutralized by the free alkaline (basic) elements, particularly the sodium in plasma. (This sodium comes from sodium bicarbonate. When sodium combines with an acid, the remaining bicarbonate is converted into carbon dioxide which is breathed out.) Other acid-eliminating reactions also occur.

Symptoms. Weakness, nausea, and vomiting are common in acidosis. The breath may have a sweetish fruity odor. Drowsiness may proceed to coma in which a characteristic breathing pattern is seen.

Treatment. Treatment requires hospitalization for proper chemical determinations which are guides for fluid and (electrolyte) alkali replacement. In diabetic acidosis and coma, insulin, fluids, sodium, potassium, and other substances must be given promptly.

ACID STOMACH   The term acid stomach is misleading. The stomach (gastric) juice should be—and normally is—acidic. The acidity is actually an aid to digestion; indeed, lack of gastric acidity can lead to definite complications.

The phrase, as used in everyday speech, is applied to a sense of burning, irritation, or distress felt at the lower edge of the "wishbone" (sternum); this minor gastrointestinal sensation may be due to regurgitation of stomach contents up into the lower segment of the esophagus. True gastric hyperacidity is another matter and is discussed in the entry GASTRITIS.

ACNE   Beginning in early adolescence, and often the first symptom of glandular change, acne is a disease of varying intensity and unpredictable duration. It can remain an insignificant condition consisting of scattered blackheads and some greasiness of the face for its entire course. Papules, pustules, cysts, and scars can develop at a very early age or appear suddenly in the late teens; recurrences after a seeming cure are not uncommon; absence of any evidence of acne in adolescence is rare. Severe eruptions are not necessarily of lengthy duration, and mild cases are not necessarily short-lived. Because it is impossible to predict with any certainty either the degree of involvement of the skin or the length of time the condition can be expected to last, it is advisable to treat even mild cases of acne in an attempt to control the eruption and minimize residual scarring.

Occurring as it does at a crucial time in the lives of young people already burdened with problems arising from rapid growth, both physical and emotional, the patient's reaction to the various degrees of unpleasantness of appearance ranges widely from feigned or real indifference to arrogant insistence on "immediate cure" to complete social withdrawal. The emotional response to acne depends more on the personality of the patient than on the severity of the condition. So, because it may be possible to avoid permanent damage to the skin and, just as importantly, to improve the immediate disfigurement with its emotional and social consequences,

ACNE

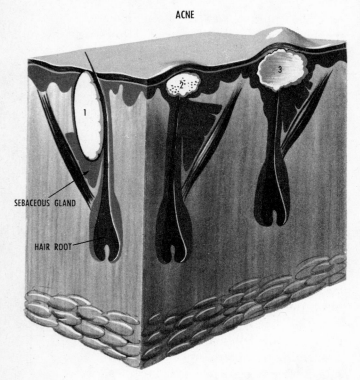

SEBACEOUS GLAND

HAIR ROOT

1 Acne usually begins as a comedo (blackhead), a blocked accumulation of sebaceous gland secretion.

2 If the comedo becomes inflamed, a prominent hard, red papule develops.

3 If the papule becomes infected, pus-filled pustules develop which finally burst.

treatment is necessary and is usually effective.

Overactivity of the sebaceous (oil) glands causes the many types of lesions comprising the acne syndrome: blackheads, whiteheads, papules, and cysts. Any of the types of lesions may occur in combination or may appear as the only manifestation of the disease. Because the sebaceous glands are so abundant on the face, chest, and back, these are the usual sites of involvement. Oiliness of the skin is also usually present as a result of the heightened activity of the sebaceous glands. Scarring is commonly the aftermath of large destructive lesions, but may follow even uncomplicated blackheads or be the result of self-induced injury (picking).

Acne of the newborn is an infrequent but nevertheless well-known condition which disappears in a few weeks with little or no treatment when the causative maternal hormones are completely excreted. A more common form of acne, and longer lasting, is that found in middle-aged women. In this condition, the lesions are usually cystic and pustular and are likely to be concentrated on the chin. Acne lesions are also found in rosacea, in forms of tuberculosis of the skin, and constitute one of the undesirable side-effects of cortisone therapy.

The fundamental cause of acne is almost certainly an imbalance in hormone secretion, the nature of which is not presently known. Adding to the difficulties of ascertaining the basic mechanisms in acne are "secondary" factors such as foods, stress, and the psyche, which often sustain or enhance or possibly even initiate the condition. The often-observed benefits of season (summer) and climate (seashore) are probably the result of the drying effect of sunlight, the freedom from stressful school situations during the summer recess, the change of dietary and sleep habits, subtle differences in metabolism, etc. The significance of menstrual-related flare-ups in girls is not clear, but this occurrence does afford a clue to the type of hormonal imbalance and a possible therapeutic approach. Similarly, flare-ups during pregnancy, and disappearance of otherwise persistent acne during pregnancy, are also suggestive of the endocrine causation of this disease.

Treatment. Mild cases can be benefited by the use of simple drying measures including frequent washing with ordinary toilet soap and with the application of drying lotions and pastes (containing resorcin, precipitated sulfur, etc.) now available "over-the-counter" in the pharmacy; dietary restrictions (avoiding chocolate, nuts, shellfish); adequate sleep; medical supervision to check on foci of infection, on anemia, on constipation, etc.

More extensive or persistent involvement may necessitate X-ray treatments to reduce the activity of the sebaceous glands; antibiotics and sulfonamides for control of the pustular lesions; vitamin A to relieve the plugging of the blackheads; surgical drainage of destructive cystic lesions; dermabrasion, dry-ice peeling or other repair of residual scars.

ACOUSTIC NEUROMA   A tumor may arise just at the point where the facial and acoustic nerves enter the temporal bone. Hearing loss, poor understanding of speech, and (later) facial weakness can then occur. The diagnosis is frequently made by the otologist, neurologist, or neurosurgeon. Even though hearing loss is involved, surgery for this problem is carried out by the neurosurgeon.

ACOUSTIC TRAUMA   Continued very loud sound or even a single extremely loud blast may lead to noise-induced hearing loss. In reversible cases there may be some tinnitus, accompanied by the sensation of "listening in a barrel." The hearing may then return. Sometimes, however, the hearing loss is permanent. Those, therefore, who are exposed to loud sounds (such as rifle or skeet shooters) should wear ear plugs as protection against noise-induced hearing loss.

ACROMEGALY   In this condition there is enlargement of the hands and feet, with marked prominence of the jaw, thickness of the lips and tongue, and unusual enlargement of internal organs. The disease develops gradually and is usually accompanied by severe headaches. It is caused by a tumor of the anterior pituitary gland. As the tumor grows there develops pressure against the optic nerves, producing defects in vision. Effects on the other endocrine glands ensue when the tumor grows to such a size that it destroys by pressure the remainder of the anterior pituitary gland. Activity of the thyroid, ad-

renals, and sex glands is depressed.

Treatment. Treatment is by means of surgical removal or by X-ray irradiation. The latter form of treatment is usually preferred and is very satisfactory—particularly where the radiation dose can be accurately delivered to the pituitary gland by modern techniques.

ACTH   ACTH is the abbreviation for *a*dreno*c*orti*c*o*t*rophic *h*ormone. It was first made available for clinical testing in 1946. This hormone is secreted by the anterior pituitary gland and stimulates the adrenal glands to secrete cortisone and other substances. It is the normal regulator of adrenal gland function in healthy people. It has been extracted from pituitary glands and in purified form is used in the treatment of some forms of arthritis, lupus erythematosus, and severe skin disorders. The beneficial effects of injected ACTH result from its stimulation of the adrenal gland cortex, which releases large quantities of naturally formed cortisone.

ACTINOMYCOSIS   The fungus *Actinomyces bovis* is ubiquitous and causes disease under conditions (devitalized tissue) favorable to its growth. Commonly present on the face in the areas of the jaws (hence known as lumpy jaw), the organism is likely to grow well in the aftermath of poor dentition and poor oral hygiene.

Symptoms. Unnoted even after lesions are produced at the site of decay or removal of a tooth, further extension along the tooth's membranous sheath finally causes the appearance of a reddish nodule under the skin. Multiple nodules enlarge to form the characteristic appearance of lumpy jaw. Pus drainage reveals yellow "sulfur" granules. Culture of the organism is not essential to diagnosis of this easily recognizable disease, but is useful. It is also possible to identify the organism on direct smear.

Treatment. Antibiotics (especially

penicillin) and sulfonamides are effective remedies when used along with surgical drainage of the lesions and supportive medical care.

ACUPUNCTURE   More than 2000 years ago the Chinese developed a system of medical treatment called acupuncture. This treatment involves the insertion of needles at specifically designated points on the body, which will then have a beneficial effect on the part of the body that corresponds with the insertion point. Some acupuncture practitioners identify up to 1000 distinctive points on the body that can be used as needle placement sites.

In the West medical authorities are most interested in applying acupuncture techniques as an element in anesthesiology and in the treatment of chronic pain. Acupuncture used as an anesthesia (frequently the needles carry a very slight electrical current) has advantages during surgery over conventional methods. Patients are conscious during the operation and they rarely experience nausea during recuperation.

How acupuncture works is not yet clearly understood. Traditional explanation maintains that the body possesses various energies that often become imbalanced. The proper placement of an acupuncture needle allows these energies to either drain or build up, thus returning the body to a normal, healthy condition. Modern explanations concerning the anesthetic capabilities of acupuncture involve the idea that stimulation of nerve fibers at specific points with acupuncture needles may block the nerve fibers' ability to send impulses of pain or discomfort to the brain.

Further research into the way acupuncture works may yield new applications for its use, such as in the treatment of some forms of hearing impairment, obesity, and narcotic addiction. In the United States acupuncture treatment is restricted to physicians who have been trained in acupuncture procedures.

ACUTE EPIGLOTTITIS   When the uppermost part of the larynx (epiglottis) becomes infected, sudden obstruction of the airway may occur. This condition is not common, but is serious, in children. (In adults it tends to be more chronic and—taking longer to develop—is not so suddenly devastating.) In three or four hours or less the epiglottis of a child can become so swollen that death may occur from inability to breathe.

Treatment. Opening of the windpipe (tracheotomy) is almost always performed when a diagnosis of acute epiglottitis is made, because the obstruction occurs with such rapidity. Antibiotics, humidity, and maintenance of fluid balance are other measures for this respiratory problem. When a young child complains of pain on swallowing and shows difficulty in breathing, he may have epiglottitis and should be seen by a physician at once.

ADAMS-STOKES SYNDROME   A patient suffering an Adams-Stokes attack loses consciousness and falls into a coma or convulsive attack, perhaps for a minute or more; the catastrophe is caused by temporary but complete cessation of the heartbeat. Its cause may be disease changes, or an inborn defect in the electrical conduction fibers of the heart which can interfere with the intermittent electrical impulse that initiates contraction of the ventricles of the heart.

Symptoms. During an attack of heartblock there is an absence of ventricular contractions, heartbeat, and blood pressure, and circulation of the blood comes to a halt. Spontaneous recovery is, however, the rule, and when the ventricles resume their rhythm, consciousness returns and the symptoms quickly disappear. Attacks occur rarely with some patients, frequently with others. If for any reason the heart fails to resume contractions, death will occur.

Treatment. Drugs can be useful in treating this condition, by speeding up the very slow heart and increasing the ability of the ventricles to resume their own rhythm.

A small electronic device, scarcely larger than a pile of three or four 25-cent pieces, has been developed which can serve as an artificial "pacemaker." Run by a tiny battery, it discharges a very small current at the same tempo as a normal heart. The device is implanted permanently under the skin, and slender wires connect it to the ventricular muscle fibers. The batteries have a life of several years, and are replaced in a minor surgical operation under local anesthesia. The presence of the implanted device creates little or no discomfort, and use of the pacemaker has freed hundreds of patients from crippling attacks of heart-block and the risk of a fatal seizure.

ADDICTION   Drug addiction is a state of periodic or chronic intoxication detrimental to the person and to society, produced by the repeated consumption of a drug, natural or synthetic. Its characteristics include: (1) an overpowering desire or need (compulsion) to continue taking the drug and to obtain it by any means; (2) a tendency to increase the dose (tolerance); (3) a psychological and sometimes a physical dependence on the effects of the drug so that withdrawal of the drug is associated with anguishing symptoms and cravings.

Addiction always involves a state of physical and psychological dependence on some drug or chemical which a person comes to crave and cannot do without. The principal addition-producing drugs are morphine, opium, hashish, marijuana, heroin, the barbiturates, and benzedrine. There is evidence that suggestion plays a part in starting an addiction, the person accepting the idea that a habit is being formed and that he is becoming an addict. Addiction may not occur when a person does not know he is being given a habit-forming drug. (See DRUGS: Drug Abuse.)

ADDISON'S DISEASE   This condition occurs when the adrenal glands are absent or completely inactive. In former years tuberculosis of the adrenal glands was a common condition, often responsible for their inactivity; recently, however, it is more common to find atrophy of the glands without demonstrable cause or to find that the glands have been surgically removed for treatment of cancer or severe diabetes. The glands are also removed surgically in some cases of Cushing's disease.

Patients with Addison's disease are constantly in a precarious state of health. If untreated, they may go into shock and collapse at any time and even die suddenly. Usually they are subject to repeated attacks of vomiting and weakness with severe drop in blood pressure. The discovery of cortisone has been life-saving to such persons. Fortunately, cortisone can be easily administered by mouth and is effective in relatively small doses. Sometimes, however, patients with Addison's disease will need to take an additional substance to promote retention of salt, which in this disease characteristically leaves the body excessively via the kidneys.

ADENOID, ADENOIDECTOMY   See TONSILS

ADENOIDS   The adenoids are masses of lymph tissue, closely related to the tonsils in position and function. They are found in the upper back part of the throat, just above and behind the soft palate; thus, they can be seen only with the aid of a special mirror.

Normally the adenoids enlarge during the fourth to the sixth year of life and may, if enlarged or infected, cause obstruction of clear nasal breathing. They may also block the adjacent inner openings of the Eustachian tubes. (These tubes equalize the atmospheric pressure on both sides of the eardrums. If the adenoids become enlarged and plug the Eustachian-tube openings, the air from the tubes becomes absorbed and the greater pressure on the outside will push an eardrum in, creating a retracted eardrum and almost always a hearing loss.

Repeated ear infections (see OTITIS MEDIA) occurring after colds are often related to enlarged adenoids. If repeated ear infections, mouth-breathing, deafness, and swollen, infected tonsils and glands cannot be controlled with conservative management and/or antibiotics, surgical removal of adenoids and tonsils before the age of seven years is a wise decision.

ADHESIVE CAPSULITIS   A syndrome in which the shoulder is limited in its motion by pain and also by fibrous capsular adhesions, adhesive capsulitis is frequently the result of bursitis in which inadequate exercise was performed and adhesions formed. It may also result from inactivity of the shoulder, as, for example, when the wrist is immobilized by a cast for a fracture and the shoulder is not adequately exercised; thus, this condition often occurs in bedridden patients who are not receiving adequate shoulder exercises. These various causes are mentioned in detail so as to stress the importance of preventing this painful, disabling syndrome.

Treatment. Treatment of this syndrome is not always completely successful. Physiotherapy, traction, and manipulation play a role in the successful management of the patient.

ADLERIAN INDIVIDUAL PSYCHOLOGY   Alfred Adler (1870-1937) was an early pupil of Sigmund Freud who broke away from his master's teachings to form his own school of individual psychology. Adler disagreed with Freud about the importance of sexual factors in neuroses and emphasized the study of ego-functioning. In his medical practice Adler had observed the remarkable ability of Nature to compensate for losses of function. Adler developed the concept of the inferiority

complex: feelings of negative self-regard which everyone experiences because of real or imagined inferiorities. Adler pointed out that persons with extreme feelings of inferiority may be severely handicapped in facing situations unless able to develop compensatory adjustments. Adler felt that a very important cause of inferiority feelings involves fears of castration or sexual impotence, called castration anxiety (see CASTRATION ANXIETY and FRIGIDITY).

One of Adler's great contributions was his style-of-life theory, referring to each person's characteristic use of psychological mechanisms in developing a strategy for satisfying his personal needs. An example would be the pampered, spoiled style, in which an only child learns to control his environment by developing temper tantrums whenever thwarted. Adler gave marked attention to such situational factors in personality development as birth position in the family. He studied the special problems of the only child, the oldest child, the youngest child, and middle children, in relation to brother-and-sister rivalry and social development. It is now generally accepted that Adlerian Individual Psychology provides an important supplement to Freudian psychoanalytic theory.

ADRENAL GLANDS   The two adrenal glands rest atop the two kidneys in "cocked hat" fashion. The glands are composed of an outer layer (cortex) and an inner zone (medulla). The adrenal cortex secretes cortisone, as well as hormones which have some masculinizing properties and are responsible for promoting retention of the chemicals which manufacture muscle in the body. Still another substance secreted (aldosterone) by the adrenal cortex regulates the body content of salt and water. The adrenal medulla is closely related to the sympathetic nervous system and secretes adrenalin (epinephrine).

ADRENALIN (EPINEPHRINE) The secretion of the inner portion of the adrenal glands (medulla) is known as adrenalin (epinephrine). It is responsible for producing contraction of smooth muscle and is therefore capable of elevating the blood pressure by constricting the small arteries. It may also produce an increase in pulse rate, perspiration, and a general feeling of fright. Its secretion helps the individual to cope with stressful experiences.

Secretion of adrenalin is increased in the body when a rare type of tumor (a pheochromocytoma) is present in one of the adrenal glands. This produces a very serious condition, responsible for episodes of rapid pulse and high blood pressure, and is treated by a delicate surgical operation.

Injected adrenalin is useful in the treatment of asthma, hives, and other allergic reactions and is usually to be found in the doctor's emergency bag.

ADRENOGENITAL SYNDROME This very important condition occurs when the adrenal glands overproduce androgen (male hormone).

In adults it may be due to benign hyperplasia (overgrowth) of adrenal cortex tissue or to an actual adrenal tumor (which may be benign or malignant).

Symptoms. Women afflicted with this adrenal disturbance develop increased body hair growth, a beard, thinning of scalp hair, loss of feminine body configuration, increased muscle strength, and deepening of the voice. Sexual interest may be increased but no homosexual (Lesbian) tendencies are noted if they were not present before.

Treatment. Treatment is by surgical removal of a tumor if one can be found, or by long continued administration of cortisone if benign hyperplasia is diagnosed by appropriate testing, which consists of measuring the adrenal secretions in a urine sample.

In children, the disorder is spoken of as congenital (prenatal) androgenic adrenal hyperplasia. It is due to a biochemical block in the manufacture of cortisone by the adrenal cortex. The hormones produced in place of cortisone are masculinizing in their effects. If they are present in prenatal life in males they produce increased growth of the normal male genitalia, which is obvious at birth. In female babies, prenatal stimulation with androgens (male hormone) affects differentiation of urogenital structures, so that at birth casual inspection may cause confusion about the child's sexual identity. Sometimes the genitalia appear so much like normal male structures that the male sex is erroneously assigned. Until recently many such individuals were considered to be true intersexes (see HERMAPHRODITISM) and were raised as boy or girl depending largely on the appearance of the genital structures. Cases are known of girls with large clitorises and scrotal appearing labia, raised as boys, and accepting the male role, until puberty when menstruation, breast development, or other evidences of femininity assert themselves. This occurrence can be a psychological catastrophe, and careful consideration must be given to the future of the individual when the true sex is made known. Some adolescents are mature enough to decide intelligently whether they wish to undergo an apparent "transformation" to their true sex (feminine), in which case appropriate plastic surgery and hormone therapy will usually permit a completely successful assumption of the feminine role. If continuation of the sex of rearing (male) is elected, the individual must be told that extensive plastic surgery including removal of ovaries and breasts must be performed, and that reproduction will not be possible, although a moderately satisfactory sex life may be pursued.

In view of the tremendous psychologic impact of a change in sex, most authorities agree that the sex in which a child is reared should not be changed unless this change can be made before the age of two and one half years, or when the individual is sufficiently mature to understand and adapt to the transformation.

Treatment. Even though adrenogenital syndrome is serious and frightening to the parents, treatment is easy and satisfactory consisting of administration of cortisone by mouth. This must usually be continued throughout life in order to prevent return of the abnormal adrenal secretions.

AFTER-BIRTH PAINS These are usually mild or moderately severe lower-abdominal pains due to the continuing contractions of the womb after delivery. They last for a few days (commonly two to three) after birth and are not as common in patients who have had their first baby. They are usually stronger while the mother is breast-feeding the baby, but respond well to relatively mild analgesics.

AFTERBIRTH (PLACENTA) The placenta is an irregularly round, flat, spongy organ attached to the inside of the pregnant uterus and connected with the baby by the umbilical cord. The placenta is essential for exchange of nourishing substances and oxygen between mother and unborn child. Abnormalities of the placenta, such as premature separation from the uterus or atrophy and fibrosis, will affect the welfare of the baby and if the function of this organ is severely impaired, fetal death will occur. The placenta is the last of the products of conception to be expelled from the womb; if parts of it are retained in the uterus after delivery, prolonged bleeding, pains, and infection may follow.

AIDS Acquired Immune Deficiency Syndrome (AIDS) is characterized by a defect in natural immunity against disease. People who have AIDS are vulnerable to serious illnesses which would not be a threat to anyone whose immune system was functioning normally. These illnesses are referred to as "opportunistic" infections or diseases.

Most individuals infected with the AIDS virus have no symptoms and feel well. Some develop symptoms which may include tiredness, fever, loss of appetite and weight, diarrhea, night sweats, and swollen glands (lymph nodes)—usually in the neck, armpits, or groin.

AIDS is spread by sexual contact, needle sharing, or less commonly, through transfused blood or its components. The risk of infection with the virus is increased by having multiple sexual partners, either homosexual or heterosexual, and sharing of needles among those using illicit drugs. The occurrence of the syndrome in hemophilia patients and persons receiving transfusions provides evidence of transmission of the virus through blood. The virus may be transmitted also from infected mother to infant before, during, or shortly after birth (probably through breast milk).

Ninety-five percent of the AIDS cases have occurred in the following groups of people:

• Sexually active homosexual and bisexual men, 73 percent;
• Present or past abusers of intravenous drugs, 17 percent;
• Persons with hemophilia or other coagulation disorders, 1 percent;
• Heterosexual contacts of someone with AIDS or at risk for AIDS, 1 percent;
• Persons who have had transfusions with blood or blood products, 2 percent;
• Infants born to infected mothers, 1 percent.

AIDS is difficult to catch, even among people at highest risk for the disease. The risk of transmitting AIDS from daily contact at work, school, or at home apparently is nonexistent. In virtually all cases, direct sexual contact or the sharing of IV drug needles has led to the illness.

Blood banks and other blood collection centers use sterile equipment and disposable needles. The need for blood is great, and people who are not at increased risk for getting AIDS are urged to continue to donate blood as they have in the past.

Casual contact with AIDS patients or infected persons does *not* place others at risk for getting the illness. No cases have been found where the virus has been transmitted by casual household contact with AIDS patients or infected persons. Infants with AIDS have not transmitted the infection to family members living in the same household.

Ambulance drivers, police, and fire-fighters who have assisted AIDS patients have not become ill. Nurses, doctors, and health care personnel have not developed AIDS from caring for AIDS patients.

The U.S. Public Health Service recommends the following steps to reduce the chances of contracting infection with HTLV-III—the virus that causes AIDS:

• Don't have sex with multiple partners, or with persons who have had multiple partners (including prostitutes). The more partners you have, the greater your risk of contracting AIDS.

• Obviously, avoiding sex with persons with AIDS would eliminate the risk of sexually transmitted infection by the virus. However, if you do have sex with a person you think is infected, protect yourself by taking appropriate precautions to prevent contact with the person's body fluids. ("Body fluids" includes blood, semen, urine, feces, saliva, and women's genital secretions.)

—Use condoms, which will reduce the possibility of transmitting the virus.

—Avoid practices that may injure body tissues (for example, anal intercourse).

—Avoid oral-genital contact.

—Avoid open-mouthed, intimate kissing.

• Don't use intravenous drugs. If you do, don't share needles or syringes.

Cases of AIDS related to medical use of blood or blood products are being prevented by use of HTLV-III antibody screening tests at blood donor sites and by members of high risk groups voluntarily not donating blood.

There is no vaccine for AIDS itself. However, there is good reason to believe that individuals can reduce their risk of contracting AIDS by following existing recommendations. Communities can help prevent AIDS by vigorous efforts to educate and inform their populations about the illness, with special emphasis on educational activities for members of high risk groups. Meanwhile, the effort to produce vaccines and drugs against AIDS continues.

Further information about AIDS may be obtained from your local or State health department or your physician. The Public Health Service AIDS hotline number is 1-800-342-AIDS. Atlanta area callers should dial (404) 329-1295.

For further information on drug treatment call 1-800-662-HELP.

AIR POLLUTION   This common phrase refers to excessive accumulation of waste products in the environmental air which may be hazardous to health and safety, may interfere with comfort, destroy property, or damage food supply. The quality and quantity of pollutants change with geographical location, the industrial growth of cities, and with technological development. Our principal air pollutants are smoke, soot, fog, motor exhausts, and radioactive materials acting individually or—more commonly—by interaction.

Medical knowledge has not yet pinpointed the specific pollutants which produce or aggravate disease (see SMOKING). Nevertheless, certain facts seem well established. Certain diseases, such as chronic bronchitis, bronchial asthma, emphysema of the lungs, arteriosclerosis, and heart disease (particularly in older and sicker patients) are definitely worsened with an increase in air pollution. Still more intriguing is the relationship of air pollution and tobacco smoking to lung cancer (see CANCER). The statistical evidence points to a definite increase in relation to both offenders.

The problem is but one aspect of man-made pollution of all the natural environment. The dumping of industrial and municipal wastes into lakes and streams has destroyed fish and other aquatic life. Noise pollution, particularly in our urban centers, is also a known hazard to health. The only effective measure against pollution is control of man-made wastes—a civic responsibility.

ALBINISM This is a rare disease in which there is an inherited inability to produce visible pigment. The condition does not necessarily result in an absence of pigment of the entire skin; but when there is a total absence of pigment, there is a concomitant absence of pigment in the retina of the eyes, which gives the pupils a red appearance. The skin is not otherwise affected.

Treatment. No treatment is available except a cosmetic covering if the areas of involvement are small. However, because the skin is unprotected from the damaging effects of the sun's rays (in the absence of pigment) it is necessary to use protective ointments on the uncovered parts of the body and to wear clothing made of materials and colors which are least likely to permit absorption of sunlight.

ALBUMIN Albumin is an important protein found in all tissues. (Egg white is a form of this substance.) The albumin in blood serum is formed by the liver from amino acids resulting from protein metabolism. The normal serum concentration is from about four to five grams per one hundred milliliters of blood. When liver cells are damaged, formation of albumin is reduced and its serum level characteristically falls. The level also falls in severe malnutrition and in some forms of kidney disease in which there is a loss of albumin in the urine.

Albumin acts as a regulator of water and salt balance between the fluid in the blood and in the tissues, thus maintaining the total blood volume in equilibrium. It also acts as a transport mechanism for many natural compounds and drugs.

ALBUMINURIA Filtration of blood plasma through the walls of the tiny blood vessels in the glomerulus of the kidney produces a clear watery liquid which passes down the kidney tubule to form urine. If blood proteins leak through, chiefly albumin, they may appear in the urine: a condition called albuminuria. Albumin is routinely tested for in all urinalyses and is an important indication of kidney disease.

ALCOHOL AND ALCOHOLISM Modern psychiatry recognizes that alcoholism is just as much a disease as the common cold, and almost as common. Alcohol has always been the poor man's antidote for emotional stress and nervousness. In spite of all the modern discoveries and the new psychiatric drugs, nothing is more immediately effective for some people in inducing feelings of well-being and alleviating nervous distress than alcohol.

Alcohol is one of the most potent and widely-used drugs known to man. From ancient times, peoples have learned to distill grain in order to produce ethyl alcohol, which has a wide range of pharmacological effects. The ancients learned to use it as a pain-killer, and it became widely used as an anesthetic. During the Middle Ages it was customary to perform amputations after getting the patient completely intoxicated.

Even more potent is the ability of alcohol temporarily to reduce mental anguish, nervous tension, and anxiety. It is well known that mental stress increases in direct proportion to the ever-growing complexities of civilized life. Neurotic disorders may be understood as emotional reactions to life's stress, and even today, many alcoholics drink to deaden themselves to the miseries of life. Alcohol has the very important effect of reducing psychoneurotic symptoms related to anxiety and tension. The more insecure a person feels in civilized society, the more neurotic symptoms he tends to develop and the greater becomes his dependence on alcohol, or some other drugs, to relieve such symptoms and produce peace of mind.

Because of its anesthetic and anxiety-reducing effects, alcohol quickly leads to addiction in insecure, inadequate, dependent personalities who require a crutch to face life. Most alcoholics take up drinking quite innocently, at first in reasonable amounts at social gatherings; only gradually does there develop dependence on alcohol for the relief of neurotic symptoms.

The unfortunate fact is that it requires increasing doses to produce these desirable effects, so that the person has to drink larger and larger amounts, to such a point that toxic effects begin to appear.

Recent research suggests an allergic factor in alcoholism. Although alcoholism does not produce changes in blood chemistry such as occur in true drug addiction, most alcoholics become very sensitive to very small amounts of alcohol which are quite harmless to the nonalcoholic but which may set the alcoholic off on a prolonged drinking spree. Each person appears to have his own characteristic threshold in developing toxic effects from heavy drinking, and even the heavy social drinker *may* become an alcoholic in time when sensitivity to alcohol and toxic symptoms develop. Alcohol taken in large amounts is a potent poison. Quick death has been known to result after consumption of less than a quart of alcohol at one time.

Symptoms. In the typical pattern of developing alcoholism, a vicious circle arises in which the alcoholic has to drink more and more in order to control progressive mental symptoms. Most alcoholics develop a pattern of continuous drinking without adequate food intake, so that serious nutritional and vitamin deficiencies quickly develop. The alcoholic usually has no insight into his condition and shows no control in limiting his excesses.

Psychologically, alcoholism has many effects in common with drug addiction. It interferes with all the departments of a person's life—causing him to lose his job, become estranged from relatives and friends, become financially insolvent, lose his health, and eventually end on "Skid Row" robbed of all social or financial resources. During this downward slide, there occurs a subtle deterioration of the personality as the alcoholic squanders his resources in order to obtain liquor. Such former traits as thrift, honesty, industry, self-respect, and honor are replaced by financial irresponsibility, dishonesty, poor work habits, loss of self-respect, and moral depravity. The chronic alcoholic is psychiatrically sick, and nothing but psychiatric treatment offers much hope for cure.

Treatment. The great error of the past was the attempt to use punishment to rehabilitate alcoholics. Most alcoholics start as neurotic, insecure, and anxious persons, already on the defensive. Any attempt to criticize or otherwise punish them for misdeeds only results in further anxiety and need to drink.

The first step in treatment is to recognize that alcoholism is always a psychological problem and can only be solved by psychiatric means. It can do no good to punish, preach, criticize, or lecture the alcoholic for his misdeeds.

The second essential is to get alcoholics off the defensive, so that for the first time in their lives they might feel accepted rather than rejected. This principle accounts for much of the success of "AA"—Alcoholics Anonymous—in which the alcoholic is handled by other alcoholics who accept him unconditionally and help him through the most difficult periods of rehabilitation. For those who can accept "AA," the movement is a source of great help and hope. The first step in the rehabilitation of an alcoholic often consists in taking him to an "AA" meeting and discovering whether he is able to accept its program.

Third, since the eventual outcome for alcoholics unable to accept "AA" or any other community alcoholic-rehabilitation service, is usually arrest and commitment to a mental hospital, most state hospitals have alcoholic wards and programs especially designed to give intensive treatment to acute and chronic alcoholics not helped by other means.

A fourth possibility for the future lies in conditioning programs directed toward abolition of the urge to drink. This is accomplished by combining alcohol with nausea-producing drugs so that the alcoholic becomes severely physically ill whenever he drinks. This acute discomfort is used to counteract the pleasurable effects of drinking, and many cures have been reported. However, the main goal in the psychotherapy of all alcoholics should be to strengthen their personalities so that they can face life without the crutch of either alcohol or drugs.

Finally, psychiatric experience indicates that before any alcoholic can be helped it is necessary for him to admit frankly that he *is* an alcoholic and that alcohol is poison to him. Unless he completely accepts the idea that he must never touch alcohol again, under any conditions, there is little hope for eventual cure.

ALIMENTARY TRACT   See GASTRO-INTESTINAL DISORDERS

ALLERGIC CORYZA   Also called allergic, or vasomotor rhinitis, this is a condition in which there is an inflammation of the mucous membranes of the nasal passages due to hypersensitivity to some substance. Animal danders (cat, dog, and others), food and house dust are among the culprits. There are two types: the seasonal (usually due to pollens and soil molds,

with symptoms appearing mainly in the spring, late summer, and fall) and the perennial type, which occurs all year round (although worse in fall and winter and usually due to foods and the presence of animals).

Symptoms. Typical symptoms of allergic coryza are: sneezing, nasal congestion, an itchy and/or drippy nose, constant sniffling, mouth-breathing, frequent throat-clearing, occasional dry coughing spells, red, itching and tearing eyes, swollen eyelids, and itchy ears.

Complications consist of nasal polyps, sinusitis, diseases of the ear, nosebleeds, loss of the sense of smell, and in some cases the development of asthma.

Treatment. The foods or animals to which the patient is allergic should be avoided. Antihistamines, eye drops where indicated, occasional use of nasal decongestants, steroids in severe cases, and hyposensitization in selected cases are also applicable.

ALLERGIC ECZEMA   See CONTACT DERMATITIS AND ATOPIC DERMATITIS

ALLERGIC REACTIONS IN CHILDREN   Allergic reactions in children are somewhat different from those in the adult. Children will show symptoms more quickly but will recover sooner. Food allergies are most common during the first two years of life.

In early childhood, allergic states are usually caused by inhalants such as dust and animal furs. As the child gets older, pollens and molds play a bigger part. By contrast, an adult tends to remain allergic to the same thing or things.

Symptoms. While adults do not ordinarily change their symptom systems, those of an allergic child tend to change frequently. Eczema may be followed by a respiratory allergy. Rhinitis and hay fever can develop into asthma, and—conversely—asthma can turn into hay fever.

Skin tests are more reliable in children than in adults.

Children do not "outgrow" their allergies but change their symptom system as they grow older. The major complications of allergy in children are sinusitis, emphysema, chronic bronchitis, bronchiectasis, deformed chests, and personality defects.

It is important to recognize an allergic disease as early as possible, because treatment will be much more effective if started at a younger age. One should suspect allergy in an infant when there are frequent vomiting, skin eruptions, excessive sniffling, diarrhea, and marked irritability. Diagnosis is based on the patient's history, physical examination, and skin tests. Continuous wheezing in an infant might indicate allergic asthma but could mean such disorders as cystic fibrosis, birth abnormalities, swollen neck glands, tuberculosis, tumors, and swallowed foreign objects. When asthma begins under the age of two the prognosis is poorer than if it starts at an older age. On the other hand, the earlier the skin manifestations of atopic dermatitis develop, the better the prognosis for complete recovery (of the skin eruption).

Most upper-respiratory allergies start between the ages of one and three years. Emotional upsets can trigger or aggravate an asthmatic attack, and such attacks may be precipitated by respiratory infections. The common inhalant causes are house dust, pollens, and molds. Some doctors feel that air-borne algae may play a part in causing asthma. Food allergy can also bring on an attack.

Children with allergic rhinitis are subject to many colds. As they get older, they may develop chronic sinusitis and nasal polyps. Their hearing may be impaired and their behavior affected. In cases of recurrent nosebleeds (epistaxis) one should consider an allergic rhinitis as an important cause.

Allergic conjunctivitis may be atopic (due to pollen, dust, or foods), contact (due to drugs or chemicals), or infectious (due to bacterial products). Corneal ulcers and impaired vision are complications.

Bed-wetting accompanied by an irritable, hostile personality may be due to food allergy. Diagnosis is established by the presence of certain cells (eosinophils) in the urine. Treatment consists of an elimination diet.

Treatment. Tonsillectomy should not be performed to cure asthma, especially since this operation will itself occasionally be followed by an asthma attack. Treatment consists of removing the cause, alleviating the symptoms, protecting against house dust, and (in selected cases) psychotherapy for both the child and the parents. Change of climate is sometimes beneficial. The child should be permitted normal activities, but not beyond the point where physical exertion begins to make breathing difficult.

The potentially allergic child is the child whose family has a strong history of allergies. Some medical authorities believe that such children should be prophylactically treated as infants. For the first nine months of life the infant should be breast fed or given heat-treated milk or milk substitutes. The earliest solid food should be barley, rice, corn, or oats. Eggs should be avoided for at least six months. Oranges, cocoa, fish, and nuts should be eliminated from the diet for at least one year. See also ALLERGIC CORYZA; ASTHMA; ALLERGIES, DIAGNOSIS OF; EMOTIONS, ROLE OF; FOOD ALLERGIES, TREATMENT OF.

ALLERGIC SKIN DISEASES The several kinds of skin disease which are caused by, or are evidence of, an allergic mechanism differ considerably. Nevertheless they have in common the important criteria implicit in the term allergic, and are identifiably different from diseases caused by dynamic mechanisms of another nature. The concept of allergy as a mechanism of the production of disease is necessary not only for purposes of describing and recording certain clinical findings, but also for purposes of seeking treatment and prevention. The adoption of the word allergy to denote a unique medical happenstance was an act of great significance in medical history and provided a basis for the study of heretofore inexplicable diseases and a working tool for an entirely new biologic field, immunology.

Allergy is an acquired, specific alteration in the capacity to react. To be the result of an allergic process, a condition must be the result of an alteration, a change—one that is not present at birth and hence is noted by the fact that the response is different on a subsequent exposure to a causative substance (an allergen) than was the response to the first exposure. Moreover, the causative substance must not only be proven capable of producing the alteration noted but must not have produced it at the first encounter, since this would indicate that the reacting person would not have had an "altered" or changed capacity to react. The alteration in capacity to react must also be acquired (not be a change predisposing to reaction by virtue of a difference in structure present at birth) and must be specific (directed at a particular chemical structure, a particular wave length of light, a particular drug, food, weed, dander, pollen, etc.). Modifications of the definition have become numerous, since the concept of the allergic mechanism has been utilized by all the biologic disciplines. But the original carefully chosen words, capable of modification as the need occurs, are meaningful, useful, and necessary in the consideration of the ever-widening situations they describe.

The allergic skin diseases are comprised of two major categories: the atopic and the nonatopic. The latter group consists of contact dermatitis, urticaria (hives),

drug eruptions, and infectious diseases of allergic mechanism. The atopic type of allergic response is evident in the skin as a dermatitis, in the lungs as asthma, and in the eyes and nasal passages as hay fever. Migraine, sinusitis, and some forms of epilepsy are considered to be some of the other manifestations of atopy. In atopic persons, there is usually both a family and a personal history of other atopic diseases; scratch and intradermal tests give positive reactions; there is a high eosinophil count of the blood; circulating antibodies are demonstrable; and the allergens (here called atopens) are usually proteins or protein-bound substances. The nonatopic allergic diseases differ from the atopic in almost every detail, except in the basic mechanism of their common causation; the acquired, specific alteration in the capacity to react.

ALLERGIES An allergic person reacts abnormally to something that does not affect the normal person, allergy itself being an altered reactivity of the tissues in various organs, brought about by previous contact with a given substance. In other words, a person becomes allergic by first being exposed to a substance, then reacting to re-exposure to it. An allergic reaction is an "immune" (immunologic) phenomenon based on chemical interaction between a foreign-acting material (antigen) and a specific substance produced against it by the body (antibody).

How does a person become allergic? One either inherits an allergy (hay fever, asthma, allergic rhinitis, atopic dermatitis, urticaria, and migraine) or one acquires it (drug reactions, contact dermatitis, allergy to infection, and physical allergy).

When introduced into the body (by contact, ingestion, inhalation, or injection), simple chemicals and complicated proteins that will stimulate the production of a specific substance, or antibody, are called antigens. The antibody is a specific protein which is produced by certain body cells (found in the lymph nodes, spleen, liver, bloodstream, and skin) when stimulated by the presence of an antigen. Immunity, in turn, is a state in which the body is protected against the ill effects of a foreign agent.

The allergic reaction will occur almost immediately if the antibodies are circulating in the blood, or will be delayed if they are confined to the tissue cells. The symptoms of allergy are due to the liberation of certain chemicals (histamine, serotonin, heparin, bradykinin, acetylcholine) when the antigen reacts with the antibody. A deficiency in two vitamin B complex chemicals (pyridoxine and pantothenic acid) seems to be responsible, as it interferes with the immune reaction and the production of antibodies. The antigen-antibody theory of allergy is not fully established and is frequently challenged. One suggested explanation is that the antigen stimulates the formation of new enzymes; these in turn produce certain "poisons," and the reaction of the body to these "poisons" is the allergic response.

One of the oldest recorded allergic reactions was the death of King Menes of Egypt in 2461 B.C. following a wasp or hornet sting. This was probably a case of an insect-allergy shock reaction (anaphylaxis). Hippocrates noted that certain foods caused stomach disorders accompanied by hives. During the second century A.D. Galen reported a case of allergy to goat's milk and nasal symptoms due to roses. In the seventeenth century, Van Helmont discussed seasonal asthma in relation to vegetation and flowers.

In the eighteen hundreds, hay fever was believed to be due to dust from new-mown hay; in 1860 the first scratch skin tests had already been performed; in 1866 hives due to physical allergy to cold were described. By 1873 certain cases of hay fever were traced to grass pollen hypersensitivity, and patch tests were first re-ported in 1895. In 1898 Dr. H. H. Curtis discussed his attempts to immunize patients to the "toxins" present in pollens. Von Picquet coined the very word allergy in 1906. In 1910 Dr. Leonard Noon discussed his technique of timothy hyposensitization. The passive-transfer phenomenon was demonstrated in 1923. It was in the year 1923 that the term atopy was introduced, meaning clinical allergies due to hereditary influences and including asthma, hay fever, and infantile eczema.

Symptoms. Allergic symptoms can involve any part of the body. The following list is an example of the types of symptoms that may be due to allergy:

Eye—Swelling lids, eczema lids, visual disturbances, increased tearing, conjunctivitis

Ear—Eczema, dizziness, hearing loss, Ménière's syndrome, inflammation of the middle ear

Nose—Sneezing, stuffiness, dripping, recurrent nosebleeds, nasal polyps, eczema

Mouth—Dry fissured lips, gingivitis, drooling, "stomach sores"

Respiratory System—Wheezing, coughing, croup, pneumonia

Digestive Tract—Colic, stomach-aches, vomiting, itching anus, constipation, diarrhea, swelling of the abdomen, bloody stool, mucous colitis, ulcerative colitis

Nervous System—Headache, malaise, irritability, restlessness, numbness of hands, tingling hands, tension, fatigue, dizziness, anxiety, fever, convulsions, encephalitis

Cardiovascular System—Extra heartbeats, flutter (auricular fibrillation), Buerger's disease, hemorrhage into the skin, anemia, low blood pressure, and rapid heartbeats

Genitourinary System—Bed-wetting, frequency of urination, painful urination, and inflammation of the vulva

Musculoskeletal System—Tremors, muscular aches and pains, backache, pain in neck and/or shoulders

Skin—Excessive sweating, pallor, circles under eyes, eczema (atopic and contact), hives, swelling of the face and lips, hemorrhage into the skin

Constant research is being done in the field of allergy. Certain diseases such as polyarteritis nodosa and ulcerative colitis are believed to be allergic in nature. Recent investigations have shown a high incidence of pollen-type allergy in peptic ulcer patients.

A new concept has developed over the last few years—"autoimmune diseases." These are conditions in which the individual becomes hypersensitive to his own body-substances. Some of these "autoimmune diseases" are: rheumatoid arthritis, rheumatic fever, thyroiditis, atopic dermatitis, dermatomyositis, and systemic lupus erythematosus.

Allergic phenomena also occur with infections. Tuberculosis, leprosy, deep fungus disease, and syphilis produce a positive skin test only during or after the infection has taken place whereas diphtheria and typhoid will give a positive skin reaction only before infection occurs and then becomes negative. Tuberculosis is an interesting example of what happens in the allergic response to bacteria. Although many people are infected with the tuberculosis organism, only a few go on to have the actual disease. Here the allergic response to the bacteria is a good one with protection against the harmful effects. Those who develop active tuberculosis do so because of an overwhelming invasion of the bacteria or a lack of proper allergic response.

ALLERGIES, DIAGNOSIS OF How does one know whether or not one is allergic to something, or is showing symptoms that are allergic in nature? Allergic symptoms can be the same as those of many other diseases. A doctor is best equipped to make this decision. He will come to a conclusion by using several diagnostic approaches. He will ask for a detailed history, perform the appropriate physical examination, have whatever laboratory studies are necessary performed, and where indicated will use skin tests.

A patient's history is probably one of the most important helps in arriving at a diagnosis of allergic disorder. When did the symptoms start? Did they occur gradually or suddenly? At what age did they begin? Are the complaints affected by emotional disturbances, by physical activity, by the weather? Is there any seasonal variation? How frequently do the complaints come on? How long do they last? What previous treatment has the patient been given, and with what results? These and many more questions must be answered to obtain a good background for substantiating a diagnosis of allergy.

Physical examination of the patient will give the physician further valuable information. The general appearance is important. A darkish discoloration about the eyes, combined with mouth-breathing, may indicate a nasal allergy. The habit of rubbing the nose with an upward motion of the hand can mean hay fever or asthma. A pinched appearance of the face can mean asthma. An eruption in the folds of the elbows and knees may be indicative of atopic dermatitis. A breaking-out on the hands may indicate contact dermatitis. Examination of the eyes will reveal whether there is redness, excess tearing, inflammation, and itching (evidence of chronic rubbing). Examination of the nose will indicate the condition of the nasal membranes: whether they are swollen, red, or pale, and whether there are any polyps or evidence of recent bleeding. Examination of the mouth and throat will show inflammation, postnasal drip, enlarged tonsils, or adenoids. Examination of the chest will pick up wheezing or any difficulty in breathing. The shape of the chest can indicate the status of the breathing habits. A swollen, gaseous abdomen may be significant of food allergy.

Laboratory studies will consist of nasal smears, complete blood count, chest X-rays, thyroid-function tests, etc. In many cases of nasal allergy a smear from the nose will reveal a preponderance of the white blood cells called eosinophils. In some cases of asthma, hay fever, atopic dermatitis, and so forth, a blood count will reveal an increase in these same cells. The blood count will also reveal any anemia or other disturbances. A chest X-ray is necessary to rule out certain infectious diseases. A thyroid-function test is given, since certain thyroid disturbances can mimic allergic states. Other laboratory procedures may be employed, depending on the individual case.

After the physical examination and laboratory studies have indicated the presence of an allergy, skin tests are employed to confirm or deny any suspicions gained from the history. There are six main types of skin tests:

1. Scratch tests. Scratches are made on the forearm or back. A small drop of the material to be tested is placed on, and rubbed into, the scratch. A positive reaction consists of the formation of a wheal within twenty minutes. (This method is relatively safe and in most cases should be the first type of test done.)

2. Intradermal tests. A small amount of a specific dilution of the extract to be tested is injected just under the upper layers of the skin. The amount of redness and whealing produced within twenty minutes indicates the degree of allergy. (The chances of reaction in a very sensitive individual are greater with this method than with scratch tests.)

3. Conjunctival tests. A drop of aqueous extract is dropped within the lower eyelid. The test is read within five minutes by the amount of redness, itchiness, and tearing. (As only one test can be performed at any one time, this test is limited to those materials which are negative on scratch and intradermal tests, yet where the case history seems to indicate that this is the substance the person is allergic to.

4. Inhalation test. The extract is sniffed into the nose and, if positive, there ensues a great deal of sneezing and watery discharge. (Although an excellent test, this is often followed by a severe generalized reaction.)

5. Electrode test. Electrodes are used with a special apparatus that carries the test material into the sweat pores. (There is no injury to the skin with this method.)

6. Patch test. The suspected substance is applied to the skin, in a predetermined concentration. It is covered with an adhesive-tape dressing and left on for forty-eight hours. The reactions are read twenty minutes after removing the dressings. Positive reactions consist of redness and blistering. (This test is used where a contact-type allergy is suspected. It is useless if the allergy is to something inhaled or eaten.)

When it is not possible or practical to give a skin test directly to a patient because of severe apprehension, a marked allergic state, or insufficient normal skin, then one can use the technique of "passive transfer": Blood is drawn from the patient and a serum prepared. A known nonallergic individual is injected with this serum in several sites. Forty-eight hours later the test materials are injected into the previously marked serum-sites. The results are read as in the intradermal method.

ALLERGIES, TREATMENT OF   The most important aspect of the treatment of any allergy is to find the cause and then avoid it. This is possible when contact dermatitis is due to chemicals, dyes, or metals; hives are due to medications or foods; headaches to foods, and so on. However, even when the allergic cause is known, it may be impossible completely to avoid the causative agent (inhalants, bacteria, physical agents).

Most therapeutic agents in allergic diseases are used for the benefit derived from the relief of specific symptoms. The following chart lists, in a general way the different types of medications that are used for symptomatic relief:

tain other allergies (where one cannot very well avoid such substances as pollen, molds, or dust), the physician may employ a method known as desensitization or hyposensitization. The principle behind this procedure is to inject small diluted quantities of the offending substance at set intervals, in an attempt to decrease the inci-

SYMPTOMS	ORAL MEDICATION	INJECTED MEDICATION	TOPICAL MEDICATION
Nasal congestion, stuffed nose, sneezing	Antihistamines Sedatives	————	Decongestants (Sprays and local injections)
Wheezing, coughing, and difficulty in breathing	Antihistamines Analgesics Antibotics Arsenic Bronchodilators Ephedrine Expectorants Sedatives Steroids Tranquilizers	Antibiotics Bronchodilators Epinephrine Gamma globulin Steroids	Bronchodilators (atomizer or under-tongue absorptive agent) Special detergents to loosen mucus plugs
Itchy, watery eyes	Antihistamines Ephedrine	————	Epinephrine (eyedrops) Saline and boric acid eyewash Steroid eyedrops
Itchy skin	Antihistamines Analgesics Steroids Tranquilizers	Steriods	Steroids Wet compresses Drying lotions
Aches and pains	Analgesics Antihistamines Sedatives Vasoconstrictors	Analgesics Vasoconstrictors	Cold compresses
Nausea and vomiting	Antihistamines Sedatives	Antihistamines Sedatives	————

Other treatment consists of special breathing exercises in asthma and emphysema; oxygen for asthmatic attacks; surgery for intractable asthma and bronchiectasis; psychotherapy; change of climate; avoidance of cold air intake; intermittent positive pressure (artificial respiration); sucking-out of material from the lungs (bronchoscopic aspiration); and opening of the air-passage by incision (tracheostomy).

In the treatment of inhalant and cer-

dence of clinical symptoms due to that substance. This method works best in inhalant sensitivity (ragweed pollen) and most poorly in food allergy. Insect hypersensitivity of the inhalant and sting types may also be treated by this method.

There are five general ways in which hyposensitization may be achieved with the injection treatment.

1. Co-seasonal. Treatment is started during the season of highest sensitivity.

Small amounts of the diluted extracts are given every one to three days. If used properly, this can be a very effective way of treating hay fever. It does, however, carry a greater risk of reactions (sneezing, itchy eyes, itchy nose, itchy palms, hives, coughing, wheezing, and difficulty in breathing).

2. Pre-seasonal. Injections are given weekly up to the season during which the patient experiences greatest difficulty.

3. Perennial. Injections are given all year round. Seasonal and nonseasonal allergies can be treated by this method.

4. Immediate. This occasionally-used method is one in which small doses of a solution of the offending material are injected every twenty or thirty minutes over a span of twenty-four hours. Bee and wasp venom immunity have been achieved by this method.

5. Repository. The offending substance is prepared as an emulsion or as a special alum-precipitated pyridine complex. (All other methods use extracts made in water solutions.) The advantage of this technique is that fewer injections (from one to eight) are necessary to achieve apparent immunity. A great many extracts prepared in this manner are still at an experimental stage.

ALLERGIST   This term or title refers to a physician who limits his practice to the study, diagnosis, and treatment of those disorders believed to be allergic.

ALOPECIA AREATA (GENERALISATA, UNIVERSALIS)   This type of hair loss, occurring either in single lesions or in varying-sized patches predominantly on the scalp (but capable of remaining confined to another area such as the bearded portion of the face) is of unknown causation. Although considered a disease primarily of young adult life, it occurs in all age-groups, including infancy, in both sexes, and is not associated with any "disposition" on the part of the patient, inheritance, or environmental influence.

Symptoms. The appearance of an area in which there is a complete loss of hair is marble- or billiard-ball-like. The single lesion can enlarge and become very extensive; or several lesions, appearing either simultaneously or progressively, can merge with each other to form bizarre patterns. When the hair of a considerable portion of the skin surface is lost, the disease is known as *alopecia generalisata* and when all of the body hair is lost, the condition is termed *alopecia universalis*. There are usually no sensations of itching or burning in the affected areas. When there is a return of hair, either spontaneously or as a result of treatment, the new hair first appears as fine, silky, gray-white shiny threads (lanugo hair). There is a gradual replacement of this forerunner of hair with the patient's usual hair texture and color.

Treatment. Not until the advent of the cortisone drugs was treatment available for this distressing condition. While not universally effective, the variety of types of these drugs (corticosteroids) makes relief possible for a significant percentage of affected patients. Until treatment makes it unnecessary, the wearing of a wig for patients with extensive loss of scalp hair can be helpful to the patient for cosmetic reasons.

ALVEOLI   The term "alveoli" is applied to two very different parts of the body.

Alveoli are the microscopic air sacs in the lungs where the exchange of carbon dioxide and oxygen takes place. The minute air chambers are quite numerous; both lungs contain several hundred million alveoli grouped in clusters. Pulmonary disorders such as emphysema force the alveoli to enlarge and decrease in numbers, thus causing a loss in respiratory efficiency.

Alveoli are also the bony sockets of the jaws which serve to encase the roots of teeth. Following the extraction of a

34

tooth, this socket (alveolus) is normally filled with blood which clots, and the process of healing and bone regeneration begins immediately. If for any reason, a blood clot does not remain intact, the result will be a "dry socket," which may be painful and which will result in delayed healing.

AMALGAM, DENTAL   An amalgam combines mercury and other metals and is used for filling teeth. Because of its silver color, its use is usually confined to the posterior teeth.

AMBIVALENCE, EMOTIONAL   Psychiatrically, ambivalence refers to the simultaneous presence of conflicting emotions directed toward an object. Ambivalence exerts important psychological effects both upon the person who expresses the ambivalent emotions and upon the person who is the object of the emotions.

Ambivalence originates dynamically where one person has conflicting feelings toward another. For example, a mother may simultaneously show love and hate toward her child, even to the point of feeling impulses to injure the child physically. The mother may not understand the unconscious sources of her mixed emotions, and may develop intense feelings of guilt and self-accusation. Psychiatric treatment is indicated immediately in cases where a person develops such intense ambivalence as to feel impulses of harming the other person or even of suicide (because of strong guilt feelings and the unconscious need to punish the self). Psychiatric treatment of ambivalence is directed at helping the person to understand and accept the conflicting emotions, and to develop more socially acceptable ways of bleeding them off.

In psychiatric terms, the object of such conflicting emotions is exposed to what is called a double bind, being simultaneously attracted by the positive feelings and repelled by the negative feelings. A mother who simultaneously expresses love and hate toward her child may confuse and frustrate the child severely, since it does not know what is to be expected. The child may develop reactive feelings of guilt, feelings that it must have done something bad or be unlikable if the mother expresses such negative feelings.

Sexual ambivalence occurs when a person is simultaneously attracted and repelled by conflicting sexual feelings. Thus, a wife may capriciously accept or reject sex advances by her husband according to the state of her feelings at that moment. Or, a woman's sexual pleasure may be inhibited by her fears of conceiving a child. Many types of conflict may stimulate ambivalence.

Ambivalence explains many types of behavior in which a person may say one thing and do another; one example is the wife who speaks loving words to her husband while at the same moment rejecting him by her actions. The psychologically healthy person expects to meet a certain amount of ambivalence from others and handles it in normal ways. For example, he does not expect any other person to be one hundred per cent positive toward him. Recognizing that love and anger are opposite sides of the same coin, he anticipates that a certain amount of anger will be directed toward him and does not overreact to it. The best way to handle ambivalent behavior on the part of another is simply to accept it by allowing the other person to express negative feelings without retaliating in kind.

AMBLYOPIA   Dimness of vision not corrected with glasses and not arising from disease of the eye may occur because of failure to use an eye before the age of seven years, because of poisons to which the eye is sensitive, or because of hysteria.

Symptoms. There is poor vision in one

or both otherwise-healthy eyes. There is no pain, and the individual may not even be aware of the visual defect until the eyes are tested separately. When an eye crosses before the age of five years, the eye is not being used and the development of vision in the crossing eye is arrested. Vision is usually developed after the age of five and crossing after this time does not affect visual acuity. Poisons and hysteria cause a dimness of vision in both eyes. Diagnosis may be extremely difficult.

In years past, tobacco was considered to be a cause of amblyopia, but this has been disproved. Amblyopia occurring in alcoholics is due to a vitamin B deficiency and is not a direct effect of the alcohol.

Treatment. This must be directed to the cause. Amblyopia due to a crossed eye must be treated before the age of seven. Usually the better eye is covered with a patch so as to force use of the poorer eye. This method is continued until there is no further improvement in vision.

Toxic amblyopia must be corrected by identification and removal of the causative poison. Vitamin B is frequently administered.

Hysteria occurs in an individual who has a personality deficiency in facing emotional conflicts, and may require skilled psychiatric care.

AMENORRHEA   This term refers to the lack of menstrual periods. The condition may be primary, when no period has ever occurred in a woman after puberty; or secondary, when a woman who has regular periods suddenly stops menstruating.

The most common cause of secondary amenorrhea is pregnancy, and this diagnosis should be ruled out before any other cause is suspected. Other than pregnancy, the most common causes of amenorrhea are congenital or acquired abnormalities of one or more such glands as the ovaries, the adrenal glands, the thyroid, or the pituitary. Anatomical anomalies of the womb and the birth canal (vagina), as well as mixed sex (hermaphroditism), may account for some of the primary amenorrheas. Psychosomatic factors are very often the cause of secondary amenorrhea, the extreme example being the so-called "false pregnancy" (pseudocyesis).

Treatment. Treatment will depend on the cause and may be surgical, medical (hormones), or psychiatric.

AMINO ACIDS   Proteins, indispensable constituents of every living cell, are very large molecules composed of great numbers of building units: the amino acids. Although they vary in chemical structure, these units all have in common a nitrogen-containing (amino) group—NH_2—and an acidic (carboxyl) group—COOH. There are some twenty-two different amino acids found in nature. Hundreds and even thousands of amino acids are joined together in a chain-like arrangement to form the numerous proteins of the body. Proteins as varied as the hormone insulin and the critical ingredient of red blood cells, hemoglobin, differ only in the composition of their amino acids.

Food proteins are broken down into the component amino acids which are absorbed, enter the circulation, and reach the liver, where many new proteins are manufactured. The circulating amino acids then reach the rest of the body where cells extract what they need, replacing the tissue being lost by wear and tear. Some amino acids are converted into carbohydrate and fats; some may be burned for energy. The nitrogen part of the molecule is eventually split off and excreted by the kidneys as ammonia, urea, and other products.

The essential amino acids must be supplied by food. These acids are: phenylalanine, methionine, leucine, valine, lysine, isoleucine, threonine, and tryptophan. The nonessential amino acids are equally important but can be synthesized by the body. Among them are glycine, alanine, cystine, tyrosine, proline, histidine (which may be nonsynthesizable in children), and arginine.

Amino-acid solutions (made from milk or other proteins) are used in the treatment of certain nutritional disorders. The nutritional quality of a protein food is determined by its amino-acid composition; generally, animal proteins—meat, milk, eggs—supply more of the essential amino acids in a balanced ratio than do vegetable proteins.

AMNESIA   Amnesia is an inability to remember events occurring over a specific period of time. It accompanies a variety of organic brain disorders. These include the time intervals relating to a convulsion or a period of stupor or coma, a head injury, brain atrophy, severe chronic alcoholism, and other conditions. When occurring in association with head injury and concussion of the brain, a period of retrograde amnesia extends from the time of injury back to several minutes, hours, or days before the injury; a second period of post-damage amnesia extends forward for hours or days after the injury. This amnesic period is longest during early convalescence, then gradually decreases during recovery. However, a residual permanent defect in memory usually persists.

In some patients amnesia is a sympton of hysteria. The individual suddenly does not remember events of the past and he does not know his own name. This loss of memory may extend over a period of months, years, or for an entire lifetime.

Inability to remember may also be a manifestation of subconscious malingering under stressful situations.

AMNIOCENTESIS   Amniocentesis is the procedure in which amniotic fluid is extracted from the womb via the abdominal wall by means of a hypodermic syringe. The extracted fluid, containing fetal cells, is then analyzed, possibly revealing abnormalities such as rubella virus infection and congenital diseases, such as Down's syndrome and spina bifida. The determination of the sex and age of the fetus can also be made, which may be important in assessing the survival potential of the fetus if a premature birth is indicated.

When a finding is made that the fetus is abnormal, doctors may offer the woman the option of terminating the pregnancy. Amniocentesis is recommended in cases where abnormal fetal development is suspected; it is not a routine procedure. Although infrequent, complications caused by amniocentesis may include continued leakage of amniotic fluid, bleeding, injury to the fetus or placenta, and miscarriage.

AMNIOTIC FLUID   While the fetus is carried in the mother's womb, it is surrounded by the amniotic fluid contained in the fetal membranes (bag of waters). The fluid varies in amount, usually equalling one or two pints when the mother is close to term. Its purpose is to supply a sort of water bath for the free movements of the fetus inside the womb, and to protect the baby from violent external injuries. When the bag of waters breaks, the amniotic fluid leaks through the birth canal; this usually happens during labor.

ANABOLISM (PROTEIN)   Anabolism is a term meaning the build-up of tissue material. More specifically, the word is applied to the formation (synthesis) of protein. Recent investigation indicates that 30 to 50 per cent of the body's protein is undergoing synthesis and breakdown (catabolism) simultaneously. Like a bank in which money is being deposited and withdrawn at the same time, the protoplasm of cells is undergoing anabolic and catabolic reactions.

During growth, late pregnancy, or convalescence, and during physical training when new muscle tissue is being formed, anabolism exceeds catabolism. When dietary protein is less than required, or when the caloric intake is significantly reduced, body protein is broken down faster than it is being built up; that is, catabolism exceeds anabolism. These processes are often measured by nitrogen-balance studies. Nitrogen is derived from protein (see AMINO ACIDS), and the balance is measured by determining the intake and urinary output.

ANAL FISSURE   A slit or tear or crack beginning just inside the anal opening and extending to the outside is called an anal fissure. It produces slight-to-severe pain and spasm at stool, and there is often a drop or so of blood on the outside of the stool. This condition is usually caused by the passage of hard, dry stools, but occasionally may be due to an allergy (citrus, melons, peaches, berries, or chocolate). If the latter is the case, the (visible) skin in the region of the anus will be red. Diarrhea may also cause anal fissure, as may pinworms, if irritation of the area is sufficiently severe.

Treatment. If the stools are hard, they should be softened by eliminating the white foods from the diet (especially milk). A small baby fed largely on a milk diet will need a teaspoonful of dark corn syrup or prune juice (or both) in each bottle of milk per day. In addition, or instead, one-half to one teaspoon of milk of magnesia in one bottle a day may also be necessary. A bit of petroleum jelly or other lubricant pushed gently into the anal opening will soothe and cover the fissure so that the next stool will pass without irritation. If the condition persists for more than a few days, medical attention should be sought.

ANALGESIA AND ANESTHESIA IN LABOR   Obstetrical analgesia means the relief of pain during labor, while obstetrical anesthesia applies to the relief of pain during delivery. It should be clearly stated that we do not as yet have the ideal type of obstetrical analgesia; the extreme sensitivity of the fetus to strong analgesic drugs is the main reason for this. Nevertheless, every mother in labor is entitled to reasonable relief from the pains of active labor, and several ways of achieving this and at the same time protecting the baby from undue exposure to heavy sedation are available. Each patient reacts differently to pain and therefore requires an individual plan for pain relief. If we exempt so-called "natural childbirth" on the one hand, and relief of pain sensations through hypnosis on the other (both of these methods being suitable for a very few carefully selected cases), there remain two well-tested and quite effective methods of obstetrical analgesia:

1. With a combination of drugs given by mouth or by injection, the physician may achieve a safe level of sedation as well as satisfactory amnesia and relief of pain. This method is started as soon as active labor is definitely established, and may be repeated one or more times, depending on the duration of labor and the reaction of the patient. The agents used are usually barbiturates or tranquilizers for general sedation, scopolamine for amnesia, and narcotic drugs for actual pain-relief. Used at the right time and in the right doses, they offer excellent degrees of analgesia; the patient sleeps between her contractions and usually remembers very little afterward.

2. In the spinal approach (epidural analgesia and anesthesia), a single or continuous injection of a local analgesic drug is given around the nerves that supply the womb and the birth canal. The needle is inserted in the back and, if a continuous method is selected, a plastic catheter is passed through the needle and left there until delivery.

Each of these methods has its advantages and disadvantages. The second method is more effective, less harmful to the baby, and quite safe; however, it requires more personnel and involves greater expense.

As far as obstetrical anesthesia is concerned (relief of pain during delivery), there are several choices, and the type best suited for one patient will not necessarily be the best choice for another. The following are the most common types of modern obstetrical anesthesia:

Spinal. Actually a low-dosage spinal called "saddle-block anesthesia." Modifications of this method can also be used earlier, for pain-relief during labor. With it the patient is awake and fully aware of what is happening in the delivery room. She can hear and see her baby right after delivery without experiencing any discomfort. It is an excellent method of anesthesia for deliveries, although some patients have definite objections to spinal anesthesia, based on exaggerated rumors about the risks of the procedure. This method is as safe as any other form of major anesthesia and is definitely the best one for the baby.

For the saddle block anesthesia the drug is injected into the subarachnoid space and mixes with the spinal fluid. Some obstetricians and anesthetists prefer to inject the anesthetic drug outside this space in the form of an epidural anesthesia. Depending on the site of the injection, this latter method can be distinguished into lumbar or caudal type; it may also be given either as a single shot for delivery or in a continuous manner for the relief of pain during labor and delivery (combination of analgesia and anesthesia).

General anesthesia. The patient is actually "put to sleep" for the delivery. Under certain circumstances this is the procedure of choice (breech deliveries, patients with severe bleeding or high blood pressure, patients refusing spinal anesthesia etc.).

Local or regional nerve-block anesthesia (pudendal). The nerves are blocked in the appropriate general area, rather than in the spine. Pain-relief achieved with this method is not as effective as with the previous two, but for a good number of patients this is again the best method of anesthesia for delivery (well-sedated patients, patients with certain medical complications in which the other two methods are contraindicated, etc.).

It should be emphasized that the obstetrician who has kept track of the patient during pregnancy and who is familiar with her physical and emotional problems should be the one to set up a plan of analgesia and anesthesia best tailored to the patient's needs.

ANAPHYLAXIS Anaphylaxis is an immediate, severe, and potentially fatal constitutional reaction with symptoms of difficulty in breathing, generalized hives, swelling of the face and neck, and complete collapse. This type of dangerous reaction may follow the taking of any drug, serum, vaccine, or extract to which a person may be severely allergic. Today penicillin is the most common drug causing anaphylaxis. Insect-sting reaction can also cause this condition. Because of anaphylaxis risk, persons allergic to eggs should not take any vaccine prepared in a chick embryo, and horse-sensitive individuals must avoid vaccine prepared from horse serum (tetanus antitoxin).

ANDROGENS The hormonal secretions of the testes are known as androgens. These are steroid chemical substances, secreted into the bloodstream, which stimulate the muscles, bones, and skin to produce the characteristic changes associated with masculinity. Preparations of androgen are available for injection and oral use in therapy (see TESTOSTERONE).

ANEMIA This is a deficiency in the quality or quantity of red blood cells. The red cells may be depleted by loss of blood from the body because of injury, repeated bloody noses, abnormally heavy menstrual flow, bleeding ulcers or fissures, or other conditions leading to blood-loss. Diseases may also produce anemia: cancer, leukemia, tuberculosis, nephritis, rheumatic fever, erythroblastosis of newborn (RH disease) may be responsible. By far the most common type of anemia in children and babies is simple iron deficiency anemia, which is almost always due to heavy consumption of milk in the first two years of life.

Treatment. The use of milk should be decreased, iron medication given, and meat and fruit added to the diet. Special blood tests are usually necessary to determine the exact type of anemia and, of course, the specific therapy (which is nearly always iron in some form). Iron should be prescribed by the doctor; unsuitable iron medications or dosages may cause digestive trouble. Shots are occasionally advisable.

ANEURISM   If a section of artery wall becomes weakened by disease changes, it tends to thin and bulge out with each beat of the heart. After months or years, a sac-like widening finally develops at this weak point along the artery; this bulging, pulsating projection is called an aneurism. In certain infections (such as syphilis) weakness occurs in the middle, elastic coat of the vessel, the aneurism wall being made up of remnants from all three layers of the artery.

An arteriosclerotic dissecting aneurism comes into existence a little differently. First a stony-hard arteriosclerotic patch replaces a section of the innermost (intima) membrane that lines the artery. Since this patch is not firmly united at its sides, pulsations of blood tend to loosen its attachment to the lining membrane, especially when a crack or fissure develops in that line of attachment. As the fissure enlarges, blood is now forced under pressure into the potential space between the intima and the middle muscle-coat of the artery. The intima is literally peeled away

from its attachment; and the middle coat, now lacking the structural support afforded by its lining membrane, bulges outward with every pulsation of blood. The vessel slowly enlarges and so does the cavity formed between the two blood-vessel layers.

Either type of aneurism can become quite large over a period of years. Most of them occur in the aorta and adjacent large vessels, producing symptoms either because of their size or because of decreased efficiency of circulation in the vessel system distant from the aneurism. In quite large aneurisms ruptures can occur, with resulting fatal hemorrhage.

Treatment. Surgery may be indicated if the aneurism produces symptoms of pain in the chest, abdomen, or wherever it may be present; or if it prevents good circulation to the head, one of the extremities or an important organ of the body; symptoms of malfunction can come in any of these places. Surgery may also be necessary if the aneurism is so large that rupture and fatal hemorrhage seem a real possibility.

At the time of operation, the aneurism may be replaced by a section of borrowed vessel or by woven plastic tubing; the aorta in the chest and abdomen lends itself particularly well to this procedure, and it can be life-saving. Borrowed segments of artery, whether natural tissue or made of plastic, can without difficulty take over blood-vessel function for many years. The body usually builds up reinforcing tissue, surrounds the implanted vessel, and strengthens it so that it seems to function as well as a natural arterial conduit.

Sometimes a by-pass graft is used and the now-empty original vessel, with its aneurism, left in place. When this is done, blood flows through the graft that lies beside the diseased vessel. Occasionally the aneurism can be removed from the artery wall, and the original vessel repaired so that a graft is not needed.

ANGER AND AGGRESSION

Anger, fear, and love are the three instinctive emotions on which all affective life is based. The noted American psychologist John B. Watson showed that anger is expressed very early in life, as for instance if an infant's limbs are pinned down so that it cannot move. Such restriction instinctively stimulates a rage reaction: the child is thwarted and screams in anger.

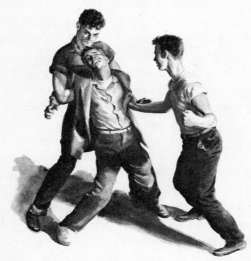

Modern psychologists recognize the importance of anger in mental life in terms of the frustration-aggression-hostility theory. This hypothesis states that a person becomes frustrated (angry) whenever he is thwarted or blocked in life. Anger stimulates aggression toward the objects seen as being thwarting or frustrating, and thereby results in overt hostility.

The whole world is organized in terms of such opposites as hot-cold, life-death, etc.; and love and hate are opposite sides of the same coin. Every person should therefore expect to encounter his share of negative emotion both in himself and in others. All major social upheavals are inevitably associated with a great deal of frustration and anger expressed as hatred of those who are seen as thwarting or frustrating. Similarly we may expect underprivileged children and others to show a great amount of antisocial aggres-

sion in expressing their frustration.

Treatment. In the past, it was customary to cope with aggression in terms of the primitive "an eye for an eye" principle. However, increasingly severe punishment to control serious aggression is a doubtful procedure. There is little evidence that punishment is at all effective as a cure for hate and aggression. On the contrary, the moment when a person is being most aggressive is the very moment when it is necessary to be gentle and forgiving in order to express understanding and help. Modern psychiatric treatment utilizes the principles of unconditional acceptance and love in helping the patient face and control the causes of aggression within himself.

ANGINA PECTORIS

Distinctly a disease of people past middle age and rarely seen earlier, angina pectoris (breast choking) gets its name from the severe pain convulsion with which it is associated. An attack usually is brought on by physical exertion or emotional stress, and generally disappears after a minute or two of adequate rest. Angina pectoris may imply that permanent changes have occurred in the anatomical structure of the coronary arteries (see ARTERIOSCLEROTIC HEART DISEASE).

The occurrence of angina pectoris in many members of one family and few in another suggests that there may be a hereditary factor involved in its development. Among ethnic groups, too, there is a predisposing influence. For example, it is very uncommon in the Bantu tribesmen of South Africa, and rarely is it seen among the Navajo Indians of Arizona, although quite common among other persons in the same area.

Obese individuals have a high rate of coronary artery disease; the mortality rate from coronary heart disease being at least 40 per cent higher in them than among standard-risk persons of average weight. It is also believed that a diet which is very high in fats can lead to coronary artery disease even though the individual on that diet may not be excessively overweight.

Symptoms. If during physical exertion, the heart muscle needs more blood than the width of the coronary arteries can provide, the resulting lack of oxygen (anoxia) and accumulation of metabolic waste products stimulate the sympathetic nerve fibers that surround these arteries. This nerve stimulation can cause pain that is quite severe—a pain usually felt under the breastbone. At the same time, it may spread down the left arm even into the little finger and the one next to it; it sometimes fans out into the neck or jaw, the right arm, or even into the abdomen. The pain usually has a constricting or "squeezing" character.

An attack of angina pectoris is usually brought on by effort, either physical or emotional, and may be relieved in a short time by either sitting or lying down. In some individuals, a large meal can create enough extra heart work to bring on an attack of angina pectoris. Pain may be rather mild and of seconds' duration, or so severe that the person suffering the attack is sure that death itself must be near.

Angina pectoris may be present for years without the existence of serious organic changes demonstrable by routine laboratory tests. On the other hand, quite an advanced stage of heart disease may actually exist even with the mildest of pain attacks.

Ordinarily, the pain of angina pectoris is caused by a temporary spasm of one of the heart-artery branches. The spasm causes enough narrowing of the vessel for the flow of blood to heart-muscle fibers served by that particular artery to be restricted, falling short of the constant requirements of muscle tissue for oxygen and nourishment. No permanent damage is done to the heart muscle, for as soon as the spasm passes, normal blood flow to the area is restored and the deficit in tissue requirements can be slowly corrected.

Sooner or later most patients involved in attacks of angina pectoris will develop a clot that plugs one of the main coronary arteries, and a segment of heart muscle will then incur an injury that is not reversible. Pain that is experienced at the time of vessel blockage may not be very different in character from that experienced during attacks of angina, with one important difference: pain does not disappear after complete rest or even after taking the medication that had always provided relief of pain when vessel spasms alone had caused it.

Treatment. Most patients with uncomplicated angina can, if necessary, carry out light manual work, but any physical activity that increases the frequency of attacks or that causes pain directly must be avoided. A diet is usually advised that does not include rich foods and large meals. Excessive intake of fatty foods should be avoided. Alcohol in moderation does not seem to be harmful.

Drugs in the nitroglycerine group, when held under the tongue, can often avert an impending attack of angina pectoris. Rest-producing medication can be of great value, especially in the period after the acute attack of pain has subsided.

Surgical removal of the blocking patches within the coronary arteries has seemed to restore the ability of those vessels to provide an adequate blood supply to the heart musculature, bringing complete disappearance of the painful attacks in many patients, even after prolonged physical exertion. Operations for the relief of angina pectoris are considered when X-ray studies of the coronary vessels demonstrate partial plugging in one of the main trunks. Modern surgical techniques have made these corrective procedures relatively safe, and for that reason many

42

individuals with coronary artery disease now are being studied to determine whether a direct surgical attack can be made on these anatomic changes.

ANGIOMAS Blood vessel tumors (hemangiomas) of several types, including both superficial and deep lesions, may be seen at birth, but are more often noted several days to weeks after birth. They occur on any part of the skin, can be single or multiple, and each tumor can comprise several types of vessel growth. Almost all types of angiomas are said to be capable of spontaneous disappearance. Almost none of them are of medical significance except for their interference with function and cosmetic deformity depending on their size and the part of the skin involved.

Symptoms. The superficial hemangiomas (strawberry marks) appear as intensely red elevated lesions grouped like berries, grow by extension, and tend to clear irregularly in the center. The color of the lesions becomes intensified on coughing or crying and can become quite dusky and purple. About 25 per cent of the superficial angiomas are accompanied by deep (cavernous) lesions of much larger size, the superficial lesion appearing to "cap" the dome-shaped deeper lesion (cavernous hemangioma). Cavernous tumors can be present with no covering superficial lesion, are irregularly dome-shaped, purplish in color, and of varied size. The rate of growth of the tumors often determines the advisability of active treatment or of awaiting spontaneous disappearance. The lesions rarely bleed or ulcerate. Another type of hemangioma, the port-wine stain (nevus flammeus) is discussed under a separate heading.

Treatment. Many factors play a part in determining the type of treatment most effective for a particular lesion at a particular site. Most cases of strawberry angioma disappear without treatment, but for the rapidly growing ones, radium may be used. Children under two years of age should not be given radium treatment for strawberry angioma, since this usually disappears itself. Dry-ice applications, radium, injection of sclerosing solutions, simple excision, and plastic repair are the most frequently used means of treatment for cavernous hemangioma. Both the dry ice and sclerosing methods are used to initiate involution rather than to destroy the lesions, and therefore are likely to leave little residual scarring. Because of opportunity for much radiation (sun, occupational, medical), radium should be reserved for situations uniquely suitable. Simple excision of very small lesions can successfully forestall growth, but is usually done with reluctance because of the size and age of the patient. Although there is a considerable body of evidence demonstrating the disappearance of these tumors, to permit a tumor to grow in the hope of eventual disappearance and then to be faced with an atypical situation—nondisappearance of the lesion—becomes regrettable for the patient, the parents, and the physician.

ANOMALY Anything which, in the process of development, exceeds a permissible range of variation, produces an anomaly or malformation. Since the blueprint for the body is determined in the early weeks of development, most anomalies—including dental ones—have their origin at this time. Nonetheless, some anomalies are not predetermined, but result entirely from environmental influences in the postnatal period. Deciduous teeth begin developing at about six weeks, and the permanent dentition at about six months, after conception—the process continuing after birth until the complete formation of the permanent third molars (at approximately twenty years). A listing of some of the more important and/or common dental anomalies follows:

Anodontia—Complete lack of development of any or all of either the primary or the permanent teeth

Supernumerary teeth—The development of extra teeth

Mesiodens—The development of supernumerary teeth located between the central incisors of the upper jaw (maxilla)

Peg laterals—A peculiar shaping of the lateral incisor teeth, in which the crown resembles a peg

Mulberry molars—An anomaly of the biting (occlusal) surfaces of molar teeth, resulting in a mulberry-like appearance

Natal teeth—Prematurely erupted teeth present at birth. Occasionally an infant is born with erupted mandibular incisor teeth, either supernumerary or normal. In either case, it may be necessary to remove them if they interfere with nursing or if there is danger of their being sucked into the lungs.

Fusion of teeth—The fusion of the crowns alone, or the entire crowns and roots, of two teeth

Mottled enamel—The development (on the crowns) of spots which are originally white but later darken through staining

Micrognathia—Underdeveloped jaws

Macrognathia—Overdeveloped jaws

Microdontia—Teeth that are smaller than normal

Macrodontia—Teeth that are larger than normal

Ankyloglossia—("Tonguetie") restricted movement of the tongue due to size or location of the frenular attachment

Tori—An excess growth of bone usually located in the midline of the hard palate and/or on the tongue side of the lower arch. Tori are usually asymptomatic, but may interfere with the wearing of artificial dentures.

ANOREXIA NERVOSA (PATHOLOGICAL LOSS OF APPETITE)

This condition involves neurotic loss of appetite and self-induced aversion to food. Occur-

ring primarily in hysteria-prone personalities, this loss of appetite appears to operate symbolically as an attempt to solve psychic conflicts by self-destruction via starvation.

Symptoms. Anorexia nervosa is most common in young women who seem incapable of assuming a normal sex role. Marriage or childbirth often seem crucial events, in reaction to which a young woman stops eating, vomits after intake of food, and develops various somatic complaints, including a low basal metabolic rate. If the condition is left untreated, weight may go down disastrously, leading to progressive starvation and death.

Treatment. Patients should receive psychiatric care as soon as self-induced starvation symptoms become apparent. Treatment should be not only physical, to maintain life; but should also involve psychiatric measures directed toward uncovering the emotional conflicts and personality difficulties which cause the disorder.

ANOSMIA

Anosmia is loss of smell. It may be congenital or acquired. Temporary anosmia is most common in nasal conditions such as the ordinary cold, sinus infection, polyps, and catarrh. Brain lesions involving the olfactory tract may result in one-sided anosmia which is of diagnostic significance in tumors of the underside of the front of the brain. One- or two-sided anosmia may result from frontal fracture of the skull. Tumors of the temporal portion of the brain may result in olfactory hallucinations. Disturbed sense of smell is not uncommon in psychoses and is sometimes seen as an aura in epilepsy. Treatment for anosmia is that of the underlying cause.

ANTIHISTAMINICS

Antihistaminics comprise a wide group of drugs designed to block the effects of histamine, a substance released by the tissues at the time of an allergic reaction. Theoretically, the antihistaminics are supposd to compete with histamine at the target-cell level—the skin in eczema or the nasal mucosa in hay fever—and prevent excessive outpouring of secretions. In actual practice, benefical effects are limited and antihistaminics' usefulness is greater in diseases such as hives or hay fever than it is in asthma or eczema. Antihistaminics usually produce some side effects.

ANTITOXIN   Literally against poison, an antitoxin is a substance which forms within the human body when certain toxins from without gain entrance into the organism. The toxins may come from germs, plants, or other animals. The antitoxin, therefore, is an antibody. Many of them are secured by introducing toxins in gradually increasing doses into horses. Then serum is taken from these animals and used (as hypodermically injected medication) to provide immunization in humans against specific toxins.

ANUS   The anal canal is the final portion of the rectum and large intestine (colon). The anus is guarded by the anal sphincter, a circular muscle which surrounds the canal. Piles (hemorrhoids), fissures, proctitis, and other common disorders of the region are discussed under their appropriate headings.

ANXIETY AND FEAR   Psychiatrists distinguish between fear, which is conscious, and anxiety, which is unconscious. The primitive cause of fear is withdrawal of support or security. The behavioristic psychologist John B. Watson produced unconditioned fear in infants by dropping them and making loud noises. This led to typical fear reactions, very similar to some neurotic reactions to modern life. All emotions have both psychological and physiological components. Under conditions of civilized stress living, every person to some

degree experiences reactions of fear and insecurity which may assume neurotic proportions; that is, reactions which are actually incapacitating.

Fear and anxiety reactions may be observed at all periods of life. Psychoanalytic evidence indicates that many infants begin to develop anxiety reactions as early as the first weeks of life if they are not fed and handled properly. The neurotic infant manifests anxiety by finicky eating habits, irregular bowel habits, sleep disorders, crying, and general irritability.

Many factors in early infancy and childhood can stimulate anxiety reactions. Anything which threatens the child's physical or emotional security tends to stimulate fear reactions revealed by a wide variety of behavior problems, including bed-wetting, eating and sleeping disorders, lying, stealing, masturbation, nervousness, and other symptoms of anxiety. In adults, symptoms may be even more diversified, it being widely understood among psychiatrists that anxiety states interfere with normal functioning of all the systems of the body.

Anxiety reactions are the commonest form of psychoneurotic states, almost as frequently met with in the general population as the common cold. Almost every person shows some degree of anxiety, and it has been estimated that at least twenty million people in the United States are more or less incapacitated by neurotic anxiety reactions. The commonest pattern of neurotic anxiety reactions is the anxiety tension state.

Symptoms. Among the common symptoms of the anxiety state are overall feelings of weakness, tension, and nervousness; band-like headache; muscular pain in the back of the neck; dryness of the mouth and difficulties in swallowing food, as though there were a lump in the throat; irregular "sighing" respiration, as though the individual could not take a deep breath; fast and irregular pulse (often with dropped heart beats and a feeling of faintness); cramps and "butterfly" feelings in the stomach; diarrhea or constipation, often with abdominal discomfort; menstrual irregularities; and feelings of generalized tension and shakiness throughout the body. The sufferer will often complain of peculiar, bizarre sensations, such as knife-like pains in the head, twitching of muscles of the scalp or face, crawling sensations underneath the skin, and atypical pains and aches. These symptoms vary widely from patient to patient, with no standard pattern, and with emotional instability as the only common element.

Where anxiety and fear become extreme, the symptoms become exaggerated in what is known as a panic reaction—an extreme state of anxiety in which the person feels that some terrible thing is about to happen. There are very frightening body sensations suggesting imminent death or insanity. Such panic states may occur in the form of horrible nightmares, in which the person dreams that some terrible tragedy is occurring. Patients commonly complain: "I feel I'm going to die. I feel I'm choking to death. My heart is pounding terribly. I have a feeling of impending doom, as if something terrible is going to happen to me."

Treatment. It is extremely important to recognize anxiey states as psychological reactions, to be treated by a psychiatrist. A common diagnostic error consists in mistaking some of the physical signs of emotional upset for symptoms of organic disease. Such functional symptoms are always of psychological origin.

Since the average patient is convinced of a physical cause for his symptoms, the first step in treatment is to teach the patient that emotional upsets can produce bodily disorders. The patient is taught to trace back to what caused the upset and so gain an understanding of the true causes of his trouble.

A further part of treatment consists in training the patient to accept and cope with anxiety. No one can live completely anxiety-free, so that it is necessary to teach young children how to compensate for their insecurity and inadequacies.

AORTA   The largest artery in the body, the aorta receives all the blood from the left ventricle; it serves as a transport line and reservoir of all newly oxygenated blood. Branching from the aorta are the supply arteries to the head, arms, legs, and —ultimately—every body tissue.

The aorta, like other arteries, has three definite layers in its elastic walls. The in-

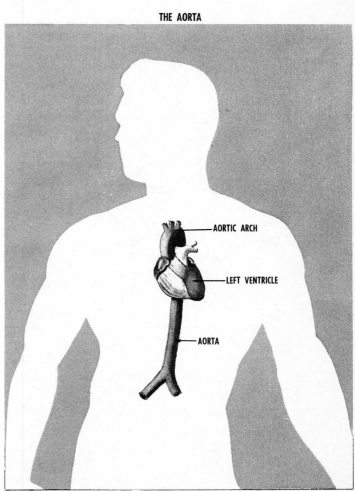

THE AORTA

AORTIC ARCH

LEFT VENTRICLE

AORTA

tima is the lining membrane—a layer of cells about as thick as heavy wrapping paper. The middle coat is relatively thick, composed of a highly elastic membrane that serves to maintain blood pressure between the heart and the peripheral arteries in between heartbeats. The outer layer (adventitia) is a bed or framework of fibrous tissue, fat, and blood vessels that separates the blood vessel from surrounding tissues, and gives it freedom to expand and contract.

AORTA, COARCTATION OF THE A constriction that narrows and may almost completely obstruct the aorta in the upper chest, is called a coarctation. A birth defect, it obstructs the flow of blood to the lower half of the body in the usual case, yet spares the circulation to the head and arms because vessels supplying these areas branch from the aorta prior to the point of narrowing.

Symptoms. Although extensive narrowing in the aorta will cause death shortly after birth, most patients with the abnormality survive for many years, often with no symptoms at all. Blood pressure in the arms may be extremely high but in the legs, can be very low. It is this disparity of blood pressure that often leads to the suspicion of an obstruction within the aorta, and the coarctation can be demonstrated by an X-ray angiogram.

Treatment. When the diagnosis has been confirmed, surgical removal of the constricted portion of the vessel is considered in every case to relieve the constant strain on the heart that must maintain an abnormally high pressure in the aorta just to squeeze blood through the point of coarctation to put blood in the lower body vessels; in addition, relief of the high pressure in the head arteries removes the ever present danger of death from cerebral hemorrhage.

In case the obstruction is not severe, the blood pressure elevation is in modera-

tion and surgical relief is usually deferred until about the age of school attendance, sometimes even a longer period of time.

AORTIC ARCH MALDEVELOPMENTS Curiously, there are two aortas in the very early development of the baby prior to birth; the right aorta disappears and the left aorta remains throughout life. If, however, any of these right-sided blood vessels do not wither away but grow either with or without the usual left system, a number of derangements are possible (depending upon how many of the abnormal vessels persist) because the right arch components invariably lie behind the swallowing (esophagus) and breathing (trachea) tubes instead of in front of them, almost completely closing off the channel within either one or both of these vital conduits. When the child attempts to take nourishment, a severe choking attack (dysphagia lusoria) can occur and even cause fatal suffocation.

Treatment. If the choking attacks are severe, or breathing is labored, surgical relief will be required. As soon as the constricting vessel is cut and tied to prevent bleeding, a normal passageway is restored for passage of air to the lungs, or food to the stomach. Meanwhile, other vessels in the area immediately take over the function of the divided artery.

APHAKIA This is the optical condition which follows removal of the lens in cataract surgery. A powerful convex lens is required, and inasmuch as accommodation for near vision is not possible, there must be increased power for close work, which is usually provided for by a bifocal lens.

APHONIA This form of aphasia is marked by loss of speech function. It may be organic in origin but often occurs as a phenomenon of conversion hysteria (a form of psychoneurosis), particularly when the conscious stimulus is a frightening one. In the latter instance, it is assumed that the speechlessness is a reaction to an unconscious emotional conflict.

Treatment. In the absence of organic factors, immediate restoration of speech can be obtained through hypnosis. However, this is not a "cure"; to avoid repetition of hysterical aphonic attacks or equivalent neurotic reactions, psychotherapy must be instituted.

APOPLEXY Apoplexy is a sudden decrease or loss of consciousness, sensation, and voluntary motor power caused by rupture or obstruction of an artery of the brain. The outstanding finding is usually paralysis of one arm and leg. Occasionally only one extremity, or all four extremities, may be weak or paralyzed. The patient may be drowsy, confused, or completely unconscious. Associated findings include speech disorders, partial blindness, double vision, facial paralysis, or difficulty in swallowing.

APPENDICITIS Surgical removal of the appendix (appendectomy) because of an infection (appendicitis) is one of the more common abdominal operations. Appendicitis is most often seen in the ten-to-thirty age group, although it may strike at any age. Its incidence has been decreasing rather dramatically in recent years, a decline ascribed to the more liberal use of antibiotics. The causes of acute inflammation of this organ are not entirely clear; however, since it is a dead-end tube, substances which enter the appendix may find difficulty in leaving; obstructions are thus thought to occur, with subsequent swelling, inflammation, and finally bacterial invasion. Hardened pieces of intestinal contents lodged in the appendix for long periods of time are a common cause of obstruction. Occasionally, intestinal worms may also cause obstruction.

Symptoms. The usual combination of symptoms is classical, hence, diagnosis is not particularly difficult; there are, however, enough variations to make proper diagnosis extremely challenging. Normally, the typical attack is characterized at an early stage by intermittent or colicky pain, either throughout the abdomen or around the navel (umbilicus). This pain gradually becomes localized in the right-lower abdomen. Onset of pain is often followed by nausea and vomiting, and loss of appetite is common. After the pain has settled in the right-lower abdomen, it tends to become constant rather than cramping, and is increasingly severe. Occasionally the pain becomes extremely severe, then suddenly ceases. This is the "calm before the storm," as it often means that the appendix has ruptured and that peritonitis will ensue. The fever ordinarily does not exceed 101° F. Constipation is often a symptom. It is extremely important not to give cathartics or enemas to anyone suspected of having appendicitis.

While the above-mentioned are the usual symptoms, there are many variations; also, because of the mobility of the intestine, the appendix may often be found in the *left*-lower abdomen, and if it is far to the rear of the cavity it may mimic the pain usually associated with kidney stones. Other conditions which must be differentiated from appendicitis include: intestinal obstructions, femoral hernia, and—in the female—inflammation of the pelvic organs. In fact, almost any disease that may affect the abdominal cavity has been mistaken for appendicitis, and vice versa.

Particularly today, with modern techniques and treatment readily available, it is probably the wisest course to have an exploratory operation if appendicitis is at all suspected, since the mortality after delay is great. In addition to peritonitis, complications of acute appendicitis may include abscess-formation, intestinal obstruction, and (occasionally) a fistula or infected opening into a surrounding structure such as the bladder. It must be remembered that in the very young, the elderly, or in people who are chronically ill from other conditions, the classical signs of appendicitis may not be present, and in these instances the doctor must very carefully evaluate abdominal pain.

Treatment. The treatment is surgical removal as soon as the diagnosis is firmly established or cannot be ruled out. There may be rare instances in which for one reason or another surgery is not feasible. In these cases, massive doses of antibiotics and careful observation may suffice; but the instances are few where this course of action is considered prudent.

APPETITE AND HUNGER Appetite and hunger are not the same. Appetite is largely the conscious psychological aspect of the desire for food. It is conditioned by past experiences, cultural customs, and habit. Thus, the urge to eat a tempting dessert (appetite) may exist long after the more physical sensation—hunger—has been appeased by an excellent meal. Hunger itself is not modified significantly by the past experience of the individual.

There are centers in the hypothalamus, a part of the base of the brain, which regulate feeding. One center regulates appetite, or the desire to eat; the other acts as a brake to prevent overeating and is called the satiety center. The nutritional roles of appetite, hunger, and the hypothalamic centers are currently under extensive investigation.

ARTERIES The arteries are tubes that carry blood from the heart, through an elaborate branching system, to all the capillaries of the body. With every heartbeat, a jet of blood is pressed into the arterial system, which, by its built-in elasticity, insures a constant flow of blood from its smallest branches (the arterioles) into the capillaries, where chemical exchanges are

made. (From the capillaries, blood returns to the heart through a separate system of vessels, the veins.)

ARTERIOSCLEROSIS Usually thought of as "hardening of the arteries," arteriosclerosis causes more circulatory disease after middle age than any other single cause. Arteriosclerosis is nevertheless occasionally seen in young persons of both sexes and, conversely, many elderly people have little significant involvement with the condition; it is therefore an oversimplification to say that the condition is always the result of stress and wear in the arteries, especially the result of the aging process.

Although high blood pressure is quite commonly a complication of "hardening" (sclerotic) arterioles, it may or may not be present in persons with arteriosclerosis. Diabetes can facilitate the development of arteriosclerotic changes; even young patients with diabetes may be severely involved in arteriosclerosis—especially when the diabetes has not been well controlled over a long period of time.

Arteriosclerosis can cause disease changes in specific organs, such as serious kidney disease. Cerebral arteriosclerosis may lead to crippling mental infirmities. Sometimes changes in one or more organs are quite severe, while the rest of the artery system seems to show little significant disease, if any at all.

Theories about the causes of arteriosclerosis often center about the individual's type of diet, his hereditary background, the amount of exercise he has had in proportion to his caloric intake, and the question of whether or not he has consumed excessive amounts of fat. There may, in fact, be more than one factor that can lead to arteriosclerosis; certainly, there are no unquestioned causes of this sclerosing process of blood vessels, so widespread today among most of the peoples of the civilized world.

ARTERIOSCLEROTIC HEART DIS-EASE

The most common cause of heart disease in patients beyond middle age is arteriosclerosis, which causes (or precipitates) more deaths in the United States than all other diseases combined. Heart-failure is more frequently caused by arteriosclerosis than any other disease process. The failure may be mild and may persist for many years before death comes as a final manifestation.

Any narrowing of the internal diameter of the arteries of the heart through arteriosclerotic changes can diminish the amount of blood flowing to the heart muscle fibers. Replenishing the vital chemicals constantly needed to energize the heart, blood flow should increase—even if only for a few minutes—every time there is a new demand for intense heart action. (Because of the efficient arrangement of the capillaries in heart muscle, almost no available oxygen remains in the blood after its passage through the heart itself, and there-fore additional oxygen can be supplied only by a proportionate increase in blood flow through the coronary arteries of the heart.)

Symptoms. Arteriosclerotic narrowing of the coronary arteries can produce several varieties of symptoms. The patient may contract angina pectoris or the involvement may be so complete that permanent changes occur in a segment of heart muscle which then becomes non-contractile and functionless (coronary infarction). Degenerative changes in the "heart-triggering" conduction system ("bundle of His") can be the result of arteriosclerotic changes that have deprived this system of oxygen and nutrients needed for its life processes. When these changes are firmly entrenched, serious disturbances may occur in the orderly, rhythmic contractions of the heart chambers such as Adams-Stokes attacks and cardiac arrests.

ARTERIOVENOUS FISTULAS

An arteriovenous fistula is an abnormal open-

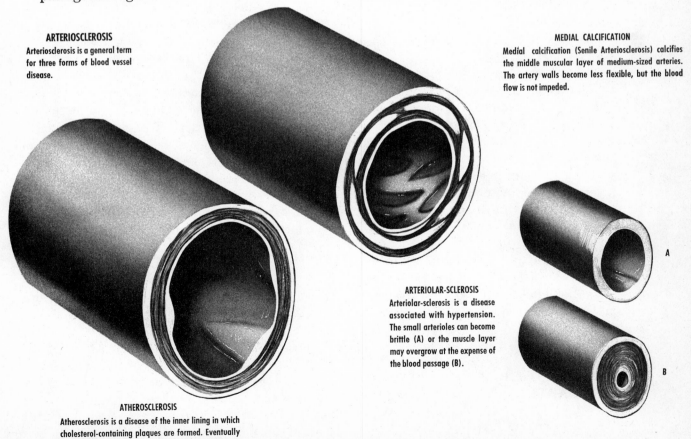

ARTERIOSCLEROSIS
Arteriosclerosis is a general term for three forms of blood vessel disease.

MEDIAL CALCIFICATION
Medial calcification (Senile Arteriosclerosis) calcifies the middle muscular layer of medium-sized arteries. The artery walls become less flexible, but the blood flow is not impeded.

ARTERIOLAR-SCLEROSIS
Arteriolar-sclerosis is a disease associated with hypertension. The small arterioles can become brittle (A) or the muscle layer may overgrow at the expense of the blood passage (B).

A

B

ATHEROSCLEROSIS
Atherosclerosis is a disease of the inner lining in which cholesterol-containing plaques are formed. Eventually the blood flow is impeded by the enlarging plaques.

ing between an artery and a vein. It may be inborn—a defect present at birth—or it may be acquired during life. Usually an acquired arteriovenous fistula is caused by an injury. If a wound should occur in an artery wall, as sometimes results from a knife or bullet injury, the injury may also involve the vein lying next to the artery. These two wounds may then unite the artery and vein walls, tightly fastening them together as the healing proceeds and through this attachment an opening for blood may slowly develop. Blood in the artery, under pressure, can then leak through the opening into the vein by way of the newly formed fistula.

If the opening lies between a large artery and vein, a great quantity of blood may flow out of the artery and return via the vein to the heart without having supplied any of the tissues. This functional leakage can be so large in extent that additional work on the heart may eventually cause heart-failure. On rare occasions, a bacterial infection will develop at the site of the fistula and result in "germs in the blood" (bacteremia), or even blood poisoning (septicemia).

Treatment. Surgical correction is the only cure for an arteriovenous fistula. In almost every instance, the opening in the artery wall can be closed by fine sutures and the vein moved aside and similarly repaired. A piece of tissue is sometimes placed between the two vessels to prevent a reforming of the abnormal pathway between the two vessels as they heal in such proximity to one another.

ARTHRITIS   The term arthritis as used by the orthopedist refers to conditions of the joints characterized by varying degrees of pain, swelling, stiffness, and loss of motion. There are innumerable causes of such conditions.

ARTHRITIS, DEGENERATIVE, OR OSTEOARTHRITIS   Degenerative ar-

thritis is the most common form of arthritis in the United States. It is due to the wear and tear of ill-matching (incongruous) joint surfaces rather than to a specific inflammatory disease, as rheumatoid or gouty arthritis. When generalized, osteo-arthritis is a manifestation of the aging process; when localized in one joint, it is usually the result of previous deformation of the joint. For example, osteoarthritic involvement of one hip may be due to old Perthes' disease, while osteoarthritis of a knee may be the result of a severe knock-knee deformity.

Symptoms.   Osteoarthritis is usually manifested in the weight-bearing joints of the body, since these joints are subject to far more wear and tear than the joints of an upper extremity. The osteoarthritic patient complains of joint pain which is worse on awakening in the morning than later in the day. If he has pain in the hips or knee, he will experience great difficulty in getting out of low or soft chairs. When loose bodies are present within the joint, the patient will note crackling sounds and locking of the joint.

Treatment. Treatment includes rest of the acutely painful joint and pain-reducing (analgesic) medication. There are no specific drugs now available to treat this mechanical condition. Treatment today is preventive in the early stage, protective during acute flareups, and reconstructive in the advanced degenerative stage.

Any patient with a tendency toward osteoarthritis should keep his weight under control, since obesity places added strain on the already-taxed joints. A cane is very helpful in taking stress off involved limbs. With hip pain, the cane should be used on the opposite side, but may be more comfortable on the same side in cases of knee pain.

ARTHRITIS, GOUTY   This condition presents essentially the same symptoms as infectious arthritis, but is due to increased

COMMON FORMS OF ARTHRITIS
AND
THE JOINTS INVOLVED

There are three main types of arthritis:
1. Osteoarthritis
2. Rheumatoid Arthritis
3. Gouty Arthritis

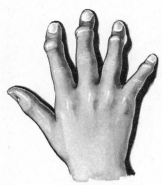

OSTEOARTHRITIS

The most common form of arthritis, occurring most frequently in elderly people, is due to the wear and tear on bones. Thickening of the bones can cause deformity. The joints nearest the finger tips are favorite sites.

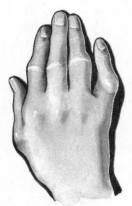

RHEUMATOID

This is a chronic, severely disabling inflammatory disease marked by deformity and union of bones.

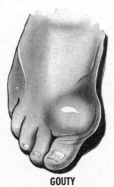

GOUTY

Gouty arthritis is caused by excess uric acid in the blood. Uric acid deposits in the joints interfere with movement and form enlarged, painful tophi (deposits of sodium urate) around the joints.

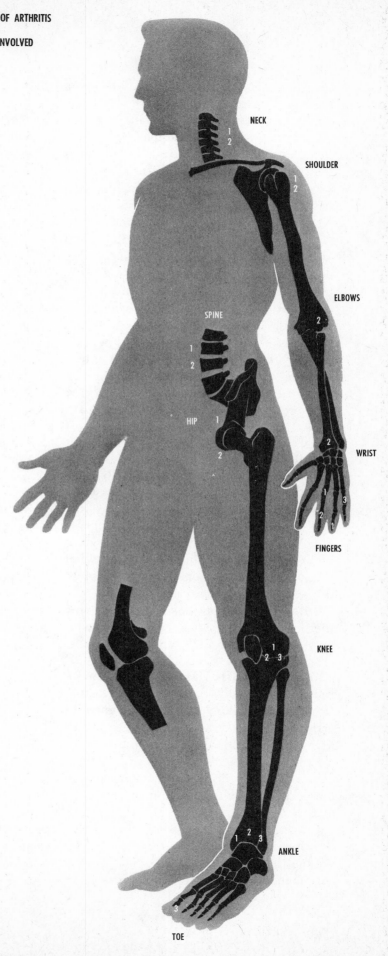

NECK

SHOULDER

ELBOWS

SPINE

HIP

WRIST

FINGERS

KNEE

ANKLE

TOE

uric acid in the bloodstream, not to an offending bacterial organism.

Symptoms. Gout is far more common in men than in women and most commonly involves the big toe; however, all other joints may also be involved. In many cases there are extensive, easily palpable, soft-tissue deposits of uric-acid salts (urates) which are called tophi.

Treatment. Treatment is carried out along several lines: anti-inflammatory drugs are used in acute flare-ups, and in the quiescent periods specific drugs such as Zyloprim® are used to lower the circulating uric-acid level. Dietary control is also of great help during the quiescent periods. Gouty patients should restrict their intake of fish, meat, and alcoholic beverages, since these contain large amounts of uric acid precursors.

ARTHRITIS, INFECTIOUS This type of arthritis is due to bacterial involvement of a joint. The joint is acutely hot, swollen, and painful. If not rapidly treated, the offending organism will destroy it and lead to ankylosis.

Treatment. Treatment includes antibiotics, joint immobilization, and either suction (aspiration) or drainage. Before the antibiotic era, the result of infectious arthritis was always catastrophic, but now there is a fair chance of healing with preservation of normal joint function.

ARTHRITIS, RHEUMATOID An inflammatory condition of unknown cause, like the other collagen diseases rheumatoid arthritis appears to be related to the body's immune mechanisms. The blood of rheumatoid arthritis patients contains abnormal amounts of certain proteins, among them a fairly specific substance known as "rheumatoid factor."

Symptoms. In classical rheumatoid arthritis, joint involvement tends to be symmetrical and intermittent. The patient may complain of painful swelling of both wrists or pain in both ankles which begins at much the same time. The symptoms will then abate, only to recur in the future either in the same or in other joints; in severe cases most of the joints of the body will be involved to some degree. Along with the joint swelling, fibrous scarring of the joint capsule and overgrowth (hypertrophy) of the joint's lining wall (synovium) takes place. If untreated, the joint becomes markedly deformed with time.

Treatment. Aspirin has traditionally been used to treat rheumatoid arthritis and even now provides the mainstay of treatment. It acts to relieve pain and to minimize the inflammatory response around the involved joints. In the past decade cortisone and the other steroids have been widely prescribed for their anti-inflammatory effect. There is some evidence now that the steroids do not affect the progress of the disease, but rather only control the acute symptoms.

An acutely painful joint should be splinted. As soon as the pain and swelling abate, the joint should be vigorously exercised to regain strength and mobility. Physical therapy plays an important role in the overall management of the arthritic patient. Heat in various forms is used to relieve pain and spasm, and gentle manipulation is prescribed to overcome early contractures. Paraffin baths are very helpful in increasing the mobility of rheumatoid hands and may be self-administered by the patient in the home.

Various surgical operations are being developed to reconstruct involved joints and restore motion to stiffened arthritic limbs. Surgery now has much to offer the severely incapacitated arthritic patient and will presumably play an important role in the total care of such patients in the future.

ARTIFICIAL KIDNEY The artificial kidney is a collection of tubes and filters which run through a carefully regulated bath of the proper chemical composition.

It is used as a temporary kidney substitute when connected to the veins and arteries of the patient, and may often be life-sustaining while a self-limiting injury or disease is healing. It is not usually used in patients with advanced incurable kidney disease.

An increasing number of centers are being created for use of the artificial kidney, which requires a well-trained team of physicians, round-the-clock nursing care, and technicians. Very recently the artificial kidney has been used to sustain life in patients with chronic kidney disease. Such patients are provided with tubes (catheters) permanently implanted in their arteries and veins, so they may easily be connected to the "kidney" for a treatment (dialysis). Sometimes it is considered advisable to remove diseased kidneys from the body because they produce poisonous chemicals. The artificial kidney is successful in maintaining a reasonably good state of health in such cases. The cost of treatment with the artificial kidney is very high, but costs are being reduced by treatment in the home setting and by the use of simplified, cheaper machines. In some cases the transplantation of a single kidney is a viable alternative.

ARTIFICIAL RESPIRATION See FIRST AID AND EMERGENCIES also FIRST AID AND LIFE SAVING, PLATES F1-F8.

ART THERAPY This is a form of occupational therapy in which mental patients are encouraged to express themselves in all kinds of art work. Psychiatrists have discovered that mental patients should be assigned a full program of work and recreational activities, resembling normal life as much as possible. Artistic activities have great psychological value because many patients are able to express in their art designs conflicts and other problems which ordinarily they would not be able to talk about. Frequently the patient reveals his mood by the selection of colors to use in his painting, and may also express the contents of his psychological problem in the artistic forms produced. Psychiatrists are often able to diagnose psychological problems by interpreting the significance of the patients' artistic productions. Art training also broadens the mental patient's view on life and gives him new interests.

Art therapy is an important part of the rehabilitational programs of mental hospitals in the attempt to get patients interested in things outside themselves and also to help them experience the actualization of personality resources. It is also used in outpatient treatment to stimulate the person to develop fulfilling hobbies.

ASBESTOSIS A disease of the lungs that is caused by breathing in minute particles of asbestos. The disease is often contracted by persons who work with the material.

ASEPSIS The absence of bacteria and other disease-producing microorganisms or germs. The care of the sick and modern surgical techniques are based in good measure on aseptic methods of avoiding infection. The meaning of asepsis is summed up in one word: *sterile*.

ASPIRATOR A medical instrument used to remove fluids from cysts or body cavities, such as the lungs, by the process of suction.

ASTHMA This word comes from the Greek meaning panting. This disease is known all over the world, and may affect any person, regardless of age, sex, or race. In the United States it is estimated that there are about five million asthmatic patients. Together with chronic bronchitis and emphysema (see OBSTRUCTIVE LUNG DISEASE), it is responsible for the loss of about thirty-five million work days annually. A great deal of confusion attends the definition of this disease, and the word asthma often becomes a catchall for many ill-defined respiratory diseases.

Broadly speaking, asthma may be due to either extrinsic or intrinsic factors. Extrinsic asthma (also called allergic asthma) is due to external offenders which sensitize ("set up") the organism to subsequent exposures to the same agents. Let us use pollen as an example. During certain seasons, pollen is carried by the wind and inhaled into the respiratory system, without causing awareness or discomfort in most individuals. In some persons, however, due to the presence of genetically inherited characteristics, a reaction will be established between the "stranger" (pollen), thereafter called an antigen or allergen, and the host body-tissue cells. The latter will not "recognize" the antigen and react by producing defensive substances, called antibodies, which will close around the antigen and create an inflammatory reaction. From then on, every time this particular antigen reaches the body, an encounter takes place in the form of an asthmatic attack. In this instance, the target-cells for the encounter are in the mucous membrane (mucosa) of the respiratory tract. The same allergic phenomenon may express itself in any other part of the body, such as the skin (eczema), and the bowels (diarrhea). Most asthmatics have a past history of allergic episodes of one kind or another.

Basically, the allergic reaction stems from a mechanism of defense set up by the body against intruders, but which in the allergic individual is carried too far and becomes deleterious. The mechanism is a sort of protective "memory" recollection. For instance, after having passed through measles in childhood, the body develops antibodies against the causative virus; if it is again exposed to measles, antibodies are summoned and quietly deter the invader. The antigens capable of producing asthma are large in number and widely distributed. Many physical agents, such as foodstuffs, animals, clothing, cosmetics, and emotional stimuli have been found to be potential allergens. The search for the particular offender in a given person is always difficult and often fruitless.

Intrinsic asthma, on the other hand, is a term coined for the type of asthma which usually starts later in life, for which no obvious allergen can be detected, and which often develops in the wake of a severe respiratory tract infection. Thus, intrinsic asthma is sometimes called infectious asthma. Regardless of the specific cause, the mechanism of the asthmatic attack is always characterized by marked obstruction of the small bronchial tubes. This obstruction is the result of a combination of factors: (1) thickening of the inner bronchial walls (edema) due to increased outpouring of fluid; (2) active constriction of the muscular circular coat present in the walls of the tubes (bronchoconstriction); (3) production of a very thick phlegm which tends to block the bronchial airways. Under these conditions it is hard to breathe in but even harder to breath out, and excessive air accumulates in the lungs so that they become overinflated.

Symptoms. Regardless of the cause, the classical asthmatic attack has the same typical characteristics. It is manifested by an acute, severe paroxysm of shortness of breath (usually of a choking nature), accompanied by audible chest wheezes, bothersome ineffectual cough, profound exhaustion, anxiety, and fear. The lips become bluish (cyanosis) and the patient perspires profusely. Most attacks develop quickly, often at night, and force the patient to sit up to insure maximal use of his respiratory muscles, including the accessory respiratory muscles in the neck. The patient feels that not enough air is coming in (though the chest is held at maximal inflation) and also that it is hard to push it out. The attack may last from minutes to several days. Spontaneously, or by medical treatment, the paroxysm is reduced and improvement is commonly heralded by expectoration of small plugs of sputum. The mechanism of the attack is interpreted as due to generalized obstruction of the small bronchial tubes by a combination of factors: contraction of the bronchial wall musculature, thickening of the inner lining, and production of thick tenacious sputum. All factors combined reduce the passageway of the bronchial tubes significantly and obstruct the flow of air. If the attack lasts for more than a couple of days, the condition is called status asthma. The attacks may recur at varying time intervals. At the onset, they may be purely seasonal (e.g., pollen asthma), related to some change in the weather, due to house-cleaning (dust asthma), or the sequel to an emotionally upsetting situation. At this stage the patient may feel perfectly well during intervals between attacks. As time goes on, however, the periodicity of attacks tends to disappear, there are less defined periods of well-being, the attacks are more frequent, and chronic bronchial asthma becomes perennial. This change is attended by new characteristics: (1) shortness of breath does not disappear between attacks and becomes progressively more incapacitating; (2) chronic bronchitis supervenes, with the production of daily expectoration and recurrent episodes of upper-respiratory infection; (3) complications set in—particularly emphysema and eventually heart failure.

In other cases the attacks may repeat themselves for several years and then taper off completely, or they may reappear after several years of "cure." The course of the disease is highly unpredictable. In most cases it will last for many years with up-and-down swings in intensity. In a minority it may cripple the patient relentlessly in a matter of a few months. The popular belief that asthmatic children will "outgrow" the disease when they reach their teens is not supported by facts and may lure one into unwarranted confidence.

Treatment. Complete cure is possible when the specific offender is detected and can be either avoided completely, made harmless, or treated. For example, avoiding certain foods is feasible, but living in an environment of pure, pollen-free air is not. If the allergen cannot be avoided completely (dust or pollen), injections of such allergens can be given, starting with very small amounts to build up immunity slowly (desensitization). If, on the other hand, one can prove a definite established emotional disturbance, psychiatric treatment should be given.

A word of caution should be spoken about cures: Many of these are only temporary because the potentiality for becoming sensitized to newer allergens, either singly or in combination, is typical of an allergic individual. Moving to a new location may bring only temporary relief since new allergies may be contracted. Specific antiallergic treatment of progressive desensitization has the best rate of success in children and young adults. Symptomatic treatment of the disease can also be highly effective, though not curative. Particularly useful are the medications given by inhalation (bronchodilators), which bring quick relief and are given through small, pocket-sized "vaporizers" (nebulizers). Bronchodilators can be also given by mouth or by rectum.

During severe paroxysms, injections are required, the two most effective drugs being adrenalin and aminophylline. For the most difficult cases, steroid drugs are used. (These drugs are very potent and derived from substances present in the adrenal gland. It is best to use them only for short periods when simpler, conventional treatment has failed.) Expectorants and drugs to liquefy the sputum are useful adjuvants in treatment, as is reeducation in breathing habits by means of physiotherapy. Antihistamine preparations are of less value than is commonly believed. The patient should have adequate rest and sedation when overtired; control of respiratory infections is most important, particularly in the very chronic and elderly asthmatics.

The list of proposed treatments for bronchial asthma is endless and the tremendous suffering of patients makes them eager to try out every suggestion of treatment, old and new.

ASTHMATIC BRONCHITIS See ASTHMA

ASTIGMATISM   If rays of light entering the eye are bent unevenly, they do not all come to focus at the same point. In astigmatism the focusing is such that the rays of light entering the eye form a line instead of a point. Astigmatism may be far sighted, near sighted, or mixed (in which one line is focused in front of the retina and another would be focused behind if it did not strike the retina first). Minor degrees of astigmatism are practically universal, presumably as a result of the weight of the upper lid resting upon the eye.

Symptoms. Marked astigmatism causes reduction in either near or far vision, sometimes also in both. Intermediate amounts of astigmatism are considered to be a particularly likely cause of eyestrain, inasmuch as a slightly blurred image is seen which cannot be put in more distinct focus by accommodation.

Treatment. Astigmatism is neutralized by cylindrical lenses which refract in one plane and not in the plane at right angles. Considerable judgment is required in prescribing lenses to correct small degrees of astigmatism.

ATAXIA   Ataxia refers to unsteadiness of the arms, trunk, or legs. In the hand and arm it is manifested by difficulty in eating, writing, sewing, and performing other coordinated movements. If the arm is at rest, there is no tremor. However, a rhythmical tremor does develop with purposeful movements. Ataxia of the trunk or legs results in difficulty in walking. The individual walks with his feet apart and has difficulty with balance. He may fall due to difficulty in coordinating leg movements properly.

Cerebellar ataxia is due to failure of development, degeneration, intoxication with alcohol or drugs such as Dilantin® (dimenhydrinate), or abscess or tumors of the cerebellum. When there is involvement of the central portion of the cerebellum, unsteadiness of the trunk is a prominant symptom. A tumor or abscess involving one lateral cerebellar hemisphere will produce unsteadiness in the arm and leg on the same side.

Sensory ataxia is due to destruction of sensory pathways, chiefly those for determining the sense of position in space. The sensory fibers may be destroyed in the brainstem, spinal cord, or peripheral nerves. If the destructive process is in the brainstem or cervical spinal cord, ataxia is present either in the arms alone or in both the arms and the legs. Involvement of the lower spinal cord results in ataxia in the legs. If the damage occurs in the peripheral nerves, it may involve the legs, the arms, or both.

ATELECTASIS   This word comes from the Greek and means incomplete expansion. Commonly the term implies an airless or nearly airless lung which becomes functionless. The degree of atelectasis in any given situation varies considerably and may involve anything from a small segment to an entire lung.

Atelectasis may be caused fundamentally by any of the following three mechanisms: (1) obstruction of the bronchi or blockage of the air passages; (2) inflammation of lung tissue which takes up the space normally used for air; and (3) insufficent chest-wall expansion or lung-collapse due to filling of the pleural space by fluid or air. In any of these conditions, although the affected lung area ceases to be ventilated, the blood continues to flow through it and progressively removes the remaining air in the space. In slow, progressive atelectasis there is always suspicion of bronchial tumors.

Symptoms. The symptoms of this condition depend on the amount of atelectasis present, varying from none, to severe degrees of breathlesness, bluish color of the lips and nail beds (cyanosis), fever, and cough. Furthermore, the symptoms of the original disease (pneumonia, tumor, muscular paralysis) which lead to atelectasis in the first place will also be present. Infection of the airless lung is a serious complication because of the lack of natural drainage from such an area.

Treatment. Treatment is directed toward correcting the original cause, together with restoration of open airways by removal of the obstruction or inflammatory secretions. Artificial respiration may be needed, particularly in cases where the nervous system and muscular mechanisms are insufficient to expand the lung. Antibiotics to combat infection, and bronchiodilators to expand the diameter of the bronchial tubes, are commonly employed. Any tumors blocking the airways (either from the inside or acting by outside compression) are treated by surgical removal or by deep X-ray therapy.

ATHEROSCLEROSIS   While the term arteriosclerosis is a general one, used to describe any of the "hardening-of-the-arteries" changes, atherosclerosis is a very specific disease.

The primary tissue-change seen in atherosclerosis is found in the lining membrane (intima) of the arterial tube. While in young, healthy arteries the intimal lining consists of a layer of very smooth and glistening cells loosely adhering to the thicker, medial layer of the artery, in atherosclerosis this lining coat shows deposits of fatty molecules (lipids) as well as variable amounts of scar tissue formation, hemorrhage, and calcification.

Recent studies show that the lipids in circulating blood tend to leak across the lining membrane and be deposited in the space between it and the rather solid (yet elastic) middle layer of the vessel. These lipids change from liquid into solid form and are taken into special cells lying in that space (mesenchymal cells). This incorporation of fatty materials into the cells of the blood vessel may represent the earliest form of atherosclerosis. When fat-laden cells leak over into the middle coat of the artery, thickening can result there in addition to formation of intimal-lining deposits. This frequently happens in the larger arteries that supply the brain, the kidneys, and the lower extremities.

As the lipid-filled cells accumulate, fibrous tissue seems to be laid down, the patch of arterial lining membrane then becoming rigid and thickened, looking in the early stages like a small white scar in the normal yellowish appearance of the intimal membrane. As the patch thickens it degenerates, and tiny blood vessels—capillaries—appear within it. These are soon prone to rupture and pour out small puddles of blood within the atherosclerotic deposit itself.

A double process is thus at work: first come the fatty deposits in the cells, together with a heaping-up of these cells in one particular location with degenerative changes that turn the whole mass into a foreign-body deposit; second, there is occurrance of hemorrhage within these accumulations, adding considerably to their bulk. The space inside the vessel still remaining useful for passage of blood becomes smaller and smaller. The vessel itself is sometimes completely blocked by the process, and blood fails to flow through it beyond the affected point. Then too, a clot may form and completely close off a vessel which, while already nearly obstructed prior to clot-formation, had nevertheless been useful. Calcium may be deposited at any stage of the disease and make the atherosclerotic patch hard and brittle.

Because atherosclerosis is now the most prevalent serious human disease the world over, the problem of prevention and control has been intensified. It is thought that fats in the diet should be reduced to about 20 or 30 per cent of the average consumption. With reduction of lipids and cholesterol circulating in the blood, the precipitation and accumulation of lipids in the intimal lining of the arteries may possibly be reduced to such an extent that the development of arteriosclerosis can be held in check.

Reversibility of atherosclerotic changes in animals was clearly demonstrated many years ago. Atherosclerotic deposits in human beings seem to disappear at times in patients who undergo severe weight loss, as in incurable tuberculosis and hopeless cancer patients.

Under proper—and less drastic—conditions, the foreign fatty material that lies within the cells and spaces of blood vessels can be withdrawn. One of these happy conditions seems to be the reduction of total concentration of certain blood lipids; the total serum cholesterol is often used as an index of this concentration. Special diets, exercise programs, and careful attention to any metabolic derangements that may be present can sometimes bring about these desirable lower lipid levels in the blood. It would, however, require many months for beneficial repairs to occur in the involved arteries.

ATHLETE'S FOOT   This common ailment is caused by fungi in persons who have the type of skin (sweaty) which is conducive to the abundant growth of the fungus and who also have inadequate local immunity to the effects of that fungal growth. The common location of the eruption between the toes is due largely to the persistence of moisture in these warm and occluded areas. While sweat is almost always available for fungal growth, moisture from inadequate drying of the feet after swimming and bathing is probably a more frequent precipitating factor in the occurrence of acute attacks of athlete's foot. The communicability of this disease is largely overstated as is evidenced by the fact that bedmates do not often contract the disease from exposure to each other; and more importantly, the eruption is not uncommonly seen on only one foot, the other apparently not affording identical facilities for the growth of the fungus. It is apparent that compulsory foot baths in public pools accomplish little as compared with what compulsory drying of the feet would do for the protection of the individual.

Several species of fungi are capable of producing this disease, but only a few cause widespread fungus disease of the soles of the feet, palms of the hands, nails and other parts of the skin, and that only in an infinitely smaller number of people.

Symptoms. The eruption ranges from a slight scaling between the fourth and fifth toes to redness, oozing, and cracking of the spaces between all the toes and extension of the eruption to the adjacent areas of the feet. Secondary infection and bleeding of the cracked and fissured areas result from inattention to the earlier lesions.

Treatment. It is essential that the feet be kept dry. It may be necessary to institute a regime of frequent change of socks and shoes, and sometimes it may become necessary to wear sandals or perforated shoes to permit both the lessening of sweat production and the evaporation of the irreducible amount of sweat present. Minor attacks can be controlled by sponging the feet with rubbing alcohol to insure final drying. The application of foot powders, while theoretically sound, nevertheless often induces further maceration of the skin by the swelling of the powder on mixing with sweat and the forming of irritating masses. Antifungal ointments should be applied at night, when the foot is not encased in occlusive footgear. During the day, use of moderately effective tinctures like mercurochrome, iodine, and other dyes is less likely to produce the undesired effects of ointments and powders. For more severe involvement and for oozing eruptions, cold wet soaks will relieve the subjective symptoms and reduce irritation and swelling. Plain cold water is both available and satisfactory, although the well-known potassium permanganate, boric acid, Burow's solution compresses, or soaks can be used if not too inconvenient.

The fungal antibiotic griseofulvin is a very effective remedy. Because of both the recurrences and the persistence of this disease, the use of an antibiotic should be reserved for either acute and disabling attacks, or for cases in which more simple remedies fail. A recently released, very potent antifungal agent, Tinactin®, is available in lotion and ointment form and is considered the drug of choice by many dermatologists; application should continue a while after visible lesions clear.

ATOPIC DERMATITIS   This is an allergic skin disorder belonging to the atopic group of diseases which are characterized by a high incidence in members of the same family; a tendency for the afflicted to have more than one form of the disease, occasionally simultaneously but not infrequently in succession (hay fever, asthma, migraine); and a persistent high "eosinophil" count (a greater than usual number of this type of white blood corpuscle), present also in other diseases and significant only as a diagnostic aid.

Symptoms. The disease begins in infancy with a reddened scaly eruption of the face and extremities, and often associated with cradle cap, a greasy scaling of the scalp. The condition improves with or without treatment. A great number of patients have no further indication of this condition but may develop the other forms later. In those in whom the condition persists the next attack occurs at about two or three years of age and usually takes the form of flexural eczema with some reddened thickening at the bends of the elbows and knees. The nape of the neck may also be the site of red papules, thickening and crusting. At six years of age, recurrence is again noted, and at puberty the disease takes on the appearance and distribution commonly seen in the adult. Since the incidence of atopic dermatitis is so low in adults, and even in adolescents, as compared with its incidence in infancy and childhood, it is apparent that a very high percentage of the afflicted young undergo some immunologic or other alteration making them nonsusceptible to further dermatitis of this type. In the adult the disease may be confined to the elbows and knees, but is more often generalized and involves the body and the face as well. The skin becomes markedly thickened and ridged, with a grayish hue, and no matter how well treated, presents the scratch marks of persistent itching. Atopic dermatitis can persist through early adult life, but is extremely uncommon after forty years of age. In pregnant women the condition has been known to both worsen and improve during the period of gestation. If a remission is noted in early adult life, it is likely to be permanent.

In all the stages of the disease the lesions can become infected, and in young children this is almost the rule. In the young, too, the disease is more moist and the lesions consist of greasy crusts, easily removed with some resultant bleeding. The older patients have lesions that are dry, thick, leathery, and ridged.

The allergic responses in these patients are myriad, often fleeting and changing, but always persistent. Removal of an allergen (food) known to cause flare-up of the eruption or immunization to a known inhalent allergen (dust, pollen) does not often result in improvement—probably because still another allergen or group of allergens will constitute the provocative agents and sustain the disease. However, removal of known or suspected allergens can be useful, especially if these substances are not essential to a person's diet or environment. Attempts at desensitization are less useful but nevertheless worth trying in some selected cases. Change of environment can cause dramatic improvement. The change can be a small one (within the same city, for instance), or it can be one to a place which differs greatly in temperature, humidity, in grasses and trees, and in elevation (usually the higher the altitude, the better). For patients with relatively mild cases of this disease, seeking a "cure" by measures which are disruptive to their personal and family lives is unfortunate since no prediction can be made of either the place or the time of "cure." In patients with extensive involvement of the skin who cannot function in their usual activities, seeking relief by means of change of environment, by immunization procedures, or by psychotherapy may be rewarding if local and systemic treatment have failed. With the presently available drugs such as antihistamines, cortisones, and antibiotics, the need for such measures has lessened considerably.

Treatment. In addition to the elimination of, and immunization to, the usual causative allergenic substances, treatment consists largely of reducing the itching (soothing baths, lotions, oral antihistaminic drugs), sedation (aspirin, tranquillizers) and reducing the inflammatory process (one of the cortisone drugs locally applied or given in "courses" by mouth, or in aggravated cases, by injection). If the flare-ups are notably seasonal, and a pollen is the likely major causative allergen, temporary removal to an area known to be free of the pollen is obviously essential. In

cases in which the attacks are related to the menstrual cycle, the nature of that relationship should be studied endocrinologically for the possibility of suitable treatment. Sympathetic understanding of the patient's distress and reassurance as to the ultimate outcome will permit the patient to seek available symptomatic relief.

ATROPHIC RHINITIS When this condition develops, the mucosa becomes flat with loss of cilia and is replaced by skinlike tissue. Without the normal mucosa and its function, the airway is too large and dry, and becomes crusted. Frequently a foul odor emanates from the nose and the patient loses the sense of smell. The direct cause of this uncommon disease is unknown. Removal of the crust and use of oils and hormones have been helpful. Surgery has been used with occasional success.

ATTRITION Attrition is the normal wearing-down of the surfaces of teeth due to the mastication of food. This occurs primarily on the biting surfaces.

AUDITORY CANAL, BLOCKING OF THE EXTERNAL The accumulation of wax (cerumen), bony growth, foreign bodies, or closure of the canal by swelling can all result in significant hearing loss. The canal must be entirely closed before hearing loss occurs, for even if a pinhole remains from the sound source to the eardrum, the hearing loss may be negligible. This is why hearing loss tends to result after water enters an ear partially filled with cerumen: the water fills the places between the wax and completely occludes the canal.

It is a very poor idea for a person to try to clean his own ear canal. The old rule that "nothing smaller than your elbow should be put in the ear" is a good one. Wax in the ear is desirable, as it is a special secretion which prevents the thin skin from drying and tends to prevent foreign particles from reaching the eardrum. This function is further aided by the hairs on the outside of the ear canal.

Only if the wax in the ear occludes hearing or becomes hard and painful should it be removed—and then only by a physician. Sometimes the services of an ear specialist (otologist) are required. He may irrigate the ear with a special syringe, or use tiny hooked instruments to remove the wax. It may even be necessary to soften the wax prior to cleaning the ear canal. The correct cleaning technique can be selected only by a physician who is able to look into the ear and properly interpret what he sees.

Sometimes young children place small objects in their ear canal. If these objects cannot be easily removed at home, they too should be extracted by a physician. Since it is possible for the child to impair his hearing seriously by pushing foreign bodies into the ear, this practice must be strongly discouraged by the parents. Occasionally an object must be removed under general anesthesia, and sometimes an incision must be made in order to remove the offending object. Parents are not in possession of the instruments or skill to remove either wax or foreign objects; this job always belongs to the physician.

External otitis is a common ear disease affecting the skin of the external auditory canal. It ranges from mild irritation (with the sole symptom of itching) to severe purulent infection (with hearing loss and excruciating pain). The cause of external otitis is frequently the fault of the patient. Getting water in the ears, or scratching the ear canal with sharp objects or finger nails, can cause external otitis. Since wax need not be removed from the ear canal except for reasons of pain or hearing loss (and then only by a physician), there is no reason to wash the ears beyond the pinna. Nor is there any need to put bobby pins, hairpins, paper clips, Q-tips®, pencils, safety pins, or washcloths into the ear canal.

If the "elbow rule" is followed and no water is allowed in the ear (particularly when showering, bathing, or washing the hair), most cases of external otitis can be prevented. Cotton plugs in the outside of the ear, shower caps, and ordinary care will prevent water from injuring the ear. Swimming may not be a hazard, although the ears of some people are much more sensitive to the effects of water than others. If the ears are as much as possible cleared of water after swimming, and if diving is not overdone, most people can enjoy the sport without worry. If, however, a person is subject to "swimmer's ear" (which is only external otitis occurring after swimming) the doctor may be able to prescribe drops to use after each day's swimming to serve as a preventive.

Moisture in the ear canal is like water in a narrow-mouthed bottle; not easy to get out. The moisture makes the canal skin susceptible to bacterial infection. This, in turn, results in swelling of the skin which here adheres very closely to the underlying cartilage and bone. With little room for expansion, the swelling causes severe pain, often requiring narcotics for relief.

Treatment. Treatment is not by home remedy, and a physician (preferably an ear specialist) should treat this condition. Frequently, local medications are enough to combat infections and swelling. Cleaning the ear by swab and suction can bring the condition under control. Long-standing chronic cases with relatively little pain (except for acute flare-ups) require more and longer treatments. After long-standing irritation, the skin actually undergoes changes and long-term therapy is required before the skin reverts to normal.

AUDITORY OSSICLES, MALFUNCTION OF THE

The three tiny ear bones (ossicles) may be the cause of hearing loss because of noncontinuity, fixation, or absence. Infection, injury, developmental defect, or otosclerosis are the most frequent reasons for these defects.

When the ossicles are not connected and no longer carry the sound vibrations to the ears' fluid system, the eardrums' vibrations are not effective and the patient experiences a moderate to severe hearing loss. Following infection of the middle ear (otitis media), parts of the ossicles may be destroyed. A blow on the head may cause dislocation of the incus and stapes, while developmental defects before birth may result in failure of one or more of the bones to form. Otosclerosis can cause conductive hearing loss by fixation (immobilization) of the stapes (the most common cause of hearing loss in young and middle-aged adults). These are among the more common examples of how difficulties with the auditory ossicles can bring on hearing loss.

Fortunately, if the eardrum is intact and the auditory nerve good, results of surgical repair are highly successful. Ninety per cent of these cases can have their hearing restored by the newer surgical techniques.

AUTISM, INFANTILE Autism refers to phantasy thinking such as occurs in daydreaming or revery. Freud early pointed out that most autistic thinking is wish-fulfilling, the person imagining pleasant events which do not ordinarily occur in real life. Daydreaming is a normal phenomenon during all periods of life and particularly in childhood when the child imagines all kinds of things which he could not realistically accomplish.

Autistic thinking and excessive daydreaming become abnormal when used to escape from real life and avoid unpleasant tasks. Withdrawal into autistic thinking may occur in children whose real-life situations are so unhappy or conflict-filled that the child seeks pleasure in daydreaming.

Some authorities believe that excessive daydreaming may be an early symptom of schizophrenia, in which the person literally withdraws from an intolerable reality into a more satisfying world of make-believe. Diagnosis of schizophrenia, however, cannot be made on the basis of this symptom alone, because many gifted people spend long periods in daydreaming that may be completely normal. Daydreaming becomes abnormal in direct proportion to its delusional and completely unrealistic nature.

AUTOEROTICISM According to the sex psychologists this, and not masturbation, is the preferred term to describe a normally secret practice. It can be defined as the practice of friction or vibration of erogenous areas (mostly the penis or clitoris) to produce pleasurable sensations. In older people, of course, autoeroticism goes beyond this to an inverted imitation of the sex act; but such is not often the case in very young children or even in adolescents. The practice is mainly carried out for the physical pleasure it generates (see MASTURBATION).

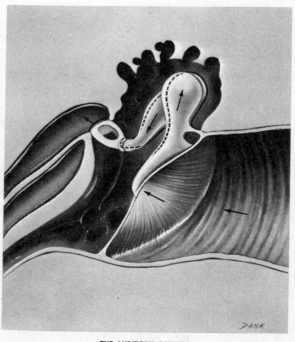

THE AUDITORY OSSICLES

When sound waves cause the eardrum to vibrate, the chain of bony ossicles also vibrate. Thus, sound waves are transmitted to the fluid-filled inner ear.

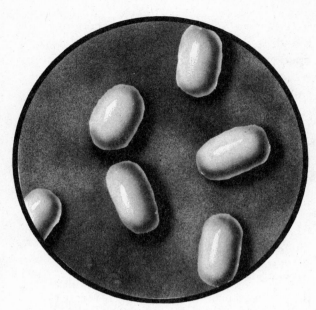

ELECTRONMICROSCOPE VIEW OF
SHIGELLA DYSENTERIAE

AUTONOMIC NERVOUS SYSTEM

The autonomic nervous system is that part of the nervous system which supplies those motor structures which are primarily not under voluntary control. These structures include smooth muscle (e.g., the intestines), heart muscle, and glands. Fibers of the autonomic nervous system are distributed to the smooth muscles of all parts of the body.

The autonomic nervous system is subdivided into the sympathetic and parasympathetic divisions. Anatomically, the sympathetic outflow is from the middle (thoracic and lumbar) parts of the spinal cord, whereas the outflow of the parasympathetic division is from the top and bottom (cranial and sacral) portions.

The autonomic nervous system serves as a balance-adjusting (homeostatic) mechanism to preserve the internal stability of the body. Control over peripheral autonomic mechanisms is maintained by centers located in the cerebral hemispheres, hypothalamus, and brainstem.

The autonomic nervous system controls the muscular tone of blood vessels and regulates the activity of the viscera. A large part of the control of bladder and bowel function is a function of the autonomic nervous system. The control of respiration, heart rate, and body temperature are also under autonomic control.

BACILLARY DYSENTERY

Bacillary dysentery is an acute infection of the bowel caused by bacteria (bacilli) of the *Shigella* group, and characterized by frequent passage of stools containing blood, pus, and mucus, accompanied by abdominal cramps and fever.

The *Shigella* are worldwide in distribution. The infection is spread from person to person. Contamination of food and other objects by human waste matter spreads the disease, and flies may also be occasional carriers. Dysentery epidemics occur among overcrowded populations having inadequate sanitation; the disease is particularly common in younger children living in areas where the disease is prevalent.

The dysentery bacilli ingested with food and drink pass into the intestines. There they produce an inflammatory disease characterized by ulcers. In the adult, the disorder is usually limited to the lower half of the large intestine.

Symptoms. In children, the disease may develop suddenly with fever, irritability, loss of appetite, nausea, diarrhea, and abdominal pain. Within a few days the characteristic stool findings will be noted. The patient loses weight and becomes dehydrated, and the disease may end fatally.

In adults, most of the infections are not accompanied by fever and there may be blood or mucus in the diarrhea. Attacks of abdominal pain, vomiting, and diarrhea recur, mixed with episodes of apparent recovery. Mild cases last about a week, severe cases perhaps a month. A chronic form is recognized in tropical areas.

The finding of pus in the stool is strongly suggestive of bacillary dysentery. The diagnosis is proven by the isolation of *Shigella* from the stools.

64

Treatment. Fluid and salt-solution (electrolyte) administration is essential, particularly in young children. A number of antibiotics have recently been shown to be quite effective. The nutritional state must be carefully maintained. The diarrhea is also treated symptomatically.

Good sanitation—the elimination of flies and protection of food from contamination—is of primary importance in the prevention of this disease. Proper hygiene is the basic protective measure; there are no satisfactory methods of immunization.

BALDNESS (MALE, PATTERN, ALOPECIA PREMATURA) This common type of male baldness is the result of an inherited characteristic which determines not only the fact of loss of hair, but also the distribution of the loss and the time of loss with a high degree of predictability. The hair can begin to thin at age seventeen or eighteen years, worsens steadily so that at twenty there is considerable attrition at the margin of the forehead and some thinning at the crown of the scalp. The pattern of hair loss varies in different families and in different individuals in quantity of loss, in the time span over which the loss takes place, in the areas involved, and in the final type and extent of the baldness. There is no known cause either for the condition itself or for its inheritance. Nothing presently known can alter the course of the baldness. Not even the clearing up of any co-existent condition such as dandruff has any beneficial effect on its unremitting course.

Treatment. The most appropriate course for the patient to pursue is to do nothing but "to accommodate his ego to his destiny."

BALLISTOCARDIOGRAPHY The physical effect of each beat of the heart on the arteries of the body, taken as a single unit, can be traced on paper. The ballistic forces (recoil and impact) are associated with heart contraction and ejection of blood followed by deceleration of blood flow through the large blood vessels. The patient to be studied lies on a board—sometimes rigid, sometimes nearly free-floating—and a recording instrument is then attached which records on slowly moving paper the thrusts that heartbeat and blood-thrust into the large arteries give to the entire body.

There are differences in the character of these whole-body pulsations or waves from person to person, and significant changes occur in special situations of cardiovascular disease.

The ballistocardiogram is often an additional means of diagnosis but is rarely the only laboratory study that will reveal significant abnormalities of the circulatory system.

BARTHOLIN'S GLANDS Found in the female, these structures are located, one on each side, at the entrance of the birth canal (vagina). They often become infected, whereupon they become swollen and tender. Treatment is incision and drainage, or complete removal of the inflamed glands.

BASE This is a layer of dental cement-like material placed in the deep parts of a cavity to serve as insulator and medication (sedative) for protection of the pulp.

"BASIC SEVEN" Everyone recognizes the importance of a well-balanced diet. A handy guide to this balance is the establishment of seven categories of food products. Some food from each group of the "basic seven" should be represented in the daily diet.

Group 1. Leafy green and yellow vegetables
Group 2. Citrus fruits, tomatoes, raw cabbage
Group 3. Potatoes and other vegetables and fruits

THE RESPIRATORY AND DIGESTIVE SYSTEMS

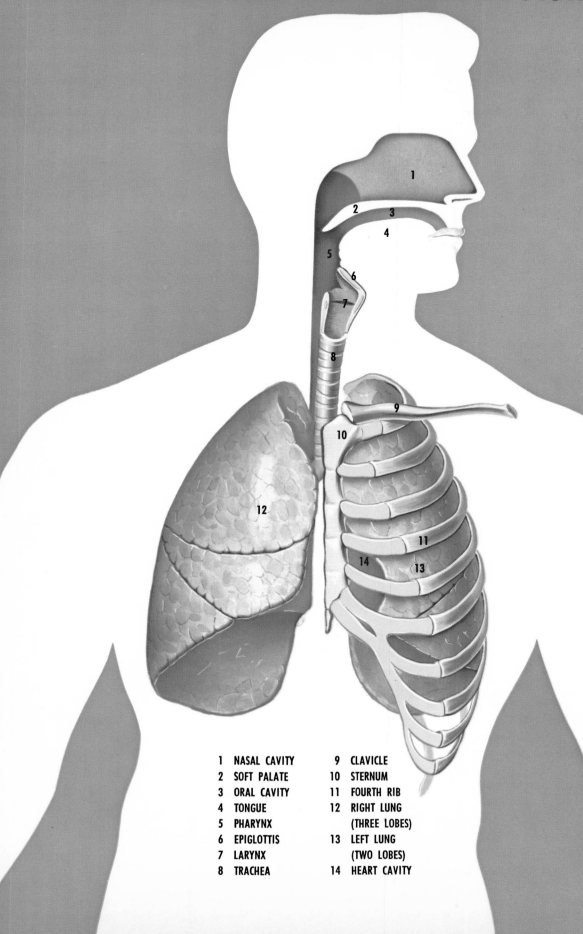

1	NASAL CAVITY	9	CLAVICLE
2	SOFT PALATE	10	STERNUM
3	ORAL CAVITY	11	FOURTH RIB
4	TONGUE	12	RIGHT LUNG
5	PHARYNX		(THREE LOBES)
6	EPIGLOTTIS	13	LEFT LUNG
7	LARYNX		(TWO LOBES)
8	TRACHEA	14	HEART CAVITY

RESPIRATORY MOVEMENTS

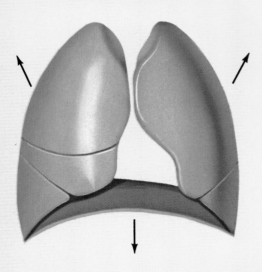

INSPIRATION

As the rib cage rises and the diaphragm falls, the lung area enlarges.

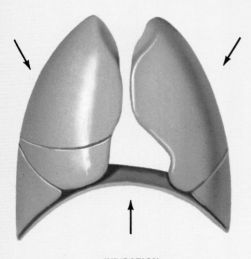

EXPIRATION

As the rib cage falls and the diaphragm rises, the lung area is decreased.

THE BRONCHIAL TREE

1 TRACHEA
2 LEFT BRONCHUS
3 SMALLER BRONCHUS
4 BRONCHIOLE
5 ALVEOLI

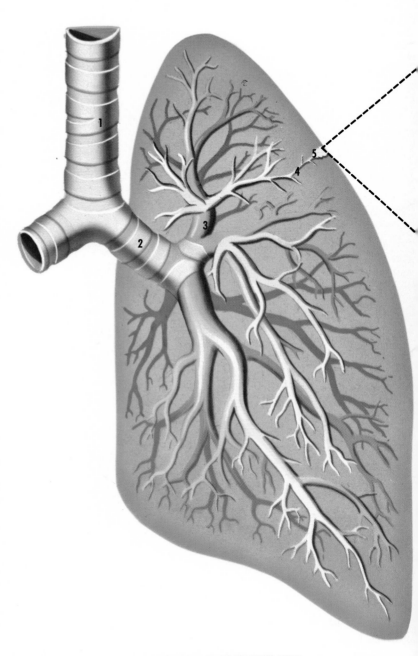

FUNCTION OF BRONCHIAL TREE

The bronchial tree is a system of branching hollow tubes whose function is to convey air to and from the alveoli (small hollows). Not shown are the companion arteries and veins which follow the branchings of the tree. At the level of the alveoli, these blood vessels become a capillary network embedded in the alveolar wall.

THE ALVEOLI
(IN CROSS SECTION)

Plate A3

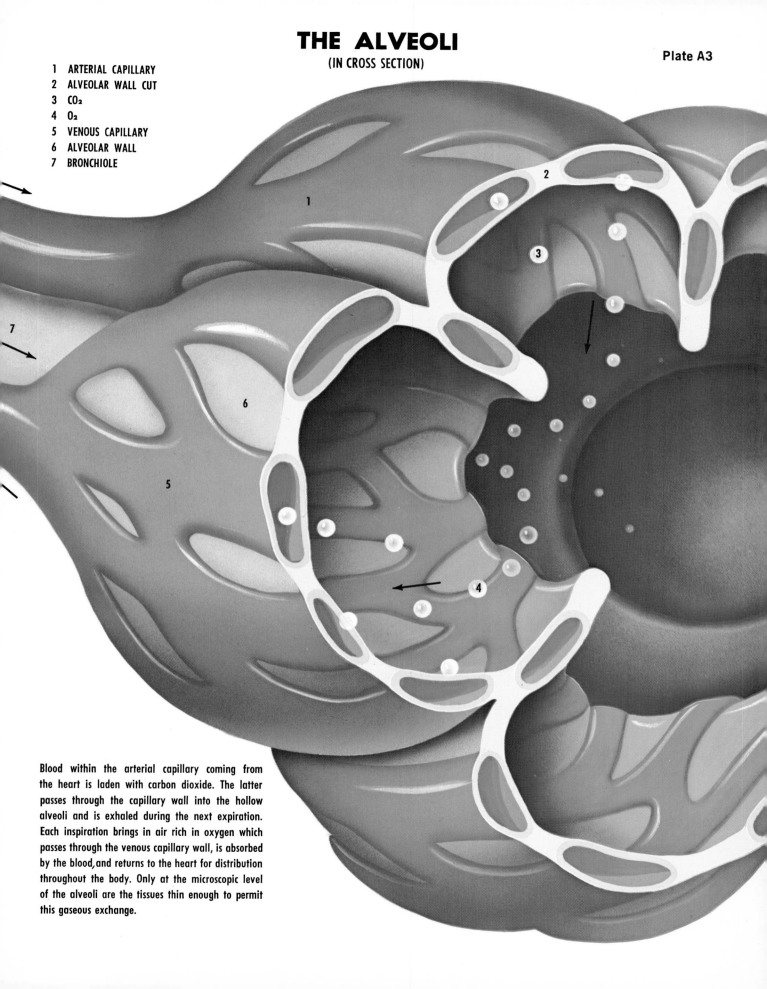

1   ARTERIAL CAPILLARY
2   ALVEOLAR WALL CUT
3   CO₂
4   O₂
5   VENOUS CAPILLARY
6   ALVEOLAR WALL
7   BRONCHIOLE

Blood within the arterial capillary coming from the heart is laden with carbon dioxide. The latter passes through the capillary wall into the hollow alveoli and is exhaled during the next expiration. Each inspiration brings in air rich in oxygen which passes through the venous capillary wall, is absorbed by the blood, and returns to the heart for distribution throughout the body. Only at the microscopic level of the alveoli are the tissues thin enough to permit this gaseous exchange.

THE DIGESTIVE SYSTEM

Plate A4

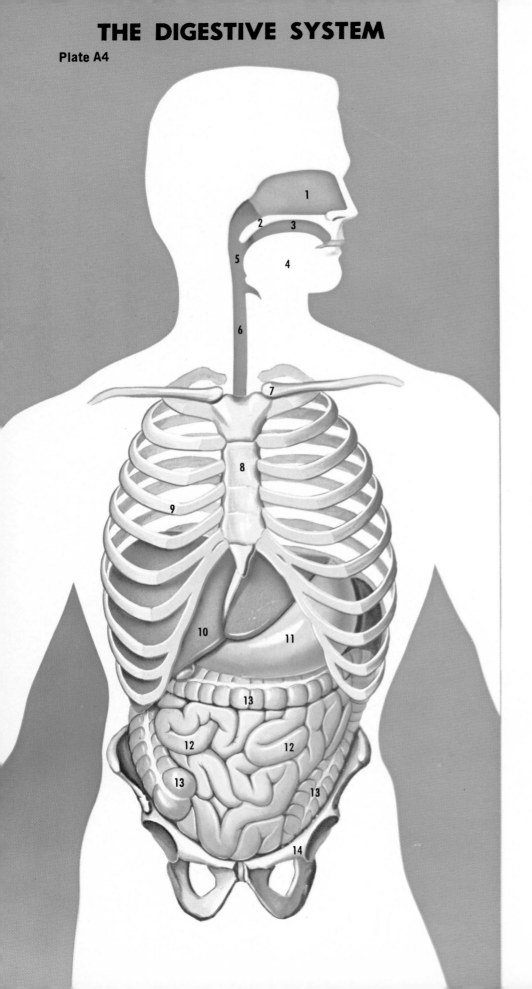

1   NASAL CAVITY
2   SOFT PALATE
3   ORAL CAVITY
4   TONGUE
5   PHARYNX
6   ESOPHAGUS
7   CLAVICLE
8   STERNUM
9   FOURTH RIB
10 LIVER
11 STOMACH
12 SMALL INTESTINE
13 LARGE INTESTINE
14 PELVIC BONES

THE MECHANICS OF DIGESTION ▶

Digestion involves three simultaneous processes: mechanical passage of food through the continuous, hollow tube called the digestive tract; the chemical breakdown of the food; and absorption of the food.

To propel food forward, the muscular walls of the various portions of the tract undergo rhythmic contractions called peristalsis.

After being masticated by the teeth, the tongue pushes the food down the esophagus into the stomach. Successive waves of contraction beginning at mid-stomach travel down its muscular walls, churning the food. In the small intestine, two types of peristalsis occur: nonmoving, segmental contractions that occur 10 to 30 times a minute and mix the food with secretions from the liver and pancreas; and waves of peristalsis that propel the food forward. The large intestine has infrequent waves which move the undigested waste into the rectum where it is stored until elimination.

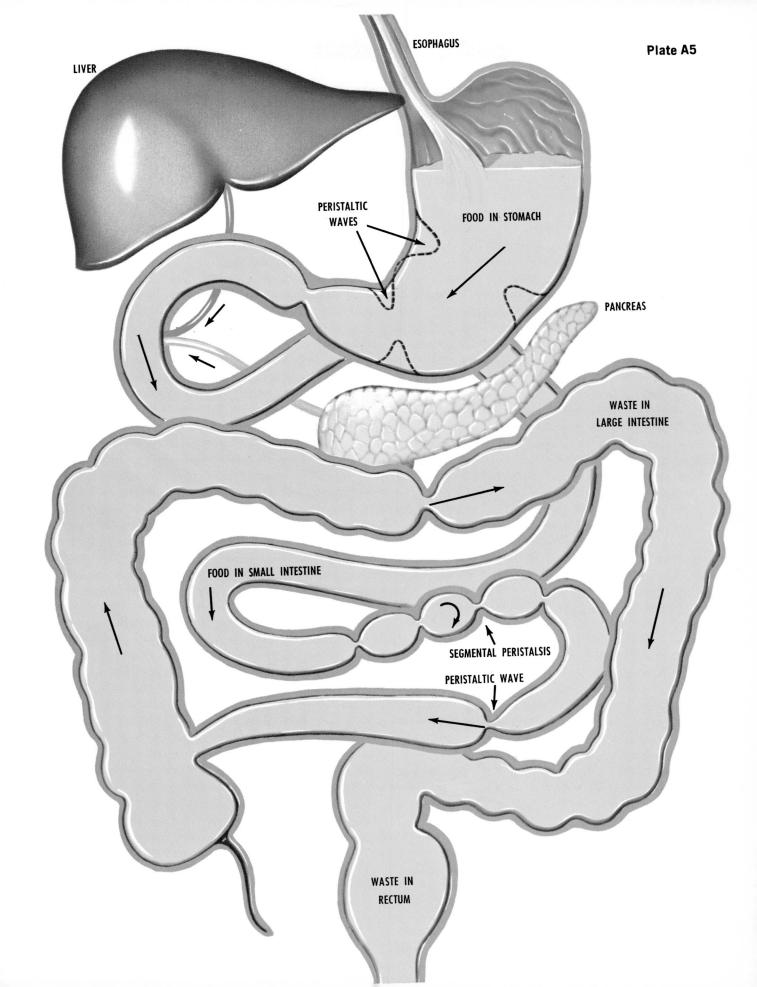

ESOPHAGUS

Plate A5

LIVER

PERISTALTIC WAVES

FOOD IN STOMACH

PANCREAS

WASTE IN LARGE INTESTINE

FOOD IN SMALL INTESTINE

SEGMENTAL PERISTALSIS

PERISTALTIC WAVE

WASTE IN RECTUM

THE CHEMISTRY OF DIGESTION

During their passage — through the composite digestive tract shown on these two pages, —foods are broken down by the action of enzymes secreted by the digestive glands. Each enzyme breaks down a specific food type: sugar, fat, or protein.

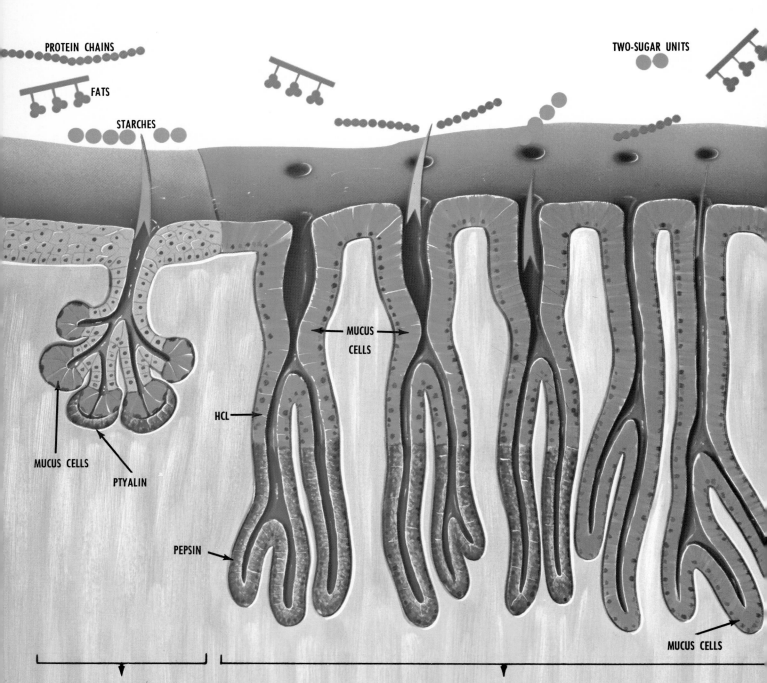

PROTEIN CHAINS

TWO-SUGAR UNITS

FATS

STARCHES

MUCUS
CELLS

HCL

MUCUS CELLS

PTYALIN

PEPSIN

MUCUS CELLS

MOUTH AND ESOPHAGUS

Three salivary glands in the mouth secrete mucus to moisten food, and ptyalin which splits off two-sugar units from the starch chain. Fats and proteins are not affected. The esophagus has a few isolated mucus-producing glands.

STOMACH

The stomach has two types of glands; the gastric glands and the pyloric glands. The gastric glands secrete mucus, pepsin, and hydrochloric acid (HCI). The latter two break protein chains into shorter segments. Fats and sugars are unaffected. The pyloric glands produce mucus only.

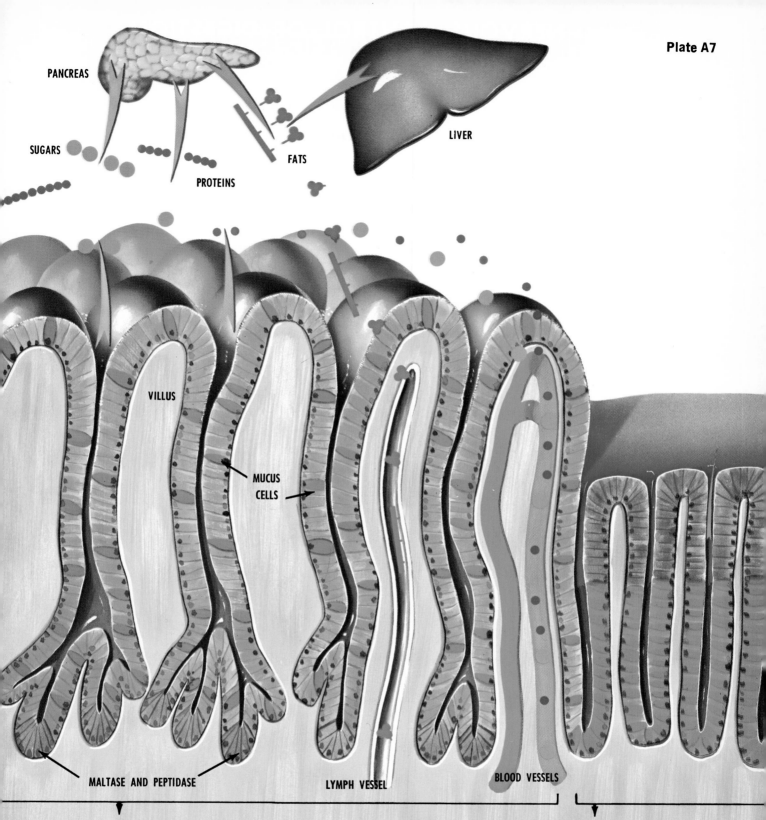

PANCREAS

SUGARS

PROTEINS

FATS

LIVER

VILLUS

MUCUS CELLS

MALTASE AND PEPTIDASE

LYMPH VESSEL

BLOOD VESSELS

SMALL INTESTINE

LARGE INTESTINE

The pancreatic secretions emptying into the small intestine contain three powerful enzymes: amylase, trypsin, and lipase. Amylase splits off two-sugar units. Trypsin splits proteins into shorter chains. Lipase, in conjunction with liver bile, decomposes fats into their simplest units. The intestinal glands located between villi produce mucus and two enzymes: maltase and pepitidase which complete the breakdown of sugar and protein, respectively. All absorption takes place in the lower small intestine. Fats are absorbed into the lymph vessels, sugars and proteins by the blood vessels. The large intestinal glands secrete mucus to lubricate the undigested food in its passage to the rectum.

NERVOUS CONTROL OF DIGESTION

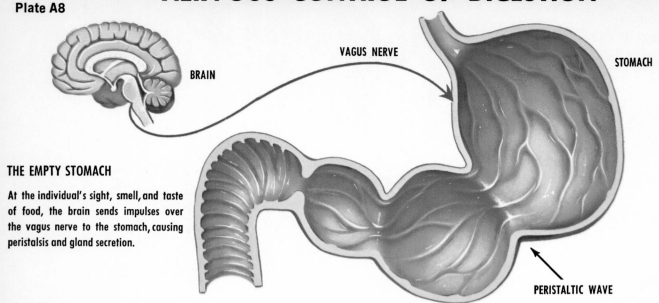

BRAIN

VAGUS NERVE

STOMACH

THE EMPTY STOMACH

At the individual's sight, smell, and taste of food, the brain sends impulses over the vagus nerve to the stomach, causing peristalsis and gland secretion.

PERISTALTIC WAVE

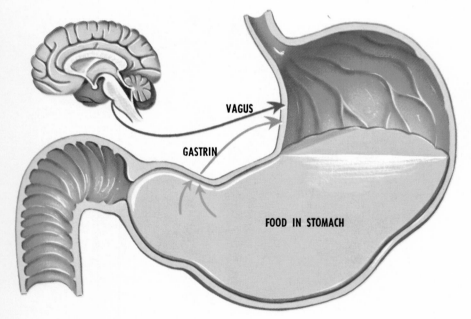

VAGUS

GASTRIN

FOOD IN STOMACH

FOOD IN THE STOMACH

During filling, peristalsis decreases. The stomach walls relax to accommodate the food. When filled, stomach peristalsis increases via vagus nerve control. The food itself stimulates the release of gastrin which travels to the gastric glands, increasing the secretion of gastric juices.

FOOD IN THE INTESTINES

If too great a food bulk reaches the duodenum, stomach peristalsis (still under vagus control) is slowed down. Food itself stimulates the release of gastrin (to stomach) and secretin which stimulates pancreatic secretions.

Food in the small intestine causes the secretion of enterogastrone which travels to the stomach and inhibits gastric gland secretion.

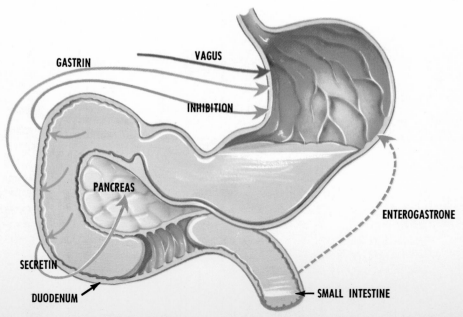

GASTRIN

VAGUS

INHIBITION

PANCREAS

ENTEROGASTRONE

SECRETIN

DUODENUM

SMALL INTESTINE

(Two items to be selected from this group)

Group 4. Milk and milk products

Group 5. Meat, poultry, fish, eggs, nuts

Group 6. Bread, flour, cereals

Group 7. Butter and fortified margarines

BCG VACCINE See TUBERCULOSIS

BEDBUG BITES The bedbug (*Cimex lectularis*) resides in the crevices of furniture, including the seams of mattresses, and emerges for purposes of feeding. It punctures the skin, producing a usually visible puncture mark around which develops a small but persistent hive, probably the result of a deposition of insect fluid.

Symptoms. The insect bites are usually grouped in a line or in an arc shape made up of three lesions. Most commonly affected sites are the ankles, buttocks, and parts of the body usually covered by night-clothes. Diagnosis is occasionally made difficult by the absence of skin lesions in one of two people sharing a bed. This lack of response may be the result of the person's immunity to the insect toxin, or due to some metabolic substance in the person's skin which either rejects or "detoxifies" the offending material.

Treatment. Eradication of the bedbugs by fumigation* will eliminate further skin response since the bedbug does not live on the body. The existing lesions can be treated with soothing lotion (calamine) and the itching minimized with the orally administered antihistaminic drugs.

BEDSORES These lesions appear in areas of persistent pressure to the skin of chronically ill or debilitated patients as a result of poor circulation in the mechanically restricted area.

Symptoms. First noted as an area of

---

*Check with local authorities about available legal methods.

redness, the skin becomes macerated, denuded, and ulcerated. Pustular infections, including boils, are common. Similar lesions can occur under restrictive dressings, such as casts, in an otherwise healthy person.

Treatment. Frequent movement of the patient in whom bedsores can be expected to occur, and the use of air mattresses to provide more resiliency, will afford some protection. The skin should be kept dry and dusting powder applied to the sheets to reduce friction against the linens. The sores or ulcers are treated with antibiotic lotions and ointments.

BED-WETTING (ENURESIS) Enuresis is the term given to persistent bed-wetting (also called nycturia). Most children acquire enough bladder control and capacity to stay dry after the age of three years. However, there is no specific age at which all children should be expected to remain dry through the night; some children obtain control and retention capacity more slowly than others. Enuresis is less common among girls. In many cases a family history of the problem is present.

Physiological causes for enuresis can be discovered by means of laboratory tests. Kidney or bladder disease may be uncovered by routine urinalysis or urine culture and (if necessary) by kidney X-rays. Sometimes an obstruction where the bladder joins the urethra may cause uncontrollable dripping during daytime and at night. If it is determined that the child has no problems holding urine and emptying the bladder while awake, then structural malformities or infectious diseases can usually be eliminated as causes.

In girls, local irritation due to uncleanliness may contribute to enuresis. A small percentage of children wet the bed because of food allergy (milk, wheat, eggs, citrus fruit, etc.), but such a condition is easy to determine; if a child wets nightly and the offending food is removed from the diet for one day, the child will not wet the bed that night.

Psychiatric theories that attempt to explain bed-wetting include the idea that enuresis is a form of aggressive behavior, and that the child may unconsciously use bed-wetting as a means of "getting even" with his or her parents for some real or imagined wrongs. In cases where the bed-wetting is not a chronic problem, the cause may be emotional stress or anxiety that temporarily affects the child. Although it is true that many emotionally disturbed children will wet the bed, not every bed wetter is emotionally disturbed.

Some medical authorities believe that enuresis occurs simply because some children mature more slowly with regard to bladder control and capacity than others. Research into the various levels of consciousness during sleep may reveal that bed-wetting children sleep so soundly that they are unable to control bladder function.

Treatment. Attempts to cure enuresis have incorporated different approaches. Those that believe that sleeping on the back causes pressure to build in the kidneys have tied bulky objects to the patient's back so that the bed wetter sleeps on his or her side throughout the night.

Also popular are methods that awaken the bed wetter as soon as urination begins. This can be accomplished by using a wire mesh connected to a battery and bell. With the first drops of urine the electrical circuit is completed and the bell sounds, awakening the bed wetter. If possible the child would then finish emptying his or her bladder in the toilet.

Restricting or prohibiting fluids at least two hours before bedtime may help some children. Making sure the child urinates, if at all possible, immediately before retiring may also lessen the chance of bed-wetting. Some parents may decide to impose earlier bedtimes and then wake the bed wetter in the late evening so that the bladder may be emptied. The child then returns to bed with

the risk of bed wetting greatly reduced.

A technique for children over eight years of age attempts to increase gradually the child's ability to retain urine in the bladder. During the day the child drinks frequently and is encouraged to refrain from urinating for as long as possible without becoming unduly distressed. The child then measures the amount of urine passed each time he or she urinates and marks a chart that will periodically be shown to the doctor. Some children have increased their holding capacity from three to fifteen ounces within six months. (A child may produce about eleven ounces of urine in one night.) This method also enables some children to become more sensitive to a full-bladder sensation while asleep.

For the chronic bed wetter the best of all medicines is parental love. Harsh punishments and ridicule usually make the problem much worse. Parents should understand that the condition corrects itself with time, patience, and love.

BENDS, THE (CAISSON DISEASE)
The bends occurs among divers and those who work under high air pressure in caissons (airtight boxes for working on river bottoms). Unless the change from high to lower (normal) surface pressure is gradual, an individual may develop paralysis, also known as "diver's paralysis."

Symptoms. Indications of caisson disease do not manifest themselves until the subject has emerged into normal air pressure at which time he complains of joint pains; these are rapidly followed by paralysis, dizziness, headache, vomiting, confusion, and convulsions. In severe cases, breathing decreases and coma ensues. Patients frequently recover, but some of them may remain paralyzed for life.

Treatment. Prevention is the best treatment. Men who apply for work involving high air pressure environment must pass rigorous physical examinations. Emergence from high pressure areas is through air locks in which the pressure is gradually reduced.

BERIBERI Beriberi is the name given to the clinical state produced by deficiency of thiamine (vitamin B_1). The disease takes two forms—the type called dry beriberi, in which there is primarily a disturbance in the nerves of the arms and legs (peripheral neuritis), and wet beriberi, a form of heart disease with accumulation of fluid (edema). Early symptoms of thiamine deficiency include loss of appetite, fatigue, nausea and vomiting, irritability, vague fears, and depression.

Symptoms. Early signs of nerve disorder are burning of the soles of the feet and numbness and tingling of the feet and legs. This may be followed by hypersensitivity and, later, loss of sensitivity in the toes. Shooting pains in the legs, muscle cramps, tenderness of the calves, weakness of the muscle, and abnormalities in the reflexes may also be observed, and the heart itself is enlarged.

In wet beriberi, the heart rate is rapid. There may be pain and shortness of breath on exertion, and the lips and nail beds may be somewhat bluish. Certain heart murmurs and disturbances in rhythm may be detected; the electrocardiogram shows characteristic findings. There is enlargement of the liver, and local accumulation of fluid—particularly around the ankles—is frequently observed.

Infantile beriberi occurs in breast-fed infants of mothers who have thiamine deficiency. Although this has not been seen frequently in the United States, it is quite prevalent in Japan and other Far Eastern countries. There is loss of appetite and vomiting, rapid pulse and respiration.

Treatment. In these forms of beriberi, the response to large doses of vitamin B_1 (usually by injection, occasionally by mouth) is often dramatic.

Other clinical forms of thiamine deficiency may also be found. One of these, known as Wernicke's syndrome, is characterized by weakness or paralysis of the muscles moving the eyeball. Lack of muscular coordination and mental disturbances are occasionally seen. Thiamine and other members of the vitamin B complex have been valuable in the treatment of delirium tremens and other acute psychotic diseases associated with alcoholism. The susceptibility of the nervous system to a deficiency of this vitamin is explained by the central nervous system's dependence on glucose (carbohydrate) metabolism and by thiamine's role in this metabolism.

BERLOQUE DERMATITIS The result of a unique type of photosensitization, this deep brown hyperpigmentation occurs in sharply defined bizarre configurations in sites of deliberate or accidental application of substances containing essential oils such as oil of lemon, oil of orange (rind), and the most frequent offender and common ingredient of perfume, oil of bergamot. The areas affected are usually those to which perfume and perfume-containing preparations are applied and which are ordinarily exposed to light.

Symptoms. The back of the neck and forehead (from hair preparations running onto the skin), sides of the neck, anterior chest, upper arms and bends of the elbows (from perfume, toilet water), demonstrate spherical, elongated, or splattered brown lesions with no apparent preceding redness or swelling or blistering. The eruption fades gradually, although remnant stains have been known to last for years.

Deliberate experimental sensitization of this type has been difficult to produce and the mechanism of this occurrence is not known.

Treatment. Avoidance of light will prevent further darkening of the affected sites. Avoidance of the application of the offending oil at least to exposed areas of the skin will prevent recurrence. Treatment to the lesions is unnecessary.

BICUSPIDS (PREMOLARS) These are the eight permanent posterior teeth, located behind the cuspids, which replace the eight deciduous molars.

BILE Bile, a secretion of the liver, is a thick greenish-yellow fluid; its chief components are salts, pigments resulting from the metabolism of broken-down red blood cells, cholesterol, and fat. Bile is primarily a collection of materials to be excreted into the intestinal tract and discarded, except for the bile salts which aid in the splitting and digestion of fats. Bile is collected in liver tubules which lead to the bile ducts which in turn carry the bile to the gallbladder. There it is stored and concentrated until the presence of food in the small intestine causes it to be discharged. In cases of severe vomiting, bile may be regurgitated into the stomach and subsequently found in the vomitus.

BILIARY COLIC See Gallstones

BILIOUSNESS This is a rather imprecise term which pertains to a feeling of nausea or uneasiness, usually after meals. There may be heartburn or vague pain in the right-upper abdominal region. The symptoms may be early signs of infection of the gallbladder, but ordinarily subside spontaneously and do not recur with any regularity. Avoiding overindulgence and highly seasoned foods, eating meals in a pleasant unhurried atmosphere, and chewing food well are often all that is required to relieve these symptoms.

BIOTIN Biotin (formerly known as vitamin H) is one of the B-complex vitamins. It is probably an essential nutrient, but it is widely present in food and is synthesized by the bacterial flora in the intestinal tract. It is unlikely that biotin

deficiency, as such, is of significance in human nutrition; however, raw egg white contains a substance—avidin—which combines with biotin, making the latter unavailable to the body. Experimental biotin deficiency can thus be produced by feeding large amounts of raw egg white. The symptoms are loss of appetite, muscle pains, and a dry, scaly skin condition (dermatitis). The role and importance of biotin to man is largely unknown.

BIRTH CERTIFICATE All states require that a birth certificate be prepared by the physician after each delivery and promptly submitted to the local municipal or county authorities. The information is also sent to the Bureau of Vital Statistics in Washington, D.C., where valuable data are obtained and coded. Statistical analysis of these data offers valuable records for medical, socio-economic, military, and other purposes.

BIRTH INJURIES The most common birth injuries are those involving the largest part of the baby—the head. Lumps noticed on the head at birth are most often caused by blood serum or superficial blood beneath the scalp; these are almost always harmless and disappear early. Blood may also collect beneath the outer layer of the scalp and/or within the brain. These more serious injuries should be treated by a doctor. Fortunately, many of them will be absorbed or will heal—but surgery nowadays is occasionally required.

Other injuries, less common today than they used to be, involve fractures. In young bones, however, many of these are not total; a collar bone, for example, is more often cracked than broken, although nerves may be stretched in the neck or shoulder.

Oxygen deprivation to the brain at the time of delivery can cause injury as serious as that of a traumatic blow on the head. There are many reasons, including too much anesthesia, which account for this trouble in a baby. Some of the spastics or "hypermotor" infants may be due to this.

BIRTHMARKS See MOLES; ANGIOMAS

BITES See FIRST AID AND EMERGENCIES

BLACKHEAD   A blackhead is formed from the oily material (sebum) secreted by the sebaceous gland and the horny keratin which lines the opening of the gland. The resulting waxy substance becomes blackened on oxidation and gives the classic appearance of a blackhead. Often this pluglike material causes further overactivity of the sebaceous gland and irritation which results in redness, papule formation, and pus characteristic of the acne lesion.

Blackheads are most frequently found on the face, chest, and back. They are less prevalent but often of much greater size in the ears, where they cause scarring and painful infection. They can exist as the only manifestation of acne or in association with the several other types of lesions. Scarring can result from mechanical distention of the skin by the plug, or as the result of secondary infection.

Treatment. Drying agents (lotions) exert a peeling effect on the orifice permitting extrusion of the plug; vitamin A taken orally is known to alter the putting down of keratin and permit the flow of sebum without opportunity to harden at the surface; proper removal (lifting out) of the horny plug prevents further distorting and possible scarring. Lack of cleanliness is no factor in the production of blackheads, though frequent washing with soap and water exerts a drying and gentle peeling of the skin and releases the blackhead.

BLADDER, URINARY   This round structure lies just behind the pubic bone and connects directly to the exterior of the body through the urethra. It is the collecting and storage sac for urine, which comes to it through the ureters from the kidneys. The urinary bladder is quite distensible and may hold as much as two or three quarts of urine; ordinarily, however, a sense of urgency to urinate occurs when four to eight ounces of urine are present.

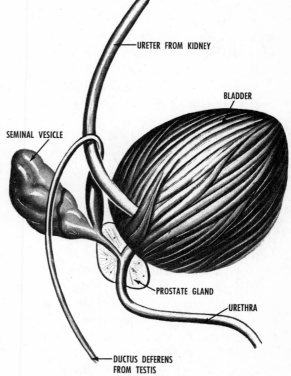

THE BLADDER AND THE PROSTATE GLAND

URETER FROM KIDNEY

BLADDER

SEMINAL VESICLE

PROSTATE GLAND

URETHRA

DUCTUS DEFERENS FROM TESTIS

BLASTOMYCOSIS   Caused by the fungus *Blastomyces dermatitidis* in the United States (few reported cases in Canada) and by the fungus *Blastomyces brasiliensis* in South America, this "deep" mycosis affects the skin and other organs, most notably the lungs. North American blastomycosis differs substantially from South American, and is most characteristically located on the face, hands, arms, and feet.

Symptoms. The small papule or tumor enlarges, becomes pustular, ulcerates, and becomes crusted. On enlarging peripherally, the central portion heals and leaves thick scars. Multiple lesions can coalesce forming arc-shaped lesions. Concomitant lung involvement is usual. Diagnosis can be confirmed by biopsy examination of the skin lesion and by culture of the fungus.

Treatment. Small early lesions can be excised surgically to avoid extension of the disease and consequent disfigurement. Treatment with iodide has been largely displaced by stilbamidine injections. Although somewhat difficult to administer and with toxic properties largely attributable to degradation of the drug, stilbamidine is effective in the treatment of blastomycosis. Related and possibly less toxic compounds are also available for patients suffering from liver and kidney damage.

BLEEDING IN PREGNANCY Vaginal bleeding after the sixth month of pregnancy is particularly significant because at this stage the fetus is usually viable, and the bleeding might endanger the baby. Vaginal bleeding, at any stage of pregnancy, should be thoroughly investigated. There are two abnormalities of the placenta which may cause severe bleeding and endanger the life of the mother as well as the fetus:

1. Premature separation of the placenta (abruptio placentae), the partial or total separation of the afterbirth from the womb before delivery of the baby. This may occur during or in the absence of labor.

Symptoms. This condition results in the loss of large amounts of blood, usually becoming evident in the form of severe vaginal bleeding. The patient experiences sudden severe abdominal pain, the uterus becomes tense and irritable, and the patient is continuously uncomfortable. Vaginal bleeding usually follows. The baby may die or be seriously compromised because of lack of oxygen.

Treatment. Caesarean section is often performed for the sake of the baby, the mother, or both. If more than 30 per cent

of the placenta becomes separated, the baby usually succumbs.

2. Placenta previa, the implantation of the placenta over the mouth of the womb. Here the placenta may cover the opening of the cervix entirely (total placenta previa) or partially (partial placenta previa). This abnormality results in vaginal bleeding, ranging from slight to very profuse and usually appearing in the absence of labor (when labor starts the bleeding becomes worse). The dangers for the fetus and the mother are not as severe as with abruptio; nevertheless this is a very serious complication of pregnancy and caesarean section is almost always required for the delivery of the baby.

BLINDNESS This term includes not only absence of all sight but may be applied to conditions in which vision is so reduced as not to be useful. As defined by industry and the Internal Revenue Service blindness is considered to be vision of less than 20/200 (see VISION, MEASUREMENT OF) in both eyes with the best possible glasses, or contraction of the visual field within twenty degrees of the point of fixation. There are about 350,000 blind persons in the United States, and approximately 35,000 are blinded annually.

Information concerning the blind may be obtained from the American Foundation for the Blind, Inc., 15 West 16th Street, New York, New York 10011, or from the local state agency for the blind.

The causes of blindness vary markedly in different parts of the world, with trachoma, a virus inflammation of the eye, the most common one. However, this disease can be cured by use of sulfonamide medications and is no longer a serious problem in the United States. The chief causes of blindness in the United States are glaucoma and senile cataract. Systemic diseases such as diabetes and disorders of the blood vessels which cause destruction of the retina are the second most common cause. The third most common cause are birth defects arising from failure of the eye to develop normally during the period of growth in the womb. Inflammations of the eye, injuries, poisoning, tumors, and unknown causes account for the remaining cases.

BLINKING Spontaneous blinking occurs in each person because of a number of factors relating to moisture of the eyes, external lighting, fatigue, and the like. Frequent blinking, particularly in children, is seldom serious and many times appears to be an attempt on the child's part to attract attention.

Frequent forcible closure of the eyelids occurs as a result of eye or nervous disease and may be extremely disabling. Treatment must be directed to the cause, but is frequently disappointing.

BLISTER Caused by the seeping of serous fluid within the skin, usually under the epidermal layer, a blister can exist as an integral part of a complex reaction comprising a disease entity (poison ivy dermatitis, pemphigus, cold sores) or result from local trauma (friction, burn).

Depending on the mechanism of production, a blister can remain small and uninfected until it is finally absorbed, leaving a brownish crust which falls off spontaneously if left alone; or it can become enlarged to almost any size or shape, drain, refill, become jellylike, peel off, become infected, etc.

Treatment. Aside from blisters which are present as part of a skin disease, treatment will vary according to the site affected, the number and size of the lesions, and the discomfort and disability of the patient. Small blisters dry up quite rapidly if treated with applications of cold water, either by immersion or by compresses. Large lesions can be emptied by ripping with an alcohol-sterilized needle. If the blister is not opened adequately, it will

refill. The opened lesion should be dressed with an antibiotic ointment such as bacitracin or neosporin. It is often useful to apply cold water compresses to opened or spontaneously draining blisters at intervals of three or four hours, following each wet dressing with drying and with the application of an antibiotic ointment.

BLOOD CIRCULATION The design for circulation of blood to all the tissues of the body centers around the pumping action of the heart, through which all blood passes. As the word circulation implies, the process is a closed and repetitive cycle.

The Heart System. Venous (vein) blood returns to the heart by passing through two major trunks: the superior vena cava, which passively draws blood in from the head, upper arms, and part of the trunk; and the inferior vena cava, which gathers returning blood from the remainder of the body, including all of the abdominal organs.

Through gateways at its upper and lower margins, blood flows into the heart's receiving chamber (right auricle). This chamber serves as a supply depot and also as a contracting chamber which efficiently moves an exact amount of blood into the right ventricular pump chamber for transmission to the lungs.

With heart contraction, the right ventricle squeezes this measured amount of blood into the pulmonary arteries supplying the lungs. Within the lungs, vessels divide and subdivide hundred of times, the heartbeat of blood ultimately passing through hundreds of miles of vessels so small that the blood cells must "wiggle" through, almost a single cell at a time. (The diameter of the pulmonary capillaries is scarcely more than the thickness of a single red blood cell.)

The lung capillaries might be said truly to float in the air we breathe, lying as they do against the cells of the terminal air sacs (alveoli) of the lungs. As red cells pass through them, carbon dioxide escapes from them into the air about to be exhaled, while oxygen from the air just breathed in passes through the capillary walls and fastens to hemoglobin located within the red blood cells.

Refreshed, the blood now flows into larger and larger collecting veins and finally arrives, by way of the pulmonary veins, into the collecting chamber (left auricle) of the left side of the heart.

This measured amount of blood arriving in the left auricle is moved by a single heartbeat into the waiting left ventricular pumping chamber. The ventricle then contracts in systole, and pushes this segment of blood into a large, elastic artery, the aorta, which carries blood away from the heart and supplies the arterial branches which reach into all the tissues.

With each pulsation, the left ventricle ordinarily moves the same quantity of blood from the heart into the body at large as does the right ventricle from the heart into the lungs. Because of this balance, blood is not trapped in the lungs and the volume of blood there remains the same from minute to minute, for each heartbeat empties as much blood from the lungs as is pumped in. If any imbalance does come into existence and the lungs become abnormally engorged with a large quantity of blood, failure of the left side of the heart to evacuate this "stagnating" blood can lead to one type of congestive heartfailure.

The Vessel System. Blood circulates from the heart to all the tissues through the arteries of the body. Vessels from the heart branch from the aorta — the main trunk of the body's arterial system — at its origin just outside the final valve of the heart, the aortic valve. (This valve prevents arterial blood from slipping back into the heart.)

As the blood reaches the smallest arteries (arterioles), it next flows into the capillaries, whose walls are only single,

flattened tissue cells and hence extremely thin; it is through these cell membranes that oxygen and fluid nutrients pass into the tissues. Accumulations of carbon dioxide and fluid waste products are gathered from the tissues after crossing these same capillary walls, and are then swept through the veins to the lungs and excretory organs where they are disposed of.

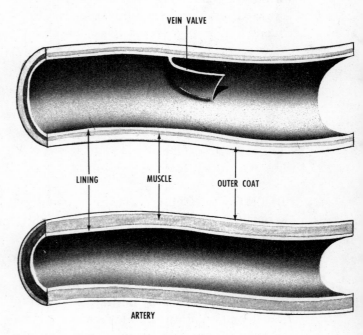

VEIN VALVE

LINING   MUSCLE   OUTER COAT

ARTERY

VEIN AND ARTERY

BLOOD PRESSURE   With each heartbeat, freshly oxygenated blood is pumped from the heart and flows under pressure into the largest vessel of the human body, the aorta. At the end of each heart contraction, a valve at the exit of the pumping chamber (left ventricle) snaps off. It is at this precise moment that pressure in the aorta reaches its highest peak. As the aorta waits for the next burst of blood from the left ventricle, pressure within it gradually drops, because blood is continually filtering out of the arteries into the capillaries.

The large aorta, with its extremely elastic walls, holds a tremendous supply of refreshed blood. It serves as a supply reservoir that, between heartbeats, insures a constant flow of blood into even the smallest vessels, far distant from the heart. Pressure that builds up at the end of ventricular contraction (called systole) is known as the systolic pressure; it does not ordinarily exceed a pressure of 150 to 160 millimeters of mercury.

Between heart contractions, pressure in the aorta falls, reaching its lowest reading while the ventricles are refilling themselves during the diastolic phase of the cardiac cycle. During diastole, the between-beat (diastolic) pressure drops to 90 millimeters of mercury or even below.

Blood pressure rises and falls as the demands of the body for oxygen change from moment to moment, a rise in pressure speeding additional blood to the tissues. With exertion or emotional stress, blood pressure rises to supply greater amounts of blood to the capillaries lying next to those cells which urgently need oxygen refreshment to satisfy the demands of added effort.

Your physician may advise you to buy your own blood pressure measuring device—a sphygmomanometer—and to monitor your blood pressure at home one or more times a day as a means of helping him regulate medication.

By keeping careful records of your pressure, indicating the date and time of the recording, the name of the drug, the dosage,

LIFE-SHORTENING IN UNTREATED HYPERTENSION

Measurement of blood pressure is the most important factor used by insurance companies in predicting life expectancy.

How dangerous is untreated high blood pressure? A study involving 4,000,000 policy holders in 26 large life insurance companies showed that at any given age the higher the blood pressure, the lower the life expectancy.

	MEN		
Age at First Reading	Blood Pressure	Expected Longevity	Loss in Life Expectancy (in years)
35	120/80	76½ years	—
	130/90	72½	4
	140/95	67½	9
	150/100	60	16½
45	120/80	77	—
	130/90	74	3
	140/95	71	6
	150/100	60	11½
55	120/80	78½	—
	130/90	77½	1
	140/95	74½	4
	150/100	72½	6
	WOMEN		
45	120/80	82	—
	130/90	80½	1½
	140/95	77	5
	150/100	73½	8½
55	120/80	82½	—
	130/90	82	½
	140/95	79½	3
	150/100	78½	4

YOUR BLOOD PRESSURE RECORD

Date	Time	Pressure Reading Systolic/Diastolic	Medication	Doctor's Instructions

the time taken, and the nature of your activity before the time the recording has been taken, you can tell him much more than if your pressure were taken only on visits to the office.

Furthermore, blood pressure readings in the physician's office often are higher because of anticipation and fear. In your own home, you become accustomed to it and no longer are tense.

Drugs ordinarily are prescribed on the basis of the blood pressure readings recorded in the doctor's office. Recordings at home permit the doctor to make medication adjustment. When the blood pressure increases, the dosage of drugs can be increased or more potent ones used. When the pressure declines, the dosage can be reduced and the more potent ones discontinued.

You soon learn through home measurements that mental and physical stress will elevate blood pressure and that rest and relaxation will lower it. Thus, you learn to avoid those factors that drive pressure up and promote those factors that bring lower pressure. Regular readings at home also can serve to remind you to take your medication.

BLOOD PRESSURE IN PREGNANCY
See TOXEMIAS OF PREGNANCY

BODY ODOR The term body odor invariably refers to unpleasant body odor and can be a problem in both health and disease. Among the diseases giving rise to perceptible and unique body odors are diabetes, gout, pemphigus, typhoid fever, and scurvy. Foods and drugs can give a body odor on being excreted in the sweat (garlic, onions, asparagus, arsenic). But more commonly, unpleasant body odor is derived from the apocrine sweat glands of the armpits, long considered the source of the "scent" of our species (as it is in other animal species). Recently it has been demonstrated that armpit odors are probably due solely to the luxuriant growth of bacteria in the presence of much sweat (apocrine). Hence efforts at preventing body odor should be directed not only at reducing the sweat, but more importantly at removing the bacteria. This is accomplished by shaving off the hair which harbors the bacteria; using antibacterial soaps containing hexachlorophene; and the local application of antibiotic remedies.

BOILS This term refers to intensely red, tender, painful nodules which are initially hard and finally soften, rupture, and drain. Variously called furuncles, carbuncles, boils, depending on their size and number, the infection may be single or multiple, chronic or recurrent. The causative bacteria are usually staphylococci, but streptococci may be present. The many predisposing factors may not be present in an individual case, but must be considered when ordinary care does not result in cure. Included among the conditions thought to contribute to the recurrence or persistence of boils are diabetes, anemias, malnutrition, obesity, poor hygiene, excessive sweating (occupational or athletics), and drugs (iodides and bromides). Boils also occur as a secondary problem to already-existing skin conditions such as insect bites, scabies, louse infestation, and eczemas.

Treatment. Antibiotics (notably penicillin) and sulfonamides are effective for the individual attack of boils and may also be useful in attempting to prevent recurrences. Locally, the application of hot-water compresses and local antibiotics until there is spontaneous drainage, or until surgical incision is indicated, are helpful in hastening the course of the lesion. Treatment of any predisposing causes and restriction of diet (chocolate, nuts, shellfish) and the halogen drugs (iodides and bromides) in addition to improving the hygiene by washing with hexachlorophene soap, may avert the occurrence of new lesions. When excessive sweating is a predominant factor, as in athletes, at least temporary interruption of sweat-inducing activity may become necessary.

BONES AND JOINTS   Bone provides the rigid supporting structure for the human body. It consists of an abundant calcified "scaffolding" (matrix) which encloses the true bone cells (osteocytes). The long bones consist of an outer shell of dense cortical bone surrounding and enclosing the spongy cancellous bone which, together with the marrow, fills the interior. Surrounding the bone is the periosteum, a fibrous sheath responsible in part for nutrition of the bone and in part for appositional bone growth. Even though bones appear superficially to be rocklike, they are actively live organs and even in their most dense areas have an excellent blood supply.

There are 206 bones in the human skeleton, and they are classified according to shape—flat, irregular, long, and short. (An example of a flat bone would be a rib.) With increasing age bones tend to become more brittle, and scientists are currently discovering some new reasons for this occurrence.

Athough bones serve primarily as a support structure, they protect some vital organs, such as the skull's covering the brain. Bones also provide points of attachment for muscles; acting as levers, they make movement possible.

Joints are the articulations between bones. The contour of the joint determines the function it performs. For example, the shoulder joint is a ball-and-socket and therefore allows motion in all directions,

SACROILIAC JOINT

The sacroiliac is the joint between the sacrum and ilium.

ILIUM

SACRUM

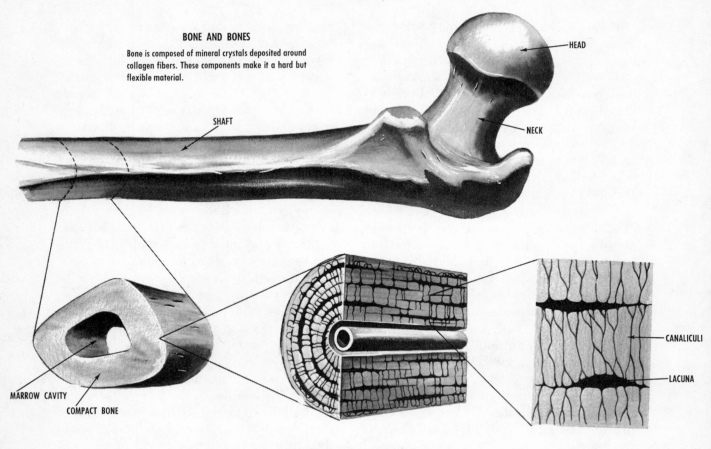

BONE AND BONES

Bone is composed of mineral crystals deposited around collagen fibers. These components make it a hard but flexible material.

HEAD

NECK

SHAFT

MARROW CAVITY

COMPACT BONE

CANALICULI

LACUNA

ENLARGED SECTION OF BONE SHAFT

The hollow construction reduces weight and frees the marrow for blood-cell production.

ENLARGED SECTION OF COMPACT BONE SHOWING PART OF A HAVERSIAN SYSTEM

Concentric layers of bone are applied around a center containing a capillary.

ENLARGED SECTION OF THE HAVERSIAN SYSTEM

Bone cells live in the lacunae. The connecting canaliculi transport nutrients from capillary to the cells.

BASIC BONE SHAPES

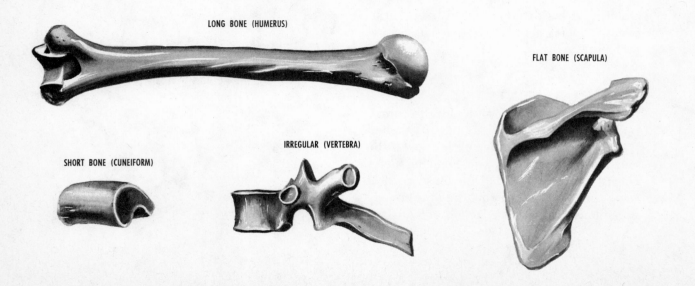

LONG BONE (HUMERUS)

FLAT BONE (SCAPULA)

SHORT BONE (CUNEIFORM)

IRREGULAR (VERTEBRA)

THE CLASSIFICATION OF JOINTS

IMMOVABLE

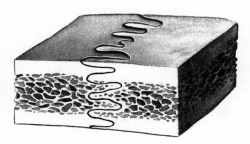

Bones are united by a thin layer of fibrous tissue. The sutures of the skull are typical.

SLIGHTLY MOVABLE

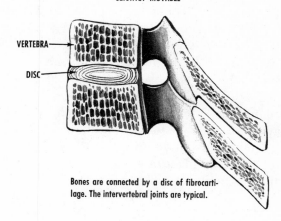

VERTEBRA

DISC

Bones are connected by a disc of fibrocartilage. The intervertebral joints are typical.

FREELY MOVABLE

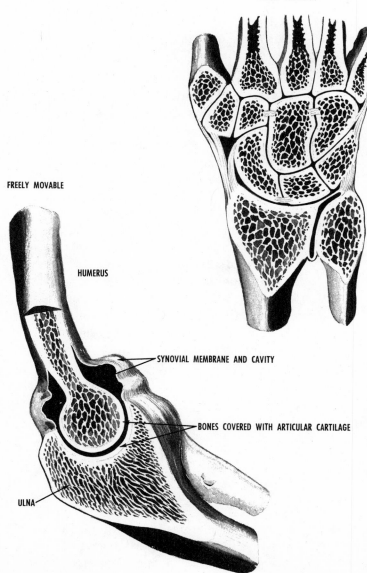

Gliding joints (the carpal bone joints are typical) permit gliding movement only.

FREELY MOVABLE

HUMERUS

SYNOVIAL MEMBRANE AND CAVITY

BONES COVERED WITH ARTICULAR CARTILAGE

ULNA

Hinge joints (the elbow or humero-ulnar joint is shown) permit only forward and backward movement.

FREELY MOVABLE

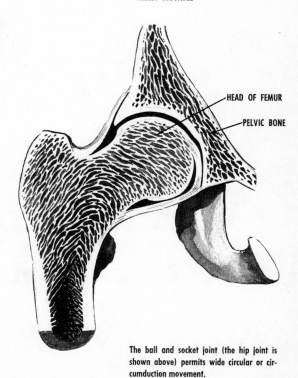

HEAD OF FEMUR

PELVIC BONE

The ball and socket joint (the hip joint is shown above) permits wide circular or circumduction movement.

while the finger joints are hinged and allow only flexion and extension. The joint surfaces of the bones are capped with cartilage, a slippery, smooth tissue magnificently able to bear weight and allow gliding motion. The joints contain a small amount of lubricating fluid which is secreted by the synovium, the lining wall of the joint. Surrounding the joints and binding them in place are the joint capsules and ligaments.

BOWEL OBSTRUCTION Obstruction to the passage of the intestinal contents may result from a variety of causes. The obstruction may be partial or complete and may occur anywhere along the course of the small or large intestine. Common mechanical causes include a kinking (or volvulus) of the bowel, adhesions as a result of previous abdominal operations, pressure from a tumor of neighboring tissue, strangulated hernia, impacted stool or foreign bodies, or strictures or tumors of the bowel-wall. A particularly serious type of obstruction follows the plugging of a large blood vessel supplying a segment of intestine, and the resulting death of that portion of the bowel. Often after surgery or during the course of peritonitis the bowel may become temporarily paralyzed.

Symptoms. Symptoms of bowel blockage vary according to the cause, duration, location, and completeness of the obstruction; but usually include intermittent crampy pain, vomiting, and abdominal distention. If the obstruction is in the large intestine, the pain is usually less severe. Vomiting may not be prominent and there may instead be occasional passage of bloody stools. In the paralytic type distention is prominent and the pain steady rather than colicky. X-rays of the abdomen will usually reveal the diagnosis.

Treatment. The treatment is directed at relieving the cause of the obstruction and often requires surgery. Early recognition is vitally important.

BOWLEGS In this condition the legs assume an outward curving. Most babies are born thus. A normal baby's legs appear a little bowed in the first ten months of life, but after he begins to walk they rapidly become straight if the bones are normal, and at the age of three years about 80 per cent of all babies are, in fact, knock-kneed.

Some persons feel that the use of bulky diapers is responsible for bowlegs, but this is hardly possible. It was undoubtedly more common years ago when rickets was prevalent; babies would stand up while the bones in their legs were still soft, and the bones would naturally bend outward. Most early cases of bowlegs will improve or become normal after the age of six.

BRAIN The brain is the portion of the central nervous system which is contained within the skull. It includes the cerebrum, the brainstem (medulla oblongata), and the cerebellum, and is the central organ which directs voluntary and involuntary bodily functions. It is the seat of memory, consciousness, emotional expression, and learning. The brain enables the individual to control voluntary musculature. Nearly all of the brain substance is composed of nerve cells and nerve fibers, which have specific functions. Therefore, damage to any segment of the brain results in disorder of function. The site of damage determines the type of resultant disability.

BRAINSTEM The brainstem is that portion of the brain which remains after the cerebral hemispheres and cerebellum have been removed. It is located inside the lower part of the skull. Through it pass all of the sensory and motor tracts connecting the cerebrum and cerebellum with the spinal cord, and most of the cranial nerves arise from nuclei in the brainstem. Certain pathways in the upper portion of the brainstem are related to consciousness. Vital functions of heart rate and respiration are

THE BRAIN
(CROSS SECTION)

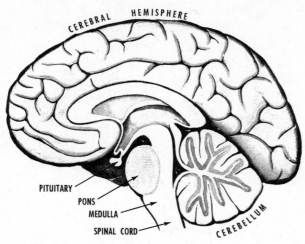

CEREBRAL HEMISPHERE

PITUITARY
PONS
MEDULLA
SPINAL CORD
CEREBELLUM

also controlled by mechanisms located in the brainstem.

Damage to a relatively small portion of the brainstem results in pronounced deficits in neurologic function. Extensive damage to the brainstem is often fatal.

BRAIN TUMORS Brain tumors may develop in the cerebral hemispheres, cerebellum, or brainstem, and occur both in children and in adults. Such tumors may spread to the brain from tumors elsewhere in the body, or they may be primary in the brain itself. Some tumors are encapsulated, while other (cancerous) ones invade nervous tissue. The cause of tumor cell growth is not known.

Symptoms. Tumors of the brain may produce symptoms due to local compression or due to invasion of nervous tissue. Other symptoms are due to generalized increase in pressure within the skull. If a tumor arises from the optic nerves, early loss of vision may occur; similarly, a tumor may compress the acoustic nerve and produce deafness. Convulsions occur as a first symptom in many tumors arising in a cerebral hemisphere. These convulsions may be associated with progressive weakness, numbness, or language difficulty. With involvement of the cerebellum, the gait becomes unsteady. Headache, nausea, and vomiting occur with increased intracranial pressure.

Treatment. X-rays of the skull may be used to locate brain tumors. The primary treatment is surgical. Encapsulated tumors are removed. If the tumor is invading nervous tissue (i.e., is cancerous), the neurosurgeon removes as much of it as is deemed advisable; subsequently, invasive tumors may be treated with X-ray therapy.

If an encapsulated tumor is successfully removed, permanent cure is usually accomplished, although regrowth of tumor may occur. The treatment of invasive tumors by operation and X-ray therapy is usually followed by recurrence of tumors after a period of months or years. Surgical therapy for tumors which have spread to the brain from elsewhere in the body is usually effective only for periods of months.

BREAST AND BOTTLE FEEDING Human breast milk is more digestible than cow's milk. If a normal infant nurses the mother's breast at reasonable intervals (every three or four hours) the amount of milk taken will not ordinarily exceed the digestive capacity of the infant. Cow's milk, however, is not so digestible. There are several factors involved. Fat curds in cow's milk are tougher and larger. To overcome this, cow's milk is "soured" with lactic acid to render it more digestible, and this acidified milk may be given in the same amount as the mother's milk, without diluting it. Undiluted sweet cow's milk given to an infant up to its stomach's capacity may cause distress. Although some babies are able to take sweet milk undiluted to the point of satisfying the appetite, such milk should, generally, be diluted if a baby's digestive capacity is limited.

A normal, healthy baby initially receives an adequate diet when nursed by a normal, healthy mother. Human milk provides all necessary food elements and furnishes energy in the form of calories—twenty to the ounce. Human milk is germfree (when the mother is healthy), easily digested, and reaches the infant at the proper temperature. In addition, certain immunity factors are passed from mother to child.

Breast milk is of especial value during the first weeks of life when the baby's digestive capabilities are small and he is susceptible to intestinal infections. Many women refuse to nurse, claiming that this will result in misshapen, flabby, or over-developed breasts. These fears are contrary to clinical fact. To the contrary, nursing serves to maintain firmness of the breasts and psychologically is a boon for both mother and child. Given a healthy mother and a normal child, there is no allergy to milk or inability to digest it. If a baby does not do well on breast feeding or there is insufficient breast milk, supplemental feeding is indicated. Where a bottle is added after breast feeding, such feeding is known as complemental; a replacement of breast feeding is supplemental feeding. The baby that does poorly on the milk of a normal mother usually fares well on artificial feeding.

A mother whose milk is insufficient or who is in poor health should not be permitted to nurse a normal, healthy infant. No mother with a severe chronic illness or active tuberculosis should be permitted to nurse her infant, and the child should not be brought into contact with her. In the event of an acute illness or surgical emergency involving the mother, the baby is weaned and the mother's breasts may have to be emptied by pump or hand until she can resume nursing her infant.

To estimate how well a baby is doing on breast feeding, the physician instructs the mother to weigh the child daily, at the same time, usually naked or wearing a diaper. This enables the doctor to determine if the amount of milk secreted is sufficient in quantity. A small gain in weight, or no gain, or even actual loss of weight indicate that the child is not receiving adequate feeding. Stools are smaller and may be less frequent; they may be frequent and green. Starvation diarrhea must be differentiated from overfeeding diarrhea. Insufficiently fed babies are fretful, cry a great deal, and suffer from colic. Such an infant may suck at various objects, or his fingers. This leads to air swallowing which may cause vomiting.

Sometimes a normal infant receives insufficient milk from a healthy mother because of inverted nipples. This defect is easily corrected by a breast shield. The baby who nurses at 4-hour intervals seldom suffers from overfeeding. On occasion a baby may consume too much milk from a mother who secretes more than is required. This overfeeding may easily result in vomiting or in loose bowel movements. The remedy is simply to shorten the nursing time.

As the infant advances, his breast-fed diet must be supplemented with other necessary elements. These are prescribed by the doctor who designates the substances, the amounts, the times of administration, and the method of giving them to the baby. The infant who receives breast milk exclusively for six to twelve months becomes flabby and anemic because of insufficient protein and iron. Bottle and breast feeding are supplemented, beginning with about the second month by orange juice (vitamin C) and a protein-rich cooked cereal. Soon thereafter, meat broths, vegetable purées, vitamin preparations and fruit purées are added as the doctor prescribes. These are necessary because milk does not provide the required protein and iron. There is nothing to be gained by continuing breast feeding after the first year; in fact, there are potential psychological hazards (overdependence, etc.). Weaning is done gradually; a bottle is substituted for a breast feeding the first day, and the substitution is continued steadily until the bottle completely replaces breast feeding.

When bottle feeding is required—whether immediately after birth or sometime thereafter—the physician is able to calculate and prescribe a diet, the basis of which is cow's milk which furnishes all the necessary food elements and minerals. In the presence of allergies or chronic disorders, milk other than cow's may be used (goat's milk, for example). When traveling or where refrigeration is lacking, dried milk is suitable. Condensed milk is also convenient; this is whole cow's milk evaporated to one-half of its volume and preserved by the addition of cane sugar. Also available are various modified milks; one example is a diluted skimmed milk to which is added milk sugar (lactose) and vegetable and codliver oils. It provides the necessary elements and, like mother's milk, has twenty calories to the ounce.

BREAST ENGORGEMENT   One or two days after delivery, mothers usually notice considerable swelling of their breasts, which at the same time become warm and sore. Contrary to popular belief, this is not due to abundant milk-production and storage, but to obstructed blood- and lymph-flow from the breast. This condition should not be confused with mastitis, which is an actual infection of the breast, with much higher fever, and which may occur a week or more after delivery.

Treatment. Treatment of engorgement consists of proper support of the breasts and application of ice bags. Aspirin is usually all that is necessary to relieve the pain.

BREAST, THE IMMATURE FEMALE Often, immediately after birth, the mother or nurse may notice a definite swelling of the female baby's tiny breasts. This is quite common—and almost never important. It is the result of the mother's hormones (probably the lactogenic, or milk, hormone) still being active in the infant's blood. The condition—also occasionally seen in boys—is generally self-limiting, lasting only two or three weeks.

Female breasts during childhood are completely unimportant and nonfunctional. They grow very little until the begin-

ning of adolescence, at which time they undergo marked sudden growth and engorgement. During this time they may be painful—upsetting to the child, especially if she develops large breasts at any early age. This is most often an almost normal adolescent engorgement, and should seldom be treated by radical measures. Restriction of fluids and salt, ice packs, well-fitting, snug brassieres, (perhaps to be worn at night), and mild pain pills (aspirin) will usually suffice.

Lumps in the immature breast should always be examined by the doctor, but will seldom require anything but conscientious observation. In certain cases, a surgical specimen may have to be taken for examination (biopsy), but this will be rare; cancer in the immature breast is very rare indeed. Little hardenings under the nipple areas may also be noticed in one or both breasts. These also are seldom serious, but should be shown to the doctor.

There is generally some slight milky, grayish-appearing discharge, present even in small breasts, especially as adolescence is approached or entered. Occasionally this may appear spontaneously, and unless accompanied by pain or lumps—or especially if it is blood-tinged—it requires no particular attention. A blood-tinged discharge should always be checked by the doctor.

Because of the present furor with regard to glamorous bosoms, very small breasts have become a source of concern among unwise mothers, with the concern transmitting itself to their children. Consequently teenage girls become seriously worried about an "underdeveloped bust." Some of them seem to be convinced that their entire sexual future, even their marital and maternal potential, depends on an opulent bosom. A child in such a predicament can be helped if the mother does not try to keep up with the Joneses.

BREATHING DIFFICULTY   The most

common causes of difficulty in breathing are infections, tumors, paralysis of the vocal cords, foreign bodies, spasms of the muscles of the larynx, and abnormalities of the larynx. (See ACUTE EPIGLOTTITIS; L.T.B. [Laryngo tracheobronchitis]; DIPHTHERIA; TUBERCULOSIS; SYPHILIS; LARYNX, TUMORS OF THE; VOCAL CORDS, PARALYSIS OF; LARYNX, INJURIES; LARYNGOSPASM; LARYNX, ABNORMALITIES OF; FIRST AID AND EMERGENCIES.)

BREATH, SHORTNESS OF Everyone experiences breathlessness now and then. Usually it is a burst of exercise such as running, that causes the consumption of more oxygen in the muscle fibers than the circulation is able to supply during the time of exertion. The heart rate quickens, blood going through the heart increases in volume per minute, and the rate (as well as depth) of breathing increases becoming much faster than the usual fourteen to eighteen per minute.

Causes other than extraordinary physical activity can bring about shortness of breath. Even with little exertion disorders of the heart or the circulatory system frequently cause breathlessness; it all depends upon how efficiently blood can run its circuit from the tissues and through the lungs. If for any reason the tissues build up an oxygen deficiency that cannot be corrected quickly, shortness of breath will usually persist until corrective treatment is supplied.

The fault will sometimes be in the lungs rather than the circulation of blood. If, for example, a stab wound of the chest collapses one lung, breathlessness will be experienced because there is not enough exposure of blood to inhaled air, the useful surface of membrane for oxygen-transfer having been halved by the airlessness of the collapsed lung. (Blood still passes through the collapsed lung and re-enters the arteries, but is not refreshed by new oxygen.)

Hemorrhage, severe bleeding, and anemia can also cause breathlessness; for, although the circulation of the blood may be within normal limits, the number of red cells in the fluid blood may be too small to satisfy the tissues' demands for oxygen. This can be very distressing if the anemic patient has need of additional oxygen in his tissues, no matter whether the increase in demand is due to a little exertion, fever, or tissue-needs after an accident or operation (which may have caused the anemia in the first place).

Occasionally the accumulation of waste products (especially carbon dioxide) in the tissues can produce additional efforts in breathing to bring about efficient elimination of these products. This sort of breathlessness can occur in metabolic acidosis of diabetic kidney, or other origin.

BREECH Approximately 3 per cent of all babies are delivered with the feet or the buttocks coming first. This is known as breech presentation. There are two main varieties of breech: the footling breech, in which one or both feet come first through the birth canal during delivery; and the frank breech, in which the buttocks appear first. Before the onset of labor, a breech baby can always turn headfirst and vice versa, but once active labor is established, this is highly unlikely. Breech deliveries are, as a rule, more difficult for the physician (the mother will not notice any difference) and require more skill and experience than normal deliveries do. This is the reason a few obstetricians prefer to deliver all full-term breeches by caesarean section, especially if the breech is the patient's first baby. This is not generally recommended, however—at least not in places where such good hospital facilities are available as prompt anaethesia, sufficient and well-trained personnel, a blood-bank, etc.

A warning of particular importance to the patient who knows that she is carrying a breech baby is to watch for rupture of the bag of waters, whether she is in labor or not. If this occurs, she should immediately be taken to the hospital, because of the increased danger of prolapse of the cord (see CORD, UMBILICAL). In such cases an immediate operation will usually be required for the delivery of the baby, if alive.

BRIDGE, DENTAL   A bridge is an artificial appliance used to replace one or more missing teeth. The remaining teeth are utilized for support and retention, and the appliance is intended to restore the function and appearance of the lost teeth. A fixed bridge is one which usually is cemented in place by the dentist and which cannot readily be removed by the patient. A removable bridge is one which is designed to be easily removed by the patient. (It is sometimes referred to as a removable partial denture. It is axiomatic that any artificial replacement of teeth or their parts requires continued and scrupulous care by both the patient and the dentist. (See DENTURES, PARTIAL.)

BROMHIDROSIS See BODY ODOR

BRONCHIAL ASTHMA See ASTHMA

BRONCHIECTASIS   Bronchiectasis is a disease characterized by extensive anatomical damage to the bronchial tubes, leading to their dilatation and to formation of ballooning pockets which become the seat of chronic infection and suppuration.

The causes of bronchiectasis are multiple and, in some instances, remain unknown. In children, the condition may develop after whooping cough or measles, or may be due to the accidental swallowing of a foreign object which "goes the wrong way" and lodges in the airways instead of in the stomach. Occasionally, in debilitated or alcoholic patients, a large amount of vomited material may be partly sucked

back into the lung and cause the disease. In many other instances bronchiectasis is the end result of a respiratory infection (tuberculosis, pneumonia, influenza) which did not resolve completely.

The common denominator of bronchiectasis seems to be the presence of foreign material which becomes "trapped" in the lung. Patients with such conditions are easy prey for infection which cannot find its way out through the normal airway channels. The infection roots itself in the bronchial walls, which become progressively more damaged and tend to dilate and lose their normal characteristics. Damage to the bronchus alters the protective function of the cilia, hairs which normally clean out the foreign material that lodges in the airways. (See RESPIRATORY TRACT INFECTION.)

Symptoms. The most characteristic symptom is the coughing up of quantities of purulent material. This is the result of chronic bronchial irritation and continuous formation of such material. Cough characteristics will depend on the degree of infection and virulence, the season of the year (outbreaks are more common in winter), the position of the body, etc. Often the cough comes in paroxysms, or following laughter. The sputum is usually yellow or greyish in color and frequently foul-smelling; red streaks or frank bloody expectorations are common. As a consequence of the chronic infection, the patient may lose his appetite, and may weaken and waste. The disease characteristically runs in "ups and downs" over a prolonged course marked by frequent lingering "colds," pneumonia, and bronchopneumonia.

Treatment. It is difficult to clear the pockets of infection completely. Medical treatment is aimed at the following objectives:

1. Identification of the type of bacteria present and institution of repeated and prolonged courses of antibiotics.

2. Liquefaction of the expectoration (if thick and tenacious), to facilitate its discharge through abundant fluid-intake, steam-inhalation, or expectorants.

3. Best utilization of the normal pathways of bronchial discharge by postural drainage. According to the area of involvement, the patient is advised to assume certain body positions to facilitate bronchial drainage. For the lower lung areas, for example, the patient should lie down with his chest and head hanging down over the side of the bed and also turned over according to the side involved.

Moving to certain geographical areas, particularly to a dry and warm climate, can be useful.

When the disease is circumscribed to a definite lung area, surgical excision may be the treatment of choice.

BRONCHITIS   Bronchitis may be described as inflammation or irritation of the inner lining (mucosa) of the bronchial tubes. The disease may run an acute or chronic course, the implications of each being quite different. Acute bronchitis is usually a benign, self-limiting disease which often develops in the course of a severe cold or a generalized inflammation of the nose, throat, larynx, and trachea. (See Respiratory Tract Infection.) Chronic bronchitis, on the other hand, is a protracted, insidious, progressive disease, prone to exacerbations and remissions and fraught with many complications.

In recent years a complete reassessment of the serious implications of this disease has taken place. Chronic bronchitis has been recognized as an extremely common disease in the United States, but its exact prevalence is not yet adequately known. It is fair to assume that it is essentially similar to the better studied "English bronchitis" which is known to be responsible for about one-fourth of all male illness, producing the loss of twenty million work-days annually and causing about thirty thousand deaths per year. There is no single cause of chronic bronchitis, and many irritants of the bronchial mucosa have been described. The most common irritants are cigarette smoking and air-pollution. Certain diseases, such as repeated upper-respiratory infections, allergy, sinusitis, or influenza are usually discovered in the background history of such patients. Eventually, with progression of the disease, bacterial infection also takes place, becoming chronically imbedded in the respiratory tract and giving rise from time to time to acute exacerbations of the disease as well as to severe complications.

Symptoms. Cough and expectoration are the outstanding symptoms, and when present daily for a period of more than six months, establish the diagnosis. Unfortunately, these symptoms are readily dismissed by most people as "smokers' cough" or "morning cough." The patient may not seek medical attention for many years, and then usually only after some complication has arisen. Expectoration can be variable in amount, character, and color. At the beginning it is clear, scanty, easy to raise, and noticeable only upon arising in the morning. As time goes on, sputum volume increases; the color changes to yellow, greyish, or blood-tinged; and the sputum itself is raised through paroxysms of cough that last progressively longer. The presence of phlegm and inflammation of the bronchial tubes commonly lead to audible respiratory wheeze produced by the passage of air through the narrowed bronchi. This wheezing is sometimes improperly ascribed to asthma, and as a result the confusing expression asthmatic bronchitis has been coined (see Asthma). Concomitantly, shortness of breath insinuates itself progressively until it severely limits the patient's activities. Another common feature is development of protracted, lingering episodes of "colds" of progressively longer duration. Unfortunately, this symptom develops slowly over a period of several years, and most patients adjust subconsciously to the changing symptoms and signs which come to be accepted as part of their normal routine. At some time a severe cold which cannot be "shaken off" will appear, and severe, persistent incapacitation will develop. If such a state has been reached, complications are to be expected—particularly the development of chronic pulmonary heart disease or heart failure secondary to lung disease which marks the appearance of the last stage of the condition.

Treatment. Due to the chronicity of this illness, there is great variation among patients in terms of degree of reversibility of the disease, which bears a relationship to the time when they seek medical attention. With increasing awareness on the part of the public of the meaning of chronic, "innocent" cough, earlier treatment can be instituted and serious incapacitation and complications avoided. Treatment can be divided into hygienic, symptomatic, and specific. Important in hygienic treatment are: avoidance of respiratory irritants (particularly cigarette smoking); of dust in all forms; of fumes, fog, smoke, excessive cold and dampness, and other types of air pollutants. During the early stages of disease, and before severe incapacitation or complications have set in, these hygienic rules alone can effect a remarkable improvement and sometimes even a complete cure. Symptomatic treatment is directed toward: (1) facilitating sputum-expulsion by bronchodilator drugs (opening up of the constricted bronchi) and by liquefaction of the sticky, heavy phlegm; (2) reducing the excessive cough; (3) vigorously treating the complications—particularly the respiratory infections. Moderate physical activity is helpful and should be allowed, according to the breathing comfort of the patient; obesity should be avoided. Specific treatment can be effective in cases where the primary offender is known (allergy, tuberculosis, fungal dis-

eases, etc.), or by surgical approach in the few cases where the disease is well-localized. Great emphasis has recently been placed on the use of antibiotics, either for short-term treatment at the time of acute respiratory infections; or as long-term treatment, particularly throughout the winter months.

BRONCHOGRAPHY   This term is applied to X-ray visualization of the bronchial tubes after they have been filled with contrast material (iodine dyes). By this procedure any section of the bronchi and their branches can be observed in detail. Bronchography and bronchoscopy may complement each other for diagnostic purposes: the former affords more detailed examination and reaches down to far smaller bronchi in caliber; the latter cannot go as deep, but allows a direct examination and/or obtaining of tissue for analysis.

BRONCHOPNEUMONIA   This is a type of lung inflammation similar to pneumonia, but involving much smaller lung areas (usually only millimeters to a few centimeters in size). It also differs from classical pneumonia in that it principally affects individuals whose defenses have already been weakened by other diseases or by toxic conditions. Also, it is more common at the extremes of the age-range: elderly people and children. (See also PNEUMONIA.)

Bronchopneumonia can be caused by many bacteria, fungi, viruses, parasites, and by physical agents either as inhalants (toxic fumes) or droplets (oil). It is important to remember that many of these agents are normal inhabitants of the upper respiratory passages and attack the lung only after some disease or condition has weakened the organism, for example, during measles or whooping cough in children, or in the course of chronic bronchitis, after surgical operations, or with malnutrition in the elderly.

Symptoms. The onset is less sudden than in pneumonia, but the main symptoms are the same: marked increase in cough and expectoration (which turns yellow or greenish), moderate rise in temperature (this may be deceptively low or even normal), and general malaise. The patient does not exhibit the markedly "hard-hit" (toxic) appearance characteristic of pneumonia. If bronchopneumonia develops in a patient already affected by chronic bronchitis, the diagnosis may at times be difficult because of the similarity of symptoms. In such cases, one should become suspicious of a relative increase in frequency and severity of the "normal" cough and expectoration.

Treatment. Treatment is essentially similar to that described for pneumonia, modifications being due to the fact that bronchopneumonia often affects previously weakened individuals, so that complications are more frequent and the rate of relapses much higher. By the same token, prevention of bronchopneumonia in such persons is extremely important and depends on continuous proper care of the basic disease or condition that first attacked the patient.

BRONCHOSCOPY   This is a procedure which allows direct visual inspection of the respiratory tract down to the level of the larger bronchi. It is performed with a long metallic tube—the bronchoscope—which is passed through the throat, larynx, trachea, and right or left bronchus. Thus the physician can methodically observe these areas, obtain secretions or tissue samples for analysis, and introduce medicines directly to any particular diseased area. Bronchoscopy is usually performed under local anesthesia and in skilled hands is a safe and easy procedure. The indications for bronchoscopy are many, particularly for diagnosis of suspected malignant disease.

BRUXISM   The gritting and grinding of the teeth while sleeping (medically referred to as bruxism) may cause excessive, premature, and abnormal wearing-away of the biting surfaces of the teeth. The unusual pressures created are generally injurious to the supporting structures.

BRUXOMANIA   This is the unconscious habit of gritting and grinding of the teeth while awake, usually during times of nervous tension. (See Bruxism.)

BURSITIS   This condition is due to inflammation of the gliding surfaces (bursae) which are placed around the joint. Occasionally an acute calcium deposit is also present.

Symptoms. The patient awakens with acute throbbing pain localized at the shoulder and radiating down to the elbow. The shoulder may be a little warm and swollen. All motion of the shoulder is painful and the patient cannot lift the arm from the side. If X-rays reveal a calcium deposit as the cause of the difficulty, needle suction of this material may completely relieve the pain. Rest in a sling is usually prescribed while the pain is acute; as the pain subsides, vigorous pendulum and figure-eight exercises are useful in restoring motion to the inflamed shoulder: the patient bends forward and toward the painful side, swinging the arm through ever-increasing pendulum arcs for two minutes; then, after a period of rest, the arm is swung through figure-eights for a few minutes. This exercise is repeated three times a day.

CAESAREAN SECTION   About 3 to 5 per cent of all pregnancies are today terminated by caesarean section for the benefit of the baby, the mother, or both. Caesarean section actually means the delivery of the baby through surgical incision of the wall of the abdomen and the womb. The term "caesarean" is derived from the Latin verb *caedere* (to cut) and not—contrary to popular belief—because Julius Caesar was delivered in this manner. The operation, as performed in our modern hospitals by well-trained obstetricians, with all proper surgical facilities at their disposal, is a relatively simple technical procedure, and the overall prognosis for the mother is excellent. Babies delivered by caesarean section have generally higher mortality rates; this, however, is not due to the operation per se, but to the many and often serious pre-existing complications which make the section mandatory. In fact, many of these babies would perish unless delivered promptly with the help of surgery. Everything else being equal, babies delivered by caesarean section have the same chances for survival and normal development as the ones delivered vaginally.

Indications for caesarean section are numerous, some of them permanent and some temporary. The most common ones are: contracted maternal pelvis—always in correlation with the size of the baby (see CEPHALOPELVIC DISPROPORTION); previous caesarean sections; distress of the baby in the womb (in either the presence or absence of labor); excessive bleeding from the afterbirth before the delivery; prolapse of the umbilical cord; an abnormal position of the baby inside the mother's womb; and tumors of the womb and ovaries.

The choice of anesthesia will depend on the general condition of the individual patient and the indication for caesarean section. In most cases, spinal anesthesia is indicated and is perfectly adequate for the operation, but occasionally the patient has to be put to sleep through general (inhalation) anesthesia. On the average, the patient is ready to leave the hospital in seven to ten days after the operation.

Should a patient who has been delivered once by caesarean section always be delivered in the same manner? This is still a matter of considerable controversy among obstetricians, and the opinion given here is only the author's own, which happens to coincide with that of the majority of specialists in this field. Everybody agrees that whenever there is a permanent indication for the original caesarean section—and the only permanent indication is small maternal pelvis—subsequent pregnancies should also be terminated by caesarean section. Whenever the original indication is temporary (such as vaginal bleeding, abnormal position of the baby, prolapsed cord, etc.) the majority of obstetricians will allow the patient to go into labor and have subsequent babies vaginally, always under close medical observation, however. There are numerous studies and reliable statistical records to back up this approach and, no matter how safe a caesarean section in general can be today, we should not forget that it is still a major surgical procedure and should not be utilized lightly in place of a more natural and safer alternative, that is, vaginal delivery.

Unless there are special indications for the termination of pregnancy before term (such as diabetes or Rh disease), the patient with a previous caesarean section should be allowed to advance as close to term as possible. The best way to achieve this is to let the patient go into early labor, then repeat the operation. This is the only way to avoid delivering a large number of premature babies by elective repeat caesarean section. Occasionally, because of lack of proper hospital facilities in close vicinity to the patient, or because the obstetrician estimates beyond any doubt that the baby is large enough to be delivered, a repeat caesarean section may be planned and performed before labor begins.

How many caesarean sections can a patient have? Actually, a patient may have as many babies by caesarean section as she wants. It should, however, be realized that with each subsequent pregnancy and operative delivery the patient is assuming the same and probably increased risks and possible complications. This is the reason why, after three or four caesarean sections, patients are advised to undergo surgical sterilization. The decision always rests with the patient.

CALCIUM   Calcium is an essential chemical element (a mineral) largely concerned with the structure of bones and teeth; a small portion is involved in blood-clotting and transmission of impulses from nerve to muscles. Absorption of calcium in the diet is enhanced by vitamin D. The element circulates in the blood where its concentration in the plasma is carefully maintained, in part by parathyroid hormone, at about 10 milligrams per 100 milliliters. Lack of calcium in the diet leads to a form of "leaching out" of bone mineral contents (osteoporosis), and when vitamin D is deficient, the condition known as rickets occurs.

Milk and cheese are essentially the only foods that supply large amounts of calcium. The precise dietary requirement for this element is not known but is generally accepted as being between 0.6 and 1.0 gram per day (one pint of milk supplies 0.68 gram). The woman who is pregnant or breast-feeding her baby may need perhaps twice this amount to protect her from the fetus's or baby's drain on her tissues.

Severe calcium deficiency (usually not dietary alone, but related to a deficient supply of vitamin D and deficient parathyroid hormone metabolism) results in tetany, a state of muscle spasm. Significant calcium excess (hypercalcemia and deposits in certain tissues) does not occur from dietary intake alone; it depends on excess vitamin D or excessive parathyroid secretion.

Calcium salts are occasionally used therapeutically, independent of the dietary intake.

CALCULUS (TARTAR)   A hard deposit of calcified material usually found on the crowns or roots of teeth, calculus is believed to be precipitated from the saliva or other secretions and is usually found in greater amounts on teeth which are located nearest the openings of salivary glands. There are two main types: that which begins forming on the visible surfaces of teeth and is usually sand-colored (supragingival [above-the-gum] calculus); and that which begins forming beneath the gum line and is usually black (subgingival [below-the-gum] calculus).

Either type acts as an irritant to the supporting structures of teeth, and should be periodically removed by the dentist. Calculus is one of the major contributing factors in periodontal disease.

CALLUS   This abnormal thickening of the skin is the result of chronic and repeated friction to the affected part. It occurs most commonly on the feet, but can be produced on almost any other part of the skin. Callusses of the palms (in laborers, tennis players) and of the finger tips (violinists), or of the knuckles, ankles, and knees may differ somewhat in appearance, but are produced in the same way as those of the feet.

Treatment. Removal of the friction causing the thickening will result in spontaneous disappearance of the callus. Application of salicylic acid plasters and lessening the thickening by cutting with a razor blade will afford some relief. For callusses of the soles of the feet, properly fitting shoes and thick socks to minimize friction are essential for continued improvement and cure.

CALORIE   The calorie is defined as a unit of heat energy which raises the temperature of 1 kilogram (2.2 pounds) of water 1 degree centigrade ($1\frac{4}{5}°$ Fahrenheit). Because the source of our energy is food, and because energy can conveniently be expressed in terms of heat, it is in calories that we measure the energy supplied by our food.

Both by direct and by indirect means, we know that a gram of carbohydrate furnishes 4.1 calories, a gram of protein 4.1 calories, and a gram of fat 9.3 calories. For practical purposes we use the values 4, 4, and 9 calories, respectively.

To maintain body weight during health, the caloric intake must equal the caloric output. For growth or repair of tissue after injury or starvation, the caloric intake must be higher. Physical work or exercise per-formed has much to do with the caloric output; it is evident that obesity is frequent-ly due to a caloric intake greater than such output. (Reducing food-consumption and increasing activity help reset the balance.)

The caloric values of foods differ considerably, largely because of the varying amounts of fat present. Thus a gram of butter yields 8.6 calories, a gram of rice 3.5 calories, a gram of potato 1 calorie and a gram of lettuce 0.2 calories.

Cancer

CANCER   Cancer is today the second leading cause of death in the United States. (The first is heart and circulatory disease.) Estimates for 1982 indicate that 430,000 Americans will have died of some form of cancer. If national trends continue, some fifty-three million Americans now alive will contract cancer sometime during their lifetime. Of this immense number, approxi-mately one-half will die of cancer, despite a medical effort to cure and prevent cancer amounting to the greatest scientific assault on a single disease in history.

Since the turn of this century the problem of cancer has increased. In 1900, the disease accounted for only one death in every twenty-five. Today it is the cause of one death in five. Some of this increase is simply due to the fact that people today live longer. The longer a person lives, the more likely some form of cancer will manifest itself. In addition, some medical authorities believe the increased rate is due, in part, to an increased exposure of Americans to cancer-causing agents (carcinogens) in the home and in the work place.

This upward climb in the rate of deaths due to cancer has not been uniform for all types of cancer. Some varieties have re-mained more or less constant, while other varieties, such as cancer of the stomach, have actually shown a decline. Similarly, cancer of the uterus has shown a steady decrease since 1936. In contrast, cancer of the lungs has literally skyrocketed due to cigarette smoking.

Perhaps the saddest aspect of all in the figures that document the rise of deaths due to cancer is the realization that a large portion of these deaths could have been prevented. Although 45 percent of the detected cases of serious cancer are curable, an increase of 5 percent in the last ten years, it is obvious that measures can be taken to increase the cure rate and also prevent the onset of various cancers.

Cigarette smoking alone has been estimated to be a contributing factor in approximately 30 percent of all cancer deaths. Early detection procedures, such as the "Pap smear" test, if made use of by larger numbers, could also help prevent death, especially reducing the fatalities due to cancer of the uterine cervix.

Many other types of cancer have cure rates that could be improved by detection and treatment at an early stage, before "regional involvement" occurs; that is, before the disease spreads to the lymph-node system in the area of the original tumor. After cancerous cells have dispersed into other regions of the body, the control or

	MALES %	FEMALES %
ESTIMATED PERCENTAGE INCIDENCE OF CANCERS FOR 1982, BASED ON NATIONAL CANCER INSTITUTE FIGURES (excluding carcinoma-in-situ of the cervix).		
Lung	22	8
Colon/Rectum	14	15
Urinary	9	4
Leukemia and Lymphomas	8	7
Prostate	18	—
Ovary	—	4
Uterus and Cervix	—	13
Breast	—	27
All other	29	22

termination of the cancer is made more difficult, if not impossible.

The Nature of Cancer. Cancer has been aptly described as the growth of cells gone wild.

To understand what cancer is, we must first consider the complex nature of growth as it normally occurs in our tissues. The many and varied bio-chemical reactions that produce and control normal growth are so delicately balanced that it is a wonder any of us escape the abnormal growth process called cancer.

To understand the mystery of growth, we must begin with a single microscopic unit of life, the cell, for it is from the single cell that each and every form of plant and animal life, including man, originates. Once formed, the cells multiply and a living organism grows. Something like a minimum of ten trillion cells must be formed to make the fully grown human body.

Not all cells are identical. Beginning with the single cell at conception, there ensues a process called differentiation, which insures that different types of cells are formed for the multitude of different tasks required for the proper functioning of a living organism. Thus, for example, as a human embryo develops, the cells that come together to form the liver have different traits from those that form the brain or the lungs.

Furthermore, growth does not end when the body reaches adult size. There must be additional, and continuous, production of fresh cells for repair and maintenance, because the wear and tear of everyday life destroys many cells. The skin, for example, would be worn away entirely in a very short time if there were not a constant supply of new cells replacing those rubbed or sloughed off.

A study of the regulated production and replacement of cells leads quite naturally to some very important questions:

How do cells multiply?

How do they differentiate to form harmoniously organized tissues and organs?

How do cells know when to stop making more of their own kind?

Exactly what mechanisms trigger the *unregulated* production of cells, which produces abnormal tissue?

When we are able to answer such questions thoroughly, we will be at the threshold of solving the biological riddle that is cancer, for cancer is simply the name given to a family of diseases marked by the failure of coordinated cell growth. Cancer is, in short, the inability of body tissues to maintain a commonwealth of cells obedient to the biological requirements that govern the health of the whole body. It is as if cancerous cells and tissues decide to go their own way, growing without restraint, at the expense of neighboring healthy tissue, which ultimately may end in the destruction of the victimized organism.

The term tumor has come to denote any abnormal new growth (neoplasm). Some tumors are benign, which means they do not usually spread into adjacent healthy tissue. Benign tumors are often surrounded by a covering of fibrous tissue. In contrast, some tumors are malignant and possess the capacity to spread and affect the functioning of one or more healthy organs.

Malignant cancerous growths are particularly dangerous because each new cancer cell retains the capacity for disorderly growth, even if it breaks off and becomes separated from the parent mass of cancerous tissue.

Such a spreading—the medical term for it is metastasis—results in the establishment of "colonies" of related cancerous cells. These colonies continue a career of rampant multiplication at a site distant from the

What increases your chances of contracting cancer?
. . . . Here are a few considerations:

1. AGE: The older you are, the higher the possibility of having cancer.

2. TOBACCO: Cigarette smokers are ten times more likely to contract lung cancer. Pipe and cigar smokers, and snuff users, have an increased risk of lip, mouth, and larynx cancers.

3. WORKPLACE: Exposure to carcinogenic substances such as asbestos, radioactive wastes, chromate, and vinyl chloride increase the chances of cancer.

4. SUNSHINE: Sunbathing for extended periods or prolonged work under the sun can increase the risk of skin cancer.

5. HEREDITARY FACTORS: A family history of cancer may indicate a predisposition towards contracting certain forms of cancer.

6. DRUGS, ALCOHOL, AND HORMONES: Drugs that are now discontinued, such as D.E.S. taken during a pregnancy, have increased the chances of cancer in offspring. Alcohol, especially combined with smoking, heightens the chances of cancer with excessive use. Long term doses of estrogen in the treatment of menopause problems may increase risk.

original formation of the disease. It is interesting that a pathologist can determine the original site of a cancerous growth by examining cancer cells in distant sites. For example, a cancer tumor of the thyroid that has metastasized into the bone may not only have a similar cell structure, but may even produce thyroid hormone as well.

The ability to metastasize, that is, to spread and establish new cancerous growth at a distance, makes cancer the very deadly disease it is. Metastases, or secondary tumors, are created when a cell or fragment of the original growth breaks away to be carried either by the bloodstream or by the lymphatic system to another area of the body. If cancerous tissue is not eliminated by surgery or destroyed by radiation or other means, before metastasis, a cure becomes extremely difficult.

Because so much of the outlook for cure depends upon the degree to which metastasis has occurred, much stress is laid on early cancer detection.

Causes of Cancer. When considering the factors that might contribute to the initiation of cancerous cell development, it is interesting to compare the incidence of various cancers throughout the world. It is evident, for example, that in countries, such as the United States, where cigarette smoking is widespread, the frequency of lung cancer is high. However, factors unknown at present indicate that cancer of the liver is relatively more frequent in regions of Asia and Africa than in other areas of the world. Too, stomach cancer is more common in Japan and Scandinavia than it is in the United States—but breast cancer is more of a problem in Europe and North America than it is in Japan.

Reasons for these geographic differences are being researched. Perhaps certain cultural or environmental factors (such as tobacco smoking, exposure to radiation, or industrial pollution) are mostly to blame.

Despite all that is known about the distribution and frequency of various cancers, the biological mechanisms that set in motion cancerous growth processes are yet to be fully understood, We have, in the last decades, learned much about *how* certain cells turn traitor to the coordinated activity of a healthy body, yet we have a great deal to learn concerning *why* these cells behave in the way they do.

A number of hypotheses have been offered to account for the causation of cancers. A few of these theories are as follows:

First, contact with known carcinogenic substances: This would include contact with cigarette smoke, radioactive materials, asbestos, overexposure to X-rays, and other substances including some drugs and pesticides.

Second, a constant, prolonged irritation: This would include cancers caused by overexposure to sunlight, cancer of the lip due to pipe smoking, or the development of a cancerous growth at the site of a mole rubbed by clothing.

Third, viral causation: Research is being done to discover whether certain viruses may be to blame for certain human cancers.

Cancer and Cell Mechanisms. Because cancer is essentially a derangement that affects the reproduction of cells, it seems certain that whatever produces cancer must act by upsetting the cellular mechanism that controls division into new cells. This mechanism lies concentrated within a small body of matter at the center of the cell, the nucleus. Within this nucleus there are curled a number of elongated structures, the chromosomes, which are responsible for each cell's capacity to divide into new cells. Chromosomes also determine what function and activity the cell has within the larger organism.

The carcinogenic (cancer producing) properties of such radiation as X-rays and ultraviolet rays, as well as of certain chemical substances—such as coal tar derivatives and some constituents of tobacco—

appear to rise from the effects produced on the chromosomes. The precise ways carcinogens work their damaging effect is still imperfectly understood. The study of how carcinogenic agents influence chromosome development is a major area of medical research today.

Only a few decades old is the major discovery of the chemical composition and structure of chromosomes themselves. Through research conducted by biologists Francis Crick and James Watson, chromosomes were found to consist largely of DNA (deoxyribonucleic acid), which is coiled in a pattern similar to a circular staircase, or what is now called a "double helix" structure. It is now certain that the arrangement of four basic amino acids—adenine, cytosine, guanine, and tyrosine—constitutes a code that spells out the reproductive details and functional destiny of the cell. Apparently, then, carcinogens can bring about cancer by disrupting or changing the instructions of the DNA code. Carcinogens might also alter the DNA itself, or influence the way coded "messages" are carried about within the cell.

Cancer and Viruses. Because it has been shown that viruses are composed of nucleic acids that can invade cells, it is quite possible that viruses may cause human cancer. Certain virsues have already been identified in animal tumors. Up to the present time, no causative cancer virus has been found in humans. However, this does not mean that such a virus does not necessarily exist. As early as 1911, a virus was shown to be the cause of a cancerous growth in chickens (the Rous sarcoma). Since then, more than a dozen viruses have been linked to various experimental animals in a cause-and-effect chain. The evidence is such that it would be surprising if viruses were not factors in the production of cancer in humans. The intensive research now going on in this field is exploring the possibility of developing vaccines to combat any viruses that might be causative agents in human cancer.

Cancer and Hormones. Hormones are chemicals produced and released by glands in the body and transported by the bloodstream to other areas of the body where they stimulate certain activity.

The hormones produced by the male and female sex glands (testicular and ovarian hormones); by the adrenals located above the kidneys; and by the pituitary gland at the base of the brain, are the ones most obviously related to the development of cancer among humans. The sex hormones and many of those secreted by the adrenal glands are closely related, belonging to the chemical family of steroids. The hormones produced by the pituitary include several substances that in turn control the output of hormones from a number of other, subsidiary endocrine glands, including those that produce steroids.

Interrelationships among different types of hormones and their production are extremely important in regard to the origin of certain animal tumors. They also have a marked effect upon the course of certain human cancers. That such complex substances as the hormones should influence cancer is not surprising. The nature of their action is one of growth-stimulation of various bodily tissues; improper stimulation or excessive stimulation could conceivably spark a cancerous response from a cell.

Types of Cancer. Cancer is most broadly divided into two classifications, carcinoma and sarcoma. Carcinomas are those types of cancer that develop from the epithelium—the bodily tissues that make up the skin and the membranes lining the body cavities and hollow organs. Sarcomas, in contrast, evolve from nonepithelial tissues—bone, muscle, and nervous-system structures are examples.

Sarcomas are rare as compared with carcinomas. Their most common points of origin include fatty tissue (liposarcoma), muscle (rhabdomyosarcoma), cartilage (chondrosarcoma), bone (octeosarcoma), and lymph nodes (lymphosarcoma).

Carcinomas are by far the most common forms of cancer and within this class there are two subdivisions; squamous-cell carcinoma, which originates from surface epithelium such as the skin, and adenocarcinoma, arising from the ducts of glands such as the breast. Of the more than a hundred subtypes of these two forms of carcinoma that may occur, a scant six account for more than half the cases of cancer recorded annually. These main six subtypes originate at the following sites: lungs, large intestine and rectum, breast, stomach, prostate gland, and uterus.

Of these, cancer of the lungs has become perhaps the most rapidly increasing of all. Lung cancer was the cause of some 18,300 deaths in 1950, compared to estimates of 111,000 deaths for 1982. The increase of female deaths due to lung cancer is most distressing. If trends continue, the age-adjusted death rate of lung cancer among women may soon rival that of breast cancer. It is not surprising that this increase in deaths due to lung cancer among women parallels statistics concerning the rise of cigarette smoking among women.

Fortunately, the percentage of cures achieved in the six subtypes mentioned above can be markedly increased if early detection and curative treatment are utilized.

The Seven Danger Signals. Because the public must be alerted to the first symptoms that may mean cancer, the American Cancer Society has placed great emphasis on its "Seven Danger Signals."

They are:

1. Unusual bleeding or discharge
2. A lump or thickening in the breast or elsewhere
3. A sore that does not heal
4. Change in bowel or bladder habits
5. Continued hoarseness or cough
6. Continued indigestion, or difficulty in swallowing
7. Change in a wart or mole

Any one of these may be a warning of cancer's impending assault. Any symptom that persists for more than two weeks should be brought to a physician's attention. Unusual bleeding or discharge is one of the major symptoms of cancer of the uterus, especially when it occurs after menopause. A lump or thickening is one of the classic signs of cancer in general, not only in the breast but in other parts of the body as well. A sore that does not heal, or a change in warts and moles, may mark the onset of skin cancer. A change in bowel habits may be a sign of cancer of the intestinal tract, whereas a change in bladder habits may relate to cancer of the bladder itself, the prostate gland, or the kidneys. Persistent hoarseness frequently indicates cancer of the larynx (voice box), and a cough that lasts for any extended time without being related to some already-identified respiratory complaint, may signal the presence of lung cancer.

Precautionary Measures. When cancer symptoms do appear, the cancer may have already reached an advanced state of development. For this reason precautionary measures are necessary.

Sometimes an individual can actually prevent the onset of cancer by his or her own efforts. Perhaps anywhere from 75 to 90 percent of all lung cancer can be eliminated by avoiding cigarette smoking. Skin cancer, too, can be considerably reduced by limiting excessive exposure to the ultraviolet rays of the sun. Overexposure to X-rays should also be avoided.

A woman can and should take preventive action against breast cancer. This can be done by examining the breasts with the fingers to detect the presence of lumps or masses. The technique of breast self-examination has been described in brochures and films available through the American Cancer Society. Because breast cancer is quite common (one in twenty women eventually contracts it), and since it is so difficult to cure, precautionary measures should be of concern to all women and physicians.

The most vital precaution of all is the annual physical examination. A physician is often able to detect cancer at an early stage, even when no physical symptoms or complaints are experienced. The physician also relies on a medical case history, which may offer important clues for further investigation. Background information concerning the incidence of cancer in one's family may be of particular help.

The physician also has at his or her disposal a battery of instruments, tests, and methods of inspection that enable the searching out and examining of many parts of the body where a cancerous growth might otherwise go undetected. Among the best known of these techniques is that of X-ray examination. Today physicians are able to inspect the structure and configuration of "soft parts" such as the intestines, the blood vessels, and the kidney and urinary system. Often X-ray procedures making use of "contrast media," such as barium, can make exploratory surgery unnecessary.

For the female patient part of the annual physical examination consists of an examination of the breasts. As an impartial and highly skilled examiner, the physician may find abnormalities that have escaped notice by the patient. The physician may also teach the breast self-examination procedure to the patient to be carried out on a monthly basis.

The detection technique that makes use of X-ray examination of the breasts is called mammography. The picture produced is called a mammogram. Often a mammogram can spot cancerous growths too small to be felt by manual breast examination. These growths may be smaller in size than a pea. Studies have indicated that the use of mammography finds six additional cases of breast cancer for every one case found by the manual technique. Although unnecessary X-ray exposure should be avoided, for many women over the age of thirty-five a mammogram might be recommended.

A detection technique that avoids X-ray radiation is the thermogram. This technique detects some cancers due to the increased temperature that they produce in the breast. However, a thermogram is not as exact as is an X-ray.

The Papanicolaou ("Pap") Test. A microscopic cell-examination technique known as exfoliative cytology is best known through its use in the "Pap" test, which is used in early detection of uterine cancer. Perfected by Dr. George N. Papanicolaou, this technique is based on the normal and constant shedding of worn-out cells from the body, a process similar to the falling of autumn leaves.

Exfoliated cells normally fall away or are expelled from the body unnoticed. Because of the anatomical structure of the uterus, however, cells shed from its lower end (the cervix) accumulate in the vagina. A simple and painless collection of secretions by syringe-suction or swabbing enables the physician to obtain a sample of these cells for microscopic examination.

This cytologic test is so sensitive that by means of it the medical specialist can detect cancer long before any symptoms appear, while the disease still involves only a relatively small number of cells. Treated at this stage of development, cancer of the cervix has a cure rate approaching 100 percent. Thus, early detection by means of a "Pap" smear can save lives.

"Pap" smear test results are usually classified into five different categories. The most frequent result is Class I, a negative determination of cancer. Classes IV and V are given the determination of a positive finding of cancer. Of every 1000 women tested, forty-five have a result other than Class I. However, many nonnegative results are caused by an infection that is not cancerous. Often an attempt is made to treat the infection and then follow up with a second "Pap" smear to see if the result has become Class I.

Cytological examination of cells ob-

What patients might ask their doctors:

1. If a tumor, lump, growth, or cyst has been found, is it benign or malignant?

2. If it is malignant has the cancer spread to other areas of the body?

3. Is surgery a possibility? Are radiation treatments to be used? What are the risks involved?

4. What is the cure rate of cancer cases similar in nature? Have new methods of treatment proven effective?

5. If drugs or radiation is used in treatment, what are the side effects?

6. What agencies, institutions, and support groups are available in the community that offer emotional, material, or financial assistance?

7. What kind of physical restrictions, if any, should be followed during and immediately after treatment? Will work activities be affected?

tained from the mouth, lung, stomach, and intestines can also often reveal cancer. The accuracy of the exfoliate method varies with the availability and accessibility of cell specimens. In this regard, the uterus remains the most convenient site for this purpose.

Treatment of Cancer. A sure diagnosis of cancer must be established before treatment is begun. No one should be subjected to the radical, extensive operations, or heavy radiation, or doses of drugs unless the diagnosis is proven. Fortunately, there are means available that provide the necessary proof. One such method is the biopsy.

A biopsy is the removal of a piece of suspected tumor tissue for microscopic inspection. A negative biopsy report does not always mean that no cancer exists, because the cells removed may not be the deranged cancer cells. A positive report, however, justifies the initiation of cancer treatment. It is, of course, essential to begin treatment as soon as cancer is detected. Any delay gives the cancer opportunity to grow and possibly metastasize into vital areas of the body.

The only sure curative means of treating cancer are through complete removal of the tumor by surgery, or by its total destruction by radiation. In both methods the aim is the complete removal of all cancer cells in the body.

Surgery for cancer is somewhat different from that for noncancerous conditions. A number of special operations have been devised for the solution of surgical problems associated with cancer. One of these is the removal of lymph nodes from sites adjacent to the cancer. These nodes, the cancer itself, and a wide margin of surrounding tissue, are removed when possible. The removal of the nodes is often an important procedure because metastasizing cancer cells often are transported through the lymphatic system.

Radiation therapy is largely restricted to the treatment of cancer. Although uncontrolled radiation has been found to produce various cancers, radiation in controlled and focused exposures provides a powerful

THE CIRCULATORY SYSTEM

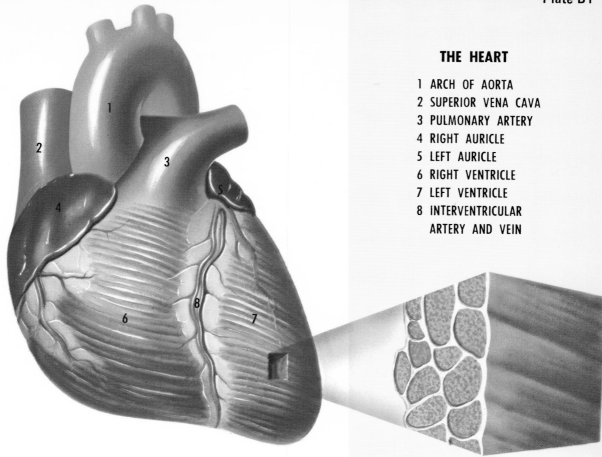

ANTERIOR VIEW OF HEART

THE HEART

1 ARCH OF AORTA
2 SUPERIOR VENA CAVA
3 PULMONARY ARTERY
4 RIGHT AURICLE
5 LEFT AURICLE
6 RIGHT VENTRICLE
7 LEFT VENTRICLE
8 INTERVENTRICULAR
 ARTERY AND VEIN

VENTRICLE WALL

CROSS SECTION OF HEART

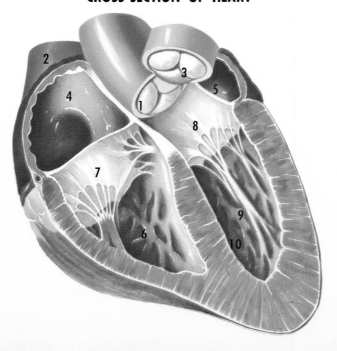

1 AORTIC VALVE
2 SUPERIOR VENA CAVA
3 PULMONARY VALVE
4 RIGHT AURICLE
5 LEFT AURICLE
6 RIGHT VENTRICLE
7 TRICUSPID VALVE
8 BICUSPID VALVE
9 PAPILLARY MUSCLE
10 LEFT VENTRICLE

ILLUSTRATED BY

LEONARD D. DANK

ST. LUKE'S HOSPITAL
NEW YORK CITY

CARDIAC CYCLE

HEART SOUNDS

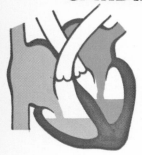

Both auricles fill with blood and contract. Blood flows through the open atrioventricular valves into the ventricles.

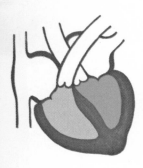

As the ventricles begin to contract, the atrioventricular valves snap shut.

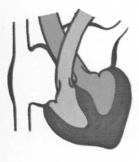

As the ventricles continue to contract, the semilunar valves are forced open. Blood is pushed into the aorta and pulmonary artery.

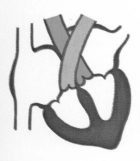

When all the blood is gone, the ventricles relax. Blood is prevented from returning to the heart by the semilunar valves.

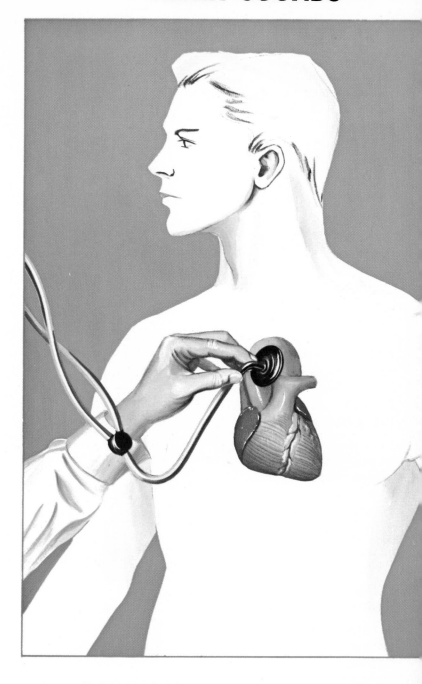

Sounds produced by the valves enable the doctor to form an impression of the cardiac cycle. The typical lub-dub sounds are produced by the closing of the atrioventricular and semilunar valves. If any valve does not close properly, a murmuring after-sound results.

Four regulatory centers in the medulla of the brain control the circulatory system. Their action can best be explained by three conditions described below.

1. A RISE IN BLOOD PRESSURE (Red Arrows)

The carotid sinus is stimulated by the rise in pressure. It sends warning impulses to the cardioinhibitor and vasodilator centers. These centers send impulses to the heart causing it to slow down, and to the arterioles of the stomach causing them to enlarge. Both actions rapidly lower the blood pressure.

2. A FALL IN OXYGEN WITHIN THE BLOOD (Blue Arrows)

A node of tissue in the aorta, stimulated by low oxygen levels sends impulses to the cardio-accelerator and to the vasoconstrictor centers. The centers send impulses to the heart causing it to speed up, and to the stomach arterioles causing them to constrict. Both actions raise the blood pressure, thus insuring an adequate supply of oxygen to vital organs.

3. DURING SUSTAINED EXERCISE (Dotted Blue Arrow)

The right auricle is stimulated by a high venous pressure. It sends impulses to the cardioaccelerator and vasoconstrictor centers. Together with impulses from the aorta due to low oxygen, the carotid sinus protective mechanism (see above RISE IN BLOOD PRESSURE) is blocked. Thus a necessary sustained high blood pressure can be maintained.

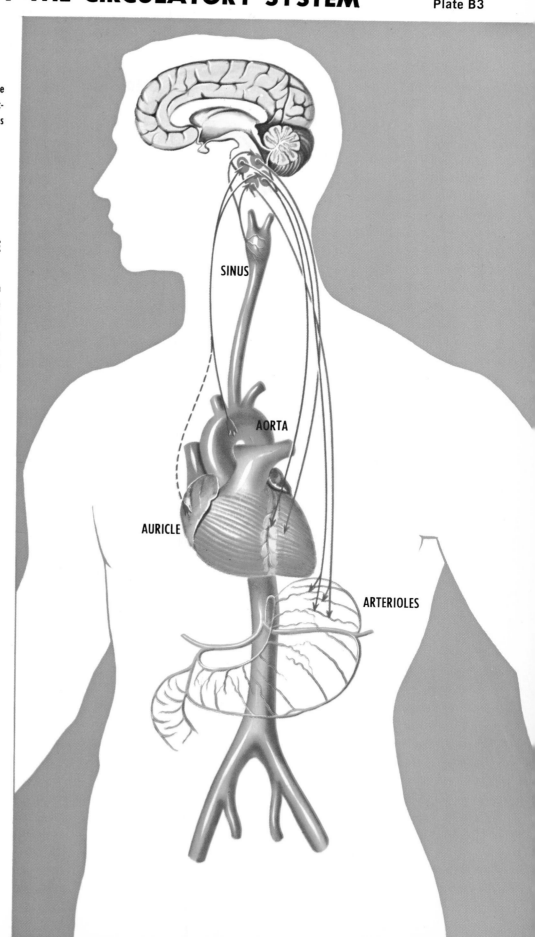

SINUS

AORTA

AURICLE

ARTERIOLES

THE BLOOD VESSELS

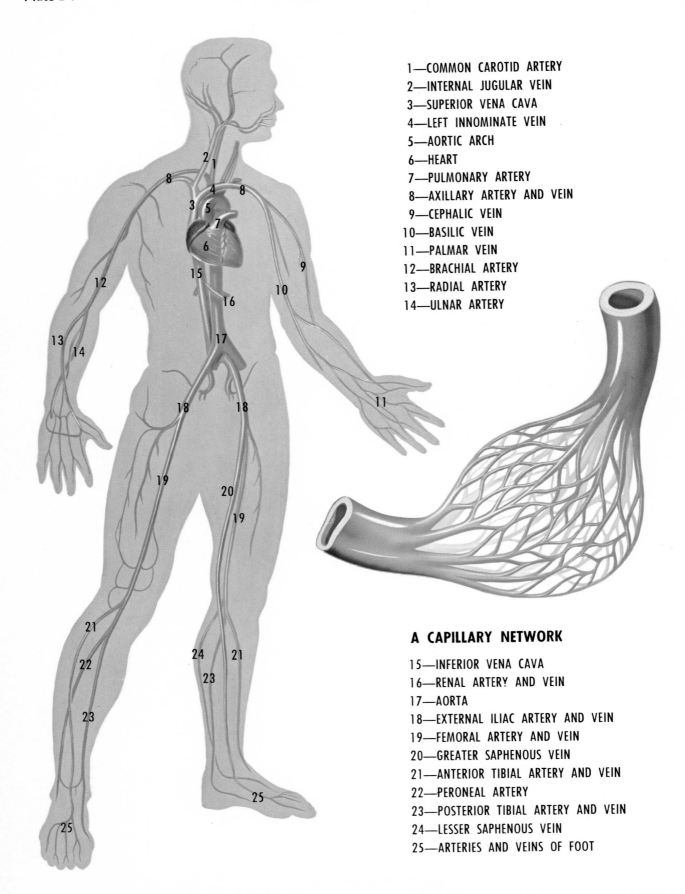

1—COMMON CAROTID ARTERY
2—INTERNAL JUGULAR VEIN
3—SUPERIOR VENA CAVA
4—LEFT INNOMINATE VEIN
5—AORTIC ARCH
6—HEART
7—PULMONARY ARTERY
8—AXILLARY ARTERY AND VEIN
9—CEPHALIC VEIN
10—BASILIC VEIN
11—PALMAR VEIN
12—BRACHIAL ARTERY
13—RADIAL ARTERY
14—ULNAR ARTERY

A CAPILLARY NETWORK

15—INFERIOR VENA CAVA
16—RENAL ARTERY AND VEIN
17—AORTA
18—EXTERNAL ILIAC ARTERY AND VEIN
19—FEMORAL ARTERY AND VEIN
20—GREATER SAPHENOUS VEIN
21—ANTERIOR TIBIAL ARTERY AND VEIN
22—PERONEAL ARTERY
23—POSTERIOR TIBIAL ARTERY AND VEIN
24—LESSER SAPHENOUS VEIN
25—ARTERIES AND VEINS OF FOOT

THE COMPONENTS OF BLOOD

ERYTHROCYTES
(5 Million per cu. mm)
CARRY OXYGEN
AND CARBON DIOXIDE

LYMPHOCYTES
(1200-2300 per cu. mm)
IMPORTANT IN COMBATING
INFLAMMATION

NEUTROPHILS
(3000-6000 per cu. mm)
IMPORTANT IN RIDDING THE
TISSUES OF BACTERIA

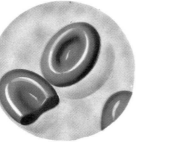
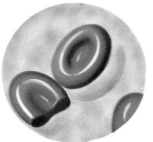
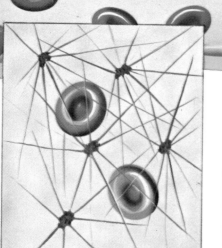
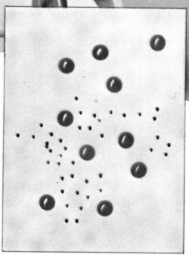
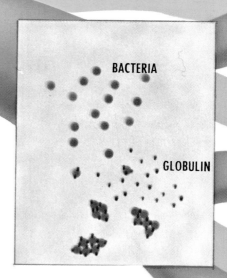

BACTERIA

GLOBULIN

PLATELETS
(250,000 per cu. mm)
IMPORTANT IN THE
CLOTTING MECHANISM

PLASMA PROTEINS
(7 per cent of plasma)
ALBUMIN REGULATES THE FLUID
LEVEL OF BLOOD

FIBRINOGEN IS IMPORTANT
IN CLOTTING MECHANISM

GLOBULINS CONTAIN ANTIBODIES

GAMMA GLOBULIN
(2.3 per cent of plasma)
CONTAINS ANTIBODIES WHICH
CAUSE BACTERIA TO AGGLUTINATE

THE ANCIENT CONCEPT OF CIRCULATION

ACCORDING TO GALEN (129-200 A.D.)

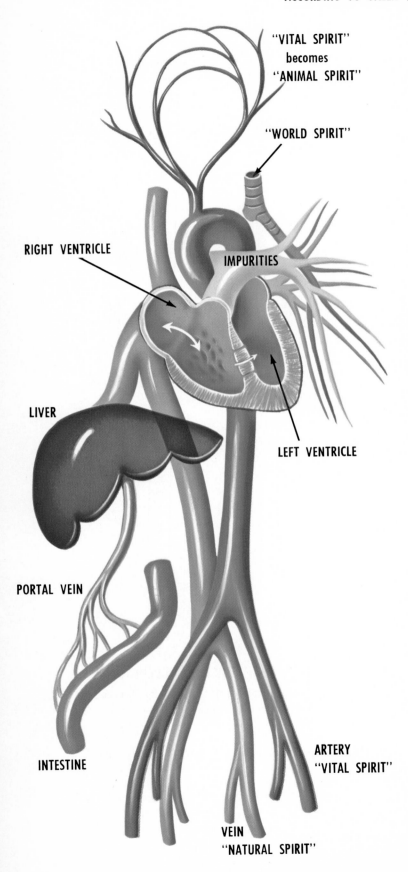

"VITAL SPIRIT"
becomes
"ANIMAL SPIRIT"

"WORLD SPIRIT"

IMPURITIES

RIGHT VENTRICLE

LEFT VENTRICLE

LIVER

PORTAL VEIN

INTESTINE

ARTERY
"VITAL SPIRIT"

VEIN
"NATURAL SPIRIT"

GALEN'S THEORY

Galen's theory of circulation dominated men's minds and actions for 1,400 years. He believed that dissolved food, transported from the intestines to the liver by the portal vein, was transformed into venous blood to which was added "Natural Spirit." The liver distributed this venous blood throughout the veins in which it ebbed and flowed.

When the venous blood reached the right ventricle, impurities flowed out of the pulmonary artery to the lungs and then these impurities somehow found their way into the bronchi and were exhaled.

"World Spirit" was inhaled, traveled to the bronchi and found its way via the pulmonary vein into the left ventricle. Here "World Spirit" encountered some venous blood that had seeped through the interventricular septum. "World Spirit" mixed with venous blood and became "Vital Spirit" which was distributed throughout the arteries.

"Vital Spirit" upon reaching the brain became charged with "Animal Spirit" which flowed out through the supposedly hollow nerves.

"Natural, Vital, and Animal Spirits" were the cornerstone of physiology until the seventeenth century.

THE MODERN CONCEPT OF CIRCULATION

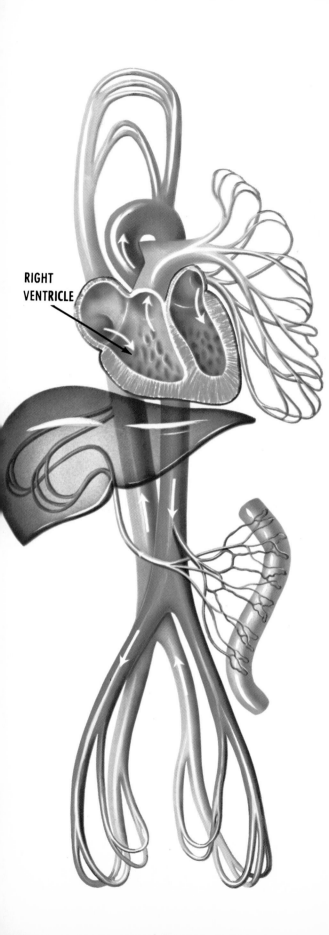

RIGHT
VENTRICLE

THE PULMONARY CIRCULATION

The right ventricle pumps carbon dioxide- (CO_2) saturated venous blood into the pulmonary artery which branches repeatedly, finally becoming a capillary network surrounding the alveoli of the lungs. The carbon dioxide is exchanged for oxygen (O_2). The oxygen-saturated arterial blood returns to the heart for distribution to the body.

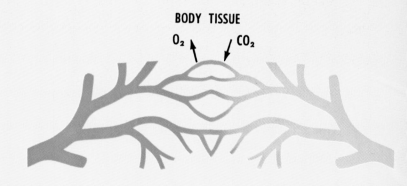

LUNG TISSUE

CO_2 O_2

ARTERY

VEIN

SYSTEMIC CIRCULATION

The left ventricle pumps the oxygen-saturated blood to all parts of the body. In the body tissues, the arteries (red) branch repeatedly until they become a capillary network surrounding the cells. Oxygen is exchanged for carbon dioxide. The carbon dioxide-saturated veins (blue) return the blood back to the heart to go through the pulmonary circulation.

BODY TISSUE

O_2 CO_2

THE PORTAL CIRCULATION

Venous blood carrying dissolved foods from the intestines takes a special route: the portal vein, to the liver. In the liver, the portal vein again becomes a capillary network. Excess dissolved food is stored. The veins regroup again to join the main veins just before they enter the heart.

BLOOD TYPES

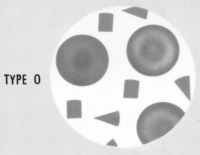

TYPE O

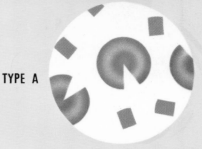

TYPE A

TYPE O CELLS CONTAIN NO ANTIGENS
TYPE O GLOBULIN CONTAIN A & B ANTIBODIES

TYPE A CELLS CONTAIN A ANTIGEN
TYPE A GLOBULIN CONTAIN B ANTIBODIES

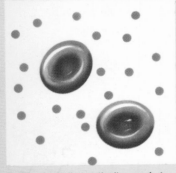

Gamma globulin antibodies agglutinate foreign red cells just as they do with bacteria. Red cells also have chemicals (antigens) which react with antibodies.

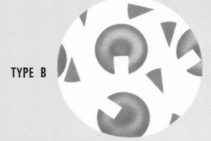

TYPE B

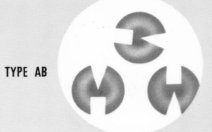

TYPE AB

TYPE B CELLS CONTAIN B ANTIGEN
TYPE B GLOBULIN CONTAIN A ANTIBODIES

TYPE AB CELLS CONTAIN A & B ANTIGENS
TYPE AB GLOBULIN CONTAIN NO ANTIBODIES

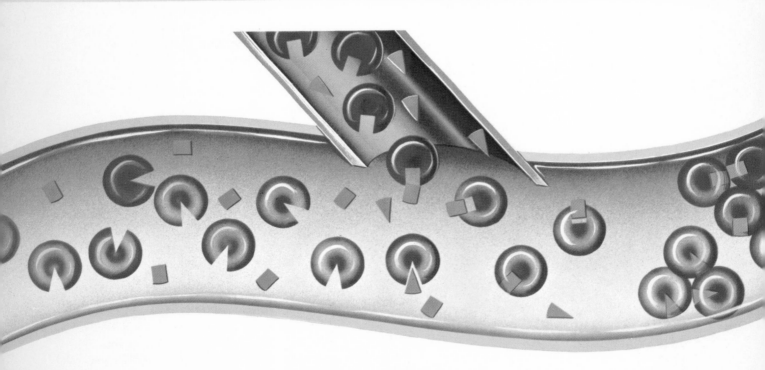

If type B blood is transfused into type A blood, the cells of both types will agglutinate. The clumps of red cells may block small capillaries, leading to shock and possible death.

weapon against cancer.

There are three general sources of radiation used in therapy, two being known before the turn of the century, the third being a product of the atomic age:

1. Naturally radioactive elements, such as radium
2. Machine-produced radiation such as that generated by X-ray machines and linear accelerators
3. Artificially radioactive isotopes, produced by exposure of nonradioactive elements to atomic reactions

The effect of these three radiation sources is the same, destruction of the cancer cell through penetration and interference with its chemical components.

A crucial problem inherent in irradiation of cancer is the difficulty of destroying all cancerous cells without causing irreparable damage to adjacent healthy tissues. The use of multiple paths of entry, or of rotation of the radiation sources around the patient, are techniques utilized to minimize this undesired damage. Thus, the cells in front of and behind the tumor receive less radiation. By carefully moving the source so that the tumor is at the intersection point of distinct beams, or so that the tumor lies at the center of a circle traced out by the source, the cancerous growth receives more radiation than does the surrounding tissues.

The use of internally placed radiation sources in the form of pellets is another method of concentrating the power of radiation where needed. By taking radioactive substances and implanting them within body cavities, tissues, or the tumor itself, the full force of the radiation is directed at the cancer and damage to neighboring healthy tissue is reduced.

Radioactive isotopes have made the concentration of radiation far more flexible than formerly possible. The isotopes are simply variations of normal chemical elements, differing from their nonradioactive counterparts only in weight and in their ability to emit radiation. Some radioactive isotopes, such as iodine-131 and phosphorus-32, have special characteristics. These isotopes can be used to treat thyroid and bone cancers respectively, because these elements naturally gravitate to these sites, rather than circulate throughout the body.

When different sources of radiation are utilized, variations in the degree of penetration into tissue and the localization of the radiation can be accomplished by adjusting voltage. The higher the voltage the deeper

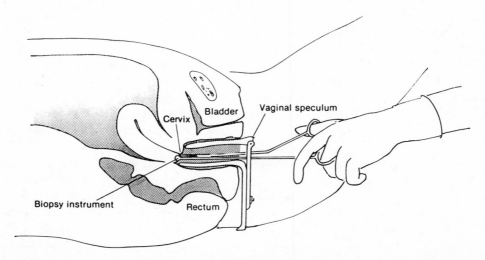

Biopsy of the cervix. The doctor uses an instrument to perform a biopsy or remove a small piece of tissue from the cervix.

into the tissue the radiation can go.

Although the cobalt "bomb" is perhaps the best-known supervoltage source of radiation, many other supervoltage sources have been developed. The linear electron accelerator, which is increasing in popularity, is capable of producing radiation of about six million electron volts. Among the most powerful machines yet devised for treatment (in terms of electron voltage) is the betatron, which can generate 10 or more million electron volts.

Chemotherapy, the treatment of cancer with chemicals and drugs, is largely a development of the post-World War II era. In one type of rare cancer, choriocarcinoma, chemotherapy has apparently produced a cure. Choriocarcinoma arises from a tissue developed during pregnancy. This cancer, which attacks the uterus of the mother, is extremely malignant and prior to the use of chemotherapy was almost always fatal. Three different chemical agents have been discovered that have produced what seem to be lasting cures for this cancer.

Other chemotherapy treatments, applied to other types of cancer, have been used to control and decrease tumor growth, but they are not expected to be cures. More than twenty different agents have been developed that either ease pain or temporarily reverse cancer cell activity. Some of these agents have been used in cases of leukemia, a cancer of blood-forming tissues. Unfortunately, cancer cells often become accustomed to a given chemical and a new one must be substituted. By a systematic changing of drugs, it is sometimes possible to maintain the patient's life for extended periods.

Many times a program of chemotherapy produces side effects that severely discomfort the patient. These side effects include intense nausea, loss of hair, general weakness, and loss of appetite.

One variety of chemotherapy consists of administering steroid sex hormones. As might be expected, this type of treatment is generally used in cases of cancer of organs related to the sex of the patient. Thus, for cancer of the female breast, a male sex hormone may be given, and for cancer of the male sex organs or the prostate, a female hormone is sometimes used. A more drastic procedure is the removal of the sex glands (the ovaries in women, the testes in men), which exert a strong influence on sex-hormone production.

The search for new and more powerful chemotherapeutic agents continues. One problem in the development of chemotherapy is extremely troublesome, discovering chemicals that will attack cancerous cells more readily than normal tissue. With our growing knowledge of synthetic compounds, the future is promising.

Worthless Cancer Remedies. One of the reasons that cancer causes so many deaths is that patients have delayed treatment. This delay may be caused by ignorance of symptoms, reluctance to face the facts, or putting off regular physical examinations. Another cause for delay is a particularly distressing one, placing one's trust in worthless cancer remedies and programs of treatment.

Why patients reach for unproven or experimental drugs and treatments stems in part from their perception, whether justified or not, that conventional methods are ineffective. In 1975 the drug Laetrile (amydalin) was termed "worthless" by the Food and Drug Administration, yet many cancer patients spent money and valuable time using this drug. Some even believed they benefited from the drug.

Controversy has also centered around the claims made for the industrial solvent dimethyl sulfoxide (DMSO). Some physicians are using this substance in treatments going beyond the recommendations set by the FDA. Not until definitive research is completed should excessive hope be placed in unproven drugs. What is claimed a "cure" may only be a means to separate patients from their money. The "cancer cure" offered

A TABLE OF SELECTED CHEMOTHERAPY AGENTS

Figure 1

GENERAL TYPE:	SPECIFIC AGENT:	TYPES OF CANCER AGAINST WHICH COMMONLY USED:
Alkylating agents (general "cell poisons" which act against the nucleus and inhibit cell multiplication, especially in rapidly-reproducing cells)	Nitrogen mustard ("HN2")	Leukemia; lymphosarcoma; carcinoma of lung, ovary, breast; miscellaneous carcinomas
	Chlorambucil	Leukemia; lymphosarcoma; carcinoma of testis
	Cyclophosphamide Thio-TEPA TEM	Leukemia; carcinoma of lung, ovary, breast; used when resistance to other agents has been built up in cases of these and miscellaneous carcinomas.
	Busulfan	Leukemia
Antimetabolites (act by cutting off some particular reaction or chain of reactions necessary for cell life and multiplication)	Amethopterin	Choriocarcinoma*; leukemia; carcinoma of the testis; used in treatment of regional carcinomas
	6-Mercaptopurine ("6-MP")	Leukemia
	5-Fluorouracil ("5-FU")	Carcinoma of ovary, colon; sometimes used in conjunction with surgery or radiation in treatment of other cancers
Hormones (affect general growth of sex-related tissues or organs, and at times other structures as well, though less directly)	Androgen (male hormone, natural or synthetic derivatives)	Cancer of female breast
	Estrogen (female hormone, natural or synthetic derivatives)	Cancer of prostrate, cancer of female breast
	Progesterone (an ovarian, pregnancy-maintaining, hormone)	Cancer of the uterus
	Adrenal (steroid) hormones	Cancer of the female breast; miscellaneous carcinomas
Miscellaneous agents (individual modes of action, but with anti-cancerous properties)	Actinomycin D (an antibiotic)	Choriocarcinoma*; cancer of testis
	Vinblastine (a plant extract)	Choriocarcinoma*
	Vincristine (a plant extract)	Leukemia
	o, p'DDD	Carcinoma of the adrenal gland

*to date, the only type of cancer in which true cures have apparently been achieved, through the use of amethopterin, actinomycin D, and vinblastine.

may be something as primitive as an amulet or a poultice. But then again, the explanation may be deceptively "scientific," a matter of mysterious serums, chemicals, or machinery.

False "healers" can sometimes be recognized by the following characteristics:

1. They guarantee a cure for every case, or they ignore serious, potentially fatal consequences.
2. They explain their fringe status by saying that the established medical profession is jealous of, or plotting against, them.
3. Their "cures" are secret and are based on some "natural" principle overlooked by everyone else.
4. They are frequently overly interested in the patient's ability to pay for treatment and may offer elaborate payment plans.
5. They can present "testimonials" from "satisfied customers."

How is it that the self-announced "miracle man" can produce testimonials to his treatment's effectiveness? There are three answers: (1) the testimonial-writing patient may never have had cancer in the first place, for not all tumors or swellings are cancerous; (2) many cancers are slow growing and may even undergo temporary improvement as a natural part of their development; (3) the delayed effects of previous treatment with X-rays or with useful drugs may be the actual explanation for an apparent improvement.

Perhaps it is the fear that the very word "cancer" inspires, or the still-mysterious details of its origin, that causes some cancer patients to seek out treatment that has exaggerated claims of success. Whatever the reason, the treatment of cancer seems to attract an unusual number of fraudulent and deluded "healers." Medical societies, governmental health agencies, and the American Cancer Society attempt to protect the public by distributing information and monitoring medical practices. However, too many people are still misled; too much money is wasted; and precious time is lost, all because of the cure that never came true.

The Family Faces Cancer. A family can do much to protect itself from cancer, either by taking preventive measures, or by correcting precancerous conditions in the environment.

Skin cancer can be prevented by avoiding excessive exposure to the sun's direct rays. Sunbathing, therefore, should be practiced in moderation. Protective clothing should also be worn by those whose occupations require prolonged periods of work in the sun.

Lung cancer, first among all cancer killers in the United States, could be reduced through the avoidance of cigarette smoking. All parents should know that, according to the American Public Health Association, "more than one million teenagers now living will die of lung cancer before reaching age 70." Parents should also realize the special influence their own smoking habits have upon their children. If the mother smokes, for example, her daughters are far more likely to smoke as well. Because studies have shown that the earlier the smoking habit begins the greater the hazard to health becomes, cancer can be prevented if all family members avoid or break the smoking habit.

Family members should be alert for symptoms that might mean cancer. Prompt treatment or removal of any precancerous lesion can minimize or forestall cancer's attack. The removal by a physician of brown or black moles that start to grow, ulcerate or are subject to continued rubbing or irritation may be a sound preventive measure. Similarly, the presence of white patches in the mouth or on the lips should prompt a visit to the family physician.

When a definite diagnosis of cancer has been made, both the patient and the family are immediately confronted with a host of problems. Unfortunately, the mere word "cancer" produces in some persons an overwhelming shock. This response may be due to the erroneous assumption that cancer is an automatic death sentence. If the realization that a family member has cancer only gives rise to despair or panic, there may be a delay of treatment, a delay that jeopardizes the health and life of the cancer victim.

Once cancer has been discovered, two temptations must be resisted: (1) to pretend that the diagnosis is incorrect; (2) to fall prey to useless, "unorthodox," or unproven cancer remedies.

Another problem families must often face with loved ones who have cancer is whether "to tell or not to tell" the patient the nature of the disease. In most cases the patient already has an idea concerning the true nature of his or her condition. Whether to tell or not depends largely upon psychological and economic factors, such as the state of the patient's morale and mental stamina, and practical considerations for the future with regard to business and provisions for dependents.

Physicians differ in their opinions concerning this subject. Some doctors offer candid appraisals of a patient's condition only if directly asked to do so. Others feel obligated to speak frankly about the course of a patient's illness, even if the report will be very difficult for the patient to accept.

Many patients do not want to be told that they have cancer. They would rather be deceived. To confront this type of person with proof positive may create added psychological trauma, causing great distress in the name of honesty.

There are cases, of course, when it is best to tell the patient the nature of the disease. When a person genuinely wants to know the possible consequences of his or her condition, facing and sharing the problem among family members, physicians, and friends may increase the solidarity and morale of all concerned.

The question of concealment is a particularly delicate and poignant problem in childhood cancer. Regrettably, many of the forms of cancer prevalent among the young are very severe. Their personal response to their illness may be fraught with confusion, in addition to the pain and discomfort of the disease itself. The child may pass through a stage in which the parent is blamed for not stopping the painful symptoms. However, annoyance directed at parents generally passes and is succeeded by curiosity in treatment procedures. Because children are highly sensitive to the behavior of their parents, it is important for parents not to unduly fuss over or spoil a child with cancer.

Practical Problems in the Home. One of the chief difficulties associated with cancer is that treatment is often long and expensive. Family income may be drastically reduced and the life-style of the family may be changed due to the details and requirements of cancer treatments.

There are, however, means of reducing the hardship that accompanies a family's fight against cancer. Almost every community offers help through agencies, private and governmental, that can cushion the blow. Certain hospitals throughout the country are able to supply treatment at greatly reduced rates, or free in cases of dire need. The cancer stricken family should acquaint itself thoroughly with the resources available through official agencies. Inquiries may be directed to health and welfare departments on the state or local level.

The one voluntary agency that deals with the total problem of cancer is the American Cancer Society which, in addition to its widespread programs of education and research, provides various services in many communities. The Society is largely decentralized, operating in state and community units. Many of these units make available assistance in the form of sickroom supplies, dressings, and transport facilities. In certain communities the Society's service program may also include the support of part-time home nursing or homemaking service. A letter or telephone call to the nearest unit office will not only supply details, but will also set in motion provision of whatever services are locally available.

Future Prospects and the "Magic Bullet." The search for a substance or treatment method that can zero in on cancer cells, destroy all of them, yet cause little or no damage to adjacent healthy tissue is the objective of most cancer research. Such a hypothetical drug or program of treatment is often referred to as a "magic bullet" capable of hitting only cancerous cells.

One example of a promising field of inquiry is immunotherapy, which is essentially an attempt to make use of the body's own defense systems to combat cancerous growth. Interferon, a naturally produced protein in almost all human cells, was isolated first in 1956 and is now the object of intensified research. The main difficulty, however, is that interferon is an extremely rare substance and researchers have not had quantities large enough and concentrations pure enough to do conclusive experimenta-

tion. Attempts to produce interferon on a greater scale using genetic engineering techniques offer a means of obtaining amounts of interferon pure and potent enough to conduct definitive trials on humans.

Summary. In conclusion, the specific biological mechanisms that cause cancerous growth are still not completely understood. However, the scientific investigation for cancer cures continues, emphasizing areas such as research into roles played by viruses, hormones, and carcinogenic substances. Improved surgical techniques, anti-cancer drug therapy, and radiation technology are being sought out, tested, and implemented. The proportion of curable cancers will undoubtedly increase, just as it has over the last half-century. Yet, although the treatment of cancer is the responsibility of the medical profession, much of the effort to cure individual cases depends on early detection; and early detection largely depends upon an informed and concerned public.

PERCENTAGE OF PATIENTS FREE OF CANCER AT VARIOUS SITES FOR AT LEAST FIVE YEARS AFTER TREATMENT

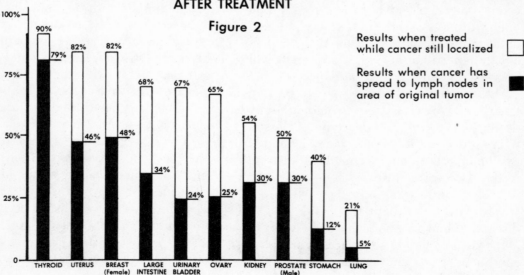

Figure 2

NOTE: The figures presented were obtained from actual records and are *not* "theoretical." Under ideal conditions, if patients were all to have annual physical examinations and were to go to their physician at the first suspicious sign, the survival figures at the localized stage would be much higher. This is most markedly true of cancer of the uterus, theoretically close to 100% curable.

Where to get more information about cancer:

1. The National Cancer Institute can be a source for free pamphlets about various cancers and cancer treatments. Write:

   Office of Communications
   National Cancer Institute
   9000 Rockville Pike
   Bethesda, MD 20205

2. The American Cancer Society has local units in many communities, which offer educational materials. One can also write for information. Write:

   American Cancer Society
   77 Third Avenue
   New York, NY 10017

3. The Cancer Information Service maintains a toll-free, national telephone number, which can be used to obtain information about cancer and related sources. The number is: 1(800)638-6694.

CANKER SORES   The scientific name for canker sore is aphthous stomatitis or aphthous ulcer. Canker sores most commonly occur in the mouth and may be caused by such things as jagged teeth, ill-fitting dentures, or the irritation to mucous membrane caused by an improper "bite" of the jaw. Emotional stress, reactions to drugs, and foods such as chocolate, walnuts, and citrus fruit may trigger canker sores in some individuals. When canker sores appear on mucous membrane surfaces other than the mouth (e.g. vagina), menstrual difficulties and gastrointestinal disturbances should be looked into as possible causes.

A canker sore is usually between an eighth of an inch to an inch and a quarter in diameter. It is circular or oval, has a bright red circumference, and is greyish-white. The sore begins in the tissue of the mouth and eventually works through to the surface to appear as a small punched-out hole. Often pain is felt before the sore appears.

Women are more susceptible to canker sores than men. Usually, if one member of the family has canker sores, other family members have them as well. Yet, unlike fever blisters, which are caused by the herpes simplex virus Type 1, canker sores are not contagious.

Treatment of canker sores may include the administration of an antibiotic under the direction of a physician. Nonsevere cases usually heal in ten to fourteen days without treatment.

CAPILLARIES   At the termination of an artery anywhere in the body, a capillary receives fresh blood. A short tube that lies in intimate contact with living cells of the body, the capillary has a wall or membrane made of a layer of thinned-out single cells attached to each other like quiltwork. The cell wall constitutes that semipermeable membrane which permits gas- and fluid-exchange from tissues to the fluids of blood, and vice versa.

The diameter of a capillary will permit the passage of red blood cells lined up in single file. A passive tube with no muscular control of its diameter, it discharges blood into a connecting vein (or veinule) for eventual return to the heart by way of the venous system.

"CAPS"   This is a colloquial term to describe artificial crowns placed on individual teeth, which closely resemble the natural teeth in shape and color. (See CROWN.)

CAPUT SUCCEDANEUM   This is an area of swelling in the baby's scalp, formed during labor as a result of the pressure of its head over the mouth of the gradually opening womb. The swelling is absorbed and disappears very promptly after birth.

CARBOHYDRATES   Carbohydrates are the main energy fuel of the body. Chemically, they are compounds containing carbon as well as hydrogen and oxygen, the latter two in the same proportion as in water. With but few exceptions, carbohydrates are of plant origin. They compose the group commonly known as sugars and starches.

Carbohydrates are synthesized by green plants from the carbon dioxide contained in the atmosphere and the hydrogen in water in the presence of sunlight in the process of photosynthesis. Life as we know it on earth depends on this process, for the carbohydrates of the plant kingdom are the major energy fuel on which the animal kingdom and man both exist.

These substances are classified according to their chemical structure as:

1. Monosaccharides. These are the simple sugars composed of six carbon atoms in a ringlike structure. Glucose and dextrose are examples.

2. Disaccharides. These more complex sugars are formed by condensation of two monosaccharides which can be split by the body. An example of this is sucrose, or common table sugar.

3. Polysaccharides. These large complex molecules are the end product of the condensation of many monosaccharides. An example of this is starch, or glycogen in animal tissue.

When ingested, carbohydrates are split through the action of enzymes in the saliva, stomach, and intestine. The complex sugars are broken down into monosaccharides such as glucose, galactose, and fructose, which are then absorbed in the small intestine. From there these sugars are carried to the liver; some continue through the bloodstream to individual cells in the body where they are burned as a source of energy. Carbon dioxide, which we throw off in breathing, and water are the end result of this process. Other carbohydrates in the liver are stored in the form of aggregates (glycogen) to be reconverted into glucose when the need arises.

In this country, about 50 per cent or more of our total energy requirements are met by carbohydrate. This varies depending on taste, economic factors, dietary habits, and so on. The foods largely concerned are rice, potatoes, cereals, flour products (bread, cake, etc.), legumes, and vegetables. Since these foods are generally considerably cheaper than meat, eggs, fish, and dairy products, which are the primary sources of proteins and fats, there is a tendency for the less economically favored as well as those living in underdeveloped areas to eat a high-carbohydrate diet. In addition, the ready availability of high-carbohydrate foods makes them popular with those who do not plan their meals adequately. It is believed that such a diet may predispose to obesity. Insulin is necessary for the proper metabolism of carbohydrates, and when there is an impairment in this function, the clinical condition known as diabetes results.

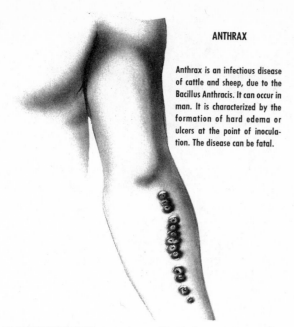

ANTHRAX

Anthrax is an infectious disease of cattle and sheep, due to the Bacillus Anthracis. It can occur in man. It is characterized by the formation of hard edema or ulcers at the point of inoculation. The disease can be fatal.

CARBUNCLE   A carbuncle is caused by the staphylococcus germ. It is like a furuncle or boil except that it penetrates to deeper tissues. It is larger than a boil (usually it is several boils that have coalesced) and may go on to extensive sloughing of tissue. It heals slowly and a large scar may ensue. Prevention and treatment are the same as for a boil. Occasionally, surgical incision of a deep and/or extensive lesion is required.

CARDIAC ARREST   The term cardiac arrest can be applied to any sudden and unexpected cessation of heartbeat. It can occur at all ages, and in hearts apparently free from evidence of disease.

Circumstances involving any type of stress seem to precipitate an attack. It may occur with severe exertion, during or after a surgical operation, and even without an exciting cause. If heart or lung disease is present, the occurrence of cardiac arrest may be more frequent, even if apparently unrelated to the coexistent disease states.

Diagnosis is made by noting the absence of pulse or blood pressure. Patients under stress of an accident, an operation, or disease are frequently attached to a cardiac-monitoring device. This electronic machine incorporates a special adaptation of electrocardiographic principles; dis-turbances in heart rate and rhythm are signaled by a visual or auditory alarm mechanism incorporated in the device.

Treatment. When a cardiac-monitoring device is arranged to trigger an electrical stimulus to the patient's heart at every prolonged pause in heartbeat, episodes of cardiac arrest can often be terminated automatically. In many instances, however, it may be necessary to open the chest with a surgical incision and massage the heart directly until heartbeat is re-established. This procedure has proven a life-saving measure when promptly employed, no matter what the primary circumstances of arrest. Some patients with cardiac arrest associated with acute coronary thrombosis have been saved from death by this technique of open-chest massage.

If the arrest occurs suddenly, a special technique of intermittent manual pressure on the breastbone—closed-chest massage—can often compress the heart artificially and give enough movement of blood through the heart to produce a spontaneous return of heartbeat.

Sometimes electroshock is needed to break up ventricular trembling (fibrillation) before an effective beat of the heart will return. A few drugs are known that will assist and reinforce returning heartbeat. If cardiac arrest is not recognized promptly, permanent brain damage may result from lack of continuous flow of oxygenated blood.

CARDIOVASCULAR SYSTEM   The organs and vessels that enclose fluid blood and cause it to move throughout the body comprise the cardiovascular system. Important components of this system include: (1) the heart; (2) the blood vessels (arteries, capillaries, and veins); (3) the lungs and their respiratory membranes; and (4) the nervous-system networks that regulate respiration, blood-flow, and distribution as required by the tissues of the body.

CARDITIS   The term carditis applies to any of a number of inflammatory states afflicting the heart. These various inflammatory diseases are ordinarily categorized according to the specific heart tissue involved. A number of such types of carditis are listed below:

Pericarditis. An inflammatory disease of the sac (pericardium) that snugly encloses the contracting heart within fibrous membranes lined with a very smooth surface lubricated by crystal-clear fluid

Epicarditis. Inflammatory changes in the membrane that covers the heart chambers and envelops the superficial coronary arteries

Myocarditis. Inflammatory changes in the heart muscle itself

Endocarditis. Inflammation of the inner membrane of the heart that lies in contact with the blood contained in the cardiac chambers

Valvulitis. Inflammatory disease that involves the valves of the heart. (The muscle component or the endocardial lining may also be involved.)

Pancarditis. An inflammation of all of the heart components, although usually one may show much more severe changes than the others

CASTRATION   Castration is the removal of the testes in the male or the ovaries in the female. Castration in the male is today practiced only for the removal of tumors and the treatment of cancer of the prostate gland. Since most prostate cancer is dependent on androgen (male hormone) for its growth, removal of the testes removes most of the source of androgen. In the female, castration often accompanies womb-removal (hysterectomy). It is now often performed in the treatment of spreading (metastatic) breast cancer in order to remove the source of estrogen which supports the growth of some of these tumors.

CASTRATION ANXIETY   According to Alfred Adler, a primary cause of inferiority complexes was fear of sexual impotence or castration. Adler believed many young girls develop feelings of insecurity upon discovering sex differences in the external genitals. He believed that all young girls develop penis-envy because they do not have male genitals and that this may be a source of lifelong inferiority feelings.

Psychiatric studies show that among the uneducated (including nurse maids), it still is common to punish a child by threatening to cut off or injure these organs. Children who have been so threatened are believed to develop castration anxiety. Since sexual potency is very highly regarded in almost all cultures, any threat of castration is unconsciously very threatening and a potential source of neurotic conflict in later life. Parents should therefore *never* punish a child by threatening to cut off or injure the genitals.

CATARACT   The crystalline lens of the eye is located directly behind the colored iris that surrounds the pupil, the central circular opening of the eye. Ordinarily, the lens of the eye is wholly transparent. The term cataract is applied to any loss of this transparency, whether slight or marked. A cataract is not a growth, but solely a loss of transparency of the lens. An entirely opaque lens is "ripe," while one that retains some transparency is "immature."

The most common cause of cataract is aging (senile cataract). Cateracts present at birth are called congenital, and may occur because of a hereditary tendency, or because of illness of the mother during the first three months of pregnancy. Other causes include injury from a blunt or penetrating blow to the eye, exposure to heat or X-rays, inflammation of the interior of the eye, and diabetes mellitus. Markedly lowered blood calcium and rare skin and muscle diseases may also be associated with cataract.

Symptoms. The chief symptom of cataract is a gradual dimming of vision that is not associated with pain or redness of the eye. In the early stages, there may be double vision in one eye only, but this disappears with further decrease in vision. Vision is frequently better in a dim light which permits dilation of the pupil. When one looks at a bright background such as the sky, there may be spots that do not dart about but remain in one position.

The diagnosis of cataract is based upon direct observation of the loss of transparency of the eye lens. When the cataract is very far advanced, the pupillary area is gray or white rather than black. Less advanced cataracts are diagnosed by special instruments.

Treatment. Nothing can restore the original transparency of the crystalline lens. During the period of dimming vision, wearing accurately prescribed spectacles will often maintain vision at a functional level.

Physical examination should be made with careful attention to the possibility of diabetes mellitus or reduced parathyroid gland activity. Examination of the eyes will usually indicate if the cataract is due to injury or inflammation.

Surgical removal of a cataract is indicated when the cataract itself causes glaucoma or an inflammation of the eye or when the defect in vision interferes with one's daily activities. As long as there is good vision in one eye, cataract removal may not be recommended solely for the purpose of improving the poorer eye. Because of the improvement in contact lenses, however, many surgeons have been recommending removal of a cataract even though the other eye is good. If one is unable to wear a contact lens, then the procedure may initially produce annoying double vision.

Cataract surgery is seldom indicated when there is a disease of the front or back of the eye affecting vision, making it unlikely that removal of the cataract will improve vision.

The surgical removal of cataracts is an operation usually performed with local anesthesia. The surgeon may use extreme cold to freeze the lens to a surgical probe, thereby permitting the removal of the cataract. Another technique makes use of high frequency sound waves that "dissolve" the clouded lens, which then can be drained away.

Because the lens is one of the main focusing parts of the eye, eyeglasses or special contact lenses are required after lens removal. Some cataract patients require a bifocal lens that is much thicker and heavier than an ordinary lens. When contact lenses are worn, magnification and optical defects are reduced. If such a lens is used, an additional lens for reading may be required.

The decision to operate on the second eye, if a cataract is present, is based on much the same factors as those governing the initial removal. If cataracts are present in both eyes, the surgeon may recommend operating on both eyes in one procedure. "Ripe" or swollen cataracts usually require removal. In other instances surgery is based upon the activity and visual needs of the individual. A sedentary person may see adequately with one eye, while a more active individual may determine he or she must have the use of both eyes.

CATARACT, CONGENITAL   Any loss of transparency of the lens which is present from birth is a congenital cataract. It may be familial; due to the occurrence of German measles in the mother during the first three months of pregnancy; or due to inflammation in the eye of the infant before birth.

Symptoms. These are the same as those occurring with other types of cataract. There may be additional eye defects which require careful examination to discover. Many types of congenital cataract do not interfere with vision, do not progress, and are discovered only in the course of an eye examination.

Treatment. The degree of interference with vision governs the selection of treatment. When congenital cataracts are associated with other eye defects, even skillful surgical removal may not improve vision. Generally, if the cataract is present in one eye and the other eye is normal or nearly so, surgery is not indicated. If cataracts are present in both eyes but vision is as good as 20/70 with eyeglasses, normal schooling is possible and surgery is not recommended. If the cataract is marked in each eye, surgery is indicated and this is usually carried out in about the second or third year. In borderline conditions, surgery is delayed until vision can be evaluated carefully, usually about the fifth year.

Following surgery, correcting lenses must be worn to compensate for the loss of focusing power.

CATHARSIS, MENTAL Early in his discovery of the psychoanalytic method, Sigmund Freud found that many patients were helped by simply allowing them to talk for hours about their problems. This process of talking-out the deepest problems of one's life is known as mental catharsis. Under the crowded conditions of modern civilization, many people live so anonymously that they have no one with whom they can talk over their deepest troubles. Further study of the method proved that mental catharsis was no cure-all for mental disorders, but it still plays an important role in psychotherapy.

In psychoanalysis, catharsis is said to occur when the patient is helped by talking-out (free association) methods or by hyp-

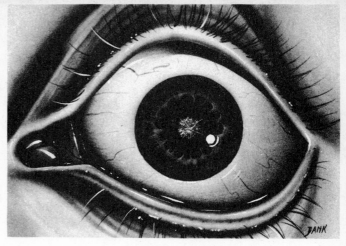

CONGENITAL CATARACT
(Lids are pulled away from eye.)

nosis, to remember forgotten or repressed ideas or experiences. When these forgotten or repressed traumatic experiences are brought back into consciousness, the patient tends to reexperience his original conflicting emotions and to relive the traumatic conditions which later gave rise to neurotic reactions. Many patients experience great relief from merely talking-out things which, until analysis, were too painful to think about.

CATHETER The catheter is a rubber or plastic tube which is inserted in the bladder to provide urinary drainage when there is obstruction of the urethra or inability to control urination. One type of catheter (the Foley catheter) has an inflatable bag at the inserted end which may be filled with liquid once the catheter is in place. The inflated bag prevents the catheter from slipping out.

CAUSALGIA Causalgia is a constant burning pain, secondary to injury of sensory or mixed peripheral nerves. It is often associated with incomplete damage to the particular nerve. A rare complication of nerve injury, it may occur immediately after the injury or after an interval of several weeks.

Symptoms. After a nerve injury (frequently of the median nerve) the patient may become aware of a constant burning sensation in the distribution of the nerve involved. Any stimulation of the skin in the area of distribution of this nerve increases the pain.

Treatment. Mild pain may disappear spontaneously after a few weeks or months; with severe causalgia, burning pain persists. Surgical treatment with sympathetic nerve block or sympathectomy may be successful.

CAUTERIZATION Cauterization or, more properly, cautery, is destruction of tissue by the application of a cauterizing agent. It is also the means by which tissue coagulation is effected through mechanical or chemical means. Among the agents used for cautery are electricity, white-hot or red-hot iron, chemicals (silver nitrate, for example), extreme cold (carbon dioxide, snow), and solar heat (as through a magnifying glass). In gynecology, the Paquelin cautery, a hollow platinum apparatus shaped like a knife, which is heated by thrusting it into a hydrocarbon vapor, is used.

CECUM The cecum is the pouch-like portion of the large intestine at its juncture with the small intestine; the appendix is attached at the apex of this pouch. Rarely, the cecum may be involved in an inguinal hernia on the right side, and conditions which affect the large intestine will also involve this portion.

CELIAC DISEASE Celiac disease is a chronic intestinal disorder of infants and young children characterized by fat in the stools (steatorrhea), loss of appetite, decreased growth rate, and symptoms of impaired nutritional absorption. The cause is unknown, but most patients seem to be unable to tolerate wheat gluten, a form of wheat protein. There are disturbances in the activity of intestinal enzymes. The disease is usually seen between the ages of six months and six years.

Symptoms. A characteristic finding is a prominent abdomen. The stool is large in size, loose, foul smelling, and often frothy. Alternating diarrhea and constipation may occur occasionally. The disease has an irregular course, improvement and relapse alternating in cycles.

Certain laboratory tests are helpful in making the diagnosis. These include laboratory examination of the stool to detect increased fat and carbohydrate. A test dose of vitamin A can be shown to be poorly absorbed by mouth. Anemia may be present.

Treatment. With adequate treatment, recovery occurs in most cases after a prolonged period of as much as several years.

Gluten-free diets, from which all products containing wheat and rye are eliminated, have been successful. Skimmed milk and the gradual addition of ground lean meat, cottage cheese, egg white, and pureed vegetables are the basis of diet therapy. Large doses of vitamins should be administered. Because they may produce a relapse, starchy foods are added last.

CENTRAL NERVOUS SYSTEM The development of human higher mental functions is directly related to the complexity of the central nervous system—CNS—both in the history of the human race and in the development of each individual. The CNS is a marvelously complex communication system which receives, transmits, associates, retains, integrates, and sends out electrical messages from all its parts, much like a telephonic communication system. It includes the brain and the spinal cord. It provides the direction and control of the activities of skeletal and smooth muscles, as well as of glands of secretion. It also controls the secretion of endocrine glands. Much reflex integration of bodily functions is carried out at the spinal cord level.

The basic unit of the nervous system consists of the nerve cell (neuron), which picks up and transmits different kinds of messages from different parts of the brain in the form of very slight electrical potentials. In general, all bodily function is controlled by a delicate balance of excitatory and inhibitory nervous control; for example, all movements are controlled by a delicate balance of excitation of one set of muscles and inhibition of opposing muscles.

The hindbrain (medulla oblongata) contains the vital centers for integrating the vegetative functions of the body—making possible swallowing, digestion, respiration, circulation, and elimination. The midbrain (thalamus and cerebellum) contains centers regulating consciousness, feelings and emotions, sleep, muscle tone, and postural coordination. The forebrain (cerebrum) controls the highest mental functions—coordinating sensations, voluntary motor actions, and associative thought processes.

The ways in which currents in nerve cells are translated into conscious mental activity are still unknown, though much progress has been made in mapping out the functions of the different brain centers and recording the small electrical discharges (brain waves) underlying brain functioning.

The action of different parts of the nervous system can be tested medically by neurological examinations which check the functioning of the different nerves and brain centers: The functioning of sensory nerves is tested by studying the normality of the senses. Motor functions are studied by checking muscular movements. The functioning of the cerebellum is tested by studying postural coordination. Cerebral functions are tested by giving complex psychological tests which measure all factors of ability.

The nervous system is subject to all the kinds of disease and injury which can attack other systems of the body. In general, damage to sensory nerves or centers produces loss of sensation; damage to motor cells and centers, loss of muscular functions; and damage to the cortex, loss of higher mental functions. The exact cause and nature of lesions (damage) to the nervous system can be determined only by neurological examination.

The functions of the nervous system can be just as easily disturbed by emotional disorders as any other organ systems. Before diagnosing disease of the nervous system, therefore, it is always necessary to rule out emotional upsets.

CEPHALOPELVIC DISPROPORTION This is a term used in obstetrics and implies that the mother's pelvis is too small in comparison with the size of her baby, and that difficulty in labor and delivery might therefore be anticipated. Such a disproportion can be due either to normal-size pelvis and an abnormally large baby, a normal-size baby and a mother with an abnormally small pelvis, or any intermediate combination of these two factors. Most caesarean sections done today are primarily performed for cephalopelvic disproportion alone, or in combination with supervening complications of labor.

CEREBELLUM The cerebellum is the lower part of the brain which lies below the cerebrum and back of the brainstem. It consists of two lateral lobes and a middle lobe. A large number of pathways connect it with the cerebrum, brainstem, and spinal cord. The cerebellum receives stimuli relating to the position of the body and parts of the body in space and regulates the coordinated control of those muscular activities which permit walking, running, sewing, and similar activities.

Disorders involving the central portion of the cerebellum produce unsteadiness in walking. If one lateral cerebellar hemisphere is involved, the arm and leg on the affected side reveal incoordination and tremor.

CEREBRAL EMBOLUS   Cerebral embolus is a bit of matter, usually a blood clot, which is carried by the bloodstream until it lodges in a cerebral artery and obstructs it. Most emboli come from clots within the heart chamber or on the heart valves and are associated with bacterial infection (endocarditis); they may, however, come from the lungs or elsewhere. On rare occasions, fat droplets entering the circulation at the site of a bone fracture; air, tumor cells, bacteria, and foreign bodies, may also produce cerebral emboli.

Symptoms. The obstruction of a cerebral artery by an embolus produces an area of tissue destruction or infarction. (For discussion of cerebral infarction, see CEREBRAL THROMBOSIS.) This results in the sudden onset of neurologic symptoms which are frequently those of weakness, paralysis, loss of sensation, or similar deficits. Partial or complete recovery usually occurs, although emboli to large vessels may be fatal. Cerebral embolus may be a fatal complication of coronary thrombosis with infarction.

Treatment. If cerebral embolus is secondary to endocarditis, drug therapy may be successful in treating the cause of the embolus and in preventing recurrence. Physical and occupational therapy and speech retraining may be of symptomatic value during the convalescent period after a cerebral embolus.

CEREBRAL HEMORRHAGE   Cerebral hemorrhage represents bleeding into the substance of the brain from a ruptured cerebral vessel. In a patient with high blood pressure, a cerebral artery may occasionally rupture without any external head injury. Also, in patients with aneurysms or vascular malformations of the arteries of the brain, spontaneous rupture sometimes occurs with bleeding into the subarachnoid space and, at times, into the brain. Severe external head injury is sometimes associated with cerebral hemorrhage.

Symptoms. Symptoms develop suddenly with loss of consciousness and paralysis. The course is usually fatal. If the patient does survive the acute hemorrhagic episode, severe neurologic deficit is frequently present.

Treatment. Occasionally a blood clot within a cerebral hemorrhage is drained surgically, with partial improvement. In some patients a ruptured aneurysm which has produced cerebral hemorrhage is treated surgically to prevent rebleeding.

CEREBRAL PALSY   Cerebral palsy includes a wide variety of conditions affecting the control of the muscular (motor) system due to lesions in various parts of the brain. The defects in brain function may occur before birth or as a result of birth injury. The precise causes of many of these palsies are not known, although some are related to infections, X-radiation of the mother during early pregnancy, and hereditary (genetic) factors.

Symptoms. Cerebral palsy produces weakness, paralysis, lack of coordination, tremor, rigidity, or spasticity which is usually noted within the first year of life and which is related to defects in those structures in the brain which control motor functions. The condition may or may not be associated with mental retardation, epilepsy, and other developmental abnormalities in the body. Approximately one in two hundred infants have some type of cerebral palsy. Severe defects in motor function may prevent walking and useful functions of the hands, such as in eating, writing, and drawing.

Treatment. Severely handicapped children, who are frequently mentally subnormal, require hospitalization for adequate care. Children who are less handicapped may be cared for at home and may attend special schools where facilities for their needs are available; these individuals need vocational guidance and training in order to develop specific skills and become productive members of society. Children with mild motor defects and normal intelligence attend regular schools. They may have limitations in motor function which prevent full participation in athletic programs; however, it is important that all of their intellectual and motor skills be developed in a productive manner. If epilepsy is associated with cerebral palsy, anticonvulsant medicines are taken daily to prevent attacks.

CEREBRAL THROMBOSIS Cerebral thrombosis is a clot of blood formed within an artery which supplies blood to the brain. Thombosis of very small arteries may produce only transient symptoms or possibly no noticeable symptoms at all. Thrombosis of a medium-size or large artery will result in a neurologic deficit which is determined partly by the site of the vessel. Damage to the portion of the brain supplied by the particular thrombosed artery is due to the resulting inadequate blood supply (ischemia). If the ischemia is transient, attacks of weakness, loss of sensation, and speech difficulty occur for from five to fifteen minutes, then clear up completely. With prolonged ischemia, death of cells in the area results. A large area of cellular destruction results in a cerebral infarction. The extent of infarction depends upon the adequacy of the blood supply available from neighboring vessels—the collateral blood supply.

The major vessels supplying blood to the brain are the two internal carotid and the two vertebral arteries. From these vessels, blood passes through a circular vascular channel to vessels within the brain. Thrombosis can occur in any of these, but approximately one-fourth of the thromboses occur in the internal carotid and vertebral arteries.

Symptoms. Cerebral thrombosis is the most common cause of apoplectic stroke or cerebrovascular accidents and may result in severe paralysis and sensory change in one arm and leg. One or all four extremities may be involved. Speech disorders, partial blindness, double vision, facial paralysis, or difficulty in swallowing are sometimes associated with it. Drowsiness, confusion, and unconsciousness may occur. With severe brain damage, death may result. In most cases, there is recovery with residual deficit although complete recovery also does occur. Cerebral thrombosis may recur in other vessels.

Treatment. Partial block of a vessel in the neck may be corrected surgically. If transient ischemic attacks recur, anticoagulant drugs will decrease their frequency. Physical and occupational therapy are of symptomatic value, and speech retraining is sometimes indicated.

CEREBROSPINAL FLUID The cerebrospinal fluid fills the spaces between the brain and its covering membrane, the spaces between the spinal cord and its covering, and also the large spaces (or ventricles) within the brain substance. This fluid enters these spaces from the arterial blood system, circulates within them throughout the central nervous system, and returns to the venous blood system. Normally the fluid is clear and colorless.

If the circulation of this fluid is blocked, the ventricles above the block dilate and this interferes with the normal function of the brain.

As a diagnostic procedure, needle puncture of the space containing cerebrospinal fluid in the lower portion of the back is sometimes done. At the time of such examination, the pressure of the fluid contained within the subarachnoid space is measured. Samples of the fluid are also obtained for microscopic and chemical examinations. In certain disorders, the fluid may be bloody or may contain pus. (Occasionally air or oils, which can be seen on X-ray films, are injected into the subarachnoid space for special procedures in the diagnosis of neurological disorders involving the brain or spinal cord.)

CEREBROVASCULAR ACCIDENTS

A cerebrovascular accident is a sudden neurologic disorder which results from thrombosis, embolism, or hemorrhage involving cerebral arteries. The term accident refers to a sudden spontaneous change in the condition of the cerebral artery. This is an internal accident and is not related to any external head injury. The most common type of cerebrovascular accident is cerebral thrombosis, or occlusion of a cerebral artery.

CEREBRUM

The cerebrum is the portion of the brain which occupies the upper half of the inside of the skull. It is divided into two cerebral hemispheres connected by large nerve-fiber bundles. Each cerebral hemisphere is divided into four lobes—frontal, parietal, temporal, and occipital.

The cerebrum is the final destination of all types of sensory information transmitted through the central nervous system from the sensory nerves. Sensory pathways for bodily sensation arrive at the parietal lobes; visual stimuli are transmitted to the occipital lobes; and auditory stimuli are relayed to the temporal lobes.

The frontal lobes are probably the site of initiation of motor impulses under voluntary control, which are transmitted through peripheral nerves to skeletal muscles.

In right-handed individuals, and probably in most left-handed ones, the left cerebral hemisphere is the site for the understanding and expression of language. Complex intellectual functions, memory, and purposeful behavior are functions in which the cerebrum plays a vital role.

Disorders of one cerebral hemisphere result in weakness, decreased sensation, and/or visual loss on the opposite side of the body. With damage to the dominant cerebral hemisphere there is frequently impairment of the ability to understand or use language, thus making a severe communication problem.

CERVICAL CANCER

Estimates for 1982 projected more than 7000 deaths in the United States due to cervical cancer. Yet, compared to other cancers, cancer of the cervix (the outer neck of the uterus) is probably the most successfully treated. Nearly 100 percent of all cases can be cured, if discovered early. Cervical cancer is currently responsible for about 30 percent of all reproductive system cancers.

Early detection of cervical cancer is usually made by means of the "Pap" smear test. This laboratory test is painless, relatively inexpensive, and can discover cancer or a precancerous condition existing without noticeable symptoms. Abnormal cervical cells resulting from dysplasia, cancer *in situ* (which involves only the first layer of cells), and invasive cancer (which has gone deep into cervical tissue) can all be uncovered with a "Pap" smear. Although cervical cancer is rare among women under the age of forty, the American College of Obstetricians and Gynecologists advised in 1980 that adult women should have annual "Pap" tests.

Symptoms. The one outstanding symptom of cervical cancer is spotting or slight bleeding between menstrual periods and after sexual relations. However, dysplasia and early cancer may not cause any noticeable symptoms. Women who have had herpes type II vaginal infections, many pregnancies, or who were pregnant at an early age have an increased risk of developing cervical cancer.

Treatment. Treatment for cervical cancer varies according to the advancement of the condition. Methods such as cryosurgery (using extreme cold), and cauterization (burning), which destroy or remove abnormal tissue, may be used for some women. Treatment of advanced cervical cancer may involve hysterectomy, or a combination of surgery and radiation and drug therapies. Women who undergo treatment should have regular checkups to detect any remaining abnormal cell growth. (See also CANCER.)

CERVICAL POLYPS

These are benign,

grapeshaped enlargements of the mouth of the womb, and can be safely removed in the doctor's office without trouble. The usual symptom is bleeding between menstrual periods and after intercourse. Again, this condition must be differentiated from cervical cancer by the physician.

CERVICITIS   This is an infection of the mouth of the womb. It is a very common infection in the adult and sexually active female.

Symptoms. This condition is characterized mainly by abnormal vaginal discharge, itching or burning, and occasional "spotting" after intercourse or between menstrual periods.

Treatment. Diagnosis of this condition is not difficult, and treatment usually consists of special vaginal suppositories, creams, or sprays and douches. Occasionally the doctor will have to resort to electrocautery (burning), which can be easily performed in the office. It is of utmost importance that this type of infection be properly treated, since it has been quite well established that repeated infections of the cervix predispose to development of cervical cancer. Spotting between periods or after intercourse in an adult female should be considered a sign of carcinoma of the mouth of the womb until proven otherwise—and the only one who can prove this is the doctor.

CERVIX   The cervix is the neck of the womb (uterus); it is located at the top of the birth canal (vagina), and connects this organ with the cavity of the womb. The cervix is a vital part of the uterus and plays a very important role both in the transfer of sperm for conception and in the maintenance of pregnancy (by remaining closed for nine months and then gradually opening when labor starts, allowing the baby to pass through and be delivered). The most common diseases of the cervix are cervicitis, cervical cancer, and cervical polyps.

CHALAZION   This is an inflammation in one of the glands in the fibrous plate (tarsus) of the eyelid.

Symptoms. There is an area of redness on the inside of the lid and an associated tenderness. The attacks tend to repeat, and between infections there is a hard pebble-like nodule in the lid which may cause a lump in the skin.

Treatment. When infected, hot compresses are indicated. Repeated infections may make it necessary to remove the infected gland.

CHAPPED SKIN   This condition results from the deliberate or inadvertent removal of oil from the surface of the skin. The usually low humidity of winter weather induces rapid evaporation of water from the skin surface and has a drying effect. Coupled with reduced production of oil, the drying can be intense enough to induce redness and scaling and a leathery feel. Use of cleaning solutions and fat solvents can produce the same effect even in the presence of normal oil production and high humidity.

Treatment. The wearing of gloves outdoors in wintertime affords protection both against evaporation of surface water and reduction of oil production because of chilling of the skin. The application of simple greases like vaseline or lanolin is useful in relieving the eruption and the burning sensation usually accompanying the reddened and roughened skin.

CHEILITIS   This term applies to any inflammation of the lips of whatever causation. The lips are subject to allergic sensitization to many substances including lipstick, mouthwashes, dentrifices, bubble gum, mangoes, fruit dyes, perfumes. Some disease processes can specifically affect the lips (lupus erythematosus, lichen planus), causing dryness, peeling, scaling, or atrophy (loss of tissue). Often, but not always, as the result of an existing disturbance of the lips, the patient is inclined to pick the free peeling edges, or to lick them to relieve the smarting sensation. Both the picking and the licking may produce further irritation. Excessive exposure to wind or to sunlight can induce inflammation with swelling and drying.

Symptoms. Except as the result of allergic reaction, a burn, or cold sores, inflammation of the lips does not often cause blistering. There is usually an intensification of the normal redness, swelling, wrinkling, peeling associated with burning, smarting, and occasional itching.

Treatment. Removal of the causative agent(s) and application of soothing ointment (vaseline, lanolin) will often suffice. Protection from excessive exposure to wind and sun may prove difficult but may be essential in chronic cases.

CHEMOTHERAPY Chemotherapy as applied to the field of mental disorders, consists in their treatment with chemicals and drugs. One of the greatest psychiatric advances of the twentieth century has involved the discovery of a large number of drugs with beneficial effects on central nervous system functions. Tranquilizing drugs have had their most successful application in the treatment of certain types of schizophrenia, the depressions, excitements, and psychoneurotic reactions. They appear to exert their principal effect by regulating emotional reactions.

Outstanding examples of the success of chemotherapy in modern psychiatry have been the great advances in discovery of new drugs for the control of epilepsy. Drugs are now available whereby grand mal, petit mal, and psychomotor epilepsy can be almost completely controlled.

So far, the only form of chemotherapy specific to a particular disease is that for the treatment of central nervous system syphilis. However, it is to be anticipated that scientific advances will produce chemical treatment for schizophrenia.

CHICKENPOX (VARICELLA) Chickenpox is an acute communicable virus disease seen almost exclusively in children. It is so contagious that almost all have had it by the age of nine or ten.

Symptoms. Chickenpox is characterized by the gradual onset of red, discrete, small bumps. On the first day there is usually a mild headache and a fever of about 100°. The following day there are new bumps, and the old ones have become water blisters. On the third day the blisters have become pustules, and on the fourth they begin to crust over.

The only condition with which chickenpox may be confused is flea bites; but the fact that the lesions in this disease come out in crops, and that there are lesions in the scalp (humans almost never get bitten there), makes this a fairly easy disease to diagnose. An occasional child will be very sick with a fever of 104° to 105°F. for four or five days; in this situation he will invariably have lesions in his mouth and down the throat.

The virus causing chickenpox is related to that of "shingles," so contact for the former disease may also develop the latter. Once the blisters are all dry scabs the patient is no longer considered contagious. It is difficult to understand why so many schools make such a fuss about a student's returning to class with some sores on his skin, when he was most contagious the day before the initial few spots appeared.

Treatment. Treatment consists in keeping the child from contacts, making him comfortable, reducing the fever, and preventing secondary infection. The newer antihistaminics will quiet the itch, and antibiotic ointments control skin infection. The time-honored soda bath—two tablespoons of bicarbonate of soda in a shallow tub, a thorough soaking all over the skin, then patting the patient dry, not ordinary towelling—will give some relief. The small diaper-clad baby with varicella invariably gets ulcers over the crotch (perineum) and needs a heavy ointment to protect him from salty urine.

CHIGGER BITES Caused most commonly by *Eutromobicula alfreddugesi* (the red bug or harvest mite) which lives on grasses, shrubs and vines, chigger bites occur most frequently on the legs, just above the shoes and along the belt line. The lesions are produced by the larvae, which become attached to the skin for feeding. In addition to intense itching, chiggers produce large papules which persist for about two weeks.

Treatment. The intense itching can be relieved by application of ice-cold water and soothing lotion (calamine). Antihistaminic drugs taken orally are also effective for the relief of itching. Prevention is possible if insect repellants are used around the ankles and wrists before exposure. Clothing of closely woven material, fitting snugly around the ankles and wrists, is also a deterrent to the bite of the chigger.

CHILBLAINS Caused by exposure to excessive cold, and more especially wet cold, this disease affects the hands, feet, face, and ears. The lesions consist of red or purplish plaques, flat or slightly elevated. On even slight warming of the affected areas, there is considerable discomfort from the smarting, burning, and occasional itching. If the exposure is more prolonged and the cold more intense, the lesions are aggravated and resemble burns with blistering and ulceration.

Treatment. Contrary to popular legend, gradual warming of the area, either with gentle dry massage or with lukewarm wet dressings, will restore normal circulation. Rubbing with ice and snow can only induce more damage, and it is difficult to understand how this "remedy" continues to enjoy popularity. For severe cases, treatment for the general symptoms of exposure and local blisters or ulcers is the same as for severe burns.

CHILDBED FEVER (POSTABORTAL AND PUERPERAL SEPSIS) The genital canal of a healthy female adult is sterile above the inner opening of the cervix of the uterus. A woman is protected from infection by (1) the acid vaginal secretion (due to lactic acid normally secreted); (2) "policing" by the white blood cells of the circulating blood; (3) the mucous plug in the cervix; (4) during and after labor by additional safeguards such as the descent of the amniotic fluid, the infant's body, and other discharges; and (5) the diminished virulence of any pathogenic bacteria resident in the vagina. Infection is introduced from the vaginal and genital skin area by vaginal examination, by unclean hands or instruments. Ordinary douches cannot be depended on as a prophylactic measure since they do not destroy pathogenic germs and do destroy the natural safeguard of acid secretion. The most common germs that cause sepsis are the streptococcus, staphylococcus, colon bacillus, gonococcus, and the welch organism (which causes gangrene).

Symptoms. The first sign is usually a chill followed by fever which rises over the next few days. The pulse becomes rapid, there is extreme weakness, the breath is foul, and the tongue is coated. There may be a skin rash and diarrhea may ensue. The patient has a foul vaginal discharge, the vaginal lips are swollen and red. Later, infectious involvement of the uterus and its ligaments is inevitable.

Treatment. The prompt initiation of antibiotic therapy will most usually check the sepsis and prevent other complications. Antibiotics generally make local treatment (during the acute illness) unnecessary; the less examination and manipulation of the genital tract the better. Sedative and tranquilizing drugs may be given. Women who have had incomplete or unsanitary (illegal) abortions performed and fail to reveal their post-operative illness until the infection is overwhelming may require abdominal operation, for example, removal of the uterus.

CHOLECYSTITIS (GALLBLADDER INFECTION) Infections of the gallbladder may be caused by bacteria associated either with gallstones or irritation by concentrated bile.

Symptoms. The symptoms are usually moderate to severe attacks of pain (often perceived under the right shoulder blade), indigestion after a fatty meal, fever, nausea, and vomiting. A large percentage of cases of gallstones are accompanied by some degree of infection. In prolonged cases, the infection may pass upward into the ducts leading to the gallbladder and thus cause obstruction and jaundice. In severe cases the gallbladder may perforate, spilling its contents into the abdominal cavity and thus producing severe peritonitis. Occasionally the pain is difficult to distinguish from appendicitis. Many acute cases subside spontaneously with the help of antibiotics; in such cases, surgical intervention is not required. Should the symptoms increase, however, with rupture or peritonitis, surgical removal becomes necessary. Patients with frequent recurrences of acute cholecystitis, particularly when gallstones are demonstrable, should be considered logical candidates for surgical treatment. Most cases of chronic cholecystitis are associated with gallstones. In patients who have recurrent indigestion or biliousness, where function is otherwise normal and no stones are demonstrable by X-rays, the diagnosis should be questioned.

CHOLERA This is an intestinal infection caused by a comma-shaped organism also called a vibrio, which is notorious for causing epidemics of severe dysentery. In recent years a new hardy strain (El Tor) has spread from the Orient to Europe and Africa and now constitutes an international public health problem far more serious than smallpox. Cholera rapidly produces massive dehydration as pints of intestinal fluid literally gush out of the victim. Fluid therapy, by vein and by mouth, is life-saving, with antibiotics of secondary importance. Vaccination is a valuable preventive measure.

CHOLESTEROL Cholesterol is a dietary substance which is believed to play a role in atherosclerosis (hardening of the arteries, coronary heart disease, "heart attacks"). This complex molecule is a fatty substance, chemically a sterol alcohol.

Cholesterol is widely distributed in the animal body and is found in nervous tissue, blood, and in the bile. Bile salts and certain adrenal and sex hormones are derived from it. In the skin, cholesterol is the precursor of vitamin D, so that when

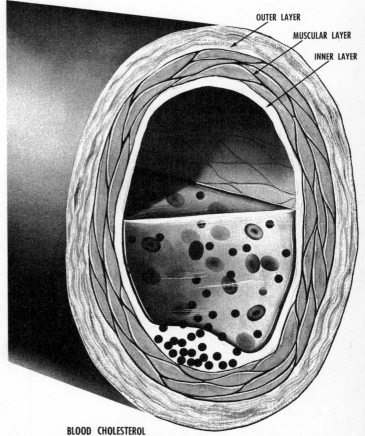

OUTER LAYER
MUSCULAR LAYER
INNER LAYER

BLOOD CHOLESTEROL
This is a cross section of a blood vessel showing the cholesterol (fat) particles invading the inner wall. A hard yellowish plaque forms which may eventually impede the blood flow.

it is irradiated by sunlight it is converted into the vitamin. Cholesterol is found only in foods of animal origin and is supplied by diets high in meats, glandular organs, and fat. However, the human body is not dependent on diet for its cholesterol supply, for it may be manufactured in the liver.

In the basic disease atherosclerosis, which causes so many deaths and so much disability in our country (through heart attacks, strokes, kidney disease, and so on,) small deposits occur on the inner lining of the blood vessels. One of the substances in the deposits is cholesterol. In addition, patients with advanced atherosclerosis often exhibit elevated plasma cholesterol levels. It therefore seems logical to conclude that atherosclerosis can be retarded by the reduction of cholesterol in the diet. So far, however, in spite of a tremendous amount of research on the subject in recent years, this point has not been conclusively proven. In point of fact, intake of cholesterol by itself has only a small effect on the plasma level. Rather, there is evidence that the quantity and quality of the dietary fat has more influence on the level of cholesterol in the blood than the cholesterol in the diet itself. In addition, there are certain personal factors to be considered. Thus two people may weigh the same and may follow the same diet over the years, yet one will develop atherosclerosis and the other will not. There may be a genetic inability to handle such a substance.

In the management of a patient with atherosclerosis or any of its manifestations, an overall program of therapy is needed, and this can be handled only by the physician. Dietary cholesterol is only one small part of this program.

CHOLINE Choline is a nitrogen-containing compound. Little is known about its importance in human nutrition. In animal experiments, administration of diets low in choline leads to a deficiency state characterized by an accumulation of fat in the liver. For this reason it has been used in the treatment of various forms of liver disease in man, but the results have not been clear-cut.

Choline is present in large amounts in the following foods: egg yolk, meat, fish, and cereals. The dietary requirements for choline are uncertain because the compound can be manufactured in the body. Human requirements are probably less than 500 milligrams daily; the average diet contains 250 to 600 milligrams of choline per day.

CHORIONEPITHELIOMA (CHORIO-CARCINOMA) This is an extremely malignant tumor, and until very recently its outcome was almost always fatal; with the discovery of a special chemotherapeutic drug (Methotrexate®) the prognosis is now somewhat better. It occurs almost always in the female, very rarely in the male (testicles). Although occasionally this cancer may develop in the absence of pregnancy, as a rule it is a rare and grave complication of pregnancy. At least half of the cases of chorionepithelioma develop following hydatidiform mole (another type of abnormal pregnancy which is usually benign). Chorionepithelioma spreads very early to the lungs, brain, and other organs.

Symptoms. The symptoms of chorionepithelioma are persistent and heavy vaginal bleeding, enlarged womb, bleeding from the lungs, and other symptoms, depending on the organs involved.

Treatment. Therapy consists of Methotrexate®, surgery, radiation, or a combination of these methods. The prognosis for survival of the patient is fair.

CHOROID, DISEASES OF The choroid is the blood-vessel layer of the back of the eye. It lines the sclera and provides nourishment for that portion of the retina adjacent to it. It extends from the optic nerve behind, to the ciliary body (with which it is continuous), in front.

An inflammation of this tissue, choroiditis, arises from a variety of causes: tuberculosis, syphilis, sarcoidosis, virus diseases, etc. It may follow injury. Many cases are probably the result of an allergy to bacteria, viruses, yeasts, or other small organisms.

The choroid is also the site of the most common malignant tumor of the eye, malignant melanoma.

Symptoms. Decreased vision, without pain, is the most common symptom of choroidal disease. It arises from two causes: (1) interference with the function of the adjacent nerve tissue, the retina; or (2) an outpouring of inflammatory cells into the vitreous cavity. Long-continued disease of the choroid may cause a cataract with even further loss of vision.

Treatment. This must be directed to identification and elimination of the cause of the inflammation. It depends upon careful examination, a number of skin tests, and laboratory examinations. Some infectious diseases may be corrected by means of specific drugs. In some instances, steroid compounds are given to reduce inflammation.

CILIARY BODY, DISEASES OF The ciliary body is located inside the eye, directly behind the outer margin of the iris. It is continuous with the iris in front and the choroid behind, and is held in position by an attachment to the outer covering of the eye, the sclera. In addition to blood vessels, it also contains the muscles responsible for the change in focusing power of the lens (accommodation).

Inflammation of the ciliary body (cyclitis) arises from the same causes as inflammation of the iris or choroid; both of which are usually secondarily involved in a ciliary-body inflammation. Paralysis of the muscles of the ciliary body is sometimes deliberately induced by the instillation of medicine in the eye, or may follow interference with the nerve supply.

Symptoms. Inflammation of the ciliary body causes a dull aching pain deep within one eye, associated with redness of the eye. If there are a large number of inflammatory cells released into the interior of the eye, vision may be reduced.

Paralysis of the ciliary-body muscles is without pain, but it is impossible to change the focus of the eye. Thus, near work is blurred, although distance vision may be unchanged. The pupil is usually dilated.

Treatment. This is directed toward identification and elimination of the cause of the inflammation. (Frequently medicines are used which dilate the pupil and paralyze the ciliary muscle.) Cortisone compounds may be used to reduce inflammation. Many of the conditions causing inflammation are self-limiting and heal spontaneously, but tend to reoccur.

Paralysis of the ciliary muscles can be reversed, if caused by medicines, by using drugs with an action opposite to those which initially produced it. When due to nerve or brain disease, treatment must be directed to the cause; however, correction frequently is not possible.

CIRCUMCISION The surgical removal of the foreskin (prepuce) from the head of the penis is known as circumcision. This procedure, routine for all Jewish male infants as a religious ceremony, has become an almost universal practice in the United States before the boy is brought home from the hospital. When performed for nonreligious reasons, it is done for the sake of cleanliness and to prevent local malignancy. (Most non-Jewish European families do not circumcise their boys.) The fact is that the circumcised penis is easier to clean, and there seems to be no record of cancer of the circumcised penis.

After the operation, the opening in the

end of the penis must be carefully watched by the mother and the doctor: a minor rash may inflame the lining cells just inside the opening and cause a narrowing (stenosis) of the opening and hence some obstruction to the flow of urine. There are well-documented cases of kidney damage due to back pressure from such a narrowed opening.

Immediately after circumcision, the head of the penis is quite raw, so that some type of ointment should be applied to prevent the wound from sticking to the diaper. A simple lanolin or soft zinc-oxide ointment is satisfactory. Urine should be forthcoming at regular intervals, and the size and trajectory of the stream carefully noted; this information is then passed on to the doctor. Bleeding after circumcision can often be safely controlled by applying pressure, sufficient to stop it, by means of clean cotton gauze or toilet tissue. If it is persistent, the doctor should be called.

CIRRHOSIS   A chronic disease of the liver, cirrhosis produces an increased amount of connective tissue and destruction of the functioning cells. This results in hardening of the organ and eventually a marked obstruction to the normal flow of blood. Although many cases are due to chronic alcoholism, this is by no means the only cause. Cirrhosis may occur after a severe case of hepatitis (infectious jaundice), long-standing malnutrition (the probable cause of alcoholic cirrhosis), untreated malaria, chronic congestion due to heart-failure, and obstruction of the normal flow of bile caused by gallstones or infection of the bile ducts. Cirrhosis may also be caused by a rare disorder, hemochromatosis (bronze diabetes).

Symptoms. Initially the liver is usually enlarged because of an infiltration of fat. Later it becomes scarred, nodular, and shrunken. The symptoms are ill-defined at first and consist of loss of appetite, nausea and vomiting, weight loss, and vague abdominal pain. In advanced cases jaundice, foul breath, red palms, abdominal swelling due to fluid in the abdomen, and gastrointestinal hemorrhages are common. Because of the many functions of the liver, the effects of cirrhosis can be profoundly serious. Abdominal fluid (called ascites) collects as a result of obstruction to the flow of blood from the intestines to the liver (through the portal vein) as well as because of a decreased amount of proteins in the blood. When severe, this portal obstruction may also cause formation of varicose veins in the esophagus and rectum (the routes by which the blood must flow when the normal channels through the liver are obstructed). Rupture of the veins in the esophagus can cause a massive and often fatal blood loss.

Treatment. The treatment of far-advanced cirrhosis is usually unsatisfactory; in early cases, however, the process can be halted or reversed by proper nutrition, strict abstinence from alcohol, supplemental vitamins, and rest. Occasionally, surgical procedures designed to relieve the pressure in the portal vein are successful in preventing hemorrhages, but careful treatment of the underlying condition is mandatory.

CLAUSTROPHOBIA   Claustrophobia is defined as pathological fear of closed places. The claustrophobe experiences extreme fear and apprehension when required to enter a closed space—such as a closet, subway car, or elevator—from which there is no easy escape. Claustrophobia is not a disorder in itself, but rather a symptom of underlying unconscious conflict which may require psychoanalytic treatment to uncover. A claustrophobe should be discouraged from paying too much attention to the symptom, and induced to seek psychiatric help to discover its unconscious causes.

Many cases of claustrophobia are caused by childhood conditioning in which the child was inadvertently confined in a closed space. Such experiences may stimulate great anxiety and continue to produce symptoms for years. In other cases, claustrophobia may develop when the child observes an older person behaving hysterically in a closed place.

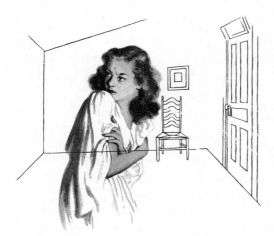

CLAWFOOT (PES CAVUS) Pes cavus, or clawfoot, or high-arched foot is a foot disorder in which the longitudinal arch is abnormally high. It is very often seen with a clawlike contraction of the joints between the toes and the bones behind them. Pain is due to pressure on the foot which is exerted on the heads of these small bones, over which calluses form. Usually there is shortening of the Achilles tendon (the tendon above the heel) which results in further weight being thrown on the front part of the foot.

Treatment. A sponge rubber bar placed across the fore part of the sole or a leather bar similarly placed toward the outer side of the sole of the shoe afford marked relief.

CLEFT PALATE Cleft palate and harelip are parts of the same congenital defect. All or part of the bony roof of the mouth may be absent, thus exposing the nasal passages and sinuses. The cleft may extend forward through the gum and the upper lip, producing the harelip.

Treatment. The only cure is surgery.

The lip is usually repaired first, so that the baby may suck. The palate is done at a time when the surgeon feels he has enough tissue with which to work so as to cover the repaired bony palate; this is best done before speech habits are established, usually between the ages of eighteen and twenty-four months. Sometimes several operations are necessary in order to free the tissues in such a way that the defect may be corrected without undue tension. The cosmetic result is not always perfect, but more often than not is very good indeed.

CLIMACTERIC The cessation of ovarian function in women and testicular function in men is called the climacteric. In women there is a gradual decrease in ovarian efficiency after the age of thirty-five. When ovulation ceases menstrual bleeding may become irregular and cause concern. Bleeding usually decreases gradually in amount, due to lowered secretion of estrogen and progesterone. Normally cessation of menstruation (menopause) occurs in the mid-forties, but may occur as early as thirty-five or as late as fifty-eight or sixty.

Symptoms. A number of troublesome symptoms may occur at this time of life. The most common complaint is "hot flashes," or feelings of warmth flooding the face and neck, often accompanied by excess perspiration. Nervous irritability is common, as are feelings of depression and fears that sexual attractiveness is being lost. Of serious import is the development of bone softening (osteoporosis) which may result in loss of stature due to collapse of vertebrae, accompanied by severe bone pain.

Treatment. When careful medical examination assures the physician that serious mental disturbance is absent, as well as abnormal causes of irregular bleeding, he may simply reassure the woman that her symptoms will be temporary. There is no basis for the fear that sexual interest and responsiveness will be impaired during or after the menopause, if sex life was previously well-adjusted.

Small doses of estrogen by mouth or by injection are often prescribed and effectively relieve menopause symptoms. Some physicians elect to continue this therapy for extended periods of time to help prevent aging of skin, muscles, mucous membranes, and bone. In the presence of osteoporosis, combinations of male and female hormone are often used, with large doses of calcium.

Of some concern is the effect on mother and child of babies born in the menopause years. It is a fact that the incidence of mongolism and other congenital abnormalities is higher in babies born during late reproductive life, probably due to aging of ova. The strain of caring for a young infant in the menopause years may prove too burdensome for the mother, causing emotional upsets.

The male climacteric is a rare event, as there is not usually a sudden decrease in sperm production during the middle years. When it occurs, however, it is associated with hot flashes, irritability, and decrease in sex drive. Response to male hormone therapy is good. Many men feel their sexual powers waning after the age of forty or fifty and become quite concerned that they will become impotent. If medical examination fails to reveal loss of sperm production and impaired hormone secretion, assurance may be given that their fears of impotence are groundless. Because successful completion of the sex act is so dependent on a healthy emotional outlook, concern about aging and the male climacteric (change of life) may actually produce psychological impotence.

CLITORIS   The clitoris is the female equivalent of the male penis. It is located in front of the entrance to the birth canal, just above the urethra (opening of the bladder) and consists of erectile tissue. Its size varies in different races, and it is an important organ for the development of sexual orgasm in the female. Except for abnormal enlargement, which is usually accompanied by other endocrinological abnormalities, diseases of the clitoris are rare.

CLOASMA (MASK OF PREGNANCY)
This condition is the appearance of irregular, brownish patches over the skin of the face and neck. It disappears promptly after delivery.

CLUBFOOT   Clubfoot is a developmental condition in which the child is born with a foot twisted both upon itself and in relation to the leg. The forepart of the foot is inverted and twisted inward, and the heel is turned downward. Treatment of his deformity is properly begun shortly after birth. By means of multiple plaster-cast changes, the foot is gradually untwisted and held in plaster casts so that, with growth, it may develop properly. Once the foot is adequately corrected, corrective shoes and braces are used to control the growing foot. In highly resistant situations, operative procedures may be necessary to release contractures or lengthen and reposition tight tendons. A properly treated clubfoot should result in a stable, supple foot which is both functionally and cosmetically excellent.

Metatarsus adductus or "one-third of a clubfoot" occurs twenty times as frequently as true clubfoot and, fortunately, is an easier condition to manage. The forefoot is turned inward so that the child walks in a pigeon-toed manner, but the rest of the foot is usually normal. A child whose feet turn inward should receive medical attention as soon as the parents recognize this situation; certainly before it stands or walks. There are many causes of in-turning of the feet in childhood and careful diagnosis is important. Treatment of the child with metatarsus adductus usually requires initial plaster-cast correction, then dynamic immobilization in a Dennis-Browne splint.

COAGULATION   Coagulation or clotting may occur in fluids as diverse as blood and milk. Blood coagulation as a physiologic process is not yet completely understood, but contemporary science believes it is a three-step process, namely: (1) activation of thromboplastin; (2) conversion of prothrombin to thrombin; and (3) formation of fibrin.

Thromboplastin is a substance derived from thrombocytes or platelets which are cells in the circulating blood. Prothrombin is a protein derivative in the blood plasma (serum) from which thrombin (an enzyme) is elaborated when blood is shed. Fibrin is an insoluble protein formed by interaction of thrombin and fibrinogen which results in a meshwork that traps blood cells when blood is shed, hence forming a clot. Fibrinogen is a protein normally present in blood plasma and other tissue fluids in the body.

COCCIDIOIDOMYCOSIS   This deep fungus infection (mycosis) is caused by the fungus *Coccidioides immitis* resident in the soil of hot dry areas and carried by dust storms. Infection of the lungs results from inhalation of the spores of the fungus, and the patient may be unaware of the infection or suffer a short febrile illness. A progressive form of the disease involving almost all of the organs, including the skin, occurs infrequently in persons of low resistance.

Symptoms. In addition to cutaneous involvement in the disseminate and overwhelming infections, the skin can be the organ of primary infection under rare circumstances of invasion of the organism at the site of injury. The skin nodules enlarge and ulcerate; the local lymph glands also enlarge, and spontaneous healing occurs in a few weeks or months with residual scarring.

Treatment. Notwithstanding the poor prognosis, progressive coccidioidomycosis is treated with supportive measures and available antifungal antibiotics.

COD LIVER OIL   Cod liver oil, as the name implies, is an oil extracted from the liver of the codfish. It is a rich, natural source of vitamins A and D.

COLD SORES   This common name for the disease herpes simplex is curious in the light of the fact that a high percentage of the afflicted have recurrent attacks on exposure to the summer sun. Of course cold sores do often accompany the common cold and other infections of the upper respiratory tract, but the disease is primarily due to activation of the causative resident virus by a "triggering" factor. In addition to the triggering agents already mentioned (infection, physical agents including ultraviolet light), both foods and drugs are not infrequent offenders. Although no food can be considered exempt from suspicion in patients in whom the triggering cause is obscure, the most commonly indicted ones are chocolate, nuts and fish. It should also be pointed out that in patients in whom the cause appears to be a preceding infection (common cold), the possibility that the medication taken for the infection has in fact triggered the cold sore must be considered.

Symptoms. The eruption consists of a small group of thick-walled blisters with very faint or no surrounding redness. In one or two days, yellowish crusting occurs, the result of some seepage of the blister serum. There is often accompanying itching, and sometimes a smarting or burning sensation.

Treatment. Local antibiotics (bacitracin and Neosporin®) are used for control of secondary infection. Prevention of the recurrent type is twofold: (1) eliminating the trigger responsible for the activation of the virus; and (2) immunization through repeated vaccination with smallpox virus (which has some cross-immunization with the virus of herpes simplex).

COLIC   This is the intermittent abdominal cramping frequently noted in infants from birth to three months of age. In the otherwise healthy, well-nourished baby it usually occurs late in the afternoon or early evening after a feeding.

Symptoms. The baby cries out with a sudden sharp cry, turns very red, draws up his legs, and despite the efforts of his mother to soothe him continues to cry out for one to six hours; he then falls asleep and may be fine all night and for the early part of the next day, but repeats the same routine the next evening.

Many theories have been proposed to explain colic but none are universally accepted. Cold hands and feet have been thought to be the cause, but actually they are the result; since the circulation has been shunted to the intestines during the cramp, there is less blood flow to the extremities and hence the skin is cold in these areas.

Some anxious mothers can apparently transmit their tensions to the baby, so propping the bottle may be the solution here. Since some babies want to eat as early as one and a half hours after a previous meal, they may suffer from hunger cramps rather than colic. Regular three- to four-hour feedings are not ideal for all babies. Then again, some babies have a very tight "anal ring" just inside the anal opening and develop cramps because they are unable to push the stool out; these cases may require the use of a stimulating suppository or a small (one-ounce) water enema for relief.

Breast-fed babies may develop cramps and colic if their mothers eat foods to which they are sensitive: fish, garlic, onions, cabbage, beans are a few of the more common gas-formers. Some babies

react violently to some formulas, and a search for the ideal milk for a certain baby may lead through evaporated milk, whole milk, various prepared powdered milks, skim milk—finally ending with goat or soybean milk. If these latter two agree with the baby, he is considered to be allergic to cow's milk; most babies outgrow this sensitivity at about six months of age but may acquire other allergies (skin and respiratory) later in life.

Treatment. Therapy for colic is finding the cause and eliminating it. If all other methods fail, most doctors recommend a sedative solution which can be given with the feeding just prior to the worst time of outbreak. Gentle rocking, a warm pad applied to the abdomen, a pacifier to suck on, and patience in the knowledge that the condition is temporary and not serious, may all help to ease the baby and his parents through this trying time.

COLITIS   Mucous colitis, or irritable colon, is a common functional disorder of the large intestine which should be clearly differentiated from the much more serious ulcerative colitis.

Symptoms. In mucous colitis, a benign but often distressing condition, the irritable colon exhibits uncoordinated, irregular contractions of its lower portion, with excessive mucous production. Constipation may occur and gas can then be trapped, causing sensations of bloating and fullness. Occasionally the spasm will cause frequent loose stools with much intermixed mucous.

Treatment. The causes are poorly understood, but successful treatment often requires relief of emotional tensions and reassurance that the condition is not serious, does not predispose to cancer, and that simple constipation does not result in the absorption of poisons, headaches, or various other diverse and unrelated symptoms. Regular meals, avoidance of straining at the stool, and general measures (dis-

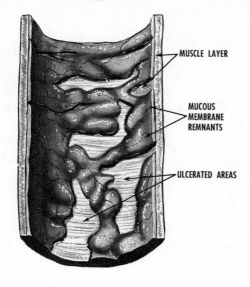

MUSCLE LAYER

MUCOUS
MEMBRANE
REMNANTS

ULCERATED AREAS

Colitis is an inflammation of the mucous membrane and walls of the large intestine, in the pathologic picture of which ulceration predominates. Ulceration generally begins in the rectum and spreads upward, eventually involving the entire colon. The symptoms are fever, malaise, prostration, persistent diarrhea, and the passage of blood, mucus, and pus.

cussed under CONSTIPATION) are of great benefit.

COLOSTRUM A yellowish fluid, colostrum is discharged from the breasts of pregnant women from the early months of pregnancy until several days after delivery. Its nutritive value is questionable; however, it acts as a mild cathartic and may provide increased amounts of antibodies for the baby.

COMA Coma is a clinical state of complete loss of consciousness of more than momentary duration. The onset may be sudden or gradual, and the coma itself may last for hours, days, or weeks. It is associated with various types of serious medical disorders, and may occur in the course of fatal or non-fatal illnesses. Among the many possible causes of coma are: severe alteration in the content of body fluids; extremely low or high blood sugar contents; kidney failure; meningitis; head injury; cerebrovascular accidents; and brain tumors.

Symptoms. Several levels of decreasing awareness are recognized, ranging from "alert," through "drowsy," "semi-

stuporous," "stuporous," and "comatose." A patient may progress in either direction through these different levels. On examination, a comatose patient does not respond to spoken commands nor look about the room (the eyes are usually closed). If an arm or leg is elevated and then released by the examiner, it will drop quickly to the bed. Strong painful stimuli, however, will increase the rate of respiration and may produce some movement of the trunk or extremities. Certain reflex responses, such as the eyelid and gag reflexes, are maintained unless the patient is in very deep coma.

Treatment. Hospitalization of the patient in coma is essential. Various laboratory tests are immediately performed. Treatment includes maintenance of adequate intake of fluids by intravenous injections, maintenance of an adequate airway for respiration, and proper care of bladder and bowel functions. Specific medical or surgical treatment depends upon the cause of the comatose state.

COMMON COLD IN INFANTS The common cold is a virus inflammation of the mucous membranes lining the nose, throat, and eyes. It begins suddenly with watery discharge from the nose, a few sneezes, a scratchy throat, and (in infants) usually some fever (100° to 104° F.) for a day or so.

A common cold is not serious and should not last more than a week. If a condition lasts longer than this, it is not simply a cold and is either a secondary bacterial infection or an allergy.

Thus, if a child sneezes and has a watery discharge from his nose and eyes for more than a week, he has probably developed an inhalation allergy and a search must be made for the offending substance.

Symptoms. A typical picture of the cold in childhood may be something like the following: A two-year-old child has had a cold for five days; just as it is about to go away, he begins to cry and develop an earache, the temperature rises to 102°F, and the discharge from his nose (which has been clear and watery) turns purulent with thick green or yellow matter. This is usually the time when the parent will seek medical advice, because now the child appears to have a treatable condition—a bacterial secondary invasion. The child may have developed pneumonia, bronchitis, or tonsillitis; or the infectious material from his nose may have caused an impetigo on the upper lip.

Treatment. The so-called "cold" is actually due to any one of a number of viruses, and at the present time we do not have precise treatments for virus-caused ailments. Aspirin (one grain for every ten pounds of body weight every four hours), steam inhalations, comfortable baths, nose-drops, decongestants, antihistaminics, rest, and fluids are the time-honored remedies for the common cold.

COMMON COLD, THE　　The function of the nose is not primarily to perceive odors, but to warm, humidify, and filter the air so that when it reaches the bronchi and lungs it is at the proper temperature, is clean, and contains the correct amount of moisture. The secondary function of the nose is to perceive odor, which also contributes heavily to the sense of taste.

As the air enters the nose, it is warmed and humidified by the turbinates. The mucus blanket picks up tiny inhaled particles and carries them away. If the air is very cold and dry, the nose has to work very hard to bring inhaled air to the correct temperature and humidity; this may cause excess mucus secretion and a "runny nose." It may be so hot and dry that the continuous mucus blanket leaves a gap of exposed mucosa. The blanket is now no longer continuous; there is a chink in its armor; viruses (tiny, submicroscopic particles which are not affected by anti-

biotics) can now gain a foothold: If the exposed area is in the pharynx, a scratchy throat may develop. Then possibly the common cold supervenes.

In such instances, the cold virus multiplies and causes some swelling of the mucosa. Its influence spreads, and the nose, sinuses, throat, and ears become affected. The mucosal lining reacts to the stimuli by producing mucus and by swelling. The temperature rises and the tissues become red—even painful. (These are all classic signs of inflammation.) Swelling of the tissues makes it difficult to breathe through the nose; excess mucus causes nasal dripping; the head feels "full"; body temperature is elevated.

Treatment. Since antibiotics do not help, what then should the patient with a cold do? The following steps and comments should be noted:

1. Bed rest. Time is saved in the long run by a few days of bed rest so that the body can fight off the virus and heal itself. If everyday activities are continued while the patient "heroically" pretends the cold does not exist, bacterial invasion of the weakened tissues can more easily occur. Bacterial complications are unpleasant and dangerous; they include pneumonia, sinusitis, and otitis media (ear inflammation). Thus, it pays to avoid the complications of the common cold by getting plenty of rest.

2. Fluids. In addition to maintaining nutrition by adequate food intake, drinking more than the usual amount of juices, water, and other fluids will make a cold more bearable.

3. Aspirin compounds. Aspirin, one of man's most versatile drugs, is effective in relieving the minor aches of a cold and in lowering an elevated temperature. One must, however, not make the mistake of assuming that if two aspirins every four hours are good, ten aspirins must be better. An overdose of aspirin can be dangerous.

4. Humidity. If a leg is broken, we set it in proper alignment and put it at rest by using a cast. When the upper respiratory system is infected, we should help make its functioning easier by providing humidity in the inhaled air (one of the functions of the nose is humidifying). Some use cold vapor and some, steam vapor; as long as sufficient humidity is provided, any of them may be used.

5. Nosedrops. Nosedrops shrink the swollen nasal lining and make breathing through the nose easier. These should, however, be used only on a physician's advice. Nosedrops should not be used for longer than ten days.

6. Antibiotics. Antibiotics have no effect on the viruses causing the common cold and should not be used unless the physician feels there are definite indications (subsequent infection, for example).

7. The celebrated Nobelist Linus Pauling created a stir in 1970 with the publication of a book asserting that large doses of vitamin C had prophylactic and therapeutic benefits for the common cold. Most of the medical profession and experts on the viruses remained unconvinced, and trials with student populations did not substantiate the benefits claimed for vitamin C. It is yet to be proved that the many viruses producing the common cold can be arrested by vitamin C.

8. "Cold tablets." These nonprescription medications may be helpful and probably cause no harm. They are usually composed of aspirin or aspirin-like compounds, together with an antihistamine and a drug that acts to make the breathing easier. It is a prudent idea to phone your doctor to make sure that it is all right to take this kind of medication.

COMMUNICABLE DISEASE See CONTAGION; INFECTION

COMPULSIONS   A compulsion is an

irresistible impulse to repeat some senseless activity. Compulsions are not disorders in themselves, but only symptoms of underlying unconscious complexes. Almost all normal people are mildly compulsive in performance of such senseless acts as avoidance of cracks in the sidewalk, repeated return to the house to check the doors, or irrational and repetitive carrying-out of rituals. A classic example is the washing compulsion: the impulse to wash an inordinate number of times a day.

Psychoanalytic theory states that compulsive behavior is usually determined by an overly strict superego (conscience). The compulsive act is interpreted as a symbolic defense against some forbidden impulse; for example, in the washing compulsion it is interpreted that the person probably feels very guilty about some fancied misbehavior and is symbolically cleansing himself by endless washing. Compulsions become pathological when their performance seriously interferes with routine duties in life. The only treatment for severe compulsions is psychiatric treatment of psychoanalytic type in order to discover the unconscious causes of conflict.

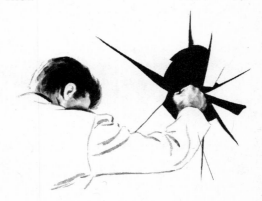

CONCEPTION   The fertilization of the ovum (egg) by the spermatozoon, a conception in the human usually occurs in one of the fallopian tubes, which the sperm reaches, through active motion,

128

from the place of their deposition. Only one spermatozoan fertilizes a given egg.

CONCUSSION, BRAIN Concussion of the brain is produced by head injury and results in transient loss of consciousness. It usually occurs as a consequence of rapid acceleration or deceleration in the motion of the head.

Symptoms. During the brief period of unconsciousness, the patient does not respond to stimulation. Reflexes are temporarily absent. After this initial period of complete unresponsiveness, the individual will respond to painful stimuli; subsequently, purposeful movements and still later volitional movements occur as consciousness is regained. After a brief period of confusion, the individual again becomes oriented and alert. Loss of memory for a brief period preceding and following the injury is usually noted. (The events mentioned above as following a head injury may occur over a period of a few seconds or during several hours.) In the days or weeks following a concussion, the patient may complain of headaches, faintness, nausea, vomiting, or dizziness.

Treatment. Patients with head injuries associated with concussion should be seen by a physician. Hospital care and observation are usually indicated. Further observation in the hospital or at home will enable the physician to exclude the possible development of an associated subdural or extradural hematoma.

CONDUCT DISORDERS As a result of studies in child psychology, it is now acknowledged that every child develops a large number of conduct disorders—lying, stealing, deceit, fighting, destructiveness, truancy, running away, cheating, etc.—in the course of normal development. Such disorders are not regarded as being very serious the first time they occur, since it is recognized that most children learn from experience and quickly pass through periods of instability as normal phases of development. Every child experiments with a large number of social and asocial behaviors to discover the limits of what society will tolerate. If the child is punished quietly but firmly he soon learns to accept social limits and becomes a mature, law-abiding person.

Symptoms. Habitual conduct disorders, repeated in spite of increasingly severe punishment, are regarded psychiatrically as evidence of behavioral immaturity or of deeper underlying neurotic disorder. Lying, cheating, or stealing may be symptomatic of deep underlying emotional insecurity, and tend to persist until needs for love and acceptance are satisfied. Fighting, cruelty, and undesirable aggressiveness often are symptomatic of underlying deep hostilities or resentments, where the child feels underprivileged or deprived.

Treatment. Where a child continues to show conduct disorders in spite of normal corrective influences, an underlying psychological problem should be suspected and the child referred to a child-guidance clinic for psychiatric evaluation. Experience indicates that neurotic conduct disorders are not improved by punishment, no matter how severe, but may actually be made worse if the punishment or rejection increase the child's inner conflicts. In such cases, the conduct should be ignored and psychiatric treatment directed toward removal of the underlying emotional conflicts or insecurities.

CONDUCTIVE HEARING LOSS See AUDITORY CANAL, BLOCKING OF THE EXTERNAL; EARDRUM, PERFORATION OF THE; AUDITORY OSSICLES, MALFUNCTIONS OF THE; EUSTACIAN TUBE, BLOCKAGE OF; EAR, MIDDLE, INFECTION OF THE

CONDYLOMATA These are warts, varying in number and size and appearing around the female genital organs (occasionally inside the birth-canal). Condylomata are produced by a virus and are common in women with poor habits of cleanliness.

Symptoms. The symptoms are usually itching, burning, and excessive discharge.

Treatment. The condition responds fairly well to treatment with application of caustic and antibiotic drugs, although surgical removal may be required for excessively large and obstructive growths.

CONFLICT, MENTAL   Modern psychiatry believes that some form of mental conflict underlies most functional (non-organic) mental disorders. The conflict may be between emotions, ideas, impulses, or any combination of these. In order to be mentally healthy, a person should be self-consistent and integrated in all the departments of his life. Conflict results in a house divided against itself, with the resultant toll of inefficiency and maladjustment, as the person struggles to resolve the inconsistent forces within himself.

This leads to an important rule for mental health, namely, that each person should strive to be self-consistent with what he considers to be the highest truths and the greatest good. Faced with many conflicting alternatives in life, every person must decide what is best for himself and strive to be consistent with this. Peace of mind depends largely on freedom from guilt, anxiety, and conflict. Antisocial behavior usually is simply not worth the cost which it entails in the form of anxiety and guilt.

It is now generally recognized that unconscious mental conflict underlies many functional psychiatric disorders, particularly the neuroses. A frequent cause of unconscious conflict is socially unacceptable impulses which are repressed from consciousness, only to appear in symptom formation; unexpressed hate toward a parent, for example, may cause psychosomatic symptoms of headache or high blood pressure. It usually requires psychoana-

lytic treatment to discover the underlying conflicts.

CONGENITAL DYSPLASIA OF THE HIPS   This is a developmental disorder in which the hip joint is underdeveloped and the femoral head is either partly or completely out of place. It may be recognized in infancy by apparent shortening of the involved leg, asymmetric skin-folds over the thighs, and relative inactivity of the involved leg. Some orthopedists feel that every child should have hip X-rays at birth; it is certainly true that every child with signs suggestive of hip abnormality should be investigated. In mild cases, double diapers or pillow splints may be adequate to reduce the malposition (subluxation) until growth properly remodels the femoral head and socket. In most complete dislocations, preliminary traction will be required to overcome soft-tissue contractures; then, either closed or open reduction may be performed. A long period of bracing follows during which the hip joint remodels itself through growth.

CONGENITAL HEART DISEASE
Congenital heart disease is present when one or more defects exist in the heart (or vascular system) at the time of birth. Almost one in every hundred live births will show these inborn defects, although discovery and accurate diagnosis may be delayed for months or years.

In its very beginning, many months before birth, the heart is a single tube. Growth causes the tube to enlarge, twist, and divide into chambers, the valves of the heart growing from the walls of these chambers. In final form the human heart has four chambers: two of these, the right auricle and ventricle, collect blood from the tissues by way of the veins and then propel it to the lungs; the other two, left auricle and ventricle, collect blood from the lungs and then move it forward through the arteries to supply every cell in

130

the body with oxygen or nourishment.

In the unfolding process from single tube to highly organized four-chambered organ, thousands of developmental steps take place in orderly sequence, timed with the passage of each hour prior to birth. Any diversion of effort in an area of growth can slow down or stop a portion of the heart's development and cause a malformation. The slowdown can be caused by involvement with virus disease (rare) or by tardy development of a terminal blood vessel that fails to supply a section of developing heart tissue with fresh oxygen and nutrition in proper time for the necessary speed and direction of growth that must occur in a normal heart.

Fright, tension, cigarette-smoking, nightmares, emotional crises of any sort experienced by the mother during pregnancy have never been proved to cause congenital deformities.

Survival rate. Almost one-fourth of babies with congenital heart abnormalities do not survive the first few weeks of life. Almost another fourth have such severe involvement that they fail to thrive and develop properly, although life is present. At least three-quarters of these latter can be helped or completely relieved by surgical procedures. A little over half do not require surgical correction until school age.

In some defects, the outlook can be grave and surgical risk enormous; but in others, notably patent ductus arteriosus, surgical correction offers perhaps less operative risk than an appendectomy, and with equally curative results.

Congenital heart disease can conveniently be classified into four main groupings:

1. Deformities that obstruct blood-flow (a) at the origin of the pulmonary artery (at or near the pulmonic valve), where blood exits from the heart into the lungs, or (b) at the very beginning of the aorta (at or near the aortic valve), where blood is squeezed from heart into the large collecting vessel, the aorta.

2. Incompletely developed chamber walls that have resulted in abnormal openings or "windows" between heart chambers. These openings permit blood to leak through, and since pressures are higher in the two chambers on the left side of the heart that squeeze blood into the entire body, that leakage passes from the left heart chambers into their counterparts on the right, which are busy forcing blood into the pulmonary artery and the lungs.

A window between the auricle chambers permits blood that has just passed through the lungs and is in the left auricle to escape into the right auricle; all this leakage must now take a second, purposeless trip through the lungs. If the leak is small, little damage will be done, but the work load of the heart is of course increased somewhat. A large leak may be disastrous and cause heart- and lung-failure early in life.

A window between ventricular chambers produces a leakage of blood with almost the same circulation difficulty as one between the auricles: some of the blood is diverted from the aorta and the systemic vessels of the body into the opposite (right) ventricle and must then make a second, unnecessary, trip through the lungs. A small opening between the ventricles can exist from birth to well past the age of seventy, with little or no harm to circulatory efficiency. A large abnormal opening, however, can rob the systemic arteries of much-needed blood volume and as a result produce extreme weakness. At the same time, blood that passes through the lungs repeatedly and without any physiologic advantage may cause early degeneration in the blood vessels of the lungs and thereby lead to complete heart failure quite early in life, unless surgical relief is provided.

3. Ductus arteriosus that persists after birth. Before birth, the lungs are dormant, airless, and are of no use to the unborn child's oxygenation system. A rather large

vessel connects the artery leading to the lungs (pulmonary artery) with that leading to the body (aorta). Thus "shunt" diverts blood which in the normally born infant goes to the lungs, into the entire body; that is, before birth, almost all the output of both the left and right sides of the heart goes into the aorta. Ordinarily, at the time of birth or shortly after, this shunt vessel obliterates itself completely; thereafter, an equal amount of blood flows into the lungs from the right side of the heart, and into the body from the left.

If this close-off process does not occur, blood will flow in a direction through this communication just opposite to the flow direction prior to birth. Why? Because as soon as the first breath is taken, the lungs expand and pressure in the artery to the lungs falls to a level less than half that in the systemic outflow of the aorta. One-third or more of the blood can escape through the open ductus arteriosus and make another trip through the lungs, for no useful purpose.

4. Double, triple, or more defects (a) in the heart itself and (b) in the blood-vessels supplying the entrance and exit of the heart. If there is a window-like defect in the wall of muscle (septum) between either the auricles or the ventricles, and in addition there is any obstructive narrowing in the outflow channel to the lungs, blood that should move into the lungs may prefer to move across the abnormal window-defect into a chamber that will pass it to the tissues of the body without its having traveled through the lungs. Blood is rather dark-blue prior to passage through the oxygenating membranes of the lungs. If a sufficient amount moves through the septum defect and is returned to the body without having been oxygenated (and reddened), the patient can show a blueness (cyanosis) of the lips, earlobes, and even of the nail beds and skin over the entire body. Babies suffering from this group of defects have therefore been called "blue babies."

The obstruction from the right side of the heart to the lungs may be caused by an improper development of the valve leaflets separating the right ventricle from the artery to the lungs (pulmonary artery). Furthermore, abnormalities can occur in the veins that supply either the right or the left auricle. Rarely, the aorta and the pulmonary artery have reversed their connections with the ventricles.

As soon as practical, a good anatomic and functional diagnosis must be made in all cases of congenital heart disease. The special techniques of cardiography and X-ray angiocardiography together with heart catheterization will supplement the examiner's diagnosis. These steps will usually give a complete diagnosis of every congenital deformity present in the patient's heart and great vessels.

Treatment. Surgical correction for cure and assistance is possible in almost every case of congenital heart disease. As soon as a complete diagnosis has been made, the safest and most satisfactory time for surgery can be selected and discussed with the patient, if old enough, and with his family. Delay in diagnosis can be responsible for many unnecessary deaths, because of delay in the optimal time for surgical correction.

Malformations in the great vessels of the aortic system can be associated with developmental defects in the heart, or can be present even when the heart itself shows no abnormality. The more frequent types of aortic malformations include aortic arch developments and coarctation of the aorta (see Aortic Arch Developments; Aorta, Coarctation of the).

CONGESTIVE HEART-FAILURE
When pumping action and the movement of the blood through one of the divisons of the circulatory system are slowed down the condition can be called congestive heart-failure. Indeed, a heart that cannot move

quite enough blood to and from the lungs and the whole body can be said to suffer from a degree of heart-failure. Inefficiency of the pumping action of the heart probably is the most common of all serious disorders that require medical care. Prolongation of a useful life can come from close cooperation between the patient and his doctor over a period of many years.

Symptoms. For months or even years, there may be few symptoms of which the patient is aware, especially if he enjoys a relatively normal life. On the other hand, if the heart incurs serious sudden damage, as from a coronary thrombosis, congestive changes in the tissues may be so severe that life may subsequently be very short indeed.

Symptoms of congestive heart-failure may occur in the the lungs: cough, shortness of breath, or even attacks that can simulate asthmatic disease. On the other hand, the symptoms may be quite distant from the heart itself—the result of sluggishness of the circulation in the more distant parts of the body. There may be swollen ankles, painful legs, numb and cold fingers, or there may be congestive liver enlargement, with loss of appetite, weight loss, and even diarrhea and jaundice.

The same basic circulatory problem affects legs, hands, lungs, liver or intestines —a lack of sufficient fresh blood to provide for tissue oxygenation and nourishment, and an accumulation in the tissues of the waste products of metabolism which, because of the impeded circulation, are unable to move on to the proper organs of elimination and excretion.

Congestive failure can occur in any person with heart disease, whenever the disease process—inborn defect, rheumatic valve incompetency, death of heart muscle from coronary occlusion, or some other heart illness—reaches such an acute stage that the heart will no longer move blood through its chambers with sufficient speed and power to refresh all the body tissues

and then call back for recircuiting every drop of blood available in the venous return reservoirs.

Inability of blood to move out of tissues and return to the heart causes a pooling of blood in the veins, with swelling (as of the ankles) or enlargement (as noted in the liver). This stagnation of blood leads to an escape of fluid into the tissues, resulting in further swelling. (Medically, such swelling is known as edema.) Most important, however, is the fact that once additional fluid appears in the tissues, it acts as a mechanical impediment to block the free passage of blood back to the heart. For this reason, edema will increase rather than decrease until corrective measures have been taken.

In addition, waste products tend to accumulate in the swollen tissues. In order to make these nontoxic and nonirritating, the body must dilute them with more water, producing additional swelling in the area. Some theorists believe that even the capillary walls themselves are injured in congestive failure, further complicating the fluid- and gas-exchange process at the cellular level.

If the left ventricle is primarily involved, the congestive failure may warrant the specific term left-sided congestive failure; if the ventricle primarily involved is the one supplying the lungs, the condition is referred to as right ventricular failure. After a few hours or days, however, both sides of the heart inevitably become involved in the malfunction.

The natural course of events in congestive failure is slow; sometimes, unless medical help is continuously provided, it progresses rapidly to a fatal conclusion. Conversely, some types of congestive failure may be resolved completely, even permanently, in a matter of hours or days, especially when failure due to anemia can be corrected by blood transfusions.

Treatment. Congestive heart-failure involves the entire field of medical practice. The heart must be supported, fluid balance restored, and the lungs and kidneys guided into satisfactory physiologic functioning.

CONIZATION, CERVICAL

Conization is the removal of a cone-shaped segment of the neck of the womb (cervix) for diagnostic and—occasionally—therapeutic purposes. This is a very valuable procedure for the diagnosis of cancer of the cervix, and can be done either in the presence or absence of pregnancy.

CONJUNCTIVITIS ("PINKEYE")

This is an inflammation of the thin, nearly transparent tissue (conjunctiva) which covers the white of the eye (sclera) and lines the inside of the eyelids. Because of its exposed position, it is liable to a variety of infections by bacteria or viruses, allergies, and irritation.

Symptoms. The eyes burn and the lids feel heavy, and there may be rapid fatigue with any task requiring intensive use of the eyes. A discharge may be present, varying in consistency from that of tears to thick, heavy pus. There may be dried pus on the eyelashes, and the lids may be stuck together upon awakening. Blood vessels on the surface of the globe may be prominent. Vision is usually not affected.

Treatment. This is directed to the cause. Many types of conjunctivitis are contagious, and in order to protect others affected persons should use separate towels and practice meticulous cleanliness. The eyes should not be bandaged. The use of dark glasses may afford some comfort, and either hot or cold compresses may provide relief from burning and/or itching. Pus should be removed from the eyelashes by means of moistened cotton applicators. If only one eye is involved, care should be taken not to spread the infection to the other eye with the fingers.

In conjunctivitis due to bacteria and some viruses, main reliance is placed upon frequent instillation of drugs to which the causative organism is sensitive. A medicine dropper and not an eyecup should be used. Penicillin and sulfathiozole are not usually used because of the frequency with which the eye is allergic to them. Conjunctivitis due to irritation from smog, smoke, chemical fumes, and the like requires elimination (frequently difficult) of the cause.

There are a number of special types of conjunctivitis. Ophthalmia neonatorum is any inflammation of the conjunctiva occurring within two weeks of birth. The most serious type is that due to the bacteria causing gonorrhea (gonococcus). The practice of instilling silver nitrate in the eyes immediately after birth has nearly eliminated blindness from this source. Other causes include many various bacteria, particularly staphylococci, and the virus which causes a mucus-discharge (inclusion blennorrhea). Gonorrheal inflammation occurs within from a few hours to a few days after birth, while the others do not cause symptoms until five or more days after birth. In all cases there is profuse discharge of pus, and medical care is indicated.

Trachoma is a chronic conjunctivitis caused by a virus. Although it is the chief cause of blindness in the world, it is rare in the United States except among Indians in the Southwest. The disease produces scarring of the conjunctiva and cornea, with distortion of the lids and reduction of vision.

Trachoma is treated with various antibiotics and sulfonamides. Currently a vaccine is being developed to immunize infants at birth.

Vernal (or spring) conjunctivitis (catarrh) is an allergic disease associated with severe itching and marked thickening of the conjunctiva. It occurs principally in the tropics, and is relieved by removal to a climate free from heat and dust. There is no specific therapy.

CONSTIPATION Healthy persons may have normal bowel movements as often as two or three times a day, or as seldom as once every four or five days. Much needless worry and consternation could be avoided by the realization that it is not essential for good health to have at least one movement a day. Ideally, perhaps, the bowels should move at least every other day, but the frequency is not so important a matter as is the difficult passage of hard, dry stools. In these times, with dieting so prevalent, it must also be remembered that a scanty diet must inevitably result in scanty stools. The habitual passage of hard, dry stools may lead to such constant use of laxatives that spontaneous movements eventually become impossible. Chronic constipation may predispose to secondary rectal trouble such as hemorrhoids, fissures, and proctitis. Injudicious use of strong laxatives and frequent "cleansing enemas" may result in loss of muscular power in the rectum and is to be condemned. Failure to respond to the urge to move the bowels, lack of exercise, improper diet, and inadequate fluid intake can all be important in causing constipation. Rectal pain due to spasm of the anal sphincter, or other rectal diseases may reduce the urge to defecate and further amplify the problem. Emotional disturbances likewise are a common predisposing factor.

Treatment. Treatment should be directed to clearing-up any underlying cause and then to reeducation, which mainly consists of setting aside a specified time of day, usually after a meal, for defecation. Avoidance of straining at the stool, responding promptly to the urge to defecate, proper exercise, diet, and adequate fluid intake are usually helpful measures. Habitual use of laxatives and enemas is to be avoided. (See also HOME NURSING CARE.)

CONTACT DERMATITIS At first largely thought of as due to contact with plants (poison ivy), contact dermatitis is now recognzed to be the result of an allergic response to literally hundreds of substances present in modern man's environment. There is no inherited tendency to this condition, and it is not associated with or related to other forms of allergy. (It would be more correct to consider this condition a contact-*type* dermatitis because some of the substances causing it can be encountered both in the external environment (causing dermatitis on contact with the skin) and on internal administration (causing dermatitis on reaching the skin through the bloodstream). Drugs like penicillin, quinine, and Benadryl® are examples of internally administered remedies capable of producing contact-type dermatitis.

Although it is usual for the causative substances to come into direct contact with the skin, the contact may be unobserved when the substances are carried in volatile materials and are deposited on the skin in uniquely susceptible areas, such as the eyelids. Thus rotogravure (printing of comics and magazines) causes a dermatitis if exposure is experienced by placing the paper in front of the patient, with no contact with the paper itself. The eyelids are affected by the volatile material emanating from the printed paper. So too, perfumes, insecticides in spray containers, room deodorizers, and the like can cause allergic contact dermatitis in the absence of obvious contact.

Some substances cause dermatitis in areas seemingly distant from application to the skin (nail polish on the eyelids and face, hand creams on the face and neck); or the dermatitis can surround the area of intended application (contact drug-allergy sparing the area treated for one of many reasons). But most commonly a substance causing an allergic contact dermatitis produces an eruption at the site of application of the substance and in the configuration in which the substance has been applied. It is for this reason that poison ivy or other plant dermatitis usually occurs in lines corresponding to the stroke of the leaf, root, or twig carrying the allergen of the causative oil. Hair dye causes an eruption around the face and neck where the hair touches, and only more rarely on the scalp, which is less susceptible to sensitization. Bubble gum causes an eruption (not always allergic) around the mouth, where the material lands after the bubble bursts; and nickel causes an eruption at the area of garters or bra hooks and on the thighs of men who carry nickels in their pants pockets. One of the common sites of poison ivy dermatitis in young boys is the penis, it being usual for little boys to use the woods for their toilet and to not wash the allergen from their hands first.

The eruption caused by an allergy to substances applied to the skin does not "spread." The lesions continue to appear over a period of time depending on the amount of substance deposited on that particular site and on the degree of allergy present. The blisters occurring in severe eruptions do not contain the causative allergen and the serum oozing from them does not cause further lesions. Only previous contacts with longer periods of development, or further contact with the causative substance, are capable of continuing the eruption of new lesions.

Symptoms. The eruption consists of a reddening of the skin and the formation of papules and finally of blisters, depending on the severity. The location and extent of the eruption depend entirely on the areas of application of the causative agent. In prolonged instances crusting and secondary infection are not uncommon. If large body areas are involved, chilliness is usual and there may be a fever. Itching is moderate to intense. In some areas the eruption gives a sensation of burning. The

course of the disease depends on the extent of involvement and on the degree of success in removing the patient from further exposure to the causative substance. Hence patients with a generalized eruption caused by an injection of a drug (penicillin, Thorazine®, dye for X-ray visualization) will continue to produce lesions until the substance is eliminated from the body. So too, patients sensitive to mangoes will continue to have a dermatitis in the anal area until the fruit is no longer present in the stool. Avoidance of continued exposure to the causative substance is sometimes made difficult by inability to determine the cause from the history or from the appearance of the eruption.

To establish a particular substance more certainly as the cause of the eruption, the patient can be deliberately exposed to the suspected allergen in a manner similar to the one causing the eruption. This is called the "use" test and is especially revealing in instances in which other testing has failed. More common in dermatologic practice is the "patch test." The suspected substances, properly prepared, are placed on the skin and covered with a patch in the center of which is an occlusive film (cellophane) to protect the substance from an admixture with the adhesive of the patch. This is allowed to remain in place for forty-eght hours (or less if the patient feels some itchiness due to an earlier response). The reaction consists of an eruption of redness, papules, and blistering similar to the original eruption. If the testing has been properly carried out, even faint redness can be significant of a positive result and means that there is a causative relationship between the substance and the eruption. A response to testing may be negative and yet not necessarily mean that the substance was not causative. The many reasons for the lack of significance of the negative reaction to a patch test are best exemplified by the finding that some substances require exposure to light (photoallergy) to produce a reaction, and when a truly occlusive patch test is applied, the substance will be absolved from blame because a reaction was not possible in the absence of light. There are instances of inadequate patch test results due to excessive dryness of the skin and an inability, therefore, for the substance applied actually to come in contact sufficiently to produce a reaction; or instances of too much moisture of the skin, with resultant masking of a reaction by another reaction due to moisture. As with all tests, an interpretation of both the method and of the result is essential for proper evaluation.

The duration of allergic sensitivity of the contact type is many years, in most instances for life. Patients tested as long as thirty years after their last possible exposure to substances to which they were then allergic give positive reactions to patch tests as before. It is clear from this that, except under extraordinary circumstances, avoidance of substances known to produce allergic contact dermatitis is essential to prevention of recurrence of an eruption.

Treatment. In addition to removal of the offending substance, treatment consists in allaying the inflammation with cold compresses (water); application of lotion (calamine); local or systemic administration of the cortisone drugs; use of antihistaminic drugs to reduce itching; and antibiotics, locally or systemically administered, for secondary infection.

Desensitization or immunization is not usually effective. While injectable material of extracts of many plants (poison ivy, poison oak) is available, only patients for whom further contact with the substances is unavoidable (farmers, florists, foresters) should avail themselves of this type of prevention, since successful immunization is usually limited.

CONTACT LENSES Contact lenses are thin, usually plastic, discs worn over the cornea and beneath the lids to correct errors of refraction. There are two main types: corneal and scleral. The corneal is a thin wafer which floats on a surface of tears covering the cornea. The scleral type overlies both the cornea and sclera and is worn with a layer of fluid between the lens and the cornea. The chief medical indication for contact lenses is irregular astigmatism caused by a corneal abnormality such as cone-shaped cornea or scarring. They should not be worn in glaucoma, nor when the cornea has been the site of a virus infection or a recent infection. They should also be avoided by individuals who have no corneal pain sensation.

CONTAGION Contagion is the spread of disease from one individual to another by direct or indirect human contact or by an intermediate agent. In the latter, for example, the anopheles mosquito, which transmits malaria to man, is an intermediate agent. A disease may be both infectious and contagious.

CONTRACEPTION There is tragic irony in the fact that the miraculous advances of modern medical science should have resulted in creating one of civilization's most serious and urgent problems—overpopulation. The tremendously increased survival rate of the newborn, coupled with the prolonged life expectancy of adults, means that the population of our planet is increasing so rapidly and steadily that the need for some kind of birth control is now almost universally accepted.

Everyone is agreed that something has to be done; but there is no uniform agreement on how the problem should be handled. There are today several highly effective methods of contraception available, even though the ideal means is not yet at hand. The ideal contraceptive method should, roughly, cover the following requirements: it should be convenient to use by every female or male; it should be temporary in its control of fertility; safe, effective, and acceptable to all religions (particularly to the Roman Catholic Church); it should be inexpensive, aesthetically satisfactory, and require no special medical follow-up; and it should neither inhibit, interfere with, nor in any way modify normal sexual intercourse. If this sounds like asking for a miracle, the answer is that in this day and age we are accustomed to expect miracles rather than merely dream of them. Moreover, since so many of our seemingly extravagant expectations no longer fail to materialize, it would not be surprising if the "ideal contraceptive" too were to be developed in the not-too-distant future. Until that time comes, however, we will have to choose one of the methods outlined below, the ultimate guide to the choice being our personal, local, or national predilections.

1. Birth control pills. These pills contain two female hormone extracts and, taken one a day as directed, prevent the ovaries from manufacturing eggs (ova) every month, so that conception cannot occur. If used properly, these pills are supposed to be 100 per cent effective. They are still relatively expensive, however, nor have they been in use long enough to provide us with sufficient definite information about their long-term effects.

2. Diaphragms and vaginal contraceptive jellies. When used together the diaphragm plus vaginal jelly is about 98 per cent effective; either one used alone is probably about 90 per cent effective. In order to do its work, however, the diaphragm must be carefully fitted by a physician, who should then carefully instruct the user on exactly how to insert it and how long to keep it in. Unless it fits properly and is kept in place for about eight hours, it will not afford sufficient protection against the sperm, which re-

main active in the vagina for some time after intercourse and which will travel into the uterus if the diaphragm is removed too soon. Vaginal jelly smeared on the rim of the diaphragm is an added precaution. Douching the following morning is not necessary, although many women prefer to douche for reasons of personal cleanliness.

The objections sometimes raised against the diaphragm are that it means an outlay of money for a doctor's visit plus purchase of the article itself; that women find it inconvenient; and that it is not particularly aesthetic. Many gynecologists and writers on marriage relations advise inserting the diaphragm every night before going to bed, making it as much a routine as brushing the teeth: this takes care of the inhibiting element of self-consciousness for both the man and the woman. Needless to say, this method of contraception could not be successfully applied to large, indigent population groups.

3. Vaginal foams. In effectiveness these are about on a par with vaginal jellies when used alone. They are considered less "messy," but otherwise the same pros and cons apply to them.

4. Intrauterine devices. These include several small plastic devices of varied shape and form which are inserted into the womb by a physician and left in place for several years. It is not yet clear how they prevent pregnancy, and the method is still in the experimental stages. Their effectiveness is in the vicinity of 98 per cent. In some women they may cause irregular or excessive bleeding, so that removal may become mandatory. Occasionally one may drop out of the womb without the patient's knowledge, which indicates a measure of unreliability. Sometimes they may also precipitate infection of the pelvic organs.

5. Condoms (prophylactics). These are fine rubber (or latex) sheaths which the male puts over the penis before intercourse. They are highly effective provided

they are of good quality. In addition to being relatively inconvenient and not always reliable (having been known to break), they interfere with the sensory contact of normal intercourse and are often rejected by both partners.

6. Rhythm method. This is the only method at present accepted by the Roman Catholic Church. It is based on the fact that most women ovulate around the fourteenth day of a normal twenty-eight-day cycle, so that if intercourse is avoided between days ten and seventeen, the chances are that pregnancy will not occur. The overall effectiveness of this method is, at best, estimated to be in the vicinity of 50 per cent. This low figure is due to the fact that, even in women with normal menstrual patterns, the time of ovulation is quite unpredictable. The rhythm method is recommended for extremely religious people as their only choice.

7. Interrupted intercourse (Coitus interruptus). With this method, it is up to the male to control the situation—he must make sure to "withdraw" and ejaculate his sperm away from his partner. This is a highly archaic, emotionally unsatisfying approach to birth control, which has little to recommend it in view of the fact that it is not even reliable, since there is always the danger of a little sperm penetrating the vagina in spite of the precautions taken.

8. Surgical sterilization of the male or female (see STERILIZATION)

9. Abortion on demand. Abortion on demand means surgical interruption of early pregnancy by scraping the womb (curettage) and removing the embryo (fetus). In recent years "abortion on demand" has been adopted as a slogan claiming that every pregnant woman has the right to decide whether or not she wants to proceed with the pregnancy. In several of the states, notably New York, essentially this state of affairs prevails. In other states illegal abortions performed out of hospitals

prevent varying degrees of risk. At worst infection leading to blood poisoning (septicemia) may result in death; in addition an inept black-market abortionist may injure the uterus while scraping it, thus causing sterility. It is not uncommon—and always tragic—to see a woman who is ready and anxious to have children discover too late that an early abortion has made her barren for life.

CONTRACTION, UTERINE Involuntary periodic tightening of the muscle of the pregnant womb, uterine contractions are experienced by the pregnant women as labor pains (see LABOR).

CONTUSION, BRAIN A contusion of the brain is a bruise following head injury. Contusions may occur anywhere in the brain, although they are frequently located in the frontal and temporal lobes. Large contusions may interrupt the function of a large part of one, or both, cerebral hemispheres. In the brainstem, contusions produce severe neurologic damage. All contusions are associated with swelling of the brain, which may result in an increase in intracranial pressure with additional neurologic deficit.

Symptoms. With severe contusion the patient may be comatose. Weakness, paralysis, or alteration of sensation on one side of the body may be present. Difficulties in speech and swallowing may occur. There may be local or generalized convulsions.

Treatment. The patient is placed in the hospital on a course of complete bed rest. Pulse, blood pressure, respiration, temperature, and neurologic status are checked at frequent intervals. (Special X-ray studies may be needed to exclude an associated blood clot.) If the patient is stuporous, intravenous medications are needed. Anti-convulsant drugs are employed to control seizures. Antibiotic drugs are used to treat specific infections if they arise. If unconsciousness is prolonged, nutrition is provided through a gastric tube.

Most of the deaths after a head injury and contusion are due to injury to the brainstem. Recovery may be complete or may be associated with residual weakness, speech disorder, or sensory disturbance.

CONVERSION REACTION   A classical form of psychoneurotic disorder is that of conversion hysteria. In psychoanalytic terms, the symptoms of hysteria are interpreted as being converted from original socially unacceptable impulses into more socially accepted overt symptoms: physical (or somatic) symptoms which, on the surface, appear unrelated to their true cause. Neurotic hysterical symptoms are capable of imitating almost every known physical and mental symptom. Thus, hysterical vomiting during pregnancy may be interpreted as a symbolic rejection of pregnancy, while "phantom pregnancy" (pseudocyesis) may mimic symptoms of pregnancy even though conception has not taken place. Conversion reactions are very common in wartime, when fearful soldiers have high unconscious motivation to escape from military service by developing hysterical blindness, deafness, loss of sensation, or paralysis. In each of these conditions, high levels of emotional conflict express themselves in terms of symptoms of physical disease. Conversion reactions can be treated only by psychoanalytic methods in the hands of a competent psychiatrist.

CONVULSIONS   This is a general term descriptive of the sudden onset of unconsciousness and generalized muscular contractions or spasms, which may or may not be epileptic in origin. In children it can be triggered by a sudden onset of fever.

Symptoms. The afflicted child may cry out, soil himself, stiffen, turn blue, fall down, and then develop twitching and jerking. When due to epilepsy, such major attacks—which are recurrent—are known as grand mal seizures. In the typical epileptic petit mal convulsion or seizure, the patient loses consciousness for only a second or so, but does not stiffen, jerk, nor fall to the floor; rather, he seems merely to stare blankly into space. Other types of seizures can vary all the way from spells of violent anger to mild, uncontrollable spasms of shaking in one arm or leg.

There are many causes for convulsions, and by no means all of them (or even most) are epileptic in nature. Tumors of the brain, blood clots on (or in) the brain substance, scars from old brain injuries, low blood sugar (or other changes in blood chemistry), high blood pressure, and certain drugs and poisons are all capable of inducing convulsive states. The vast majority, in fact, have no known cause, although in some cases a family history of convulsions can be found. It is noteworthy that children who suffer from febrile (fever-induced) convulsions do not continue to have seizures as adults—hence the idea that people sometimes "outgrow" epilepsy.

Treatment.   If at all possible, diagnosis of the underlying cause must be made. This is accomplished in most cases by an electroencephalogram (brain wave test) which will help establish the type of seizure and, if a localized lesion does exist, tell where it may be found. In the congenital cases of grand mal without discernible cause, successful treatment is difficult to attain.

When a seizure lasts more than a few seconds, the convulsing person must be removed immediately from any dangerous situation. The airway to the lungs must be opened by placing a gag between the victim's teeth and keeping the tongue out of the throat. If the victim is a child, the assumption is that there is a fever: sponging the naked skin is therefore a most important thing to do.

CORD, UMBILICAL   A glistening cord-like structure connecting the baby's navel with the afterbirth (placenta); this organ serves for the transfer of blood from the placenta to the fetus, and vice versa, during pregnancy. The cord contains two small arteries and one large vein; its average length is twenty inches, although it may vary from a few inches to several feet in length. It is vital for the normal development of the baby in the womb, and severe congenital or acquired abnormalities of the cord may result in early or late fetal death. A few days after birth, the cord dries up and falls off, leaving a button-like formation—the navel, or umbilicus—at the site of its juncture with the baby's body.

The most common complications involving the cord during pregnancy and endangering the life of the baby are: (1) prolapse, or expulsion, of the cord before

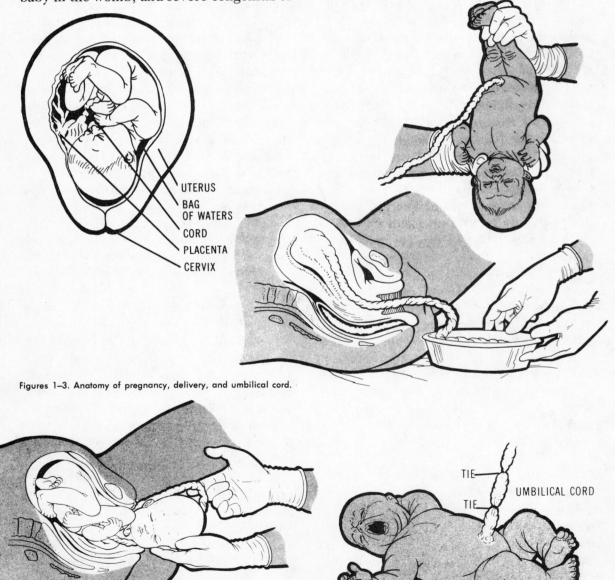

UTERUS

BAG OF WATERS

CORD

PLACENTA

CERVIX

Figures 1–3. Anatomy of pregnancy, delivery, and umbilical cord.

TIE

TIE

UMBILICAL CORD

Figure 4. Umbilical cord wrapped around baby's neck.

Figure 5. Tying and cutting the umbilical cord.

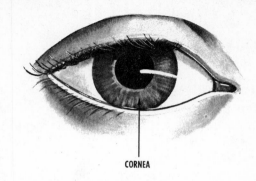

CORNEA

delivery of the baby; this usually requires immediate delivery by caesarean section in order to prevent compression of the cord between the baby and the mother's bones, which may obstruct the flow of blood to the baby; fetal deaths from this complication are not unusual; (2) knots of the cord; (3) looping of the cord tightly around the baby's neck; and (4) congenital anomalies of the vessels of the cord. In most of these conditions, the baby can be saved through caesarean birth, provided that the abnormality is detected early enough by the doctor.

CORNEA AND SCLERA The outer coats of the eye, the cornea and sclera, are fairly tough tissue approximately one-twenty-fifth of an inch thick. Five-sixths of the eye, the white (sclera), is opaque while the remaining portion, the cornea, is transparent. The cornea is the front portion of the eye through which the colored iris and black pupil can be seen. It is the main focusing portion of the eye, and the quarter-inch at its center is most important to clear vision.

CORNEA, INFLAMMATION OF The cornea is the transparent tissue of the eye which lies in front of the iris and pupil. It is liable to injury and infection because of its exposed position. Inflammation of the cornea, called ulcer or keratitis, may be superficial or deep.

Superficial keratitis includes: (1) catarrhal keratitis, due to secondary infection of the cornea by the agent causing conjunctivitis (staphylococcus is the usual cause); (2) serpiginous keratitis, an acute corneal infection caused by bacteria or other infectious agent which enters through mechanical injury; (3) dendritic keratitis, a virus inflammation of the cornea caused by the same virus that causes cold sores (herpes) of the lip; like cold sores, it tends to be recurrent, and it is triggered by injury, fever, menstruation,

and so on; (4) lagophthalmic keratitis, an inflammation which may follow exposure when the lids do not cover the eye (lagophthalmos), associated with a lack of pain sensation in the cornea.

Deep or interstitial keratitis is usually due to congenital syphilis. It occurs between ten and fifteen years after birth, and is associated with many new blood vessels growing into the cornea, with subsequent reduction of vision. Effective treatment of syphilis has made the condition rare in the United States.

Symptoms. Inflammation of the cornea usually causes a marked sensation of a foreign body in the eye. The eye waters and is markedly uncomfortable. The eye becomes markedly reddened. If the ulcer involves the line of sight, vision is reduced. The involved area may appear as grayish-white, or it may be necessary to stain the area with a special dye and observe it with a microscope.

Treatment. An eye bandage may be applied to make the eye more comfortable and hot compresses may give some relief. Eyedrops to combat infection and to dilate the pupil may be used. Skilled diagnosis is required, as drugs which aid in some conditions may cause damage in others. If the cornea has no sensation, or the lids do not cover the eye, lid surgery may be necessary to protect the globe.

CORNEAL TRANSPLANT An entire eye cannot be transplanted. However, replacement of a diseased with a healthy cornea can be carried out by transplanting either the full thickness of the cornea (penetrating) or the front two-thirds (lamellar). The operation is indicated either to improve vision, or to remove infected or injured tissue. The donor-eye is secured either by removal after death or from a donor afflicted with some disease not affecting the cornea itself. (Healthy eyes of living individuals are never used. Arrangements to donate one's eyes after death can be made with a local eye bank, information may be obtained from the local Lions' Club.) The graft always "takes," but visual results vary with the disease for which the operation is performed.

CORNS   Caused by ill-fitting shoes and more likely to occur in certain people, both soft and hard corns are the result of repeated friction. Soft corns differ in appearance from hard corns only because the moisture in the area between the toes macerates the lesions. Rarely, both types of corns are painless and do not require removal.

Treatment. Other than going barefoot, wearing shoes of proper fit is the only certain way of preventing recurrences. The corns can be lifted out. Slicing them with a razor blade is ineffective. Removal is made easier by the application of a salicylic acid plaster or ointment for several days.

CORONARY HEART DISEASE   Obstructive disease of the coronary arteries of the heart eventually leads to weakness of the heart musculature itself. It is perhaps the leading cause of chronic heart failure and of disturbances in heart rhythm.

In clinical practice, coronary disease is usually discussed in terms of the separate disease processes with which it is associated: angina pectoris (ischemia), coronary thrombosis (infarction), cardiac failure and arrhythmias of the heartbeat.

CORONARY INSUFFICIENCY   When one or more coronary artery branches are narrowed by a disease, usually arteriosclerosis, circulation to the heart-muscle segment supplied by that artery or arteries can be seriously impaired.

Symptoms. At rest, there may be no symptoms; with exertion, pain in the chest, radiating down the arm or up into the neck, may occur. Severe breathlessness may also be present. Attacks of short-windedness are sometimes the only indication of the disorder. An electrocardiogram will invariably diagnose coronary insufficiency. An X-ray study of the coronary arteries (a coronary angiogram) may be needed to confirm the diagnosis and show whether surgical techniques may be indicated to remove the arterial obstruction.

Treatment. Patients with coronary insufficiency are very numerous. With proper attention to diet and medication, life may be extended and most useful activities continued for many years, even indefinitely.

Surgical removal of the blocked points in the heart arteries is sometimes indicated, and may restore heart function to relatively normal capacity. In most cases at the present date, however, this is considered unnecessary.

CORONARY OCCLUSION   When a blood clot (thrombus) blocks the passageway (lumen) within one of the major coronary arteries, blood stops flowing through that vessel, coronary thrombosis or occlusion has occurred, the closure almost always being permanent. The area of heart muscle supplied by the vessel dies (is infarcted) because it is completely dependent for life upon the blood brought to it by that particular artery, the only supply line for that segment of muscle tissue.

Although it may occur in both sexes, coronary thrombosis typically attacks the middle-aged man. He may have had a previous heart attack or anginal pain episodes, but this is not very often the case. There is occasionally a warning chest pain and discomfort for several days, or some change in the usual pattern of the angina-pectoris attacks which the patient may have suffered for months or years.

When the coronary occlusion occurs, the patient usually feels an agonizing pain (something like a crushing sensation) beneath the breast bone; this persists for an hour or more, often in spite of the administration of pain-relieving drugs. Rest and nitroglycerine tablets alone cannot relieve the discomfort (although they will in angina pectoris). Collapse of the entire circulation usually develops, with profuse sweating, vomiting, and profound shock. Severe breathlessness may complicate the distress.

Collapse, coma, and even death may occur before a satisfactory diagnosis is possible. The blood pressure is low, there is an increase in white-cell count, and blood levels of characteristic chemical substances (enzymes) may be quite high. The electrocardiogram usually shows a typical pattern, but all of the changes may be delayed for ten days or more.

Treatment. At this time the basis of treatment is rest, followed in days or weeks by selected exercise or physiotherapy. Drugs may be needed to steady the rate and rhythm of heartbeat, and oxygen administration can diminish the work load of the heart, thereby aiding in its reparative efforts.

Anticoagulants are usually given. These substances prolong the time it takes for blood to form a clot, and for this reason it is thought that additional thromboses can be prevented and enlargement of the already-formed clot adequately curtailed.

If the patient survives the first coronary thrombosis, special attention to diet and general medical care will often result in a relatively normal life-span. Carelessness in health measures and medical attention can often drastically shorten a useful existence, or even result in untimely death.

CORONARY OCCLUSION

An obstruction in a branch of one of the coronary arteries which hinders the flow of blood to some part of the heart muscle. This part of the heart muscle then dies because of lack of oxygen supply. Sometimes called a coronary heart attack or simply a heart attack.

CORONARY THROMBOSIS
See CORONARY OCCLUSION.

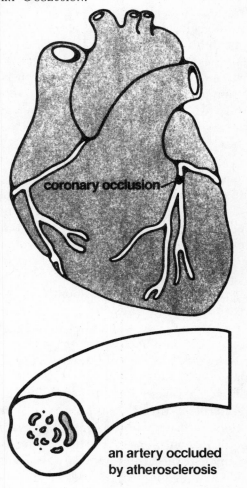

coronary occlusion

an artery occluded by atherosclerosis

CORTISONE
The most important secretion of the adrenal cortex is cortisone, which belongs to the family of substances known as steroid hormones. It is lacking in patients with Addison's disease and in those who have had their adrenal glands removed; its secretion is low in patients with Simmond's disease and other forms of hypopituitarism.

Cortisone is obviously the treatment of choice in patients whose adrenal cortex activity is either low or nonexistent. It is also used—in much larger dosage—to treat rheumatoid arthritis, lupus erythematosus, and other diseases of connective tissue.

COUGH   Cough is a sudden, violent expulsion of air following a deep intake of air, exerted against some degree of glottis (larynx) closure. It is a very common symptom observed in most persons at one time or another. Essentially, it denotes an irritation of some part of the respiratory system and is basically a protective mechanism to expel an intruding object or excessive amounts of body-produced substance.

Of no particular significance is the acute cough, which follows a common cold or upper respiratory infection and progressively decreases in intensity, disappearing over a period of two to four weeks. In contrast, a cough which appears for no particular reason or which is accompanied by expectoration unusual in character or color; or which lingers for more than a month (with or without expectoration) is considered a chronic cough and should not be dismissed lightly. This is often a symptom in smokers, and unfortunately the term "cigarette cough" is widely employed to denote what is believed to be an innocent occurrence of no significance. In fact, any degree of cough which is present daily for more than a month should be considered potentially serious and brought to the attention of a physician.

Cough can be produced by numerous mechanisms acting either directly as irritants of the respiratory mucosa or by reflex action. Thus, the stimulation to cough may be initiated by an inflammation of the nose, throat, larynx (the upper respiratory tract), or below—in the trachea, bronchi, or lungs themselves. These areas may be stimulated by local inflammation, allergy, or the presence of foreign bodies. So it is that nasal discharge may travel downward as a postnasal drip and irritate the lower respiratory tract. Excessive bronchial secretions, heartfailure, airless lung (atelectasis), chronic bronchitis, pneumonia, and pleural disease have cough as an early and prominent feature. In addition, cough (particularly dry cough) may occasionally be of psychological origin either involuntary or as a means of attracting attention.

Specific diseases of the respiratory system in which chronic cough is a prominent symptom are tuberculosis, chronic bronchitis, lung cancer, and bronchiectasis.

Treatment. There is no specific treatment of this symptom itself, but rather of the underlying disease of which cough is a feature; nevertheless, when the cough is excessive, one must artificially reduce or suppress it to insure periods of rest. The best medications for this purpose are codeine, mild sedatives (such as phenobarbitol), and certain newly developed non-narcotic cough-suppressors. It should be understood that in general it is not advisable to suppress a cough entirely, since it accomplishes the function of ridding the respiratory system of offending agents.

CRADLE CAP   See Seborrheic Dermatitis

CRANIAL NERVES   Twelve pairs of cranial nerves connect portions of the brain and the brainstem with sensory and motor structures about the head and neck. Many of these nerves have specialized functions. However, they are comparable to the peripheral nerves, which supply the remainder of the body. The numbers and names of these paired nerves are as follows:

I	Olfactory Nerves
II	Optic Nerves
III	Oculomotor Nerves
IV	Trochlear Nerves
V	Trigeminal Nerves
VI	Abducens Nerves
VII	Facial Nerves
VIII	Acoustic Nerves
IX	Glossopharyngeal Nerves
X	Vagus Nerves
XI	Spinal Accessory Nerves
XII	Hypoglossal Nerves

The sensory portions of cranial nerves supply sensory impulses including special visual, auditory, olfactory (smell), and gustatory (taste) information. Motor activities transmitted through the cranial nerves determine movements of the eyes, face, palate, and tongue.

Cranial nerves may be damaged by physical injury or by illnesses such as meningitis or neuritis.

CREEPING ERUPTION   This disease is caused by several species of roundworms (nematodes) not uncommonly found in the southern portion of the United States, and in many other parts of the world. The larva of the worm (present in the soil) can enter the skin through even slight abrasions.

Symptoms. The eruption is found on the feet of children whose barefoot habits and inattention to small scratches or cuts make them especially susceptible to the disease. At the point of entry of the larva, a small papule forms and the larva tunnels its winding way into the skin, forming more papules and blisters in the form of arcs, circles, and hyperboles. Itching is often intense. Secondary pustular infection is uncommon.

Treatment. Freezing with ethyl chloride spray, and taking care that the advancing "head" of the larva is frozen, are usually completely effective. When local freezing methods fail, systemic medication must be carried out by the physician.

CRETINISM   A dwarfed individual who also lacks a functioning thyroid gland is known as a cretin. Children with this disease may be readily recognized by a trained observer: even in early infancy, a cretin has a dull facial expression, lack-luster eyes, a runny nose, and a thick protruding tongue; the hair is dry and there is an excess of it on the skin of the body. When the child begins to walk—at a rather late age—there is a swaybacked and pot-bellied appearance. All reactions are slowed, and development of speaking, walking, bowel- and bladder-training, and self-feeding are delayed. In some iodine-poor areas of the world this condition is common, and is known as endemic cretinism. Cretinism also appears sporadically and may be due to destruction of the thyroid before birth by antibodies developed in response to material from the mother's thyroid which enters the fetal circulation. It may also be due to other unknown toxic substances.

Diagnosis of this condition is quite easy for a physician with some experience in treating children. There is no reason to confuse it with mongolism, although such confusion used to occur in the past. When there is doubt about the exact diagnosis, however, a blood protein-bound iodine (PBI) test may be helpful. Although this test usually registers low in cretinism, it may sometimes register normal; in such cases other means of verifying the diagnosis must be sought. The most helpful is an X-ray taken to reveal several centers of bone growth: these appear spotty and fragmented in cretinism. When even after all available tests there still is doubt about the diagnosis, thyroid hormone is usually administered for several weeks. If the child is not a cretin, no response will be evident. In the cretinoid child, on the other hand, dramatic changes occur after administration of thyroid hormone. In the event that the diagnosis is still in doubt, further administration of thyroid substances can do no harm, and may be of great value in the long run.

Treatment. A number of thyroid hormone preparations are on the market which are inexpensive, effective, and readily available everywhere. The hormone is administered by mouth, and may be given dissolved in milk to very young infants, or on a spoon with soft foods. It is important that the medication be given regularly and in the prescribed amounts. If doses are omitted, the child may fail to develop a normal mentality. One of the most tragic sights encountered by the physician is the child or adolescent who appears normal in all respects except for mental development, and who has a history of cretinism which remained untreated until the age of three or four. Once mental deficiency exists, it may be accurately diagnosed; but nothing can be done to accelerate the mental development of youngsters afflicted with it.

CROSS-EYE IN CHILDREN Also called strabismus, squint is the turning-in or -out of the eyes. ("Crossed" denotes the turned-in type and "wall-eyed" the turned-out.)

In the first six months of life most babies do not always use their eyes together, but at six to eight months the eyes should be working together at all times. If this is not so, the baby should be examined by an eye specialist (ophthalmologist).

Many babies have such a flat nose bridge so that the adjacent skin covers the inner corner of the eyes and the baby appears to be cross-eyed. If a baby is using one eye to the exclusion of the other, the brain "suppresses" the image it gets from the little-used one and a condition of disuse atrophy occurs. If this situation is not corrected, the eye never regains its ability to see clearly (although the squint may be cosmetically corrected by surgery.) A squint should never be ignored beyond the first eight to ten months of life on the assumption the baby will outgrow it.

CROSS-EYE (SQUINT OR STRABISMUS) Crossed eyes may be divided into those in which there is a paralyzed muscle and those in which the ocular muscles are normal. If the eyes turn in toward the nose, the condition is called esotropia; if the eyes turn outward it is called exotropia.

Nonparalytic (comitant squint) cross-eye is the most common type. The degree

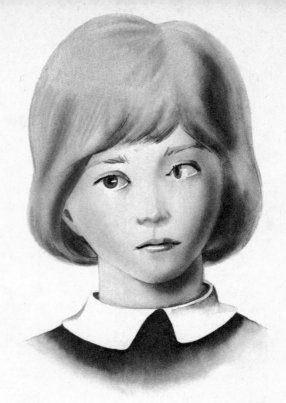

CROSS-EYE (STRABISMUS)

Strabismus is a squint deviation of one eye from its proper direction so that the visual axes cannot both be directed simultaneously at the same objective point.

of crossing is the same in all directions of gaze. It may occur because of some disease preventing clear image-formation on the back of the eye; because of disturbances in the ratio between focusing and converging for near work; or because of disturbances in the perception of images by the brain.

Paralytic crossing of the eyes arises from a disease or injury involving the ocular muscles or their nerve supply. The amount of crossing is more marked when the eyes move toward the field of the paralyzed muscle.

Symptoms. In nonparalytic cross-eye, the turning of the eye inward or outward is usually the only sign. In the early stages the eyes cross alternately, but eventually one eye is usually turned at all times. If double vision is present, the child is usually too young to describe it and soon ignores the image from the poorer eye. If an eye remains turned in or out constantly before the age of five, there is arrest of visual development in the deviating eye (amblyopia).

A paralytic crossing, if acquired after the development of binocular vision, causes the individual to see double. This, in turn, may lead to tilting of the head.

Treatment. Treatment of nonparalytic cross-eye is initially directed to tests and examination to learn whether or not there is any disease preventing normal image-formation on the retina. Far-sightedness or myopia must be fully corrected; most eye physicians believe that this can be done only after instillation of medications in the eye to paralyze the focusing mechanism. Drops which make the pupil small may be helpful in eliminating abnormal focusing mechanisms. The most important step is to prevent poor vision in the crossing eye. Usually this is carried out by covering the better eye in order to force use of the poorer. Prior to the age of seven years, patching should be carried out for at least two months before it is concluded that vision in the deviating eye cannot be improved. If there is improvement, patching should be carried out until there is no further improvement. Generally after the age of seven there is no more improvement in vision with patching.

There is a sharp division of opinion as to the value of eye exercises in crossing. Most doctors agree that the exercises are directed toward establishment of better vision and do not have any effect on the eye muscles or the development of fusion (stereoscopic vision).

To bring about a parallel orientation of the eyes, surgery is carried out. This has no effect on ability to see, although it may align the eyes in such a way that fusion is possible. Usually it has no effect upon the need for correcting lenses. The surgeon's aim is to do the minimal operation that will correct the crossing. If there is any danger of overcorrection, it is preferable to do a series of operations rather than attempt full correction in one operation. Usually six months should elapse between operations, to permit stabilization and evolution of the procedure.

The management of paralytic crossing depends upon the cause. When present at birth, it may be impossible to distinguish the paralytic from the nonparalytic type.

CROUP This is an acute infection of the larynx (voice box) which produces spasm and swelling of the vocal cords. The condition usually strikes suddenly at night during cold, dry weather.

Symptoms. The child awakens from a sound sleep as if someone were choking him. He produces a deep, barking, brassy cough followed by a prolonged, wheezy rasp (stridor) on inhaling. (This should not to be confused with asthma, in which there is a prolonged exhalation.) The condition is always worse at night, and there are apt to be three consecutive bad nights, followed by several days of loose phlegmy cough.

Treatment. As croup is often due to a virus, there is no specific medication. However, steam inhalations will allow the victim to sleep at least an hour or so between spasms. Lemon juice and honey in equal amounts is the most effective cough remedy, and if a little alcoholic beverage is mixed with this, the value of the remedy is further enhanced.

If steam and cough remedies do not induce sleep or relieve the spasm and difficult breathing, the condition is obviously more serious than simple croup and may require oxygen and vapor administered in the hospital; an occasional patient requires a tracheotomy (the cutting of a hole and insertion of a metal tube in the windpipe) because the obstruction is so great. In this latter situation the infection is most probably due to a bacterium, and antibiotics are often necessary. There are occasional patients who suffer from croup because of some allergy to food or inhalants; skin testing is usually required to determine the cause here. (See also First Aid and Emergencies.)

CROWN (ARTIFICIAL)   An appliance constructed of porcelain, gold, plastic, or other combination of substances, an artificial crown is designed to cover and form the top (coronal) part of a tooth, utilizing the natural root for attachment.

CROWNING   This is the stretching of the entrance to the birth canal (vagina) by the baby's head just before delivery. At this stage, the baby's head is visible from the outside, and the delivery is only a matter of a few more minutes.

CROWN (NATURAL)   The crown is that visible portion of a natural tooth which is covered with enamel.

CUSPIDS (CANINES, EYETEETH)
The cuspids are the four spear-shaped anterior teeth located at the corners of the mouth. A permanent set replace the deciduous cuspids.

CUTIS HYPERELASTICA   See DERMATOLYSIS

CYANOSIS   A bluish discoloration of the skin, lips, and nail beds, cyanosis is caused by insufficiently oxygenated blood passing through the tiny capillaries and vessels under the skin or mucous membrane. If the oxygen saturation in arterial blood falls below about 75 per cent (the normal is 97 per cent), a blueness of the skin and mucous membranes appears. This can be a sign of great importance. The blue color is determined by the concentration of unoxygenated hemoglobin in the capillaries of the skin. Cyanosis requires 4 or 5 grams of unoxygenated hemoglobin per 100 milliliters of blood before it can be seen with the unassisted eye. Thus when a severe anemia is present cyanosis may never appear, even though serious oxygen-deficiency exists in arterial blood, because there is simply not enough hemoglobin to produce the cyanosis. On the other hand, if hemoglobin is much higher than normal, cyanosis may be seen in a patient who is not suffering at all from abnormally low oxygen saturation. In some of the congenital heart diseases, the hemoglobin can rise to 20 grams or above. In these patients, cyanosis indicates the need for careful study of the blood count as well as the heart or lung defect that has caused this high level to appear.

The oxygen concentration of the blood determines hemoglobin saturation, for all oxygen is transported by adding itself into the hemoglobin molecule during passage through the capillaries of the lung.

There are three chief causes for cyanosis originating in the heart-lung system:

1. Decreased ventilation of the lungs. If for any reason adequate oxygen is not able to reach the lung capillaries, the oxygen-uptake of blood passing through the lungs will be very poor. This can happen in pulmonary diseases, such as emphysema of the lungs, or during an attack of choking on a foreign body lodged in the throat or windpipe that interferes with the in-and-out flow of air to the lungs.

2. Short-circuiting of blood in heart or lungs. If there is a defect in the chambers of the heart, part of the blood in the right-hand side of the heart can pass into the left-hand side and be forced into the arterial system without having taken the trip through the lungs. This is aggravated if there is, in addition, an obstruction in the pulmonary artery leading to the lungs. Occasionally, there is an inborn "short circuit" in the arteries of the lung itself, so that blood passes abnormally from artery to vein before the respiratory membrane is ever reached; this is called an arteriovenous fistula of the lungs.

3. Failure of oxygen diffusion across the respiratory membrane (alveoli). An oxygen-diffusion block can be caused by some lung diseases that thicken the respiratory membrane. Thickening or any other abnormal state, including cysts, of the membrane, can prevent oxygen-transfer

across the pulmonary membrane into the blood in spite of adequate circulation in the lungs and an adequate supply of oxygen in the alveoli of the lung. (A common example is the hyaline-membrane disease frequently seen in premature babies.)

CYCLE, MENSTRUAL Menstrual cycle is the interval, in days, between two menstrual periods and is usually twenty-eight to thirty days in length. From the gynecologist's point of view, the menstrual cycle is divided into three phases: the menstrual phase, three to five days in duration, represents the days of active menstrual bleeding; the early or proliferative phase, which on a normal twenty-eight-day cycle covers the next nine to ten days; finally the late or secretory phase which covers the last thirteen to fourteen days, just before the next menstrual period.

Ovulation (release of the egg) occurs between the early and late phase, on about the fourteenth day of the cycle. This is the optimal time for conception. (See MENSTRUATION.)

CYSTIC FIBROSIS Cystic fibrosis is essentially an inborn error of metabolism involving glands, such as the mucous, salivary, and sweat glands, which secrete an extremely tenacious mucus that produces the changes in the lungs, liver, and pancreas by obstructing the flow of air or fluids to these organs. It is familial in nature and carries a strong hereditary factor. It is the principal cause of pancreatic enzyme deficiency in children, many of the cases of cirrhosis of the liver in children, and of most of the nontuberculous chest diseases. Every two and one-half hours a child with cystic fibrosis is born. Not too long ago these infants did not survive the first year of life; with modern treatment some patients are living into adulthood. The cause of the disease is not known.

Symptoms. Pulmonary and digestive symptoms are first noted; four out of five patients present such features before the twelfth month of life. They are often misdiagnosed as suffering asthma or primary lung disease. In 5 to 10 per cent of babies with cystic fibrosis the first indication is intestinal obstruction. Rarely, infants may have prolapse of the rectum or portal hypertension (in the liver) as the initial sign. The most prominent feature is chronic respiratory disorder. Bronchial mucous obstruction makes the patient particularly vulnerable to respiratory infections that recur, each time leaving the breathing apparatus with more damaged lung tissue. Among common complications are lung collapse, lung abscess, coughing up of blood, and cor pulmonale. Sinusitis and nasal polyps are also common. Insufficiency of pancreatic enzyme production causes malabsorption, so that the affected child produces malodorous stools that are bulky and greasy. Even though his appetite remains good, he becomes malnourished. In the summer the cystic fibrosis victim suffers with abnormal perspiration which results in salt depletion of the body.

Cystic fibrosis is suspected in an infant or young child who fails to thrive despite a good appetite and normal food intake, has a chronic cough; foul, bulky, greasy stools; rectal prolapse; intestinal obstruction at birth; a sibling or first cousin with cystic fibrosis; recurrent respiratory infections; nasal polyps; excessive perspiration; stunted growth with pot belly; emphysema, and clubbing of fingers. Specific tests for salt content of sweat are extremely helpful in estabishing the diagnosis.

Treatment. Therapy is aimed at thinning glandular secretions, and by providing frequent postural drainage. A spray of 10 per cent propylene glycol and 0.15 per cent phenylephrine hydrochloride administered in a mist tent or by mask has proved to be most helpful. Mechanical suction of excessive bronchial secretions is also beneficial. The spray may have antibiotics and enzymes added. The lung collapse is treated with intermittent positive pressure therapy with the same spray. Postural drainage, exercise, and other physical methods are used. The child is taught how to increase lung intake of air by exercises that bring the diaphragm into prominent play in respiration. Diet is fortified with pancreatic enzymes, vitamins A, D, E, and K, while infants are fed a low-fat, high-protein formula. Older children usually can take a normal diet. Salt loss is overcome by salt tablets and additional salt in the food. Physical exercise and play are encouraged since they are among the best preventives of mucus in the respiratory tract.

CYSTITIS   Cystitis is a bacterial infection of the urinary bladder and almost always occurs in females. It is assumed the immature female is more susceptible because of the shortness of the tube joining the bladder to the outside of the body (urethra) and the consequently short distance from the anal opening to the inside of the bladder.   Furthermore, the secretions of the girl are more alkaline than those of the adult woman, thus making this site more suitable for bacterial growth than the more acid environment of the adult female bladder.

Symptoms.   There is usually a burning sensation and unusual frequency of urination, occasionally associated with fever or blood in the urine.   A soreness of the abdomen below the navel is frequent.   Since it is easy to see the pus cells in the urine under the microscope, rapid diagnosis can be made by bringing a specimen to the doctor.   (Clouded urine is seldom due to pus—more often to harmless crystals.)

Treatment.   Neglect of cystitis may result in the migration of the infection upward through the ureters (pyelitis) to the kidneys (pyelonephritis).   Drug-treatment may be easy if the causative bacteria

are not resistant to the medication prescribed.   Some doctors will take a culture and identify the germ more accurately, actually testing to find what medication kills it quickest.

The treatment, often a sulfa, is usually continued for ten days to two weeks at full dosage, then halved for another week or two.   If the child has more than three episodes of this disease, it may be assumed that there is something wrong with her tubing.   In such cases a more thorough investigation should be made by a urologist who will look inside and/or X-ray the urinary system, and will make cultures of the bacteria obtained.

CYSTOCELE   This is a form of hernia in which the bladder drops into the female birth canal (vagina). It is the result of a weakening of the structures that support the bladder and is usually secondary to childbearing.   It is much more common in the white race, especially in women who have given birth to several children and have lost most of the normal anatomical support for the birth-canal.

Symptoms.   Even large cystoceles may remain totally without symptoms.   A large number of them, however, will result in stress incontinence—the involuntary loss of urine under minimal stress, such as laughing, coughing, standing up.

Treatment.   Treatment is surgical, and consists of repair of the cystocele via the vaginal route, with or without hysterectomy.   Removal of the uterus will insure fewer recurrences and should be recommended to women who have completed their families.

CYSTOSCOPY   This is an instrumental procedure in which a tube with a system of lights and mirrors is inserted into the bladder through the urethra. The doctor can observe the interior of the bladder, including the openings of the ureters through which urine is discharged from the kidneys, and can evaluate the condition of the bladder wall. In men, cystoscopy makes it possible to sight enlargements of the prostate gland and to detect bladder tumors. Cystoscopy is not a painful procedure if the patient is well relaxed; it is often done in the doctor's office. Cystoscopy is often accompanied by the passage of tubes into the ureters so that opaque (contrast) material may be sent into the body (pelvis) of the kidneys for the purposes of X-ray observation.

CYST, SEBACEOUS These dome-shaped tumors range in size from that of a small pea to that of a small lemon. Occurring usually on the face, scalp, and behind the ears, they are not uncommonly also found on the chest and back. They can disappear spontaneously as the result of pressure or other injury, but it is more usual for them to persist, to become infected from time to time, and occasionally but rarely to become calcified. Multiple lesions are common.

   Treatment. Surgical excision, though curative, is not often necessary, and should be avoided if possible for cosmetic reasons. Drainage of the sebaceous material through the pluglike opening which is usually present, and removal of the sac through this opening, is likely to leave little or no scarring. In instances in which the cyst has become infected and removal of the sac is difficult, simple drainage of the lesion may cause disappearance. If the cyst is not infected or bothersome, removal is not essential.

D & C (DILATATION AND CURETTAGE) This is an operation consisting of opening the mouth of the womb (dilatation) and scraping the uterus (curettage). It is done either to clean out the womb after an incomplete abortion; or for diagnostic purposes, as in determining the possible causes of irregular vaginal bleed-

ing, infertility, or in diagnosis of uterine cancer, etc.

DANDRUFF See Seborrheic Dermatitis

"DANGEROUS AGE, THE" The decade from forty to fifty is often a perilous one for marital happiness. The wife is entering the menopause and faces the end of her reproductive years. She fears that she may no longer be attractive to her husband. (Indeed, this may be true if she is not capable of developing the special charm which maturity brings.) The husband, on the other hand, may feel his general vigor and sexual powers declining somewhat and may be secretly concerned about his attractiveness to the opposite sex. This may lead him into extramarital adventures. This so-called "dangerous age" may be weathered successfully if husband and wife learn to understand each other and if they have established patterns of compensation for difficult times.

DARK-ADAPTATION An increased sensitivity of part of the eye occurs when there is an extremely low level of illumination. The process involves the rods of the retina, which are so arranged that although form and color vision is poorer than in bright illumination, there is a marked increase in side vision and in the ability to detect movement. Sensitivity is further increased by dilation of the pupil which permits more light to enter the eye. Dark-adaptation is decreased in vitamin A deficiency, glaucoma, retinal degenerations, and many other conditions.

DEAFNESS Deafness can be either complete or partial. Complete deafness in children is unusual, and modern electronic devices are now helping many who may have thought themselves completely deaf. Congenital (inborn) deafness is usually due to damaged or poorly formed nerves which transmit the sound impulses from the ear to the brain.

It may be difficult to tell if a child is deaf until he is two years old, by which time he should be able to say at least a few words. (Since speech is dependent upon hearing, if a child has never been able to hear he will be unable to speak.)

It is important that deafness be discovered while a child is still young, because the newer techniques now used in educating deaf children are more effective if begun early.

Virus infections of the mother during the first three months of pregnancy are probably the most common cause of deafness. Acquired deafness is usually due to repeated ear infections, persistent fluid behind the eardrum, and/or enlarged adenoids.

Treatment. Ear infections should be treated quickly and adequately. If there are persistent signs of fluid or obstruction, drainage must be done by incising the eardrum, with the adenoids and tonsils perhaps being removed later.

DEAFNESS, CONDUCTION Many causes, known and unknown, are behind conduction deafness. Congenital defects of the ear or parts of the ear or of the Eustachian tube (running from the internal ear to the throat) are not unusual. Impacted wax, foreign bodies, tumors, stenosis (narrowing or constriction), perforation, inflammation, or scars of the tympanic membrane, rigidity of the small bones of the inner ear, chronic middle ear disease, otosclerosis (literally, "hardening of the ear) which does not allow the small bones of the inner ear to respond to vibratory stimuli, and blockage of the Eustachian tube are among the major causes. In children, however, the most common cause is excessive lymphoid tissue in and around the Eustachian tube's opening which clogs the tube so that proper ventilation of the middle ear cannot be

achieved. Lymphoid tissue is the same tissue that makes up "enlarged tonsils and adenoids." Otosclerosis is the most frequent cause of conduction deafness in young people, especially girls. It is most often seen in the eighteen to forty year age bracket. The cause of otosclerosis is unknown, but it seems to run in families.

Treatment. Modern surgical repair includes procedures such as fracturing the small bone known as the stapes with interposition of a vein graft and the making of a window (fenestration) if the stapes-replacement procedure fails. Hearing aids are most useful in conduction deafness, especially when surgery is contraindicated. Hearing aids with transistor tubes are extremely small, to the extent that they can be enclosed in eyeglass frames. Bone conduction aids are worn behind the ear against the skull; air conduction aids are placed in the outer canal of the ear. Specialists perform speech audiometry to ensure that the most suitable instrument is prescribed for the deaf patient. Special classes, such as lip-reading classes are most useful for deaf children.

DECIDUOUS TEETH (PRIMARY, "MILK," "BABY," FIRST, TEMPORARY) The twenty teeth of the first dentition, these teeth are usually erupted by the time a child is two years old. The last of them are shed (exfoliated) by about the age of eleven or twelve.

DEFENSE MECHANISMS Every person develops a distinctive personal style of life, involving strategies for securing ends and avoiding pain. The famous psychiatrist Sigmund Freud invented the concept of defense mechanisms to describe a variety of behavior patterns which people use unconsciously to avoid conflict. In general, the purpose of a defense mechanism is to defend the ego from critical attacks by others. A typical defense mechanism is escape, whereby a person avoids everything unpleasant; for example, a young girl who is afraid of speaking in public may, for instance, claim illness as an escape mechanism. The very insecure spend so much time escaping the things they fear that they accomplish little in life. Psychiatrists believe that the best defense is not to try to conceal fears, but to admit them frankly and learn how to cope with them.

DEHYDRATION This term, which really means drying out, describes a condition in which the body loses too much of its normal fluids and fails to retain enough for maintenance of adequate circulation, proper excretion of waste products through the kidneys, and individual cell function. Small babies show poor tolerance to dehydration, and may go into coma and die rapidly if it is not corrected.

Symptoms. The dehydrated infant becomes listless and breathes shallowly, his eyes half-closed and appearing sunken; he seems pale and shrunken and the tongue is dry. Such an infant may excrete urine which is scanty, infrequent, and very concentrated. (This usually is the result of gastroenteritis—often called intestinal flu —which produces vomiting and diarrhea; the child has vomited almost everything which he has taken in, and what little has stayed down seems to run out the other end.)

Treatment. In most cases the intestinal flu is due to a virus and is self-limiting, and the patient recovers before he loses too much fluid. Once dehydration sets in, however, treatment almost always demands intravenous or subcutaneous fluids, best given in the hospital, where proper attention can be paid to the minerals in the body, which are often too low or too high in concentration. Some patients are helped by anti-vomiting medicines given via the rectum. Other victims of fluid-loss have been saved from dehydration when given liquids by enema, for the lower intestine

(colon) absorbs fluids easily. If a baby can urinate at least twice a day, and can play and laugh occasionally, he is probably not too dehydrated. During the vomiting phase no milk should be offered; and only water (six ounces with a pinch of salt and a teaspoon of sugar), cola drinks, gelatin water, and tea are allowed. Any child who loses large amounts of fluids by vomiting or diarrhea, or both, must be quickly seen by a doctor.

DELIRIUM TREMENS Delirium tremens is a clinical disorder producing an acute psychosis associated with marked tremors. It is usually associated with abstinence for a few days after prolonged excessive alcohol intake, but it may also appear during the course of other types of brain disorder. In rare cases this clinical picture may be associated with acute inflammatory disorder of the brain or with severe vascular disease of the brain.

Symptoms. Delirium is manifested by hallucinations together with extreme restlessness and hyperactivity. The patient may be dangerous to himself and to others. Marked tremors involving the face, tongue, arms, and legs occur. Characteristic visual hallucinations include animals (such as snakes and rats), peculiar faces, and similar images which the patient may freely describe during the acute state. There may also be auditory hallucinations of voices which usually defame the individual. The patient appears extremely fearful during periods of active hallucination. Convulsions frequently occur and memory is defective. Liver disease and involvement of the brainstem and peripheral nerves may be associated with this disorder.

Treatment. Hospital care is essential. Sedative drugs are used to calm the marked restlessness and overactivity. If the patient is extremely hyperactive, restraints are necessary until adequate sedation can be obtained. Due to the patient's lack of cooperation, it is usually necessary to give medication by injection until the delirium has been brought under control. Intravenous fluids are required to prevent dehydration. Subsequently, adequate caloric intake and supplementary vitamins are important to maintain nutrition. After recovery from delirium tremens, psychiatric therapy is indicated.

DELIVERY   Delivery, or childbirth, is the expulsion of the baby from inside the womb to the outside world. More than 95 per cent of all deliveries are today done vaginally, and the rest by means of caesarean section.

Vaginal delivery takes place during the second stage of labor. We will describe it briefly here, together with some simple instructions on how to assist in an emergency delivery.

When the mouth of the womb becomes wide open as the result of uterine contractions and the baby's head (occasionally the feet or buttocks) is ready to appear, the mother will experience a 'bearing down sensation,' as though she were going to have a bowel movement. This is a sign that delivery of the baby is imminent. The person or persons helping should bear one important point in mind: Let the baby be born by itself. Do *not pull* and do *not* push on anything. Just scrub your hands thoroughly with plenty of soap and warm water, and have several clean towels ready to take care of the baby after it is born. While waiting, sterilize scissors or a knife as well as some string or heavy-duty thread.

Once the mother gets the 'bearing down feeling,' she should be allowed to push until the baby's head appears and stretches the opening of the birth canal. At this point she should be instructed to take deep breaths, panting like a dog, and thus allow the baby to be delivered *slowly*—otherwise considerable harm may result to herself and the baby. She should keep her thighs and legs wide open, and

there should be adequate space in front of her for the safe deposition of the baby after birth. Most babies are delivered face down, or turned to one side. After the head has appeared, do not be tempted to pull the rest of the baby out. The only thing you have to do now is check whether or not the cord is around the baby's neck; if it is, you should try gently to slip the cord over the baby's head and leave it there. If the cord is too tight to slip over the head, leave it alone; ask the mother to push the rest of the baby's body out; you may then unwrap the cord from the baby's neck.

Your attention now should be turned to the baby. Having wrapped a towel around its ankles, get a firm grip on its feet and raise them, letting the head and the rest of the body hang down while you gently wrap the baby's back. There is no need for the traditional slap on the bottom —most babies will cry at this time. You may then put the baby down beside the mother, making sure that the cord is slack. Using a clean (preferably boiled) piece of string, tie the cord five or six inches away from the baby's navel; then tie it again an inch or so further away and cut between the two ties with a pair of clean (preferably sterilized) scissors. Then make sure that the part of the cord connected with the baby is not bleeding; if it is, put another tie close to the first one. Wrap the baby in a warm towel and leave it alone. A normal healthy baby will need nothing else at this time.

The afterbirth is still inside the uterus, which now looks like a hard, pear-shaped mass with the top just above the mother's navel. Do *not* pull on the cord. You may, however, apply some gentle massage with one hand to the top of the womb, above the mother's navel. Do *not* push. The womb will get harder again and ten to fifteen minutes after delivery of the baby you may notice a small gush of blood coming through the vagina. This means that the afterbirth has become detached from the womb and is ready to be delivered. Indeed, soon afterward you will see it coming through the vagina and finally being expelled. Continue applying gentle massage of the womb for thirty to forty-five minutes following delivery of the afterbirth. This will help the womb remain tight, and prevent excessive bleeding.

Remove the wet and bloody bedcovers and keep the mother clean and warm. If she asks for something to drink, she may be given water or juice. The mother will need rest now; see that she gets it, and keep an eye on the amount of vaginal bleeding. If no tears have occurred in the birth canal and the mother's womb becomes nice and tight, no active bleeding should be present.

In case of a breech delivery, the course will be about the same as described above. The only difference is that one or both feet may be seen protruding through the birth canal for a considerable time before the baby is really ready to be born. The temptation to pull them is great—be sure to resist it. When the right time comes, the baby will be born of its own accord.

In general, it should be remembered that a normal delivery requires little or no help from an outsider. If something does go wrong, only experienced and qualified persons can help. The amateur is liable to cause more harm than good to both mother and baby.

DENTAL ANESTHETICS   Certain agents when injected, inhaled, applied, or otherwise administered, result in a loss of sensation in the affected area. Primary use of such anesthetics in dentistry is to prevent pain during certain procedures. There are two main types:

1. A local anesthetic. One which is injected or applied topically to anesthetize a specific area of the body (as with cocaine

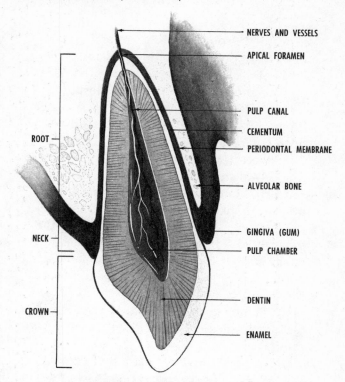

THE TOOTH AND ITS SURROUNDING STRUCTURES

derivatives)

2. A general anesthetic. One which may be inhaled, injected, or otherwise applied to render the entire body insensible: for example, pentothal sodium, which is injected into the bloodstream, or nitrous oxide ("laughing gas"), which is inhaled.

DENTAL CARIES (CAVITIES)   Early detection and correction of dental caries (decay) by the dentist is of the utmost importance. Left untreated, dental caries will deepen through the enamel and dentin to the pulp, resulting in pain and possible loss of the tooth. Early treatment of caries is simplest, less expensive, and more likely to succeed then delayed treatment.

What you can do to break the chain of dental caries:

Theoretically microorganisms may be destroyed by the use of certain antibiotics (penicillin), but this is not practical since it would also destroy useful bacteria and may result in other harmful side effects.

The soft, white deposit—plaque—found on unclean areas of teeth may be prevented from forming, or may be removed by proper brushing and the inclusion of "cleansing" foods in the diet (apples, raw carrots, cabbage, celery, etc.).

Anti-enzyme dentifrices have been proposed, but their effectiveness has not been completely established.

There are many types of carbohydrates—sugars—but some are more readily converted into tooth-destructive acids than others. It has been shown that refined carbohydrates (such as those found in the majority of soft drinks, candies, pies, cakes, cookies, etc.) are most directly related to dental caries. The between-meal use of these foods should be discouraged, especially among children and adolescents, and the amount eaten at mealtime kept to a minimum.

The most obvious method of controlling the amount of acid formed is to keep the total intake of refined carbohydrates (sugars) to a minimum at all times. Sugars ingested, or acids formed, should be removed as soon as possible after eating (preferably by brushing the teeth within fifteen minutes).

The resistance of enamel and dentin to "leaching-out" of calcium (decalcification) and eventual decay may be enhanced by the ingestion or application of proper amounts of fluorides. This may be accomplished by the following methods:

1. The teeth which are developing in the fetus during pregnancy may be aided by the ingestion of fluoride by the mother.

2. Inclusion of fluorides in drinking water

3. Direct application of fluorides to the teeth by the dentist

4. Use of some dentifrices containing fluoride

DENTAL FLOSS This is a waxed strand of cotton, silk, or synthetic fibers which is used to remove certain materials from between the teeth. The routine use of dental floss is unnecessary, unless pre-

scribed by a dentist. Improper use of this material may cause irritation to the hard and soft tissues, resulting in bleeding and recession of the gums that may be followed by gingivitis, periodontal disease, and even loose teeth. If dental floss constantly needs to be used in any one area, the cause should be sought and the problem corrected, since it is not normal for food to accumulate between teeth. Occasionally, when it becomes necessary to remove debris wedged between the teeth, a short piece of dental floss is carefully worked diagonally through the contact areas, without snapping the strand into the soft tissue (which may cause harm). The floss is then moved upward along the surface of each tooth and out through the contact area.

DENTAL HEALTH (ORAL HYGIENE)
The word oral pertains to the mouth and is derived from the Latin word *os* (mouth); hygiene is derived from the Greek word *hygieinos*, which pertains to the science of health and hence means healthful. Combining these concepts, it would be impossible to consider the healthful mouth and exclude the remainder of the body. One must therefore think of the practice of oral hygiene in relation to the general health and development of the body, as well as those structures particularly related to the oral cavity.

To develop an understanding of the oral cavity and its related structures, it is essential to consider all the influences which occur throughout life. Within the womb (uterus), the development of the oral structures is dependent upon such factors as heredity and environment. The transfer of certain characteristics from parent to offspring is understandable, since the ovum of the female and the sperm of the male transmit characteristics by genetic combination during conception; this would include such hereditary in-

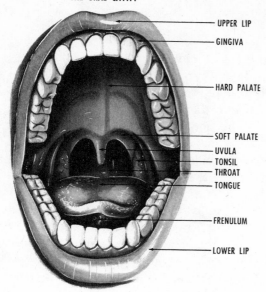

UPPER LIP

GINGIVA

HARD PALATE

SOFT PALATE
UVULA
TONSIL
THROAT
TONGUE

FRENULUM

LOWER LIP

fluences as size, shape, color, and number of teeth; size and shape of facial bones; and similar characteristics.

During the formative period of the unborn child (fetus) the "within-womb" environment is directly related to the pregnant woman, since many factors affecting her health may in turn produce an effect upon the fetus itself, even though it is enclosed by a sac in the womb. There are, in fact, conditions of the mouth which are related to disturbances of the growth and development of the fetus in the uterus. In some cases prolonged treatment of the mother with certain antibiotics (tetracyclines) may cause the first teeth of the newborn to be more yellow-gray than normal.

During formation of the embryo it is protected by a placental barrier. Substances which penetrate this barrier could produce effects in the embryo. Nature, however, has designed the barrier to be selective, thereby greatly reducing the possibility of disturbing normal growth and development.

At birth the heredity pattern has been established, and from this point on the major factor under our control is the environment. In the art and science of dentistry this control includes two elements: prevention and treatment. To this end dentistry embraces various specialties concerned with these complex concepts:

Endodontics. A branch of dentistry which has to do with the diagnosis, treatment, and correction of diseases occuring within the pulp of teeth (root-canal fillings)

Oral Pathology. A branch of dentistry which has to do with the diagnosis of diseases of the mouth in relation to all changes from the normal (benign and malignant growths)

Oral Surgery. A branch of dentistry which has to do with surgical procedures related to all physical structures of the mouth (extracting teeth and treating fractures of the related bones)

Orthodontics. A branch of dentistry which has to do with the diagnosis, prevention, and correction of abnormal or irregular positioning of teeth and their related structures, so as to maintain proper function and aesthetics (straightening of teeth)

Pedodontics. A branch of dentistry which has to do with dental care in the treatment of children (children's dentistry)

Periodontics. A branch of dentistry which has to do with diagnosis, prevention, and treatment of abnormal conditions of the structures which support the teeth (gum problems and periodontal disease)

Prosthodontics. A branch of dentistry which has to do with the functional and aesthetic replacement of missing oral structures, so as to maintain proper function and pleasing appearance by artificial means (dentures and crowns)

Public Health Dentistry. A branch of dentistry which has to do with the total relationship of dental health to the community (fluoridation of drinking water)

At birth, certain structures of the oral cavity have already developed; however, no functional teeth are normally visible. The first teeth (variously known as primary, milk, temporary, baby, or deciduous teeth) begin formation within the bones of the jaws of the unborn child and are in various stages of development beginning six weeks after conception and until they appear in the mouth.

After birth, the individual teeth continue to develop, and through the process of eruption they migrate toward the oral cavity from their positions within the jaws. This process continues throughout life; however, once the teeth of one jaw contact the teeth of the opposite jaw, the rate of eruption decreases. The lower teeth usually precede the corresponding upper teeth in erupting, and teeth usually erupt earlier in girls and in slender individuals. The teeth emerge into the mouth in a pattern of eruption which follows a normal sequence, even though there is a time variable for each individual. This applies to both primary and second teeth. In fact, a time exists when some primary and some permanent teeth are simultaneously present in both arches, indicating a mixed or transitional phase of growth and development. During one phase in growth, more than forty teeth, primary and secondary, are in various stages of development.

When the primary teeth appear, they are twenty in number: ten in each jaw, arranged to form two horseshoe-like arches—an upper (maxillary) and a lower (mandibular). This primary set consists of teeth of various sizes and shapes, depending upon location and function, which match one another in both the upper and lower arches. For convenience, the ten teeth of the upper arch may be described in terms of the five on the right and the five on the left, using the midline of the face as a dividing point; the same principle applies to the ten teeth of the lower arch. The five corresponding teeth in each of their four quadrants have identical names in relation to their position and function in the arch. Beginning at the midline in the front of the mouth and progressing backward, the primary teeth are the central incisor, lateral incisor,

cuspid, first molar, and second molar.

It is frequently thought that, since the primary teeth are shed at a relatively early age, their retention is not important since the permanent teeth will eventually replace them. Why expend time and effort retaining baby teeth when they are destined to be shed eventually. But it is a mistake to consider the premature loss of primary teeth unimportant. Normally, all of them are in use from the age of two until the age of seven. Certain ones appear as early as six months of age while others remain as late as twelve. During this latter period, children undergo rapid mental and physical changes, and their teeth are essential for their proper development. Unless the primary dental arches remain intact until these teeth are destined to be shed normally, problems of adequate space and proper position for the succeeding permanent teeth can be created. Then too, if the primary dental arches do not remain intact until the proper time for shedding, it may be difficult (if not impossible) for nature to achieve the orderly transition from the primary to the permanent teeth.

Even though all the primary teeth are lost in a definite pattern, the permanent teeth may not occupy ideal positions in their respective arches. Every tooth has a specific reason for being in the dental arch, and thought must therefore be given to the complications which may result from the premature loss of any tooth for any reason. A definite knowledge of all factors related to growth and development is essential to proper alignment and function of either the primary or secondary teeth. It is therefore advised that children should be examined periodically, beginning at an early age, in order to diagnose, treat, and prevent minor dental deformities, thus minimizing the possibility of prolonged and expensive dental procedures later on. These early visits are also valuable in that the child begins his adjustment to dentists and dental treatment without fear.

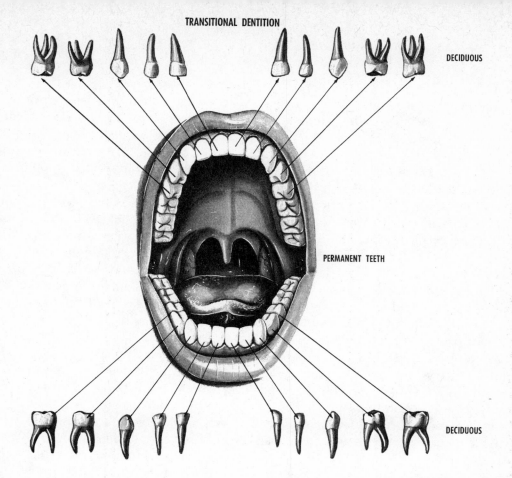

DECIDUOUS

PERMANENT TEETH

DECIDUOUS

Eventually the permanent (secondary, adult) teeth occupy positions in both arches in a normal sequence of growth and development for the individual. Primary teeth are normally shed as some of the permanent teeth assume their positions.

In addition to the twenty secondary teeth which assume the positions of the twenty shed primary teeth, the first permanent molars erupt and occupy positions behind the last primary molars (which will not be shed until about age twelve). In many cases parents may mistake these permanent first molars for primary teeth, since at this time all of the deciduous teeth are usually still present. The first permanent molars serve as "keystones" for the proper positioning of the adult teeth. If they are lost because of neglect, the child becomes a "dental cripple" at an early age (approximately six years).

It will be noted that more teeth are present in an adult than in a baby, for more than twenty permanent teeth will replace the twenty primary teeth which

are shed. The second teeth (adult, or permanent) usually consist of three additional molar teeth in each quadrant. The completed permanent dentition therefore usually consists of thirty-two teeth: sixteen in the upper arch and sixteen in the lower.

As with the primaries, the sixteen teeth of either the mandibular or the maxillary arch may be divided into two groups—those on the right (eight) and those on the left (eight)—again using the midline as a dividing point. In each of the four quadrants there are thus eight teeth which have corresponding names. Beginning at the midline and progressing backward, the permanent teeth of each arch are the central incisor, lateral incisor, cuspid ("eye-tooth," canine), first bicuspid (first premolar), second bicuspid (second premolar), first molar (six-year molar), second molar (twelve-year molar), and third molar (wisdom tooth).

To recapitulate, many events must follow in orderly sequence for adult dentition to function properly. These changes involve the formation and development of unobservable teeth in the jaws and the eruption of twenty primary teeth (by two years of age). These are in turn replaced by thirty-two adult teeth. Any disturbance in these events during this entire process of transition will result in the diminution of the functional efficiency and appearance of the entire dentition.

One may speak of a usual sequence in which individual teeth—primary or permanent—are replaced in normal individuals. Variations do exist from individual to individual, since "birth-date age" may differ from "dental age," depending upon hereditary and environmental influences. However, preceding, during, and following the eruption of teeth, their supporting structures are also developing.

In some cases it is possible to demonstrate that either the upper or the lower arch, or both, may not be sufficiently "long" to accommodate the teeth which must occupy positions within them; if an arch thus lacks sufficient room, the teeth will be twisted, rotated, crowded, and malpositioned. The same result may be observed if the teeth are excessively large or extra teeth are present.

Spacing between some of the teeth is normal and desirable in the primary dentition. Once all of the permanent teeth have erupted, however, spacing is detrimental both to the teeth and their supporting structures. Such spacing can occur either when the arch is large but the teeth are normal in size, or when there are fewer teeth present (for example, before all the permanent teeth have erupted or when some are lost). Either of the above situations may be evident in various proportions in the upper or lower jaws. Furthermore, certain habits may create problems related to the positioning and functioning of the teeth: thumb-sucking, tongue-thrusting, the biting of foreign objects, etc.

The premature loss of a primary tooth may create a problem of insufficient space, resulting in the malpositioning of the permanent tooth. An opposite possibility is that in which a primary tooth may be retained for a longer period than normal, preventing the proper sequence of eruption of permanent teeth. The premature loss of a primary tooth results in movement of the remaining adjacent teeth into the empty space, so that the permanent tooth which is in the process of developing does not have sufficient room to erupt. This is particularly serious if it is a primary molar which is lost before the first permanent molars erupt; since the latter are the first adult teeth to appear, any malpositioning of these keystones influences the positioning of all the permanent teeth. The teeth are designed to sustain themselves and their supporting structures, and any malpositioning hastens their loss.

In order to function properly during the process of chewing, the teeth of the upper arch must occupy positions which will allow them to "mesh" properly with the teeth of the lower arch, in a fashion similar to the meshing of gears. It is the lower jaw (mandible) which opens and closes, and provides the forces necessary for chewing; whereas the upper jaw (maxilla) acts as a fixed base. In the process of chewing, forces are created by the contraction of particular muscles which pull the lower jaw against the stationary upper jaw, pulverizing the food between the teeth. It is this repeated opening-and-closing action that reduces the size of the food particles between the upper and lower teeth, permitting the food to be intermixed with saliva, and swallowed. The efficiency of mastication depends upon the number of chewing strokes it takes to pulverize food particles to a particular size; if the teeth do not mesh (occlude) properly—that is, if teeth are missing, malpositioned, or badly broken-down—this efficiency is greatly decreased. More stresses

MUSCULAR AND SKELETAL SYSTEMS

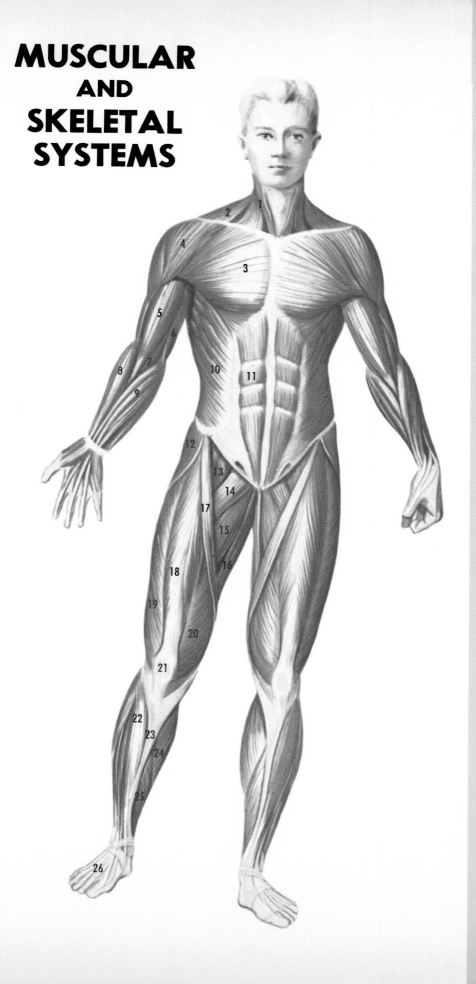

THE MUSCLES

1 STERNOCLEIDOMASTOID
2 TRAPEZIUS
3 PECTORALIS MAJOR
4 DELTOID
5 BICEPS
6 TRICEPS
7 BRACHIALIS
8 BRACHIORADIALIS
9 FOREARM FLEXORS
10 EXTERNAL OBLIQUE
11 RECTUS ABDOMINIS
12 TENSOR FASCIA LATA
13 ILIOPSOAS
14 PECTINEUS
15 ADDUCTOR LONGUS
16 GRACILIS
17 SARTORIUS
18 RECTUS FEMORIS
19 VASTUS LATERALIS
20 VASTUS MEDIALIS
21 PATELLA
22 TIBIALIS ANTERIOR
23 TIBIA
24 GASTROCNEMIUS
25 SOLEUS
26 EXTENSOR TENDONS OF FOOT

ILLUSTRATED BY

LEONARD D. DANK

ST. LUKE'S HOSPITAL
NEW YORK CITY

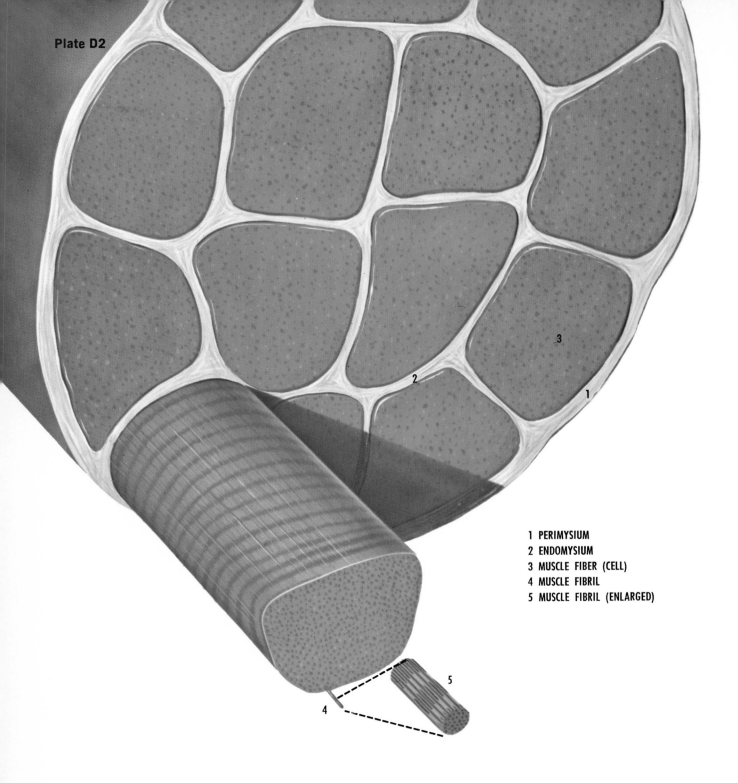

1 PERIMYSIUM
2 ENDOMYSIUM
3 MUSCLE FIBER (CELL)
4 MUSCLE FIBRIL
5 MUSCLE FIBRIL (ENLARGED)

CROSS SECTION OF A MUSCLE BUNDLE

A voluntary muscle is composed of numerous muscle bundles. Each bundle, surrounded by
an outer covering (perimysium) contains many muscle fibers (cells). Each fiber, ensheathed
in the endomysium, contains thousands of longitudinal fibrils. Each fibril is composed of
long and short filaments (5) which impart a cross-striated appearance. Since the stria-
tions of all the fibrils are in register, the fiber as a whole seems to be cross-striated. The
actual mechanism of contraction is thought to involve the sliding of the short over the long
filaments.

CONTROL OF THE MUSCLES

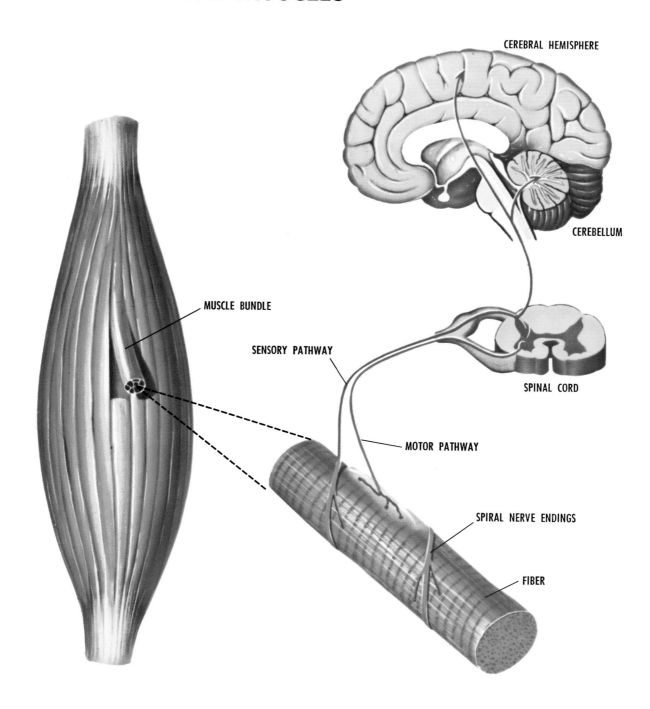

CEREBRAL HEMISPHERE

CEREBELLUM

MUSCLE BUNDLE

SENSORY PATHWAY

SPINAL CORD

MOTOR PATHWAY

SPIRAL NERVE ENDINGS

FIBER

Where fibers stretch or relax, they stimulate spiral nerve endings which send sensory impulses to the spinal cord. Motor impulses are activated and return to the fiber causing it to contract. This unconscious "stretch reflex" maintains the muscles in a state of balanced partial contraction called "tonus." If many muscles are involved, sensory impulses are sent to the cerebellum, the chief unconscious muscle coordination center. Impulses may also go to the cerebral hemispheres, to inform the conscious mind of the state of the muscles.

MUSCLE ACTION

1 SCAPULA
2 HUMERUS
3 TRICEPS
4 BICEPS
5 ULNA
6 RADIUS

In order to produce movement, a muscle must be attached to at least two bones. When the triceps, attached to the scapula, humerus, and ulna, contracts, it extends the ulna. Muscles occur in antagonistic pairs: the triceps extends, the biceps flexes the forearm.

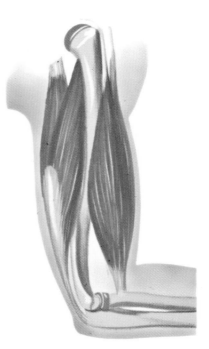

As the biceps contracts, the triceps relaxes.

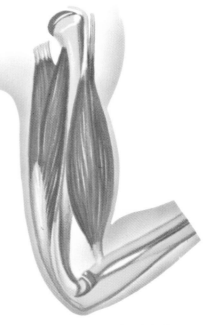

The fully contracted biceps has flexed the forearm. The triceps is fully relaxed.

ANATOMY OF BONE

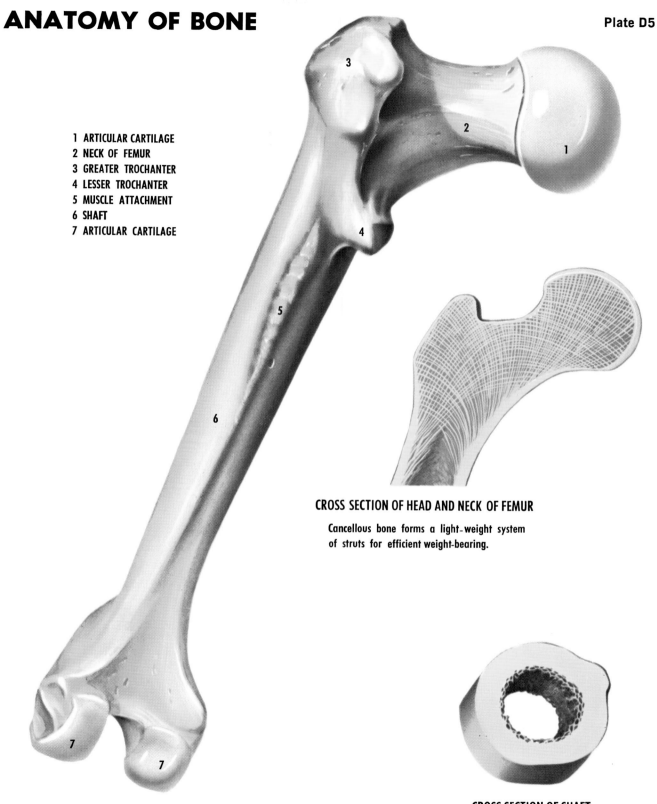

1 ARTICULAR CARTILAGE
2 NECK OF FEMUR
3 GREATER TROCHANTER
4 LESSER TROCHANTER
5 MUSCLE ATTACHMENT
6 SHAFT
7 ARTICULAR CARTILAGE

CROSS SECTION OF HEAD AND NECK OF FEMUR

Cancellous bone forms a light-weight system of struts for efficient weight-bearing.

POSTERIOR VIEW OF FEMUR

CROSS SECTION OF SHAFT

Bone is hollow to reduce weight.

SKELETON IN INFANCY

Most bones are preformed as cartilage which bone tissue gradually replaces. Some bones are not fully replaced until the late teens; the articular cartilage is never replaced.

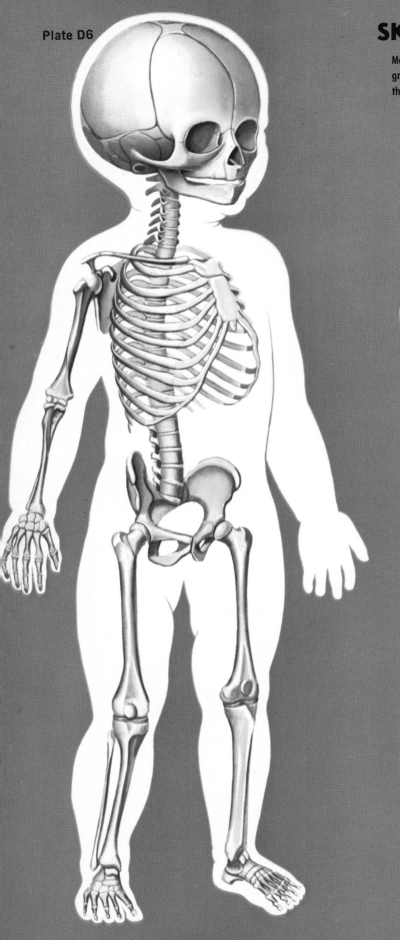

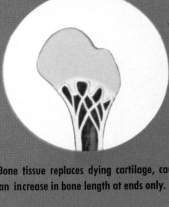

Bone tissue replaces dying cartilage, causing an increase in bone length at ends only.

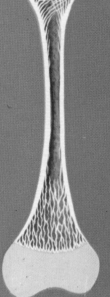

CROSS SECTION OF NEWBORN FEMUR

yellow = bone
blue = cartilage

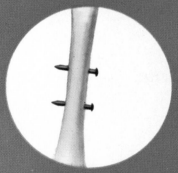

Pins inserted in femur at birth will be same distance apart in adult. Only circular growth occurs in the shaft.

SKELETON IN ADULT

Some cartilage persists in the adult. This cartilage lines the joints, and forms part of the rib cage.

GROWTH OF A BONE (Femur)

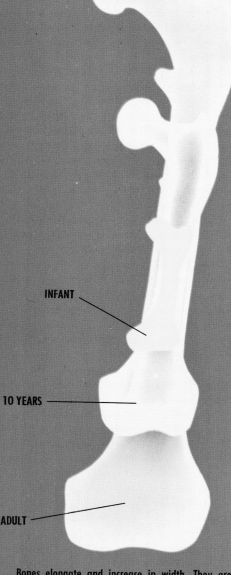

INFANT

10 YEARS

ADULT

Bones elongate and increase in width. They are also remodeled to reach final conformation.

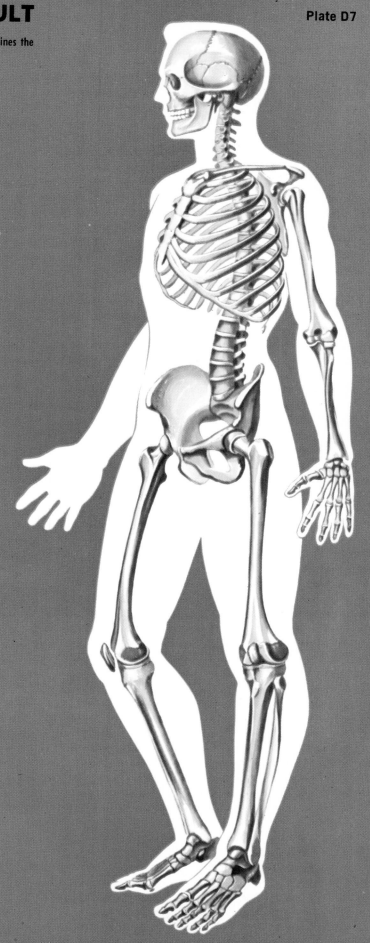

ARTICULATION OF BONE AT A JOINT

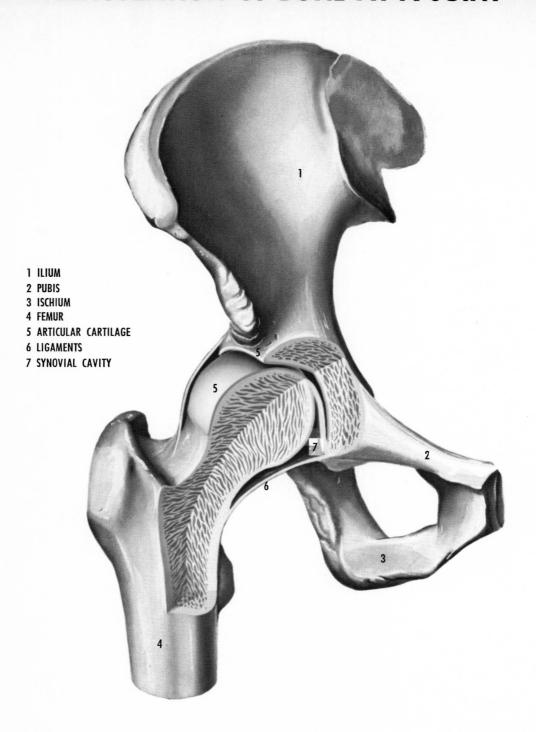

1 ILIUM
2 PUBIS
3 ISCHIUM
4 FEMUR
5 ARTICULAR CARTILAGE
6 LIGAMENTS
7 SYNOVIAL CAVITY

CROSS SECTION OF FEMERO-PELVIC JOINT

Most of the freely movable joints are of the synovial type. Both bones are covered with a thin layer of articular cartilage to reduce friction. The inside of the joint contains a mucous lubricant called synovial fluid. Various ligaments hold the joint together.

THE PERMANENT DENTITION

THE DECIDUOUS DENTITION

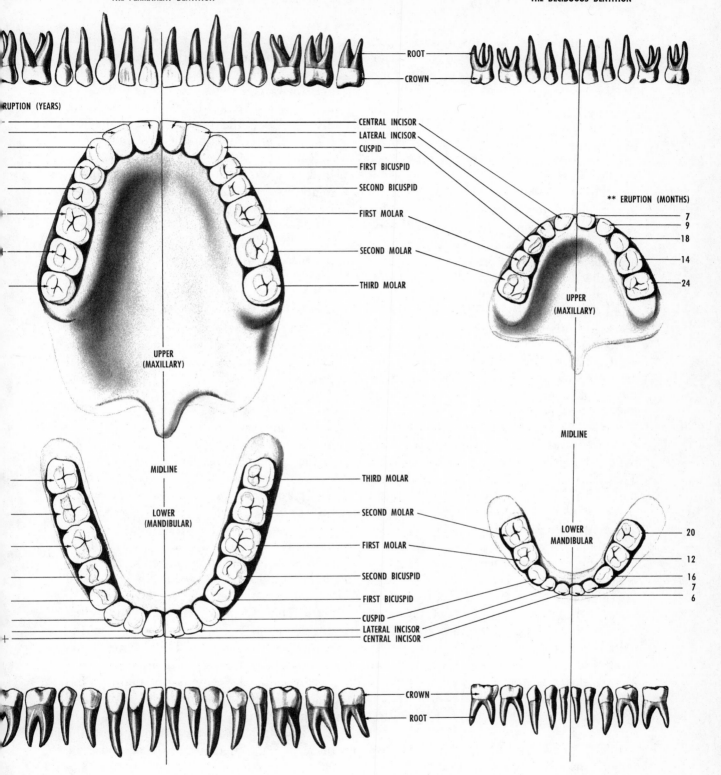

ROOT

CROWN

RUPTION (YEARS)

CENTRAL INCISOR
LATERAL INCISOR
CUSPID
FIRST BICUSPID
SECOND BICUSPID
FIRST MOLAR
SECOND MOLAR
THIRD MOLAR

** ERUPTION (MONTHS)

7
9
18
14
24

UPPER
(MAXILLARY)

UPPER
(MAXILLARY)

MIDLINE

MIDLINE

THIRD MOLAR
SECOND MOLAR
FIRST MOLAR
SECOND BICUSPID
FIRST BICUSPID
CUSPID
LATERAL INCISOR
CENTRAL INCISOR

LOWER
(MANDIBULAR)

LOWER
MANDIBULAR

20
12
16
7
6

CROWN
ROOT

* Plus or minus 1 year
** Plus or minus 1 month
All teeth are drawn to same magnification

and strains are placed upon those teeth present, and teeth that are so badly overworked and made to perform extra functions may thus be lost.

Though the primary function of the dental apparatus is mastication of food, it also functions in the production of sound and, needless to say, it is related to aesthetic appearance.

The individual teeth of both arches are designed to perform specific jobs related to their position and shape. The incisors, located in the front of both arches, are chisel-shaped and designed for cutting like the blades of scissors; the cuspids occupy a position at the corners of the arches and are spear-shaped for holding, tearing, and cutting. Collectively, these teeth are known as the front (anterior) teeth. The six front teeth in the upper arch are in a more forward position (overjet) and overlap the six corresponding lower teeth (overbite).

The bicuspids and molars are positioned at the back of the arch and are hence known as the back (posterior) teeth. These have pointed projections (pyramidal cusps) and broad biting surfaces like a potato masher, designed for crushing and grinding food. When the muscles contract and pull the lower jaw upward, the chewing surfaces of the lower back teeth make contact, in a meshing action, with large areas of the opposing surfaces of their upper counterparts. To prevent biting of the cheek and tongue, the upper posterior teeth are placed closer to the cheek than are the lower; these latter, in contrast, are placed closer to the tongue. The tops of the cheek surfaces of the lower posterior teeth thus fit into the middle of the biting surfaces of the upper posterior teeth.

The lower jaw (mandible) has two projections which rise in a more or less vertical direction from its horseshoe-shaped body. By means of these projections, the mandible is hinged on either side to the temporal bones of the skull, just in front of the ears. These temporomandibular joints, right and left, are so designed that the mandible can move from side to side and forward and backward, as well as up and down like a hinge. A cartilaginous disc between the bones of the joint permits smooth functioning during various movements. Malpositioned, lost, or badly broken-down teeth may produce problems related to the temporomandibular joints by not permitting smooth movements. Either of the joints, or both, may become painful; a clicking sound may develop; or dislocation can occur. In fact, any disease which can affect the joints of the body (rheumatism, arthritis, etc.) may produce problems in the temporomandibular joints. System-wide factors may also affect the muscles related to opening and closing the jaw. For example, "lockjaw" (tetanus) is produced by a bacterium (*Clostridium tetani*) commonly found in dirt; this bacillus can enter the body by contaminating a wound, and eventually cause spasms of the muscles of the jaw. (Tetanus shots are one of the routine immunizations given to children because, without protective measures, the percentage of fatalities is extremely high.)

To withstand all the forces related to mastication, the individual teeth have certain things in common: their composition, supporting structures, and general formation and arrangement within the jaws. Though there are many individual differences between the primary and the permanent teeth, their basic composition is similar in that each consists of four tissues—enamel, cementum, dentin, and pulp. (The first three are hard tissues and the last is soft.)

Enamel, the hardest substance in the body, is composed primarily of inorganic calcium compounds arranged in rods. Between the rods are microscopic amounts of organic cementing material which binds the rods together. It is this protective cover which is initially penetrated by dental caries (dental decay). The bulk of the tooth under the enamel and cementum is dentin, which is bone-like. The dentin, in the form of tiny tubules, contains more organic material than the enamel and is rapidly destroyed once the decay process has penetrated the enamel. For some unexplained reason, the dentin tubules transmit sensations of heat, cold, etc., from the exterior to the internal nerves of the tooth in the form of pain. Hence, repeated periodic pain in a tooth should be a warning that the protective coverings of the tooth are no longer intact. Early dental treatment can usually resolve this problem, alleviating the pain and preventing the possible loss of the tooth.

Each tooth is divided into a root and a crown. The root is usually longer than the crown and is that part which is embedded in the bone of the jaws; the crown is the part which is usually visible in the oral cavity and contacts the adjacent and opposing teeth. Since the crown is exposed to the oral environment, it is subject to destruction from wear and the process of decay. The dentin of the crown is covered by a hard mantle of enamel and the dentin of the root is covered by a thin layer of cementum.

There is a longitudinal canal in the center of the hard tissues of the crown and root which ends as a minute opening at the tip of the root (apex). The pulp occupies this canal and furnishes the blood and nerve supply. As long as the tooth is alive, it can form new dentin along the walls of the pulp canal or chamber to protect the pulp from external harm. (Enamel does not possess this ability.) If the blood supply is destroyed (either by a blow which ruptures the vessels, or by bacteria which enter the pulp via a deep cavity) the tissue will die; the tooth will not respond normally to external stimuli (heat and cold) and the pulp will be non-vital. Unless dental treatment is initiated, a health hazard exists, since bacteria can in-

fect a local area of the jaw, and from there the whole body. The tooth may have to be removed unless the root canal is cleaned, sterilized, and sealed (root-canal filling).

It has been mentioned that the crowns of the teeth vary in shape according to function; this is also true of the roots. The upper and lower front teeth usually have one root apiece, the lower molars have two, the upper molars have three, and the bicuspids may have one or two. (The cuspids, located at the corners of the arches, have the longest roots and should be retained as long as possible. These strong teeth may eventually serve as attachments for artificial appliances which replace other missing teeth.)

The supporting structures act mainly to hold the roots firmly fixed in the jaw. The portion of either jaw which provides this support is the alveolar bone, and the bony socket is called the alveolus. Fibers of a particular membrane (the periodontal) are dense and elastic, and attach the alveolar bone to the cementum of the root. This ligament not only serves as a means of attachment for the tooth but also acts as a shock absorber, cushioning the tooth and bone from the forces of mastication. Though the membrane occupies the small space between the root and the "socket," it consists of thousands of fibers which encompass the tooth from its apex to its neck. This allows the tooth to move very slightly without injuring the blood vessels and nerves which enter the tooth at its apex. If any disease or injury results in damage to the periodontal membrane, the tooth will no longer be anchored properly to the bone and will become loose.

The protective covering for the body is the skin, while in the mouth the covering is termed the mucous membrane (mucosa). The mucosa immediately surrounding the necks of the teeth is called the gingiva (gums). This tissue is subjected to considerable forces of friction and pressure during chewing. Utmost care must be taken to avoid injury to it, since such injury might eventually result in involvement of the other supporting structures.

The mucosa appears pink, since it lacks the thick layer of keratin found in ordinary skin, and thus allows the blood vessels to show through. The color of the gingiva serves as a measure of its health: normally it is pale pink, firm, and stippled, and does not bleed readily. It must fit tightly around each tooth like a collar, otherwise debris from the mouth will accumulate in this area and infection of varying intensity may ensue. If confined to the gingiva, the infection is termed gingivitis; if, however, the infection progresses to the periodontal membrane, the condition is known as periodontitis. If either of these conditions persist, the structures supporting the teeth are weakened, and even though the involved teeth may be free of caries they may eventually be lost because of insufficient support. Periodontal disease is the major cause of tooth-loss in people past thirty. (Before this age, the major cause is dental caries.)

As already mentioned, the teeth actually begin developing about six weeks after conception, and by birth the crowns of the deciduous teeth are in varying stages of completion. Those of the incisors are generally completely formed, whereas those of the molars have only begun. Usually, by the time the first permanent teeth erupt the crowns of all teeth have formed completely, the first of the deciduous teeth have completed their life cycle and are in the process of shedding. In all cases, a tooth develops beginning at the biting edge and proceeds gradually to the end of the root. The root is not actually fully formed until the tooth has been visible in the mouth for some time; this accounts (in some cases) for the mobility of newly erupted teeth, both deciduous and permanent. The life cycle of both sets of teeth is similar except for the fact that the deciduous teeth are naturally shed, whereas those of the permanent set are intended to remain in function throughout life.

A tooth actually begins forming from certain cells which line the fetal jaws. These cells begin to multiply and grow at the site of each future tooth. In this stage, the "tooth-buds" within the fetal jaw do not actually resemble a tooth but (as their name implies) are actually bud-shaped; later, the buds begin to resemble the shape of the teeth they are to form. This is the "blueprint" stage, and it is during this phase that damage to the bud may result in a badly shaped tooth.

The cells of the bud begin to specialize, each group assuming the role of forming a certain part of the tooth: some are delegated to form enamel, others dentin, and so forth. At this point the developing bud resembles only the outline, or soft framework, of the crown portion of the tooth it is destined to produce. This spider-web-like framework is then gradually filled in and hardened by the deposition of certain inorganic salts, mainly calcium phosphate. This calcification process results in the formation of the familiar hard enamel and underlying dentin of the crown and—eventually—the root. These inorganic salts of calcium are derived from: (1) the bloodstream of the mother in the case of teeth developing in the unborn child; and (2) the bloodstream of the child itself after birth. Once teeth have been completely calcified, calcium salts can *not* revert to the bloodstream of the mother; calcium in the teeth of the mother therefore cannot be removed during pregnancy to be deposited in the forming teeth of the fetus. The apparent increase in dental caries and other oral diseases during pregnancy is generally due to neglect of oral hygiene, the acid products of vomitus, poor dietary habits, and hormonal changes in the oral tissues.

The source of bloodstream calcium and other necessary minerals for calcification should be assured by adequate intake of foods rich in calcium and vitamins. The roles of vitamins A, B, C, and D in the development and calcification of teeth is well established, and these must be present in adequate amounts.

After the enamel and dentin of the crown have been calcified, the root begins to take shape through formation and calcification of the dentin and cementum that comprise it. At the time the root begins to grow, the tooth begins its movement toward final eruption into the mouth. As mentioned previously, however, the entire root is not completed for two to four years following the eruption of the tooth.

The eruptive process is essentially the same for deciduous and permanent teeth; but in the case of those permanent teeth which actually take the place of deciduous ones, the deciduous root must be resorbed or shortened before the erupting permanent tooth beneath can take its intended position in the mouth.

The precise mechanism of the forces which cause a tooth to erupt, or those factors responsible for the resorption of the deciduous roots, are not completely understood. Neither the eruption of all teeth nor the shedding of deciduous teeth can be explained by the mere fact that the root of the erupting permanent tooth is growing in such a way that its crown is causing pressure on the root of the deciduous tooth to be shed; in other words, the eruption of all teeth and the exfoliation of deciduous teeth cannot be explained solely on the basis of pressures. This is proven by the fact that occasionally a tooth without a root will still erupt, and a primary tooth may be shed that has no underlying permanent tooth to cause pressure. Deciduous teeth which do not shed, because of the lack of permanent teeth to replace them, may not resorb completely and may in this case remain in position.

Nature has been extremely lenient to man in providing him with two different sets of teeth. This doubling of organs does not occur in any other part of the body. The development and eruption of deciduous teeth, their shedding and replacement by permanent teeth, and their shape and arrangement so that they are self-sustaining, are all only a small part of the master plan and miracle of life.

DENTAL HEALTH AND BAD HABITS

There are a number of physical habits which may be detrimental to dental health. Among these are: thumb- or finger-sucking; tongue-thrust; excessive use of pacifiers or teething rings; biting on pencils, hairpins, or other hard objects; lip-biting; resting of chin in hand ("thinker's pose"); sleeping on one side of the face with constant pressures exerted in one area of the dental arch; use of a pipe in one area of the mouth; abnormal and constant movements of the jaws (biting cuspid to cuspid); bruxism and bruxomania (persistent gritting of teeth); excessive use of toothpicks or other objects for cleaning the teeth; bone-chewing; cigar-chewing; cuticle- and nail-biting; excessive use of citrus juices; excessively hard or soft diet; mouth-breathing; nail- or needle-holding; cracking of nuts or opening of bottles with the teeth; and thread-biting.

The adverse effects of some habits upon the teeth or their supporting structures are too involved to mention here. Diagnosis and correction of these habits is often extremely involved and may require the advice of professional personnel in many fields. On the other hand, some—such as thumb-sucking and nail-biting—are quite easy to detect and (in some cases) simple to correct.

As with all habits, the individual will is the deciding factor in correction. In the very young, this is of course difficult to instill, but patience and competent advice will aid in the solution of this problem.

DENTIFRICE   Any preparation used to assist the toothbrush in cleansing the accessible surfaces of the teeth is known as a dentifrice. Such preparations may be in the form of flavored liquids, powders, or pastes which contain soap or detergents. (It should be noted that some dentifrices contain sugar as a sweetening agent and therefore, at least in part, tend to defeat their purpose: that of preventing caries.)

Powders and pastes usually contain some type of abrasive. A common constitutent of pastes is a liquid, such as glycerin. The powders are generally more abrasive than the pastes and liquids, and thus might be more easily misused. The primary purpose of abrasives is to remove stains from teeth; if, therefore, teeth are not prone to staining, there is no real need for the abrasive agent. The occasional use of sodium bicarbonate with a wet toothbrush will usually prove very effective in the removal of stains.

It should be noted that the use of a toothbrush and a dentifrice should not only cleanse the teeth, but should also be beneficial to other oral structures, such as the gingiva. This involves both proper use of the brush itself and choosing a dentifrice which aids in the cleansing action. (The use of dentifrice containing fluoride compounds has proven to be effective in the reduction of caries, but the fact remains that this method alone is not the best one for applying fluorides; it is merely one technique of topical application.)

A mixture of equal parts of salt and sodium bicarbonate remains one of the best available cleansing agents, but in all cases the choice of the dentifrice, the brush, and the technique of brushing should be determined by the dentist on the basis of individual needs.

DENTURES This term is generally used to denote those removable appliances which are designed as the replacement for several or all of the missing teeth and their adjacent tissues. The artificial teeth are attached to a base which resembles the gingival tissue.

There are two main types of dentures: full (complete dentures), replacing all of the missing teeth in either the upper or lower jaw; and partial dentures, replacing some, but not all, of the missing teeth and depending upon remaining natural teeth and tissues for retention and support.

Any artificial appliance replacing a part of the body which has been gradually or suddenly lost (for example, an artificial limb or a crutch) is not readily tolerated by the rest of the body, especially the immediate area. The entire body must become accustomed to the changes necessary in its daily routine. The same is true to some degree in regard to persons adapting to full or partial dentures. This replacement (prosthetic) appliance cannot possibly be as efficient as the organ or organs it replaces, especially if these were functioning well when they were lost and replaced. Full dentures, for example, may be no more than 40 per cent as efficient as the normal teeth which they replaced. If, however, only a few teeth existed at the time of replacement, or those that were replaced were not functioning completely, the prosthetic appliance may be more efficient than the natural teeth. The final success of any dental prosthesis depends primarily upon the patient's ability to adapt to it, assuming that it has been designed and constructed with the individual's particular requirements in mind. The factors that must be considered can only be ascertained and evaluated by a dentist who has given careful study to all facets of the patient's physical and psychological traits.

In some cases, it is possible to remove the remaining teeth and replace them immediately with previously constructed dentures (immediate dentures). In other instances, the remaining natural teeth must have been extracted some time prior to the initial phases in construction of dentures; this allows sufficient time for healing and for stabilization of the process of resorption which always follows the extraction of natural teeth.

Although the gingiva and bone eventually become more physically static, the process of resorption (and other changes) invariably continue throughout life, just as other physical characteristics change. These changes require that dentures be adjusted, readapted, or remade periodically, since although they themselves do not normally change, the living parts with which they are associated do. When the physical changes reach a certain point, the dentures must be remade or altered to fit the existing condition. This "remake" or alteration (reline, rebase) requires the utmost skill and training on the part of the dentist, who is able to diagnose and prescribe the exact changes necessary to insure the proper design of the revised appliance.

The mere refilling of the dentures by the addition of material to replace the resorbed tissue is not necessarily enough to insure the proper functioning of dentures. Other factors, such as occlusion of the denture with the opposing teeth, the restoration of profile and speech characteristics, and changes in jaw interrelationships and movements must be considered and accomplished.

DENTURES, CARE OF   Although dentures are inanimate objects which normally do not change, they must be cared for properly. Dentures should be stored in room-temperature water when not in the mouth. The dentist will usually inform the wearer as to whether or not dentures should be worn during sleep; in general, they are removed at night to provide rest for the tissues upon which they lie. The dentures themselves may be cleansed either with ordinary dentifrices and a brush, or with special denture-cleaners and brushes. Care of the gums (gingiva) and

remaining teeth is of primary importance. These should be brushed to remove accumulated food particles and to provide needed stimulation. In many cases, warm salt water as a mouth wash is beneficial.

DEPRESSION   Everyone has normal mood-swings ranging from excitement at one extreme to depression at the other extreme. In a normal person these mood-swings are usually of mild degree, oscillating between mild exhilaration and mild depression or melancholy. Such cycles of emotionality are entirely normal. Under certain conditions, however, they become abnormally exaggerated, resulting in pathological excitement and depression.

Symptoms. Depression is an abnormal mental state characterized by severe feelings of melancholy, worthlessness, sadness, self-depreciation, and self-hate. The depressed person feels that everything has gone wrong in the world. He tends to lose interest in life, nothing appeals to him any more, and he derives no enjoyment from normal things; instead, he tends to brood about all the evil in the world, particularly his own sins and shortcomings. Many depressed people cry constantly and express feelings of worthlessness and self-hate.

There are two important patterns of depression: reactive and endogenous. In reactive depressions, mood-disturbance is to some degree proportionate to some real event in the person's life. A widow may become depressed following the death of her husband, and in this case there is a valid reason for her reaction, Reactive depressions are relatively hopeful as to outcome, and usually disappear within a matter of months, irrespective of treatment.

Endogenous depressions are apparently due to physical disorders of the brain centers controlling emotions. They tend to appear insidiously without any obvious cause. Psychoanalysts believe that some endogenous depressions may involve unconscious reactions of self-hate, in which the person is punishing himself for something very evil which he thinks he has done. Whatever the cause, endogenous depressions tend to show a pattern of increasing melancholy and depression until, at their height, the depressed person may feel that all is hopeless and suicide the only solution. At this point the person may lose interest even in eating and have to be force-fed.

Some depressed patients show a large hysterical component manifested by crying, agitation, and overt displays of anguish. This behavior represents an unconscious bid for sympathy and help from observers. Unfortunately, reassurance or solace does little good for those in an agitated state, since their verbalizations are largely irrational and unanswerable.

Treatment. All seriously depressed persons should be admitted immediately to a psychiatric hospital because of the ever-present danger of suicide. It is safest to consider the seriously depressed as potentially suicidal, to be kept hospitalized as long as any depressive trends remain. One of the worst mistakes is to accept reassurances on the part of a depressed person that he or she is not contemplating suicide.

Depressive states have been one of the more easily treated psychiatric conditions; most cases spontaneously recovering within six or eight months if suicide is prevented. Electric shock treatment results in rapid disappearance of symptoms in most cases, but is potentially dangerous and should not be prescribed until all other methods have failed. The recent development of many highly effective antidepressant drugs has resulted in a very high percentage of cures of depressive symptoms, and has made electroshock unnecessary in most cases.

Even though modern psychic energizers may effectively remove depressive symptoms, they should always be supplemented by psychotherapy directed at re-moving the basic causes: guilt, feelings of worthlessness, and self-hate.

Only a competent psychiatrist can render an opinion concerning the seriousness of suicidal threats, which should always be taken seriously. The old saying that "those who threaten suicide are never the ones who do it" cannot be depended upon, since such people frequently get up courage to carry out the threat. Any severely depressed person is potentially suicidal and should be placed under psychiatric observation immediately.

DERMATITIS   The word dermatitis denotes merely inflammation of the skin. It is often mistakenly used to denote a specific condition of the skin, but the word dermatitis has little meaning without a modifying word or phrase to describe either the appearance of the dermatitis (exfoliative, exudative), the location of the dermatitis (palmaris, plantaris), the causative agent of the dermatitis (medicamentosa, plant, occupational, diabeticorum), or a factor in the mechanism of production of the dermatitis (varicose, allergic, atrophic). The term is also used as part of a compound name for a specific disease caused by infecting microorganisms, as in infectious eczematoid dermatitis, dermatitis blastomycetica, streptococcic dermatitis; and by physical agents, as in roentgen dermatitis or dermatitis calorica or solare.

DERMATITIS FACTITIA   This condition is produced by the patient with the ill-conceived notion of achieving sympathy or monetary gain, of avoiding responsibility, or seeking revenge. It is almost impossible to deceive the knowledgeable and sophisticated physician for any length of time, chiefly because the patient cannot sustain the resemblance of the disease he is attempting to mimic in spite of his artistry and ingenuity.

Symptoms. The angular and bizarre configuration of the self-induced lesions;

the preponderance of lesions on the left side of right-handed patients; the sudden inexplicable worsening of lesions; the "un-physiologic" course of an eruption; and, finally, the disruption of seemingly-un-marked dressings applied by the physician are among the signs of self-induced der-matoses. Although most patients are careful not to produce irreparable harm, scarring and infection are no deterrent to a patient determined on this course of action unless he is confronted with irre-futable evidence of his activities and is further convinced of their futility.

Treatment. No treatment of the skin is usually necessary. It is often not difficult to convince the patient of the diagnosis. More important is to help the patient find a way out of his dilemma that is sensible and constructive.

DERMATITIS HERPETIFORMIS (DUHRING'S DISEASE)

Of unknown causation, this disease is most common in adults but is occasionally also present in children. It is primarily a disease of the skin and is not associated with any other condition. Many variants of the usual skin lesions and distribution of these lesions sometimes make the diagnosis difficult, and a biopsy (study of a microscopic specimen of the skin) may be necessary.

Symptoms. The lesions consist of papules and vesicles (small blisters) arranged in groups situated over the eminences of the back (shoulders and buttocks) and distributed also over the rest of the trunk and the extremities. The groups of lesions can vary considerably in size, and also in duration (weeks to months), with fresh crops of lesions appearing irregularly and periods of remission unpredictable. The involution of a lesion is often succeeded by an area of increased pigmentation which can remain for years. The condition is accompanied by severe itching.

While the cause of the disease is not known, an attack can be induced or worsened by certain foods, notably those containing free iodine (shellfish) and drugs containing bromides or iodides. A diagnostic skin test with potassium iodide is often used in questionable cases.

Treatment. The two most commonly employed remedies are sulfa drugs and arsenic (Fowler's solution). Either of these can be very effective; but treatment, because it is usually prolonged and repetitious, must be under the physician's surveillance. Avoidance of iodide- and bromide-containing foods and medicines is essential.

DERMATOLOGY

Dermatology is the science of the skin in health and in disease. Historically, dermatology is the oldest discipline in medicine, not only because its overt display of disease could be contemplated before even the crudest instrumental aids were invented, but also because the skin was available for observation over varying periods of time. This has permitted documentation of many diseases of lengthy duration and tortuous course such as syphilis and leprosy; of swift and devastating infections such as smallpox, erysipelas, diphtheria, gangrene; and of slow and unremitting conditions such as lupus, cancer, and scleroderma.

Dermatology is the oldest discipline, and the most challenging, for the same reason: its availability. One can see the disease process directly; not indirectly by a shadow cast on an X-ray film, or by looking at a blood smear and interpreting from it what the bone marrow is doing, or by testing with dyes and deducing from this the function of the liver. The dermatologist can observe the details of the disease process—then can alter the process and study it. The skin can be excised and looked at under a microscope; it can be transplanted to another site, to another person, to another species; it can be stained and observed; or chilled and observed; or heated and observed; or peeled and observed; or even treated and observed. The disease can be smelled (as in pemphigus) and in sweatiness (bromidrosis); it can be felt (leathery, nutmeg-grater-like, horny, velvety, marble-like, doughy, woody). Readily observable for study are the colors and the shades of color of different diseases, the many shapes and configurations of the lesions, each unique for each disease, or at least for each disease of similar dynamic mechanism.

And for all its availability and notwithstanding the countless recorded facts and therapeutic victories, there remain unanswered the myriad questions seemingly capable of ready answer. Why is most itching worse at night and, as a matter of fact, why do temperatures rise at night in most febrile diseases? Where in its growth does kinky hair get its kink and how does it retain it for its full growth for its entire life; how do "circles" under the eyes get to look that way; why does a person seemingly not changed in any other way suddenly develop an allergy to something he has been exposed to with no reaction for many years, as for instance poison ivy, shoe leather, or aspirin; how do warts disappear overnight after being present for years; why does nobody contract leprosy in a temperate climate; what has happened to make scabies such a rare disease when only a few years ago it was endemic?

As in other fields of medicine, so too in dermatology, the physician today practices with a host of therapeutic modalities undreamed of a few short years ago. With their causes not yet established, treatment is nevertheless now available for a great variety of both serious and inconveniencing diseases such as pemphigus, cancer, lupus erythematosus, scleroderma, vitiligo, alopecia areata among others. And diseases of known cause, such as boils, leprosy, fungous infections, erysipelas, allergies, syphilis, diseases of vitamin deficiency and of hereditary disarrangement, are among those for which cure is now possible where prevention is not possible. The science of the skin, part of the complex science of medicine, shares in the labors and in the rewards of alleviating the diseases of man.

DERMATOLYSIS (CUTIS LAXA)

This is a condition of looseness of the skin resulting in the skin lying in folds. There is no elasticity, and when the skin is stretched it does not rebound. This is in contrast with cutis hyperelastica, an inherited condition of excessive elasticity of the skin associated with hyper-flexibility of the joints, fragility of the blood vessels, and other defects including clubfoot and dental anomalies.

DERMATOMYOSITIS

This poorly understood syndrome occurs at almost any age and in both sexes. The skin lesions consist of varying-sized red plaques which are occasionally slightly elevated and hive-like. The lesions become atrophic or hardened (scleroderma-like). Concomitant changes in the muscles result in swelling, pain, and tenderness, followed by atrophy of the muscles and crippling contractures. Other changes include puffiness of the eyelids, enlargement of the liver and spleen, fever, and anemia. A significant number of patients have cancer (adenocarcinoma) of an internal organ.

Treatment. Eradication of the cancer in patients in whom this appears to be the cause of the dermatomyositis usually results in remission of the skin and muscle symptoms. For patients not affected by malignancy, the cortisone remedies afford a high percentage of remissions, some of them permanent.

DEVELOPMENT, PSYCHOLOGICAL

Research indicates that the average human brain does not achieve complete maturity of function until about fourteen years of age. During the course of life, every person passes through standard phases of development: prenatal life, infancy, childhood, adolescence, early adulthood, adulthood, change of life (the climacteric), old age, and senility.

Maturation of the central nervous system, including the higher brain functions, is ordinarily measured by observation of different types of behavior. The infant, for example, should be sitting up at six months, standing alone at twelve months, walking at twelve to eighteen months, talking at fifteen to eighteen months, and becoming toilet trained by twenty-four months. The average child learns to count at age four or five, to read at age six, and to master increasingly more difficult subjects at the times when ordinarily presented in the regular school grades. (Similar patterns of development occur in relation to emotional maturation, to socialization, self-control, and ability to maintain personality integration under increasingly stressful life situations.)

Psychologists now recognize that wide individual differences normally exist in the rates of development of different mental functions. Children of high intelligence and superior native endowment tend to show precocious patterns of development, and schooling and other developmental experiences should be adjusted to their needs. Conversely, delayed patterns of development may result from many factors, emotional instability in particular. The child burdened with emotional conflict may show all kinds of developmental retardation, starting with late talking and toilet training in infancy, reading disabilities and other forms of educational retardation in school, and a variety of conduct disorders in community life. Where extreme disorders of personality development are evident, the child should be referred to a child guidance clinic for psychological and psychiatric evaluation.

DEXTROSE Dextrose is the technical name of the biologically important sugar white crystalline powder ($C_6H_{12}O_6$), also called d-glucose. This is derived from fruit sugar and from starch. Dextrose is the form in which sugar appears in the blood. A solution of dextrose may be dripped into the vein or administered through a tube passed into the stomach.

DIABETES, BRONZED (HEMOCHROMATOSIS This is a rare disorder manifested by deposits of hemosiderin (an iron-protein compound found in all body tissues and possibly the result of decomposition of hemoglobin, the coloring element of blood). Hemochromatosis most often occurs in the liver and the pancreas. The cause is unknown; it is probably due to a deficiency in iron metabolism.

Symptoms. Hemochromatosis most often afflicts elderly males, three-quarters of whom show the classical signs of diabetes, bronzing of the skin, and cirrhosis of the liver. Other manifestations include atrophy (shrinkage) of the testicles, enlargement of the liver, and the formation of fibrous tissue in the heart muscle. Laboratory examination of the blood and/or microscopic study of a skin specimen determine the diagnosis.

Treatment. To prevent the building up of iron deposits in the tissues, weekly bleeding (usually a pint) of the patient is required until the iron in the blood serum is depleted.

DIABETES IN PREGNANCY Although most women with diabetes have a very good chance of bearing normal children, there is a definite hazard to the mother and child. Diabetes is almost invariably more difficult to control during pregnancy. Insulin requirements are more variable and diet is more difficult to regulate. Of greater importance from the long-range standpoint is the fact that the effects of diabetes on the kidneys may be aggravated by the increased burden of pregnancy.

The effect of diabetes on the unborn child is also apt to be harmful. Prematurity is common in diabetic pregnancies, and stillborn infants are more often encountered than in normal mothers. Furthermore, many babies of diabetic mothers are excessively heavy.

Ordinarily the pregnant diabetic woman with severe kidney disease and high blood pressure should undergo a therapeutic abortion and sterilization. Religious motivations may modify this recommendation in individual cases. In general, it is wise for diabetic women who know they also have either high blood pressure, kidney disease, or eye complications to avoid pregnancy.

DIABETES INSIPIDUS In this rare disorder, which is unrelated to diabetes mellitus, damage to the posterior portion of the pituitary gland causes the passage of large volumes of water due to the disruption of the secretion of antidiuretic hormone. In some cases as much as twenty-five quarts of urine per day may be excreted, compared to the normal amount of about one quart per day.

Symptoms. There is excessive thirst with afflicted individuals perhaps consuming as much as fifteen quarts of water daily. Diagnosis of this condition is sometimes difficult because people with certain nervous disorders are also inclined to drink large amounts of water.

Treatment. Treatment of diabetes insipidus is with a posterior pituitary hormone that regains the body's antidiuretic ability. This hormone may be taken by injection, in tablet form, or by blowing a powder into the nose. Treatment is usually lifelong, although some cases have improved spontaneously.

DIABETES MELLITUS (SUGAR DIABETES) Diabetes mellitus affects about 2 percent of the American population. It occurs among all age groups, but most commonly makes its appearance between the ages of forty and sixty. Studies indicate that about 10 percent of those over age sixty have diabetes mellitus. Twice as many women as men have the condition. In the mid-1970s diabetes mellitus was the major factor in more than 36,000 deaths annually.

The diabetic person is not able to produce or regulate the hormone insulin, which is produced in the pancreas. Insulin is necessary to control the level of glucose (a type of sugar) in the blood. If glucose is not properly assimilated by the body, it will accumulate in the blood and tissues, and be passed out of the body in the urine. This results in the loss of nutrients and energy the body needs in order to carry out basic activities.

There are two major categories of diabetes mellitus. Juvenile-onset diabetes appears in children or young adults and requires regular injections of insulin and strict dietary controls so that proper blood glucose levels are maintained. Juvenile diabetics have increased risk of developing degenerative changes and diseases of the eye and kidneys.

Adult-onset diabetes is generally less severe than juvenile diabetes. Sometimes the symptoms are so subtle the condition is overlooked. Usually adult-onset diabetes can be controlled with dietary restrictions alone or with added drug therapy. For adults, diabetes means a greater risk of eye disorders, such as cataracts, and greater susceptibility to infection, among other health problems.

Diagnosis of diabetes is made by the detection of sugar in the urine and abnormal amounts of it in the blood. It should be recognized that there is a normal level of sugar in the blood at all times, a level that varies somewhat, depending on the time of day and length of time after a meal. Usually, however, there should be no sugar in the urine. Diabetics may test for urine sugar by simple methods such as noting a color change when a piece of chemically impregnated paper is dipped into the urine. In some instances a sugar-tolerance test is performed at which the patient is given a measured amount of glucose solution, followed by analysis of blood and urine sugar concentrations at intervals of several hours. A number of other tests have been developed to detect diabetes in questionable cases.

Symptoms. The diabetic who is taking appropriate treatment should not normally feel ill. When treatment is inadequate, or when the initiation of the disease is sudden, acidosis and coma may result. This is a potentially serious condition and must be treated at once. It may be marked by a feeling of dullness and fatigue followed by nausea and vomiting. The senses become dulled and the patient becomes progressively more stuporous. Usually this condition is preceded by increased thirst together with increased urine output, which causes loss of large amounts of body fluids and minerals making the patient dehydrated. There is also a characteristic deep breathing described as "air hunger," as a result of the body's attempt to restore a normal balance of acids and bases.

Important late complications of diabetes are found chiefly in the eyes, kidneys, and blood vessels. The eyes may be afflicted by changes in the retina or by cataracts. If these problems are severe enough, blindness may result. Small blood vessels in the kidneys may also suffer damage, causing the kidneys to shrivel and decrease their ability to remove poisons from the circulation. Arteries may become narrower and calcium deposits may build up. This may lead to clotting in the arteries of the brain, thus producing strokes; and to the complete stoppage of arteries in the lower extremities, producing gangrene.

In children the onset of diabetes may come on suddenly with extreme thirst and increased output of urine. Itching in the genital region or elsewhere may also occur. One of the most common precursors of diabetes in adults is obesity. It is recommended that obese adults should have their urine checked for sugar at least yearly after the age of forty.

Treatment. Treatment of diabetes for the past fifty years has been primarily with insulin. During the past fifteen years, however, substances have been developed that can be taken by mouth in mild diabetes to lower the blood sugar and spare the pancreas. Attempts are also being made to manufacture synthetic insulin incorporating the techniques of genetic engineering. Currently insulin is processed from pork and beef pancreases. In any case, because the body is not able to manufacture insulin and vary its concentration, it is vital that the patient maintain a carefully regulated diet.

The balance of carbohydrates, proteins, and fats must be kept within close limits, and meals should be taken at regular intervals; each individual's dietary prescription should be worked out by the physician. The obese diabetic is put on a weight-reduction program. Exercise is carefully regulated and infections are carefully avoided. For older diabetics care of the feet is especially important. Corns and calluses should be cared for by someone acquainted with the diabetic's tendency to develop infections and gangrene. Proper footwear should be worn to prevent the development of corns, calluses, and ingrown nails. (See also INSULIN SHOCK.)

DIAPER RASH The term diaper rash is usually reserved for eruptions of the diaper area thought to be due to contact of the skin with urine and feces. Other skin diseases (moniliasis, contact dermatitis, impetigo) which are not uncommon in the diaper area are discussed under specific headings. There is no definitive evidence that urine high in ammonia content causes diaper rash, nor is it necessary to establish such a causation mechanism to explain the condition. Diaper rash is quite similar to heat rash, and is the result of the macerative effect of the moisture (both urinary and sweat), the presence of a great number of potentially infective organisms from the urine and feces, and the susceptibility of the thin and vulnerable infant skin to the damaging effects of both these factors.

Symptoms. The buttocks and groin are the site of redness, small papules, occasional pustules, and in aggravated cases, peeling of the skin. Small boils can appear on the labia or on the penis.

Treatment. Thorough drying of the skin after each diaper removal and frequent change of diapers are essential for both prevention and treatment. Starch baths (a handful of starch added to the infant's tub), soothing lotion (calamine), and when infected, antibiotic ointment (bacitracin, Neosporin®), are effective. Application of oil should be avoided because it occludes the sweat gland openings, causing heat rash and further macerating the skin.

DIAPHRAGM   This is the chief muscle of respiration and expulsion and separates the abdomen from the thorax.

Diaphragm is also the name of a birth control device. (See CONTRACEPTION.)

DIARRHEA   This term refers to abnormally frequent bowel movements of fluidlike fecal matter. Diarrhea is frequently caused by minor infections of the intestinal tract and is commonly referred to as acute enteritis or intestinal flu (no relation to influenza).

Many disorders of the alimentary canal are accompanied by diarrhea of varying severity. Colitis, regional enteritis, some liver disorders, and emotional disturbances may have diarrhea as the cardinal symptom. The term dysentery usually refers to a condition of greater severity, in which blood and mucus make up a prominent portion of the stool. (See also HOME NURSING CARE.)

DIARRHEA IN CHILDREN   Diarrhea is the frequent passage of loose and/or watery stools. The form of diarrhea most common in children is due to a virus; some

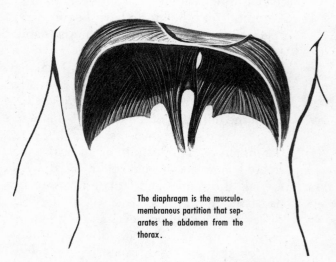

The diaphragm is the musculomembranous partition that separates the abdomen from the thorax.

sensitive children, however, show a limited type—lasting through only three or four bowel movements—after eating certain foods to which they are allergic.

Symptoms. Diarrhea may or may not be accompanied by fever, cramps, and blood in the stool. (The presence of blood often characterizes dysentery, a more serious, bacteria-caused condition.) The typical picture of the disease in the child is one in which the patient suddenly becomes ill, with vomiting which continues for from twelve to twenty-four hours and is then immediately followed by diarrhea. If the condition is severe enough, the patient may dehydrate.

Common childhood diarrhea usually continues for approximately a week. Between the spasms of cramps and loose stools, the diarrhetic patient usually feels almost normal, except for a sense of weakness.

Treatment. There is no specific treatment. Plenty of fluids are needed to guard against dehydration, and only white (bland) foods are allowed, as these have no roughage. The diet is also a low-fat one. Typically, it would consist of rice, toast, tea, banana, applesauce, gelatin, and custard. Most doctors advise stopping milk for several days and substituting only clear liquids; then, after two or three days, the milk is restored slowly, in diluted form.

DIET   What a person eats has a profound effect on his well-being, but because individuals vary so much in age, height, weight, physical activity, inherited characteristics, and so on, there is no single "normal" diet plan. Current nutritional knowledge, however, indicates that a wide variety of foods helps to insure a better diet for whatever the individual needs may be. One-sided and "crash" diets are apt to be deficient or harmful if consumed for more than a very short while. Furthermore, for many illnesses a physician's advice concerning diet is extremely important.

Caloric needs and food preferences vary widely, but there is a minimum of certain types of food (see BASIC SEVEN) which forms the basis of a normal dietary intake. Around this minimum a full diet can be planned with considerable freedom of choice of foods.

The basic daily diet plan for adults (which supplies about 1,500 calories) is briefly as follows:

Milk: 1 pint

Meat, fish, or poultry: 1 average serving (about 3½ ounces)

Egg: One

Additional protein foods: 1 egg, ½ pint milk, or 1 ounce of fish or cheese

Vegetables: 1 medium potato or 2 servings of a leafy green or yellow vegetable or 1 serving of another vegetable

Fruits: 1 serving of citrus fruit or juice, or noncitrus fruit

Butter (or enriched margarine): ½ ounce

Breads and cereal: 4 slices of enriched or whole-grain bread, or 3 slices of bread and ½ cup serving of enriched cereals

DIET IN PREGNANCY   One of the most disturbing and occasionally dangerous complications of pregnancy is excessive weight gain. The appetite in general is improved during pregnancy and, unless the pregnant woman watches the quantity and quality of her caloric intake, she may gain tremendous weight and endanger both her life and that of the baby.

The total weight gain during the entire pregnancy should not normally exceed twenty to twenty-five pounds. This can be accomplished without much difficulty provided the patient stays on an average diet of 2,000 to 3,000 calories daily. The quality of the food should be checked in order to make sure it provides more proteins and more vitamins and minerals than the average diet. Sufficient quantities of meat, fish and poultry, fruits and vegetables as well as an average of one quart of milk daily should be the basis of a proper diet for the pregnant woman. In addition, the expectant mother will require extra amounts of iron and calcium and several vitamins. All these requirements are easily met today, with special multi-vitamin and mineral preparations usually taken in one-a-day form.

Sudden weight gain during the last few weeks or months of pregnancy should be considered a danger sign, especially if accompanied by swelling ankles, puffiness of the face, and headaches, and should be immediately reported to the physician.

DIGESTIVE DISORDERS   A broad definition of digestive disorders would include any condition or disease that might interfere with the breakdown and absorption of ingested foodstuff. Impaired digestion may result from mechanical problems such as ill-fitting dentures or poor dental repair. Extensive surgery on the gastrointestinal tract may leave a shortage of absorptive surfaces. An obstruction due to tumors, scar tissue, kinking of the bowel, or a foreign body will impede the passage of food and hamper the digestive process.

Generalized infections may cause a temporary decline in the efficiency of the digestive apparatus such as is seen in the vomiting which accompanies many illnesses. Localized infections of the stomach, liver, gallbladder, pancreas, and intestine can cause disturbances in the secretion of the necessary digestive ferments or enzymes, and interference with absorption may likewise result from infections of specific portions of the intestine. In cases of diarrhea, ingested food passes through too quickly to be utilized, and in chronic cases severe malnutrition may result. Certain diseases such as sprue (lack of vitamin B_6) and celiac disease are characterized by poor absorption of fats. Voluminous greasy, foul-smelling stools may result. The treatment of these various disorders depends upon their cause.

DIGESTIVE TRACT   The digestive (alimentary) tract comprises the mouth or oral cavity, the gullet or pharynx, the esophagus, stomach, small intestine (considered to have three areas—duodenum, jejunum, and ileum), large intestine or colon, rectum, and anus. In addition to this irregular tubular structure, the digestive tract involves such food-processing organs as the salivary glands, liver, gallbladder, and pancreas.

The digestive tract consists basically of a cavity (lumen), through which nutrients pass. This is lined by mucous membrane (mucosa), behind which there is a muscular layer. Behind the muscle, in turn, there is an outer layer of connective tissue. The mucosa is lined with various cells; some produce mucus, a thick lubricating fluid, whereas others secrete digestive enzymes. Folds of mucosa called villi enable an enormous surface area to be exposed to the substances in the digestive canal.

DIPHTHERIA   Diphtheria is an acute infectious disease to which children are particularly susceptible and whose main focus is in the nose, throat, and larynx. The specific agent is a bacterium called *Corynebacterium diphtheriae,* isolated by Loeffler in 1884. This bacillus cannot survive outside the human body; hence, the human host is the only significant reservoir of the germ and the one responsible for its transmission, usually through cough. Not every person infected by the Loeffler bacillus contracts the disease; this will depend on the germ's virulence and the victim's susceptibility. Those in whom examination of the throat does reveal the presence of bacilli but who do not exhibit clinical signs of illness, are called carriers. This condition is dangerous and such individuals should be isolated and intensively treated to prevent them from spreading the germ to receptive persons.

Virulent diphtheria bacilli have the property of secreting a specific poisonous substance (diphtheria toxin) which is responsible for the local damage characteristic of the disease, as well as for distant complications in the body.

Symptoms. The incubation period is short, ranging from one to four days. The clinical manifestations depend on the anatomical site of the primary infection (throat, nose, larynx) and the severity of the infection. Throat diphtheria is described here as a typical form. Onset of the disease is abrupt, with chills, moderate fever, malaise, and sore throat. On examination the throat is dull red in color, this stage being followed by formation of a grayish, gelatinous pseudomembrane which first appears over one tonsil, then spreads to the other. The neck glands are slightly painful. When the disease is mild, these are the only manifestations. The disease may, however, continue to spread upward to the back of the nose and downward toward the larynx, creating a particularly

THE INTESTINAL TRACT
(ALSO CALLED ALIMENTARY CANAL OR DIGESTIVE TRACT)

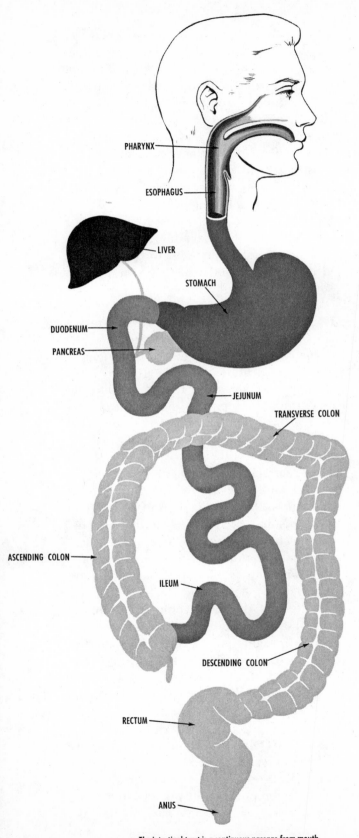

PHARYNX

ESOPHAGUS

LIVER

STOMACH

DUODENUM

PANCREAS

JEJUNUM

TRANSVERSE COLON

ASCENDING COLON

ILEUM

DESCENDING COLON

RECTUM

ANUS

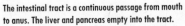

The intestinal tract is a continuous passage from mouth to anus. The liver and pancreas empty into the tract.

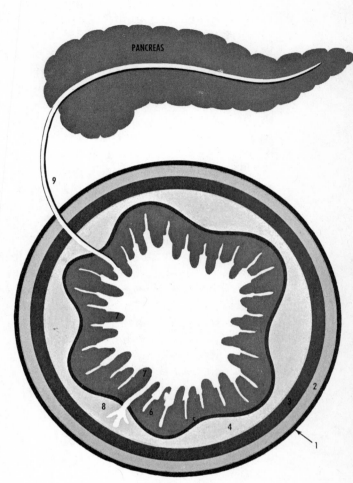

PANCREAS

SCHEMATIC CROSS SECTION

The schematic cross section illustrates the general plan of any part of the digestive system.

1   OUTER COVERING
2   OUTER MUSCLE LAYER
3   INNER MUSCLE LAYER
4   SUBMUCOSA
5   MUSCULARIS MUCOSA
6   LAMINA PROPRIA WITH GLANDS
7   VILLUS
8   GLAND IN SUBMUCOSA
9   EXTERNAL GLAND DUCT

dangerous situation (see Laryngitis).

If the disease is not promptly and vigorously treated, diphtheria toxin may give rise to serious complications, the most important being involvement of the heart (myocarditis) and of the nervous system (in the form of muscular paralysis). These complications usually appear during the third to fifth week of the improperly treated disease, when convalescence has been erroneously assumed.

Treatment. The most important step is prompt administration of diphtheria antitoxin in adequate amounts. The role of antitoxin is to bound and neutralize the diphtheria toxin and prevent further damage. Hence late administration may be ineffective if serious cellular damage has already occurred. Since the antitoxin is a foreign substance (horse serum), precautions should be taken if the patient has previously received other similar serums because of the possibility of an allergic reaction which may be extremely severe. Antibiotics may also be used if secondary bacteria are present. Bed rest is mandatory and the usual hygienic measures are helpful. A careful watch for the development of complications should be maintained.

Prevention by active immunization is feasible and practiced widely today, especially in combination with tetanus and whooping cough vaccination during infancy. Still, it should be remembered that booster doses are necessary at intervals because immunity decreases with time. If a person has been exposed to diphtheria and there is reliable evidence that he has been adequately vaccinated in the past, all that is required is a new booster dose of vaccine. If such assurance is not forthcoming, antitoxin serum should be administered.

DISLOCATION OF THE KNEECAP (PATELLA)

Dislocation of the kneecap (patella) is a condition in which the kneecap slips out of its groove in the knee joint. The child usually states that the knee went out of place and then immediately jumped back in place. This may be due to a number of causes, including abnormally shaped kneecaps (patellae), knock-knee, and misshaped knee joints. In most cases the condition is recurrent, and some children affected with it are afraid to straighten their knees for fear that dislocation will occur. Each fresh episode may inflict damage on the joint surfaces, and this in turn may lead to degenerative arthritis. Treatment of this condition is surgical.

DISLOCATIONS

Dislocations are the result of sprains of such a degree that the normally opposing bones are no longer in place. Dislocations involve greater force than sprains, since the tear is of sufficient magnitude to separate the joint surfaces and to force one or both of the bones out of the joint through a rent in the joint capsule.

Treatment. The object of treatment is gentle, non-damaging reduction of the dislocation and immobilization of the part to allow healing of the rent in the capsule. Failure to recognize a dislocation early may make manipulative reduction impossible and an open operation may be required.

Perhaps the most common complication of a dislocation is recurrent dislocation of the same part. Recurrences are due to inadequate healing of the capsular rent after the first dislocation, and as a rule require surgical repair of the deficient capsular and ligamentous structures.

DISTENSIONS

Abnormal collections of food or gas as intestinal contents may cause localized swelling and distress. Most cases are temporary and subside spontaneously. A temporary "paralysis" of the gas-

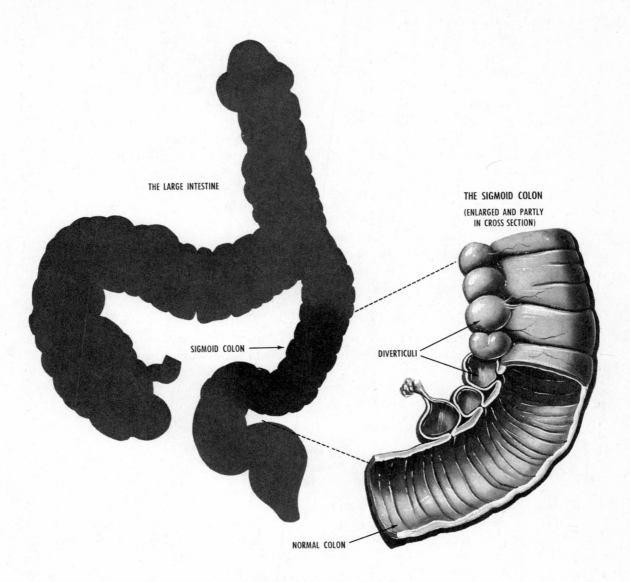

THE LARGE INTESTINE

SIGMOID COLON

THE SIGMOID COLON
(ENLARGED AND PARTLY
IN CROSS SECTION)

DIVERTICULI

NORMAL COLON

DIVERTICULOSIS AND DIVERTICULITIS

trointestinal tract is often present after abdominal surgery and acute stomach distension can be particularly troublesome. Postoperative gas pains are distressing but short-lived and are usually easily treated. Partial or complete obstruction of the bowel will cause marked distension, one of the early signs of this serious disorder. Distension of a portion of the gastrointestinal tract may also be due to peptic ulcers, gallbladder disease, infections, digestive disorders of the small intestine, as well as (more

commonly) emotional disturbances, excessive swallowed air, or constipation.

DIVERTICULOSIS AND DIVERTICULITIS   Diverticulosis is the presence of diverticula, which are small pea-sized outpouchings, usually of the lining of part of the large intestine (sigmoid colon). (These may occur elsewhere in the alimentary canal, but they are the most common in this location.) Causes for their formation are not known; ordinarily they cause no symptoms and do

---

no harm. Inflammation or diverticulitis occurs when the opening into the sac becomes obstructed, favoring bacterial invasion of local tissue; abscess formation and subsequent perforation and peritonitis may follow. Fortunately, such severe complications are rare; the usual case of diverticulitis will subside with conservative treatment.

Symptoms. The symptoms are constant pain in the lower left abdomen, slight fever, abdominal distension, and perhaps an inability to pass gas.

Treatment. Treatment with antibiotics, rest, and cleansing enemas (after being certain that no complications are present) usually suffice. The avoidance of non-digestible foods is helpful in chronic cases.

DOUCHING Medical opinion is not unanimous on whether douching should be part of a woman's hygiene during her reproductive years. Some doctors believe that frequent douching may disturb the natural (benign) flora of the vaginal region and should therefore be avoided except in some infections.

Douching should always be done in a reclining position, preferably in a bathtub. Plain vinegar (two tablespoons to a quart of warm water) is as good a douching solution as any of the commercially prepared ones, and costs practically nothing. If there is persistent vaginal discharge which continues in spite of douching, this is usually due to infection and should be treated by a physician.

DOWN'S SYNDROME See MONGOLISM

DROPSY Dropsy is one of the traditional terms applied to the body-swellings (edema) of congestive heart-failure or kidney infection (nephritis). The term usually refers to swelling of the feet and ankles often accompanying congestive heart-failure.

Drugs

DRUGS Any substance taken to cure, diagnose, or prevent illness, or any substance that affects the regular functioning of body organs, can be considered a drug. Thus, anything from aspirin for headache to vitamin C for the treatment of scurvy can be considered drugs. The term "drug" may also refer specifically to chemical substances that cause physical and psychological dependence. Alcohol, heroin, cocaine, codeine and methaqualone are examples of such drugs.

The origins of many modern medicinal drugs can be traced to folk remedies. For example, the juice of the unripe seed capsule of a poppy has for hundreds of years been known to have narcotic effects. Dried, the juice—opium—is today the source of morphine, a narcotic drug used as a painkiller. Cocaine, used at times as a local anesthetic, comes from the leaves of cocoa shrubs growing in the mountains of Peru and Bolivia. Its properties as a stimulant were known to the natives of these countries before the arrival of the conquistador Pizarro in the 16th century. The leaves of the flower foxglove were used as a heart stimulant for many centuries before digitalis, a medicine prepared from its powdered leaves, was officially introduced to the medical profession in the latter portion of the 18th century. Natives of South America also found a certain plant to be an excellent source of arrow-tip poison. The active ingredient in this concoction, curare, an extremely powerful blocker of nerve impulses, is useful today as a muscle relaxant in anesthesia.

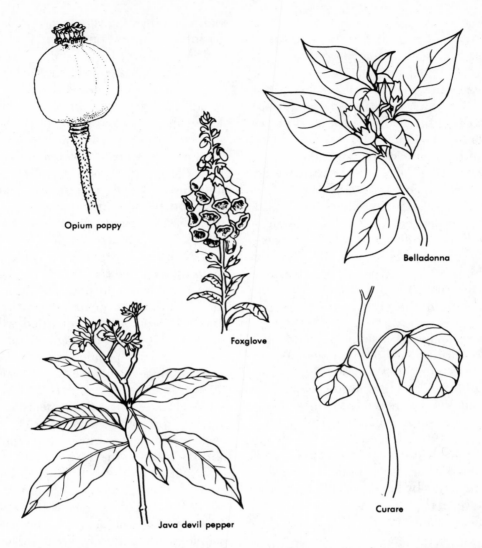

Opium poppy

Foxglove

Belladonna

Java devil pepper

Curare

Plants that are still used in medicine today: The **opium poppy** (*papaver somniferum*), known for over 3,000 years, remains the source of some of our most effective painkillers—morphine, heroin and codeine. **Foxglove** (*digitalis purpurea*) was described in the writings of Welsh physicians in 1250. It yields many currently used heart drugs—the cardiac glycosides, such as digoxin—which increase the force of contraction of the heart muscle. **Java devil pepper** (*rauwolfia serpentina*) has been used by Hindus since ancient times to treat hypertension, insomnia, insanity and even snakebite (because the plant's root resembles a snake). An extract of it, reserpine, became one of the first effective anti-psychotic drugs in Western medicine in the 1950's. While better drugs to treat the symptoms of mental illness are now available, reserpine is still used to treat hypertension. **Belladonna** (*atropa belladonna*), also called deadly nightshade, is the source of atropine and scopolamine. Preparations of belladonna were known to the ancient Hindus. In the Middle Ages they were used by poisoners to produce blurred vision and hallucinations. Today they are used mostly as eye-drops to dilate the pupils. **Curare** (*chondodendron tomentosum*) has been employed for centuries by South American Indians as an arrow poison. Doctors now use it as a muscle relaxant during shock treatment.

In many cases a natural substance, commonly a plant, has both very obvious desirable and undesirable properties. The chemist tries to manipulate the chemical structure of these substances to lessen the undesirable traits. Similar tactics—but applied to drugs originally synthesized in the laboratory—have yielded new and better forms of drugs already of proven value.

Some drugs have been discovered purely by chance. In 1928 the British bacteriologist Alexander Fleming noticed through happenstance that a substance produced by mold could literally cause staphylococci bacteria to dissolve. Fleming called this substance penicillin. His research served as the stimulus that ultimately revolutionized the treatment of germ-caused infections.

The isolation of insulin illustrates another way drugs may be discovered. When Frederick Banting and Charles Best set to work in 1922, scientists were reasonably certain that the pancreas was the most likely source of a sugar-regulating substance. Banting and Best succeeded in identifying this substance because their research methods included a means of protecting insulin from destruction by enzymes in the pancreas. More recently, efforts are being made to synthesize insulin in the laboratory for human use.

Medicinal drugs most commonly used are either prescription or over-the-counter (nonprescription) drugs. Prescription drugs should be taken only on the recommendation of a physician. Medical authorities usually recommend taking only a single ingredient drug for the treatment of a specific symptom or disorder. For example, if one suffers from headache, doctors generally recommend a single-ingredient analgesic such as aspirin, rather than a product that has caffeine in addition to aspirin. Drugs purchased without a prescription should be taken as directed on the package. Taking medications in ways different from a doctor's or manufacturer's instructions may diminish their effectiveness and lead to harmful complications.

Age also plays an important role. Newborn infants seem particularly sensitive to certain drugs because their drug metabolizing systems are not fully developed. Many drugs do cross the placenta during pregnancy, however. The barbituates that are sometimes given to women during labor may be stored in the infants' tissues for a long time, causing respiratory depression.

The new technique of mass spectrometry, which allows researchers to identify the minutest traces of a drug or drug metabolite with extraordinary precision, has been used to detect traces of about 60 different drugs in the body fluids of newborn infants. In a mass spectrometer, the chemical being studied is bombarded with electrons until it splits into fragments of varying mass, forming a specific pattern—the equivalent of a fingerprint for each molecule. Now that these drugs can be detected, scientists can begin to evaluate their effects on infants.

At the other end of the lifespan, considerably less is known about the metabolism of drugs in the aged, and the situation is further complicated by the fact that older patients often take several different medications which may interact with each other. Although more medicines are prescribed for people over the age of 60 than for any other age group, until recently nearly all drug tests on humans were carried out on healthy young volunteers. This was a mistake, since the aged may react to drugs quite differently than the young. Older people may develop toxic reactions to certain drugs when given the same doses as young people (which means that, in general, the old should get smaller doses of these drugs); yet when taking other drugs, the old may require doses that are just as big as those prescribed for the young. There may be changes in the sensitivity of certain cell receptors as people age. Barbiturates, for example, sedate young people but often cause old people to become agitated. Researchers are only beginning to tackle these problems.

In the future drugs will become safer, more potent, and more specifically geared to treat a particular symptom or disorder. (See also ALCOHOL AND ALCOHOLISM.)

Drug Abuse. The consumption of illicit substances, and the misuse of medicines and alcoholic beverages, constitute drug abuse, which may lead to life-threatening addictions. Narcotics such as heroin, stimulants such as cocaine, and hallucinogens such as mescaline and LSD (lysergic acid diethylamide) are examples of controlled substances that are abused principally because they induce euphoric or hallucinogenic states of consciousness. The abuse of prescription medicines such as appetite suppressants, pain relievers, and sedatives is also an increasing problem.

Emotional or other psychological distress may cause a person to abuse drugs. Many people erroneously believe that "medicines" can answer their problems, or provide escape from tension, anxiety, or the boredom of routine. In some situations the abuse of controlled substances such as marijuana and cocaine has become an element of social recreation among the affluent.

Often, especially for young people, experimentation with drugs is a consequence of the need to be accepted by one's peers. Such social pressure can cause young people to do things they would not normally do alone. Too, some drugs come in forms that are legal and acceptable in many social contexts, such as alcoholic beverages and tobacco (nicotine). Yet, the abuse of these substances is perhaps the most widespread, affecting the largest number of Americans. (Each year about one-half of all auto fatalities are associated with the consumption of alcohol.)

The drug abuser places in danger not only his or her own health and life, but may also jeopardize family relationships, or be led into associated criminal activities in order to support the "habit." Although it is true that the majority of people who simply experiment with various drugs do not then become regular drug abusers, there still exists a potentially health-threatening outcome with even the first drug abusing experience, depending on the type, potency, and quantity of drugs consumed. When drugs are regularly abused, the possibility of drug dependencies is greatly increased.

A psychological dependency on a drug exists when the effects of the drug become a part of the person's perception of his or her own well-being. Abusers may then be compelled to seek out and abuse drugs in order to "feel right" about themselves or their environment.

A physical dependency exists only if the withdrawal symptoms (such as nausea, vomiting, nervousness, and muscle tremors) are not psychological. In other words, through prolonged abuse of a drug or drugs the body becomes physiologically conditioned to receiving the drug's effects. Discontinuing the drug may produce severe, potentially fatal consequences.

A number of treatment programs are possible for drug abusers. For drugs other than alcohol, these programs include methadone maintenance, which consists of giving a synthetic narcotic (methadone) to a heroin addict as a substitute. About one-third of the patients in programs funded by the federal government receive methadone. Alcohol treatment programs, including nongovernment organizations like Alcoholics Anonymous (for alcoholic persons) and Al Anon (for friends and family of alcoholic persons), are available in most cities.

Criminal penalties for the possession or marketing of illicit drugs can be severe. Under the Controlled Substances Act of 1970 the United States Attorney General has the authority to classify drugs and drug-containing substances based on their potential for abuse, physiological effects, and history of abuse. The different classifications have different penalties for violations, ranging from one year/$5,000 to

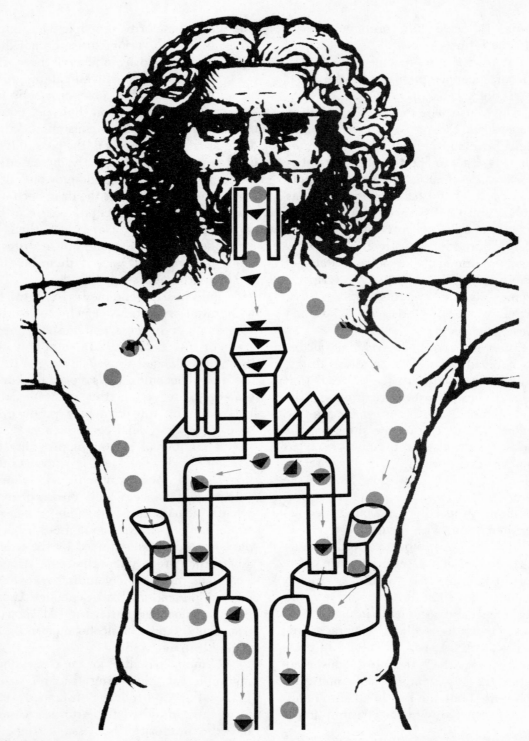

The body's two ways of dealing with chemicals: When substances are water-soluble (gray circles), they go directly to the kidneys and are excreted in the urine, unchanged. Substances that dissolve only in fat (black triangles) go to the liver, the body's main chemical-processing plant, to be transformed into more water-soluble compounds which can be eliminated in the urine.

Some commonly abused drugs:

Drug	Medical application	Common trade name	Potential for physical dependence	Possible withdrawal symptoms
Narcotics: Heroin Codeine	None Painkiller, cough suppressant	None Various including Codeine	High Moderate	Watery eyes, runny nose, irritability, panic, chills and sweating, cramps
Depressants: Barbiturates Methaqualone Tranquilizers	Sedation, sleep, anticonvulsant Sedation, sleep Antianxiety, muscle relaxant, sedation	Amytal, Nembutal, Seconal Optimil, Sopor Quaalude Librium, Miltown, Valium	High High Moderate	Anxiety, insomnia, tremors, delirium, convulsions, possible death
Stimulants: Cocaine Amphetamines	Local anesthetic Hyperkinesis, narcolepsy, weight control	Cocaine Benzedrine, Dexedrine	Possible Possible	Apathy, long periods of sleep, irritability, depression
Hallucinogens: LSD Mescaline PCP	None None Veterinary anesthetic	None None Sernylan	None None None	Not reported

fifteen years/$25,000, for the first trafficking offense. Laws and penalties for the possession of some controlled substances, such as marijuana, vary from state to state.

Concerned parents can do a number of things to prevent or stop their children from using dangerous drugs.

First, parents should be informed about the types of illicit drugs available to young people in the community. It is also important for parents to obtain and read current information about drugs so that their discussion and advice to their children is up-to-date and reasonable.

Second, parents should be aware of the signs of drug use among young people. Often the odor of alcohol and marijuana is hidden with incense, room deodorizers, or perfume. The behavior of the child may also reveal a lack of physical coordination, muddled or confused thinking, or an uncommon intolerance of frustration. If physical evidence of drug use, such as a butt or "roach" from a marijuana cigarette, alcohol containers, powders, pills, eyedrops, or cigarette rolling papers is found, parents should take action.

Third, parents should make it clear that their children will not be allowed to abuse drugs. Perhaps the strongest argument a parent can make is that drug abuse can jeopardize their child's chance of becoming a truly independent young adult.

Fourth, parents should examine their

Slang terms for commonly abused drugs:

DRUG	SLANG TERM
Amphetamines	Bennies, Chalk, Dexies, Speed, Uppers
Barbiturates	Barbs, Blues, Downers, Nimbies, Pinks, Reds, Yellows
Cocaine	Bernice, Big C, Blow, Coke, Nose Candy, Snow
Heroin	Big H, Caballo, H, Horse, Smack, Stuff
LSD	Acid, Haze, Orange Wedges, Strawberry Fields, Sugar, Window Pane
Marijuana	Acapulco Gold, Bush, Gage, Grass, Mary Jane, Pot, Reefer, Stick, Tea, Weed
Methaqualone	Quas, Quads, Sopes
Morphine	Cube, Hocus, Morf, Morphy, Mud
Phencyclidine	Angel Dust, DOA, Hog, PCP, Peace Pill
Psilocybin/ Psilocyn	Mushroom

own drug use habits. What kind of example are they setting for their children? Are medicines used indiscriminately in the household? Is alcohol abused? Parents can instruct by example, whether good or bad.

Fifth, parents should work together to build confidence and create facilities to deal with drug related problems. If twenty parents, and then two hundred parents, decide to work together to eliminate the influence of drugs in the lives of their children, then their community would undoubtedly change.

Drug Allergy. Apart from their medicinal effects many drugs can cause side effects that are undesirable. Some people are intolerant to certain drugs and will have uncomfortable if not dangerous responses to them; they might be advised to use a different medication entirely.

True drug allergy may manifest itself as conjunctivitis, asthma, rhinitis, jaundice, skin eruptions, blood disorders, or various neurologic reactions.

Anaphylaxis is an immediate, severe, and potentially fatal reaction characterized by difficulty in breathing, hives, swelling of the face and neck, and collapse. Penicillin may be the cause of an anaphylactic reaction. If there is any question of sensitivity to penicillin, it should not be administered.

Neurologic reactions to drugs consist of headaches, convulsions, behavior disorders, blindness, deafness, dizziness, and paralysis.

Blood disorders range from the lowering of the white cell count (leukopenia) to a lowering of the blood platelets (thrombocytopenia). Anemia can also be caused by a drug allergy. Usually these complications are temporary and the patient will return to normal when the offending drug is discontinued.

Drug Eruptions. The term "drug eruption" includes all skin diseases caused by drugs taken by mouth, given by injection, suppository, or inhaled. These methods of administration result in the drug being introduced into the bloodstream. Usually excluded from this group is contact dermatitis caused by the allergic sensitization to drugs applied directly to the skin.

The types of skin eruptions due to drugs are varied. Aspirin can cause hives and certain analgesics can cause bleeding into the skin (purpura). Phenobarbital has been shown to cause generalized itching as well as any number of other skin reactions (redness, scaliness). Among other possible skin reactions to drugs are pustular, tumor-like blisters; discoloration; and increased pigmentation.

Skin reactions to drugs are almost always the result of an allergy and are therefore seen only after time for the allergic process to develop (usually seven to ten days after the first dose). It is possible for the first dose of a drug to induce an allergy that is not apparent until a second dose is taken. This second or any subsequent dose may occur at a much later time and not necessarily for the condition for which the drug was first prescribed. Sometimes there is no allergic

response to a drug taken consistently or sporadically for months or years, followed by a sudden and inexplicable allergic reaction to the same drug taken under the same conditions. Because drug eruptions can mimic almost all known skin diseases, it is necessary to consider the possibility of a drug eruption if other diagnoses are unclear.

Hives, measles-like eruptions, and blistering lesions are more commonly caused by penicillin, barbiturates, and sulfonamides. Pustules and boils are the usual eruptions produced by iodides and bromides; and acne-like lesions by cortisones. Loss of hair is produced by thallium and by heparin (but probably not based on an allergic mechanism); an excessive growth of horny skin tissue (keratoses) by arsenic and mercury; seborrheic dermatitis by gold; giant hives by serum.

Unlike any other skin disease a fixed drug eruption consists of coin-shaped, purplish-red, flat lesions occurring in no particular arrangement on any part of the skin, and it may exist as a single lesion. Each time the drug is taken, the affected site develops a red halo around the previously formed lesion, and this newly enlarged lesion becomes purplish as the reaction subsides. The purplish stains persist for a long time after the last intake of the offending drug. A common cause of this type of eruption is phenolphthalein, but aspirin, penicillin, sulfonamides and other drugs have been known to cause this distinctive type of eruption.

Drug induced skin eruptions can be accompanied by reactions to the drug in other organs of the body (anemias, kidney irritation, hepatitis). Often the appearance of the drug eruption establishes the cause of puzzling symptoms observed in other organs.

Drug Reactions. Drug reaction is a general term used to describe any unusual response of the body to any drug. The reaction may vary from itching and hives in a localized area to a severe response that may

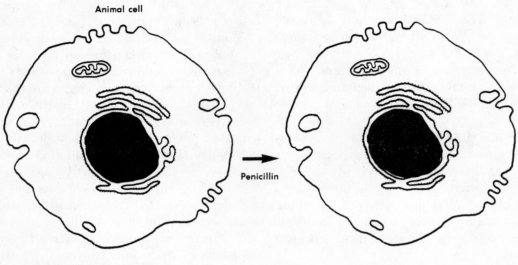

Animal cell

Penicillin

Flexible surface membrane

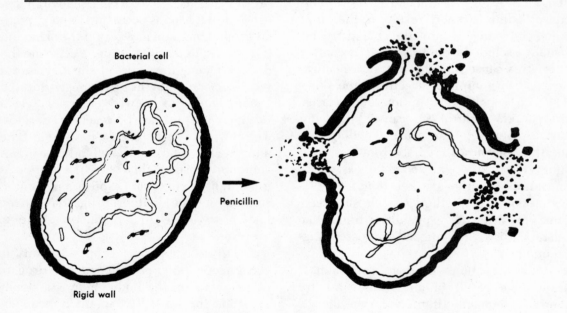

Bacterial cell

Penicillin

Rigid wall

Penicillin kills bacteria without harming mammalian cells because it prevents bacteria from forming the rigid cell walls which they need for survival. Animal cells (above) have flexible surface membranes, also called plasma membranes, and within these cells the osmotic pressure is equal to the pressure outside the cells. Bacterial cells (below) need rigid cell walls around their plasma membranes to help them maintain a higher osmotic pressure within the cells than the pressure outside the cells. When penicillin destroys a bacterial cell's ability to form a rigid cell wall, the bacterial cell ruptures and dies.

have fatal results. A patient should inform his or her doctor of any allergy or sensitivity related to food, pollens, or drugs so that the safest treatment can be employed. If any unusual reactions occur after the first administration of a drug, the doctor should be informed immediately. When sensitivity is related to a particular drug, such as penicillin, written confirmation of this should be carried with the person at all times.

Antacids. Each year Americans spend millions of dollars on medications to relieve the discomfort of indigestion and heartburn. Sodium bicarbonate, aluminum salts, magnesia salts, and calcium carbonate are the four principal ingredients, found singly or together, in nonprescription products. All these products are alkaline and their effect is based on neutralizing excess acid in the stomach.

Self-treatment of heartburn and acid indigestion is usually safe and effective; however, if discomfort persists, medical opinion should be sought. The prolonged use of antacids, or the taking of excessive doses (especially of sodium bicarbonate) can lead to heart and kidney problems.

Some Antacids:

Principal ingredient	Brand name
Sodium bicarbonate	Alka-Seltzer
Calcium carbonate	Tums
Magnesia salts	Gaviscon (liquid)
Aluminum salts	Amphojel (tablet)

Antiflatulent Drugs. The carminative drugs (relievers of flatulence) that promote the release of intestinal gas include alcohol—either alone, or as a tincture of capsicum, ginger, cloves, or cardamon—and a volatile oil such as peppermint. How carminatives achieve what is claimed for them is not certain. However, carminatives are usually irritating to intestinal mucous membranes and may be effective because they increase muscular action in the intestine, thus forcing the expulsion of gas.

Simethicone is a carminative drug often present in antiflatulent medications. It promotes the bursting of gas bubbles in the intestine, which allows the easier release of the gas in the form of flatus or belching. Di-Gel, Mylanta, and Mylicon are examples of over-the-counter products that contain simethicone.

Antimicrobial substances, including Antibiotics. One of the greatest advances in medicine occurred with the discovery that infections could be treated with chemical agents, some of which are produced by certain molds. Since then the number of sources of antimicrobial drugs has expanded and now includes bacteria, fungi, higher plants, and various animal tissues. However, thousands of antibiotics isolated from these diverse sources are of little or no practical value because they are more harmful to the host than to the agent causing the infection.

Nevertheless, an impressive array of antibiotics is available for prescriptive use. Some of these are capable of combating a wide variety of infection-causing organisms and are accordingly called wide-spectrum antibiotics. Penicillin, amoxicillin, ampicillin, and the numerous tetracyclines are examples of wide-spectrum antibiotics.

Penicillin is generally effective against infections caused by organisms including staphylococci (with some exceptions), pneumococci, hemolytic and nonhemolytic streptococci, anthrax, tetanus and diptheria bacilli, and the organisms responsible for gonorrhea and syphilis.

Tetracyclines, a group of broad-spectrum antibiotics, are particularly useful when infectious organisms become resistant to penicillin; or, when individuals are penicillin sensitive and need alternative medication.

In spite of the effectiveness and variety of antibiotics that are now available, che-

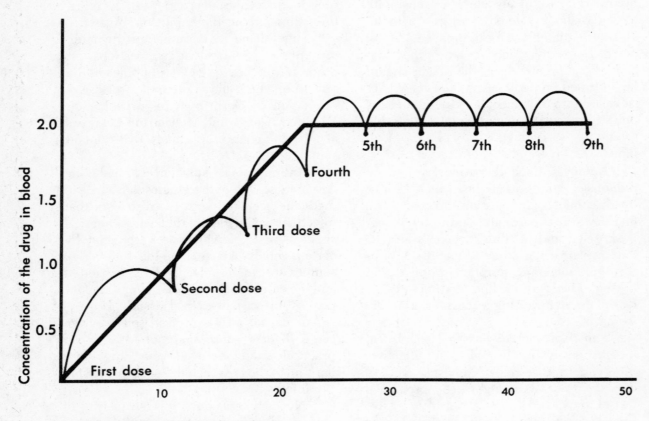

motherapeutic agents (not produced by living organisms) are very valuable in the treatment of certain infections. Sulfonamides and cephalosporins are examples of this type of antibiotic. Sulfonamides are frequently prescribed for urinary tract infections.

When taking an antibiotic it is important to follow the physician's program of administration. Even if the symptoms of an illness subside, one should not discontinue a prescription of antibiotic earlier than advised, unless instructed to do so by the prescribing physician. Levels of the antibiotic in the body must be high enough and present long enough to work a lasting effect.

The bacteria that produce disease may be placed into one of three groups on the basis of their response to a staining procedure devised by Christian Gram in 1884. Briefly, the Gram reaction is as follows: Bacteria which are Gram-positive hold the Gram stain (crystal violet) so completely that they resist decoloration by acetone or alcohol. Gram-negative bacteria, however, release the Gram stain very readily when exposed to either acetone or alcohol. A third group, called Gram-variable, reacts in an unpredictable way, which does not permit placement in either of these categories.

The Gram stain is of great practical importance because it is usually the first step taken in determining the identity of an organism responsible for an infection. Knowing the identity of the organism makes the selection of an antimicrobial agent less difficult.

Immediately upon entering the bloodstream a drug begins to lose its strength as determined by its concentration in the blood because the body begins to metabolize it. As following doses are added at regular periods, a relatively stable concentration of the drug in the blood is eventually achieved. Especially true of antibiotics, it is important that the concentration of the drug in the blood reaches a level high enough and lasts long enough to combat a specific infection effectively. Of course, each drug will have a different rate of weakening (not necessarily the rate shown on the graph) depending on its chemical qualities and on factors particular to the individual, such as weight and age.

Appetite-Reduction drugs. Weight reduction through the use of appetite suppressant drugs should probably be the method of last resort and should be undertaken only upon the advice and direction of a physician. Prolonged use of appetite suppressants (anorexiants) is probably not possible without undesirable side effects. Insomnia and nervousness are examples. Of more concern is the possibility of psychological and physical dependence, which may be followed by withdrawal symptoms when the medication is discontinued.

If obesity is associated with decreased thyroid gland function, the administration of thyroid hormone will lead to appreciable weight loss. However, the loss of weight does not depend upon appetite suppression, but rather upon the alteration of body metabolism. If thyroid dysfunction is not the cause of the obesity, then thyroid hormone will do very little to help; on the contrary, excessive sweating, insomnia, and nervousness will be induced.

Indigestable materials such as methyl cellulose, have been suggested for treatment of overweight. This suggestion is based on the erroneous assumption that the appetite can be satisfied if the stomach is filled with any material whatsoever. A dubious assumption similar to this is the idea that the intake of glucose (in the form of "candies") thirty to sixty minutes before meals will effectively inhibit the hunger mechanisms in the brain. Of course, if this assumption is sound, one could save money by simply consuming a teaspoon of corn syrup thirty minutes before meals.

Sometimes the emotional need to lose weight becomes a potentially dangerous psychological condition. *Anorexia nervosa* is an illness in which a person, usually a young woman, develops an extreme fear of gaining weight and may be so psychologically repulsed by eating that malnutrition and even starvation may result.

Current medical opinion now emphasizes regular exercise and moderate eating habits, rather than reliance on either prescription or nonprescription weight loss preparations. If additional measures are warranted, the advice of a physician should be sought.

Caffeine.   Caffeine is the stimulant drug found in coffee, tea, cola drinks, cocoa, chocolate, and as an additive in some nonprescription pain relievers. If taken in large doses caffeine can produce effects such as insomnia, nervousness, anxiety, and irregular heart function. Approximately 10 grams of caffeine, the amount to be found in 70 to 100 cups of coffee, can be fatal.

Recent research has also linked caffeine to birth defects in laboratory rats. For this reason doctors have begun to advise pregnant women to decrease or stop their intake of caffeine. Caffeine has also been found in the breast milk of nursing mothers who regularly drink and eat caffeine-containing foods.

That caffeine is a prevalent element in the American diet is confirmed by beverage industry statistics. An American consumes on the average of 33.6 gallons of soft drink and 27.8 gallons of coffee each year (compared to 24.8 gallons of milk per person per year).

Cardiac and Circulatory Drugs. A large number of drugs currently in use influence the heart and the performance of the circulatory system.

A heart muscle stimulant (often digitalis) is used in congestive heart failure in which the cardiac muscle is unable to circulate the volume of blood the body requires. Digitalis is the oldest medicine used in heart disease. It is commonly obtained from foxglove leaves, but is also found in other plants and in the venom of certain toads. The effect of digitalis is to strengthen the heart muscle action by increasing its force of contraction, which usually occurs along with a slower heart rate. Because it also acts as a depressant (as well as a stimulant), it is used to maintain normal heart rhythms. Digitalis is a powerful drug. The therapeutic dose is very nearly the same as the toxic dose, so the amount a patient receives must be carefully monitored. Yet, even under the strictest regimen patients experience occasional dizziness, headache, blurred vision, nausea, and diarrhea.

Another cardiac dysfunction is coronary thrombosis. Because the heart depends entirely on the circulatory system for oxygen and nutrients, and for the removal of waste products, when a stoppage of blood through the circulatory system occurs the heart is deprived of these requirements. Such a condition causes the symptoms of coronary thrombosis, commonly called "heart attack." Drugs such as heparin are used as anti-clotting agents (anticoagulants). Heparin acts directly on the clot-forming system; its effects are immediately evident but are of short duration.

The danger of hemorrhage is increased when anticoagulants are used. To guard against an overdose frequent testing of the clotting ability of the patient's blood is required.

Clotting may also occur elsewhere in the circulatory system. For example, a common site is a leg vein, and the resultant disease is called thrombophlebitis. The seriousness of thrombophlebitis, aside from the lack of circulation in the limb, is that very small portions of the clot may break off and enter the bloodstream, possibly to find their way to the lungs or other vital sites.

In contrast to coronary thrombosis, angina pectoris may be described as a condition of diminished flow of blood, which occurs because the internal opening of an artery or arteries has become smaller than normal. Thus it is unable to carry the amount of blood required by the heart, especially under conditions of stress.

Inadequate supply of oxygen and nutrients brings on symptoms of angina pectoris. The most frightening of these is intense pain in the chest, which may be brought on by physical exertion. The pain usually subsides quickly upon the cessation of activity simply because the heart is again allowed to work as hard as the blood supply permits.

Rest and controlled exercise are an essential therapeutic element. In some angina patients an attack, indicated by severe breath-catching pain in the chest, can be ended only with medication. An appropriate dose of trinitroglycerine, for instance, generally offers quick relief because this drug increases the diameter of the constricted arteries, thus allowing the passage of more blood.

There are drugs available in forms that are active for extended periods. These are swallowed as pills and slowly absorbed from the intestinal tract. Examples of this type include isosorbide dinitrate (Isordil) and propranolol hydrochloride (Inderal).

High blood pressure, or hypertension, is often treated with drugs. Some antihypertensive drugs are able to decrease blood pressure by relaxing or dilating blood vessels, which reduces the resistance to the flow of blood. Hydralazine (Apresoline is one trade name) is a unique drug because it reduces blood pressure and increases car-

THE GLANDS

TYPES OF GLANDS

There are two classes of glands: exocrine (with ducts) and endocrine (ductless).

SIMPLE EXOCRINE

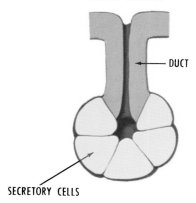

DUCT

SECRETORY CELLS

COMPOUND EXOCRINE

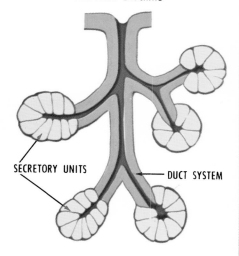

SECRETORY UNITS

DUCT SYSTEM

CAPILLARY

SECRETORY CELLS

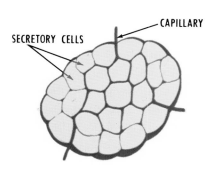

ENDOCRINE

THE MAJOR GLANDS

1 PITUITARY
2 PAROTID
3 SALIVARY
4 THYROID and PARATHYROIDS
5 LIVER
6 ADRENAL
7 GASTRIC
8 PANCREAS
9 INTESTINAL
10 TESTES
11 SKIN GLANDS

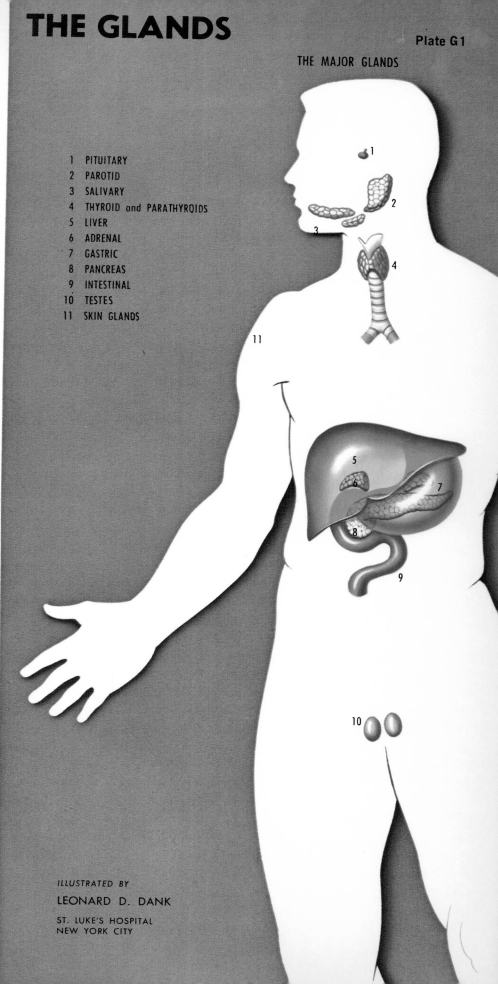

ILLUSTRATED BY

LEONARD D. DANK

ST. LUKE'S HOSPITAL
NEW YORK CITY

THE DEVELOPMENT OF GLANDS

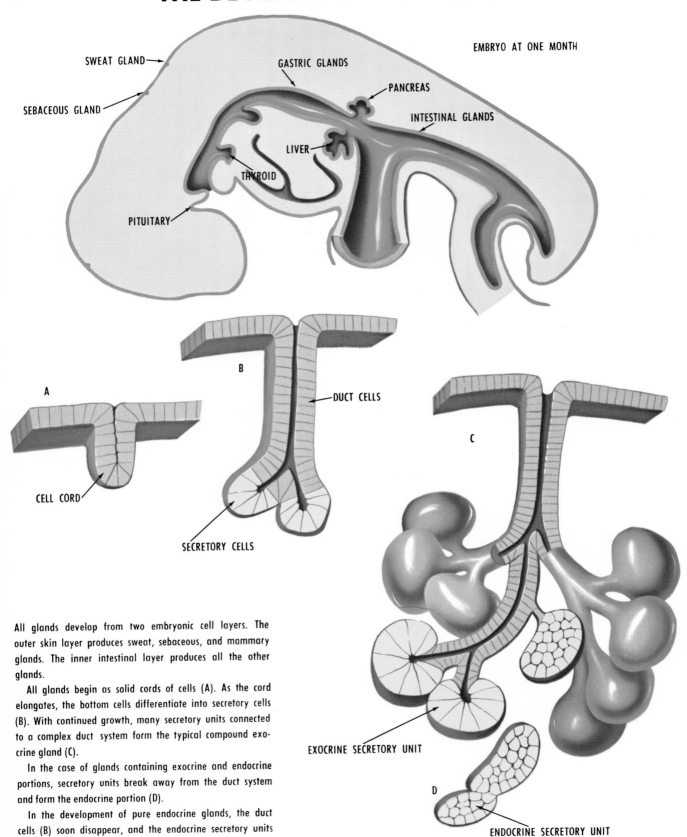

EMBRYO AT ONE MONTH

SWEAT GLAND

GASTRIC GLANDS

PANCREAS

SEBACEOUS GLAND

INTESTINAL GLANDS

LIVER

THYROID

PITUITARY

A

B

C

D

DUCT CELLS

CELL CORD

SECRETORY CELLS

EXOCRINE SECRETORY UNIT

ENDOCRINE SECRETORY UNIT

All glands develop from two embryonic cell layers. The outer skin layer produces sweat, sebaceous, and mammary glands. The inner intestinal layer produces all the other glands.

All glands begin as solid cords of cells (A). As the cord elongates, the bottom cells differentiate into secretory cells (B). With continued growth, many secretory units connected to a complex duct system form the typical compound exocrine gland (C).

In the case of glands containing exocrine and endocrine portions, secretory units break away from the duct system and form the endocrine portion (D).

In the development of pure endocrine glands, the duct cells (B) soon disappear, and the endocrine secretory units develop without any duct system.

THE EXOCRINE GLANDS

The sweat and sebaceous (oil) glands are distributed throughout the skin.

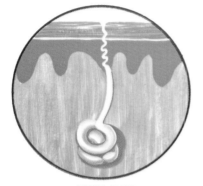

SWEAT GLAND

Numerous small glands located in the lips, tongue, palate, cheek plus the salivary glands empty into the oral cavity. All produce a complex liquid called saliva.

The esophagus has isolated mucus glands.

SALIVARY GLAND

The liver in addition to other functions produces bile, a digestive juice. Bile is stored in the gallbladder until needed.

The stomach contains an estimated 35 million gastric glands which produce digestive enzymes.

The exocrine portion of the pancreas produces the three most potent digestive enzymes.

The small intestine contains millions of glands producing digestive enzymes.

The exocrine glands are under involuntary nervous control. Sweat, sebaceous, and salivary glands, in response to local stimuli, adjust their secretory activity. For example, a temperature rise causes increased sweating.

The gastric and intestinal glands, the liver and pancreas are under both nervous and chemical hormonal control. The sequence of action and reaction between nerve and chemicals is described here in a simplified manner.

1 The sight, smell, taste of food stimulates a "hunger center" to send impulses to the hypothalamus.

2 The hypothalamus sends impulses over the vagus nerve to the gastric glands.

3 The vagus nerve stimulates the gastric gland cells and initiates secretion.

6 Food in the duodenum also causes the production of gastrin.

4 Gastric juice mixes with food.

5 Chemicals contained in all food cause the stomach lining to secrete the hormone gastrin. Gastrin travels to the gastric gland increasing the flow of gastric juice.

7 The interaction of hormones continues in the duodenum and small intestine. In brief, the duodenum produces the hormone secretin which causes the pancreas to secrete digestive juices. These juices cause the duodenum to secrete its own digestive juices.

THE ENDOCRINE GLANDS

The endocrine system is composed of widely scattered ductless glands which manufacture complex chemicals called hormones. The hormones empty directly into the blood stream, travel to their site of action and exert a powerful, long-sustained control over the body and each other.

The anterior pituitary produces a group of hormones which control the other glands, and a group which influences the body as a whole.

The posterior pituitary produces several hormones which help regulate fluid levels, blood pressure, and involuntary muscles.

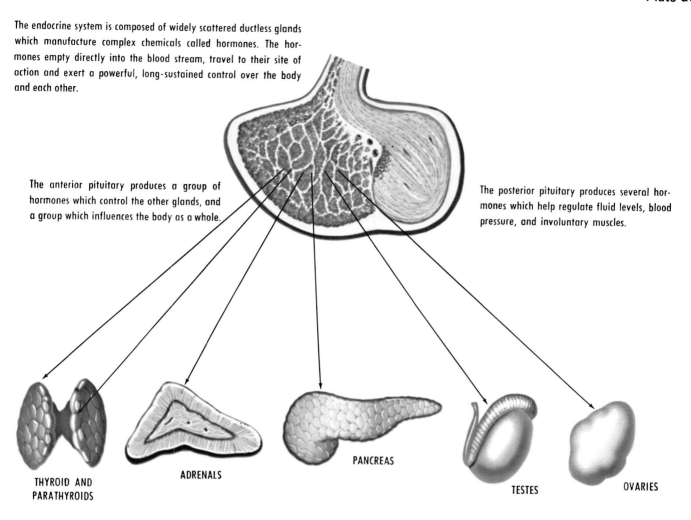

THYROID AND PARATHYROIDS

ADRENALS

PANCREAS

TESTES

OVARIES

BODY ACTIVITIES REGULATED BY THE ENDOCRINE GLANDS

ENERGY

CHEMISTRY

GROWTH

SEXUAL GROWTH

EMERGENCY

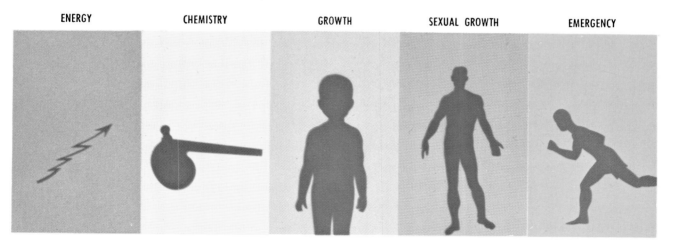

THE ADRENAL GLAND

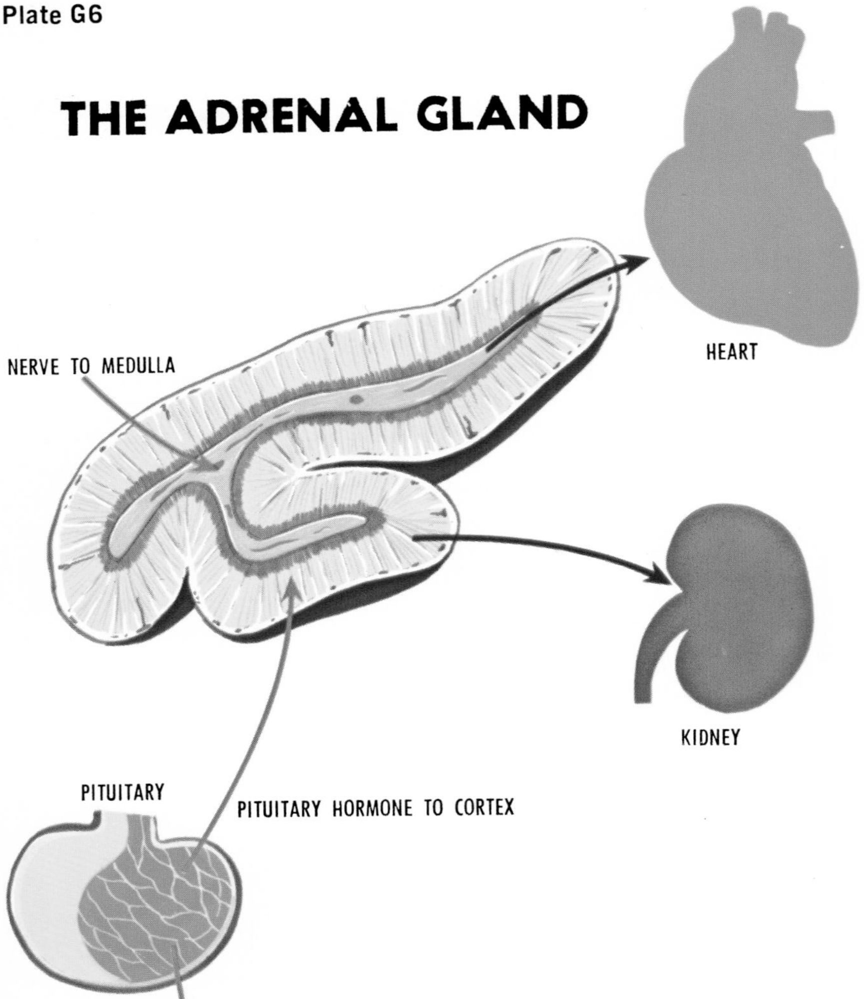

HEART

NERVE TO MEDULLA

KIDNEY

PITUITARY

PITUITARY HORMONE TO CORTEX

PITUITARY HORMONE TO ISLE

INSULIN

The core or medulla of the adrenal gland is the only endocrine under nervous control. In an emergency, the medulla releases two hormones, adrenalin and noradrenalin, which raise blood pressure and speed-up heart action.

The outer layer or cortex under pituitary control produces the steroids. These help maintain body fluid levels by acting on the kidney, and also regulate the production of sugar for energy.

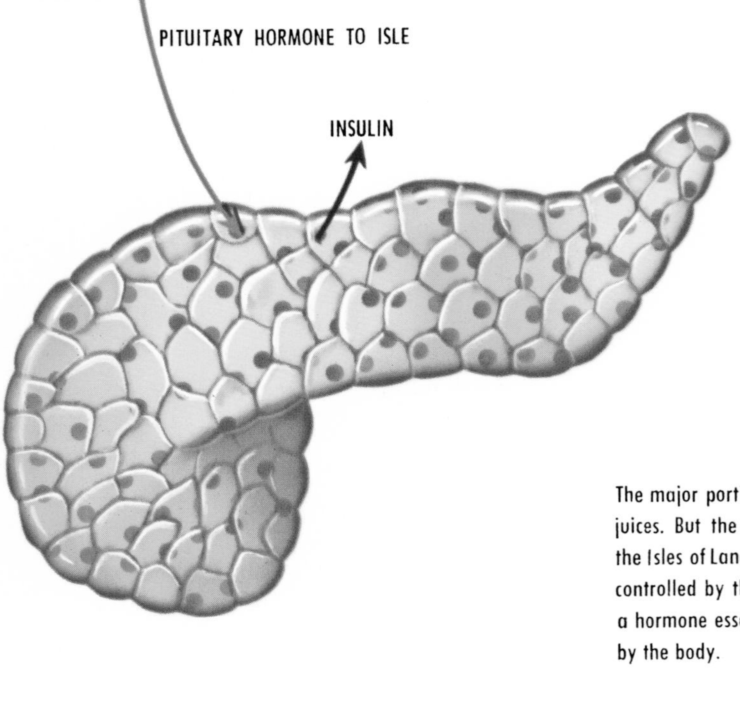

THE PANCREAS

The major portion of the pancreas produces digestive juices. But the pink scattered groups of cells called the Isles of Langerhans are endocrine in function and controlled by the pituitary. The Isles produce insulin, a hormone essential to the storage and use of sugars by the body.

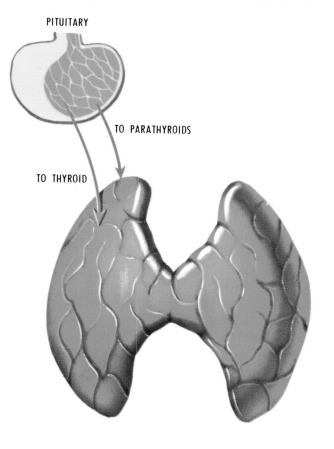

PITUITARY

TO PARATHYROIDS

TO THYROID

THE THYROID

The thyroid produces one hormone, thyroxin. Thyroxin regulates the metabolism (rate of energy consumption) and the physical and mental growth rate. The thyroid and parathyroids are under pituitary control.

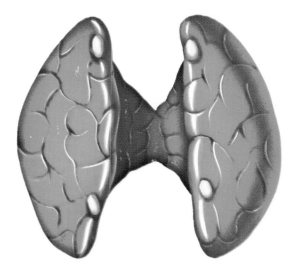

THE PARATHYROIDS

The four yellow nodes located on the back of the thyroid constitute the parathyroids. They produce one hormone, parathormone, which has the sole function of regulating the calcium balance between blood and bone.

THE TESTIS

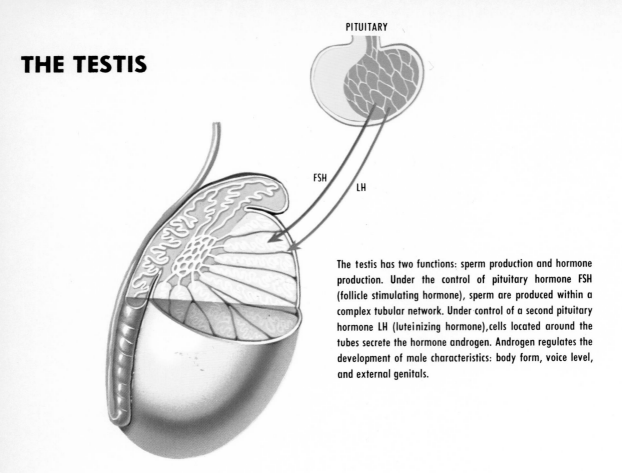

PITUITARY

FSH

LH

The testis has two functions: sperm production and hormone production. Under the control of pituitary hormone FSH (follicle stimulating hormone), sperm are produced within a complex tubular network. Under control of a second pituitary hormone LH (luteinizing hormone), cells located around the tubes secrete the hormone androgen. Androgen regulates the development of male characteristics: body form, voice level, and external genitals.

THE OVARY

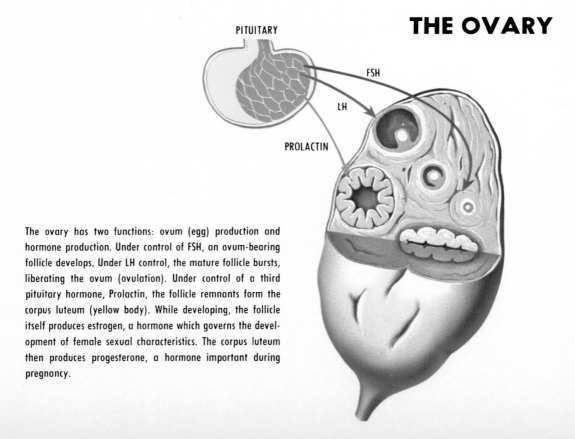

PITUITARY

FSH

LH

PROLACTIN

The ovary has two functions: ovum (egg) production and hormone production. Under control of FSH, an ovum-bearing follicle develops. Under LH control, the mature follicle bursts, liberating the ovum (ovulation). Under control of a third pituitary hormone, Prolactin, the follicle remnants form the corpus luteum (yellow body). While developing, the follicle itself produces estrogen, a hormone which governs the development of female sexual characteristics. The corpus luteum then produces progesterone, a hormone important during pregnancy.

diac output and the flow of blood through the kidneys. However, the side effects of hydralazine are numerous: headache, nausea, numbness, and dizziness being possible.

Reserpine (Hiserpia, Rolserp, Reserpoid are trade names) is one of a group of drugs obtained from the plant rauwolfia. Some of the properties of rauwolfia have been known in India for many years. Although the exact mechanism by which reserpine lowers blood pressure is not known (action in the hypothalamus is suspected), it is an antihypertensive drug of some importance.

Cough-controlling Drugs. Coughing removes material from the lungs and respiratory passages. Coughing can be a symptom of disorders ranging from the uncomfortable to the very serious.

Infections due to viruses, bacteria, or fungi may induce coughing. The common cold, measles, influenza, pneumonia, tuberculosis, pertussis (whooping cough), and histoplasmosis also are characterized by coughing. In addition, irritations to the respiratory system caused by smoke, noxious gases, lack of air moisture, and exposure to temperature extremes may induce coughing.

Allergic reactions such as hay fever and asthma can bring on coughing spells and coughing may even accompany nervousness. Establishing the cause of a persistent cough is crucial in the determination of how it should be treated. Some of the factors to consider are: Is the cough a symptom of a respiratory infection? Is it dry or is mucus expelled? How long has the cough lasted?

Anti-cough drugs (antitussives) that contain a narcotic, such as codeine, should be used only as directed and never for a prolonged period. Non-narcotic cough preparations such as dextromethorphan offer an alternative that has fewer undesirable side effects.

Many over-the-counter anti-cough medicines contain ingredients in addition to the antitussive. Some of these preparations include an expectorant, such as guaifenesin, which stimulates the increased production of fluid in the respiratory system so that matter can be coughed up more easily. However, current medical opinion tends to recommend a single ingredient drug to treat specific symptoms like coughing. Multi-ingredient drugs increase the potential for undesirable side effects, and are generally more expensive.

Depressants. Depressants are drugs used to treat insomnia, anxiety, abnormal irritability, and tension. In excessive doses depressants can produce a state remarkably similar to alcohol intoxication. Low doses produce mild sedation; higher doses, by relieving anxiety or stress, may cause a temporary state of euphoria. They may also produce mood depression and apathy. In contrast to the effects of narcotics, however, intoxicating doses invariably result in impaired judgment, slurred speech, and an often unrealized loss of motor coordination. Depressants may also induce drowsiness, sleep, stupor, coma, and possible death. Tolerance to depressants develops rapidly, extending the intake capacity, and narrowing the range between an intoxicating and lethal dose. The person who is unaware of the dangers of increasing dependence will often seek prescriptions from several physicians concurrently, increasing the daily dose up to ten or twenty times the recommended amount.

Some common depressants include chloral hydrate, methaqualone, meprobamate, and barbiturates. Depressants also are a means of suicide, if a large enough dose is available to a sufficiently despondent person. Fatalities have also occurred when depressants have been used and then followed by alcoholic drinks.

Perhaps the oldest depressant drug is chloral hydrate, which was first synthesized in 1862. Barbiturates, a group of depressants that include pentobarbital (Nembutal), secobarbital (Seconal), and amobarbital (Amy-

194

Controlled Substances: Uses and Effects

	Drugs	Schedule*	Often Prescribed Brand Names	Medical Uses	Dependence Physical
Narcotics	Opium	II	Dover's Powder, Paregoric	Analgesic, antidiarrheal	High
	Morphine	II	Morphine	Analgesic	High
	Codeine	II III V	Codeine	Analgesic, Antitussive	Moderate
	Heroin	I	None	None	High
	Meperidine (Pethidine)	II	Demerol, Pethadol	Analgesic	High
	Methadone	II	Dolophine, Methadone, Methadose	Analgesic, heroin substitute	High
	Other Narcotics	I II III V	Dilaudid, Leritine, Numorphan, Percodan	Analgesic, antidiarrheal, antitussive	High
Depressants	Chloral Hydrate	IV	Noctec, Somnos	Hypnotic	Moderate
	Barbiturates	II III IV	Amytal, Butisol, Nembutal, Phenobarbital, Seconal, Tuinal	Anesthetic, anti-convulsant, sedation, sleep	High
	Glutethimide	III	Doriden	Sedation, sleep	High
	Methaqualone	II	Optimil, Parest, Quaalude, Somnafac, Sopor	Sedation, sleep	High
	Tranquilizers	IV	Equanil, Librium, Miltown Serax, Tranzene, Valium	Anti-anxiety, muscle relaxant, sedation	Moderate
	Other Depressants	III IV	Clonopin, Dalmane, Dormate, Noludar, Placydil, Valmid	Anti-anxiety, sedation, sleep	Possible
Stimulants	Cocaine †	II	Cocaine	Local anesthetic	Possible
	Amphetamines	II III	Benzedrine, Biphetamine, Dosoxyn, Dexedrine	Hyperkinesis, narcolepsy, weight control	Possible
	Phenmetrazine	II	Preludin	Weight control	Possible
	Methylphenidate	II	Ritalin	Hyperkinesis	Possible
	Other Stimulants	III IV	Bacarate, Cylert, Didrex, Ionamin, Plegine, Pondimin, Pre-sate, Sanorex, Voranil	Weight control	Possible
Hallucinogens	LSD	I	None	None	None
	Mescaline	I	None	None	None
	Psilocybin-Psilocyn	I	None	None	None
	MDA	I	None	None	None
	PCP ‡	III	Sernylan	Veterinary anesthetic	None
	Other Hallucinogens	I	None	None	None
Cannabis	Marihuana Hashish Hashish Oil	I	None	None	Degree unknown

*Scheduling classifications vary for individual drugs since controlled substances are often marketed in combination with other medicinal ingredients.

† Designated a narcotic under the Controlled Substances Act.
‡ Designated a depressant under the Controlled Substances Act.

Potential: Psychological	Tolerance	Duration of Effects (in hours)	Usual Methods of Administration	Possible Effects	Effects of Overdose	Withdrawal Syndrome
High	Yes	3 to 6	Oral, smoked	Euphoria, drowsiness, respiratory depression, constricted pupils, nausea	Slow and shallow breathing, clammy skin, convulsions, coma, possible death	Watery eyes, runny nose, yawning, loss of appetite, irritability, tremors, panic, chills and sweating, cramps, nausea
High	Yes	3 to 6	Injected, smoked			
Moderate	Yes	3 to 6	Oral, injected			
High	Yes	3 to 6	Injected, sniffed			
High	Yes	3 to 6	Oral, injected			
High	Yes	12 to 24	Oral, injected			
High	Yes	3 to 6	Oral, injected			
Moderate	Probable	5 to 8	Oral	Slurred speech, disorientation, drunken behavior without odor of alcohol	Shallow respiration, cold and clammy skin, dilated pupils, weak and rapid pulse, coma, possible death	Anxiety, insomnia, tremors, delirium, convulsions, possible death
High	Yes	1 to 16	Oral, injected			
High	Yes	4 to 8	Oral			
High	Yes	4 to 8	Oral			
Moderate	Yes	4 to 8	Oral			
Possible	Yes	4 to 8	Oral			
High	Yes	2	Injected, sniffed	Increased alertness, excitation, euphoria, dilated pupils, increased pulse rate and blood pressure, insomnia, loss of appetite	Agitation, increase in body temperature, hallucinations, convulsions, possible death	Apathy, long periods of sleep, irritability, depression, disorientation
High	Yes	2 to 4	Oral, injected			
High	Yes	2 to 4	Oral			
High	Yes	2 to 4	Oral			
Possible	Yes	2 to 4	Oral			
Degree unknown	Yes	Variable	Oral	Illusions and hallucinations (with exception of MDA); poor perception of time and distance	Longer, more intense "trip" episodes, psychosis, possible death	Withdrawal syndrome not reported
Degree unknown	Yes	Variable	Oral, injected			
Degree unknown	Yes	Variable	Oral			
Degree unknown	Yes	Variable	Oral, injected, sniffed			
Degree unknown	Yes	Variable	Oral, injected, smoked			
Degree unknown	Yes	Variable	Oral, injected, sniffed			
Moderate	Yes	2 to 4	Oral, smoked	Euphoria, relaxed inhibitions, increased appetite, disoriented behavior	Fatigue, paranoia, possible psychosis	Insomnia, hyperactivity, and decreased appetite reported in a limited number of individuals

tal), are a frequently prescribed, and abused, medication.

These barbiturates are prescribed frequently to induce sedation and sleep by both physicians and veterinarians. Small therapeutic doses tend to calm nervous conditions, and larger amounts cause sleep from twenty to sixty minutes after oral administration, and the duration of action is up to six hours. Physicians prescribe barbiturates for purposes of sedation; veterinarians use pentobarbital for anesthesia and euthanasia.

Methaqualone, once thought to be safe and nonaddicting, is now known to have a high potential to cause physical and psychological dependence, and has caused many cases of serious poisoning. Common trade names of methaqualone include Quaalude, Optimil, and Sopor.

Meprobamate, considered one of the "minor" tranquilizers, is widely used for the relief of tension, anxiety, and as a muscle relaxant. It does not induce sleep at therapeutic doses unlike some of the barbiturates. However, excessive use can cause physical and psychological dependence. Miltown, Equanil, and SK-Bamate are common trade names.

The benzodiazepine group of depressants are considered relatively safer than other drugs used for sedation, to relieve tension, anxiety, and muscle spasms, and to prevent convulsions. These drugs have a slow rate of effect but last for a long duration. Some trade names in this group are Librium, Dalmane, and Valium. These drugs have also been abused, either through excessive doses, prolonged consumption, or when taken with alcoholic drinks.

Diabetes-controlling Drugs. There are essentially two types of diabetes patients, the juvenile and the adult. The juvenile diabetic may be a child, an adolescent, or even a young adult. The juvenile's diabetes is due to a complete (or almost complete) lack of insulin. Usually the juvenile diabetic is totally dependent upon an external supply of insulin. In contrast, the adult diabetic may be able to manage his or her condition through a carefully programmed diet. Usually the adult diabetic is not totally incapable of producing insulin. When dietary regulation becomes ineffective, two courses of therapy are possible, treatment with insulin or treatment with an oral hypoglycemic agent that stimulates the production of natural insulin in the pancreas.

The first practical oral hypoglycemic agent was a sulfonylurea discovered in 1955. Sulfonylurea drugs (such as Diabinese, Orinase, and Tolinase) promote insulin secretion. However, response to a particular oral hypoglycemic agent may suddenly cease. In some cases, treatment can be continued by changing to another sulfonylurea. It should be emphasized that the oral hypoglycemic agents available are effective only for certain diabetics; they cannot be used in juvenile diabetics.

Fluid-removing Drugs (Diuretics). Drugs that promote the removal of water from tissues are called diuretics (urine-promoters). The excessive accumulation of fluids in body cavities and tissues (edema) is usually treated with diurectic drugs of which the thiazide group of medications are the most popular. Diuril, Dyazide, Aldactazide, and Enduron are examples of prescription diuretics containing thiazide.

A common complication occurring with the use of diuretics is the depletion of potassium in the body. Often potassium supplements must be taken with the diuretic in the form of a preparation such as K-Lor, or the consumption of potassium-rich foods such as bananas, apricots or oranges. There are also special diuretic drugs developed to lessen the depletion of potassium. Aldactone and Dyrenium are examples.

Excessive fluid retention is best treated when it first makes its presence known. Mild procedures are usually effective to eliminate fluids. However, delay of therapy may make more drastic measures necessary. Patients with cardiac edema are greatly helped by diets low in salt.

Generic Drugs. Generic names for drugs are usually a shortened form of the drug's chemical name and are not under the protection of trademark laws. Pharmaceutical companies can produce a generic drug and then register their exclusive right to market that drug under a distinctive brand name. For example, Datril is the generic acetaminophen analgesic produced by the Bristol-Myers Company, while Tylenol is the version of acetaminophen produced by McNeil Consumer Products Company. In addition, a number of companies produce acetaminophen simply under the generic name.

In many instances generic products are substantially less expensive than the equivalent trademarked product. Taking the time to discover a drug's generic name with the help of your pharmacist or doctor may save money. In 1979 a report by the Federal Trade Commission estimated that some four hundred million dollars a year might be saved if consumers purchased generic drugs. However, because of patent regulations, some drugs are not yet available under a generic label.

Hallucinogens. Hallucinogens are natural or synthetic drugs that alter a person's perception of reality. They have the ability to induce sensory illusions, causing the user to fantasize and hallucinate. Hallucinogenic experiences are particularly dangerous because their effects are unpredictable; toxic responses may cause psychotic behavior, which may result in self-injury or violent behavior toward others.

Examples of hallucinogenic drugs include mescaline (derived from the peyote cactus), LSD (lysergic acid diethylamide), PCP (phencyclidine), and psilocybin (obtained from certain mushrooms). With the exception of PCP, which has limited use as an animal tranquilizer, there are no practical medical applications for hallucinogenic substances.

Intestinal Parasitic Disease Drugs. There are various drugs used in the treatment of amebic, hookworm, roundworm, and whipworm infections, and many other intestinal diseases due to parasites. Amebiasis (amebic dysentery), the infection caused by the ameba *Entamoeba histolytica* has been treated with the drug emetine. An antiamebic drug with iodine in its structure is diiodohydroxyquin.

Hookworm infections are most generally due to *Necator americanus* and *Ancylostoma duodenale*. Tetrachloroethy-

Common Over-the-Counter Laxatives:

Method of Action	Brand Name
Forms bulk in the intestine	Serutan, Metamucil, Modane Bulk
A "saline" type preparation	Haley's M-O, Phillips' Milk of Magnesia
Stimulates digestive tract with phenolphthalein	Ex-Lax, Correctol
Lubricates digestive tract	Nujol

lene has been used for treatment. It is given in the morning on an empty stomach and food is withheld for four to six hours. During treatment alcohol and fat must be absent from the intestine.

The roundworm *Ascaris lumbricoides* infects the large intestine and is one of the most dangerous of parasites. Eradication of the infection has been accomplished by using piperazine citrate. The medication rarely causes discomfort, although occasionally there may be nausea and vomiting. No purgative to expel worms is necessary.

Mild infection by the whipworm *Trichuris trichiuria* has been cured with dithiazine iodide. Heavy infestations may require more potent medications.

In addition, humans may become the host to at least four types of tapeworms. The pork tapeworm is potentially the most dangerous because it may penetrate into any organ of the body and lodge there. Most tapeworm infestations have been successfully treated with quinacrine. Oleoresin of aspidium has also been successful.

Laxatives. At one time drugs that promote the elimination of feces (cathartics, purgatives, laxatives) were considered of much greater importance than today. In fact, in the 17th and 18th centuries the enema syringe was often depicted to symbolize the medical profession. However, current medical opinion does not favor the repeated or unnecessary use of laxatives, because it is believed that nothing is accomplished by disturbing a process that functions best naturally.

There are, of course, situations when laxatives are needed. In these cases the choice of a cathartic agent should probably be the decision of a physician. There are, however, many people without any diagnosed illness who claim to feel better if they purge themselves at intervals. These people should realize that the indiscriminate stimulation of the bowels by cathartic drugs is considered dangerous.

Materials without nutritive value, but which fill the intestines, are thought to move the bowel contents by providing bulk. Bulk-forming laxatives are generally what doctors recommend. Agar, psyllium seed, methyl cellulose, and bran are bulk cathartic agents.

Agar is an indigestible material obtained from seaweed. In the Orient it is used extensively as a thickening in soup and in other foods. It provides bulk by absorbing and holding large amounts of water.

Psyllium seed when moistened forms a gelatinous mass that can be eaten as a spread on bread or crackers, or mixed into liquids. Bulk, and probably lubrication, is provided because of the gelatinous nature of the material. Metamucil and Modane Bulk are nonprescription laxatives of this type.

Methyl cellulose is a product of the laboratory. In appearance it resembles cotton and is, in fact, chemically related to it. Methyl cellulose is not digested during passage through the digestive tract. It has been used to treat both constipation and diarrhea; in the latter case it makes the stool firm and manageable.

The consumption of bran to promote bowel movement and regularity is increasing in popularity. Adding bran to muffins, cookies, cakes and breakfast cereals may be a way to provide fiber to stimulate the digestive tract. An increased percentage of fiber in the diet has also been recommended by some nutritionists as a means to maintain regularity.

Phenolphthalein is the cathartic ingredient in many over-the-counter laxatives (such as Ex-Lax and Correctol). It is generally reliable, although at times its effects are unpredictable. A dose that previously produced a stool of normal consistency may cause unexpectedly sudden elimination of the bowels or have no effect at all. Phenolphthalein-type laxatives are usually taken at bedtime, with their effects occurring the next morning.

The so-called "saline" laxatives act by drawing water into the intestine, creating very loose stools. They often react rapidly, within thirty to sixty minutes, and are therefore best taken during the day. Epsom salts (magnesium sulfate) is probably the most common saline laxative. Magnesium citrate is another, but though somewhat more violent in action. Milk of magnesia, a suspension of magnesium hydroxyde in water, is an antacid in addition to its laxative effect and serves to neutralize stomach acidity. If taken with fruit juices containing citric acid some of the magnesium hydroxide is converted to magnesium citrate, thus strengthening its cathartic action. Haley's M-O and Phillips' Milk of Magnesia are examples of nonprescription saline laxative products.

Marijuana. The psychoactive drug cannabis, commonly known as marijuana, is present in marijuana tobacco-like cigarettes ("joints") and in hashish and hashish oil. The principal agent in marijuana is believed to be delta-9-tetrahydrocannabinol (THC). Cannabis contains other chemicals, the physiological effects of which have not been determined.

The number of children, teenagers, and adults becoming involved with marijuana is increasing. In a survey conducted in 1978, one out of nine of a high school graduating class smoked marijuana every day; three out of five reported using it at least once, some before the age of twelve.

Low doses of cannabis are inclined to induce restlessness or an increased sense of well-being, followed by a state of relaxation and alteration of the senses, including a distortion of time and spatial perception. Slightly increased doses may bring on a state of intoxication that intensifies these characteristics. Higher doses can lead to the loss of self-identity, fantasies and hallucinations. The long term effects of regular cannibis consumption are still being researched. Some studies suggest that adverse effects upon heart, lung, and brain functions are possible.

Laws concerning the possession and marketing of marijuana exist in all fifty states. Attempts in some states to legalize the adult use of marijuana have achieved limited success. In some states the possession of less than an ounce of marijuana for personal use is classified as a misdemeanor, rather than a felony.

Research for medical applications for cannabis include its use in the treatment of glaucoma and to prevent nausea and vomiting that is associated with some forms of cancer chemotherapy.

Motion Sickness Drugs. It has been estimated that somewhat less than half of any group of people are susceptible to seasickness or airsickness. No method is available, however, that can predict how individuals will react to a particular motion. The common experience is that one person may be violently ill and the next person completely unaffected. In general, children are more sensitive to motion than adults.

Motion sickness is usually characterized by nausea, vomiting, retching, pallor, and weakness. These and other symptoms are relieved to some extent when the patient is in a reclining position. On board a ship the sufferer might lessen discomfort by limiting head movement and by fixing the eyes upon the stable horizon.

Drugs that counter the effects of the body's histamine are usually effective in the control of motion sickness. An example of such a drug is meclizine (Bonine, Dizmiss, and Eldezine are trade names). Generally this drug is taken one-half to one hour before exposure to possibly discomforting motion. One dose per day may be sufficient. When necessary, however, three daily doses are permitted.

Narcotics. In current usage the term "narcotic" refers to derivatives of the drug opium, or to synthetic substitutes, that produce psychological and physical dependence. Narcotic drugs have medical applications such as the relief of intense pain, the suppression of cough, and the treatment of certain cases of diarrhea.

Narcotics may also produce a temporary state of euphoria, along with other possible effects such as apathy, lethargy, constipation, and reduced vision. A large dose may cause sleep. However, the possibility of vomiting and respiratory depression is increased.

At least twenty-five organic substances can be extracted from opium, of which morphine, codeine, papaverine, and noscapine are examples having medical applications as pain relievers, cough suppressants, and muscle relaxants. Morphine is one of the most effective pain-relievers known. It is used licitly in hospitals in the form of white crystals, hypodermic tablets, and injectable preparations. It is odorless, tastes bitter, and darkens with age. Dependence can develop rapidly. Heroin, first synthesized from morphine in 1874, was introduced as a pain remedy by the Bayer Company in Germany in 1898; however, its high potential for addiction and the availability of safer pain relievers made its medical use obsolete.

Signs of withdrawal from morphine or heroin usually occur shortly before time for another dose. The addict makes complaints, pleas and demands which become more intense from thirty-six to seventy-two hours after the last dose, and then subside. The addict may yawn frequently, perspire, and have watery eyes and a runny nose eight to twelve hours after the last dose, and then may fall into a restless sleep. Restlessness, irritability, loss of appetite, insomnia, goose flesh, tremors and violent yawning occur, becoming intense by forty-eight to seventy-two hours. These symptoms progress until the patient finally becomes very weak and depressed. Nausea and vomiting, accompanied by stomach cramps and diarrhea are common. Extremes from chills to flushing, with excessive sweating, occur along with increased heart rate and high blood pressure. The physical pain progresses into the bones and muscles of the back, and muscle spasms and kicking movements become prominent. At this point an individual is likely to become suicidal. Without alternative treatment, most of the symptoms disappear within seven to ten days.

Symptoms of addiction are manifested in infants born to addicted mothers. These infants will suffer the symptoms of withdrawal when no further contact with the narcotic occurs. This places the babies in a possibly life-threatening situation, and therapy may be necessary to save the infant's life.

Synthetic narcotic drugs may be chemically similar to narcotics of natural origin, but are produced entirely within the laboratory. The synthetic narcotic methadone was developed by German chemists because of a shortage of morphine. It is used widely in the attempt to detoxify heroin addicts.

Since methadone itself can cause physical dependence, it is under strict government regulation. Addicts admitted to methadone treatment are usually over eighteen and have a long history of dependence. Many programs provide for withdrawal from methadone maintenance, once rehabilitation has succeeded. If a person does not follow the recommended dosage, he could die from an overdose.

Other synthetic narcotics with medical application include levorphan, phenazocine, and anileridine. These products have many of the same effects as morphine, but they differ in their potency and duration of action. All have the potential for addiction.

Nicotine. When tobacco smoke is inhaled, the lungs receive a dose of the drug nicotine. Nicotine then acts as a stimulant, which elevates blood pressure and increases the heart beat. If present in pure concentrations, nicotine can be one of the most toxic substances known.

Overdose. An "overdose" occurs when a person has taken a quantity of a drug that produces an acute reaction. Often an overdose causes a stupor and may induce coma. Treatment by a physician must be sought immediately. Artificial respiration and other first-aid procedures can be used until medical help arrives.

Many communities have drug "hotlines" that offer assistance over the telephone or they maintain poison control centers that can be of aid in emergencies.

Over-the-Counter, or Nonprescription Drugs. This class of drugs includes all medicines and health preparations sold without a doctor's prescription. This would include anything from medicated shampoo and acne creams to aspirin and vitamin tablets. Some 3.5 billion dollars or more are spent each year on over-the-counter drugs sold in pharmacies, drugstores, and discount department stores.

Some important factors to remember when using nonprescription medications include: (1) Read the labels and understand the directions. (2) Know what the active ingredient in the medication is and if it is the most effective for your condition. (3) Remember, over-the-counter preparations are not meant to cure disease. If the condition treated persists, consult a doctor. (4) Never prolong the use of any over-the-counter medication.

Pain Lesseners (Analgesics). Analgesics are drugs that act on the central nervous system in a way that dulls the sensation of pain. The opiates, the coaltar analgesics, the salicylates, and acetaminophen are in this category.

Although all the substances that fall into the groups named are analgesics, some also have additional properties. The opiate morphine has widespread effects on the central nervous system; salicylates, such as aspirin, reduce fever.

Although morphine is an extremely valuable analgesic, it has objectionable characteristics that make its use limited. Simply because it is so toxic and addicting, morphine is not used for ordinary aches and pains. In general it is used when there is intense pain, such as may occur in cancer patients; in cases of severe burns; and immediately following some types of surgery. Codeine, another opiate, is not as potent as morphine, nor does it induce sleep.

Aspirin and acetaminophen are the most common ingredients in over-the-counter analgesics. The yearly consumption of aspirin in the United States makes it the most used of all medicines. It is the preferred analgesic for "aches and pains" and is considered the universal antipyretic (fever lessener). Usually aspirin is more effective against pain originating in joints and muscles than pain in internal organs. Although aspirin is very common, care must be taken in its use as it causes some people to have cases of gastric irritation or allergic reactions.

Acetaminophen is less likely to upset the stomach, but it does not possess the anti-inflammatory effects of aspirin. For those who cannot take aspirin, or if a headache is accompanied by stomach upset, acetaminophen may be preferred.

Over-the-counter analgesics that contain aspirin or acetaminophen may also contain drugs such as caffeine, which have no known analgesic effect. The safest, most effective, and least expensive analgesics are usually single ingredient (aspirin or acetaminophen) products.

Sedatives. Compounds that reduce emotional tensions, producing relaxation in both mind and body, are sedatives. These drugs are generally intended for use during the day, leaving the patient awake but calm. Barbiturates have long been used as sedatives; however the potential for abuse or addiction makes their use limited and controlled. Another drug used as a sedative is meprobamate of which Coprobate, Miltown, Bamo, and Protran are trade names.

Skin Disorder Drugs. Estimates suggest that 15 percent of the patients visiting a general practitioner have some kind of skin problem. Acne, eczema, psoriasis, seborrhea, poison ivy, and athlete's foot are common complaints.

Broad spectrum antibiotics, such as

202

tetracycline, are often of help in suppressing adolescent acne. In the absence of toxic effects, such a treatment program may last several months to a year. If this is done, however, the patient should have regular health examinations. Supplementation with vitamin B complex may be necessary.

Vitamin A in the form of an ointment or solution may also be prescribed for the treatment of acne. Over-the-counter acne preparations such as Clearsil and Oxy-5 contain benzoyl peroxide, an effective antiacne agent. Of course, regular cleansing of the skin with soap and warm water will aid in the prevention of acne.

Antieczema agents are used in treatment of acute eruptions that are red, swollen, blistering, or weeping. The affected area is kept moist by application of wet compresses, or emulsions. The solutions used are physiological saline solution, fresh milk, or aluminum acetate. If the lesions are infected, a weak bath of potassium permanganate may be used. Corn-starch baths, or oatmeal baths, will soothe and soften tender, inflamed eruptions. If widespread application is necessary, then lotions or emulsions may be more suitable than compresses.

Among the newest and most effective dermatological drugs is cortisone. This drug is applied directly to the skin and is spoken of as a topical ("on-the-spot") remedy. Cortisone-derived preparations are usually safe if taken as directed; however, the overuse of cortisone in any form is never advised.

For the treatment of fungal infections, such as athlete's foot, medications containing tolnaftate are often recommended. Aftate and Tinactin are over-the-counter products that contain tolnaftate. Another successful medication for fungal infection is undecylenic acid. Products that have undecylenic acid include Cruex and Desenex.

For skin problems caused by poison ivy or poison oak, a preparation containing calamine and zinc oxide is effective. However, some people dislike this remedy because it is rather messy. An alternative is simply an equal-parts solution of rubbing alcohol and water. (Witch hazel may be a substitute for the alcohol.) Over-the-counter drugs may contain an anesthetic or an antihistamine, which is usually not recommended for typical poison ivy infections. Non prescription medications that contain zirconium oxide should not be used because some individuals have increased skin irritation after extended use.

Sleep-inducing Drugs. Methods other than drugs are usually preferred to induce sleep. When a drug is used to cause sleep it should be at the indication of a physician. Often simple adjustments in sleep habits, environment, and perhaps diet, will alleviate most insomnia. When drugs are prescribed, pentobarbital (Nembutal, Seconal, Butisol are trade names) and flurazepam hydrochloride (Dalmane) are the most commonly used. Whenever these drugs are used care should be taken that alcohol is not consumed.

Over-the-counter drugs that claim to induce sleep often contain the chemical scopolamine, along with an antihistamine. Trade names of products that contain scopolamine include Compoz, Sominex, and Sleep-Eze. These preparations should be taken with caution. Overdoses of scopolamine, as has been observed in suicide attempts, bring on excitement, confusion, and hallucinations. The potential abuse of prescription and nonprescription sleep-inducing drugs is a risk that makes their use a matter of questionable value in many situations.

Stimulants. The use of drugs or drug-containing substances to stimulate the central nervous system is a common occurrence in modern society. The two most popular stimulants are nicotine, found in tobacco products, and caffeine, a common ingredient of soft drinks, tea, coffee, and nonprescription pain relievers. Stronger stimulants include amphetamines, cocaine, and various drugs used as appetite suppressants.

The effects of stimulants can range from the "jitters" of excessive coffee drinking to the bizarre "hyper" behavior of amphetamines. The abuse of stimulants can lead to psychological dependence and damage to the lungs, heart, and other organs, or even death.

Chronic users of stimulants rely on them to feel stronger, more confident and decisive. They often fall into a habit of taking stimulants during the day and something to make them sleep at night such as alcohol or sleeping pills.

People may abuse stimulants to push themselves beyond normal limits. Some reasons might be to stay awake to drive, to study for an exam, or to do well in an athletic contest. This kind of abuse rarely leads to serious problems, but it is possible if repeated.

After protracted use of stimulants, an unpleasant feeling of depression occurs. Since this can easily be resolved by another dose of the stimulant, this pattern often becomes difficult to break. This may continue until the user injects himself every few hours, causing delirium or physical exhaustion.

Tolerance develops rapidly, increasing the probability of overdose. Psychosis often occurs from larger doses, which appears in such signs as grinding the teeth, persistent touching and picking at the face and extremities, repetition of tasks, suspiciousness and a feeling of being watched. Paranoia along with visual and auditory hallucinations characterize the toxic syndrome resulting from high doses. Sublethal doses produce such symptoms as dizziness, agitation, hostility, panic, headache, flushed skin, chest pain with palpitations, excessive sweating, vomiting, and abdominal cramps. Without medical intervention high fever, convulsions, and cardiovascular collapse may occur, possibly causing death. Fatalities have occured among athletes who have taken moderate amounts of stimulants and then increased their bodily temperature through extreme exertion.

The psychological dependence on stimulants is so strong that cronic users do not easily return to normal. There is often profound apathy and depression, and disturbed sleep up to twenty hours a day in immediate withdrawal, which may last several days. Perception and thought processes may be impaired for an indefinite period of time after the initial withdrawal. Anxiety, tenseness, and suicidal tendencies may persist for weeks or months.

Tranquilizers. Tranquilizers were discovered quite by chance when it was observed that a substance (promethazine) had a remarkable ability to calm excited patients. This characteristic effect of tranquilizers is also obtained from the preparations of the plant *Rauwolfia serpentina*, the only naturally produced material containing such properties, one known in India for hundreds of years.

Rauwolfia in both crude drug form and as the purified extract has been used as a tranquilizer. A crystaline derivative of rauwolfia, called reserpine, has been used as a major tranquilizer in the treatment of psychosis; however it is rarely prescribed currently because it has been a factor in some suicides.

Of more importance is a rather large number of phenothiazine tranquilizers. All of these compounds have essentially the same effects, but differ in their potency. Most phenothiazines are capable of suppressing nausea and vomiting, and thus are of possible benefit in the treatment of certain phases of radiation sickness and some cancers. Their peculiar tranquilizing effect may relieve itching and distress in some skin disorders.

It may be helpful to become familiar with the more commonly available tranquilizers. Thorazine is a phenothiazine used in the treatment of certain psychotic disorders. Haldol, a butyrophenone, has uses similar to Thorazine.

The following IQ Test is designed to challenge your present knowledge about drug abuse. By drug abuse we mean the use of a chemical substance, licit or illicit, that results in an individual's physical, mental, emotional, or social impairment. Like any test of this sort, it has some trick questions and multiple answers. Unlike most tests, it will not give you a rating from doper to expert. We recognize that specific information about drugs is less important than the meaning and function of drug use in our lives. No simple IQ Test can measure that.

DRUG IQ TEST

1. During which time(s) was drug abuse a problem in the United States?
   (a) During the Civil War
   (b) In the 1950s
   (c) In the 1960s
   (d) All of the above.

2. In which age group(s) is drug abuse likely to be a problem?
   (a) 12-16
   (b) 16-25
   (c) 25-45
   (d) 45 and over
   (e) All of the above

3. How do most drug users make their first contact with illicit drugs?
   (a) Through "pushers" seeking new customers
   (b) Through their friends
   (c) Accidentally
   (d) Through the media

4. Which of the following is the most commonly abused drug in the United States?
   (a) Marijuana
   (b) Alcohol
   (c) Cocaine
   (d) Heroin

5. Which of the following is not a narcotic?
   (a) Heroin
   (b) Marijuana
   (c) Morphine
   (d) Methadone

6. Which of the following is not a stimulant?
   (a) Amphetamine
   (b) Caffeine
   (c) Mescaline
   (d) Methamphetamine

7. Which of the following is not a hallucinogen?
   (a) MDA
   (b) LSD
   (c) STP
   (d) MPA

8. Which of the following drugs does not cause physical dependence?
   (a) Ethyl alcohol
   (b) Morphine
   (c) Peyote
   (d) Secobarbital
   (e) Codeine

9. Which of the following has the highest immediate risk to experimenters?
   (a) Inhalants
   (b) Marijuana
   (c) Nicotine
   (d) Heroin

10. At what point in time does a person who uses heroin become physically dependent?
   (a) Immediately (first time)
   (b) After four or five times
   (c) After prolonged use (20 times or more)
   (d) Different for each person

11. Which ingredient is most commonly found in compounds sold on the street as "mescaline"?
   (a) Lysergic acid diethylamide
   (b) Morphine
   (c) Tetracycline
   (d) Naltrexone
   (e) All of the above

12. Why is intravenous injection the most dangerous method of using illicit drugs?
   (a) Because of the rapidity with which the drug enters the system
   (b) Because nonsterile equipment and solutions are likely to cause serious medical complications
   (c) Because the amount of drug entering the bloodstream is likely to be large
   (d) All of the above

13. When a person becomes physically dependent on drugs, what is the primary reason he continues to take the drug?
   (a) Experience pleasure
   (b) Relieve discomfort
   (c) Escape reality
   (d) Gain acceptance among friends

14. Which of the following drugs has never been used to treat the narcotic addiction problem in the United States?
   (a) Cyclazocine
   (b) Naloxone
   (c) Methadone
   (d) Psilocybin
   (e) Heroin

15. Which of the following is an effective treatment method for drug abusers?
   (a) Maintenance
   (b) Detoxification
   (c) Abstinence
   (d) Psychotherapy
   (e) All of the above

ANSWERS TO THE DRUG IQ TEST

1. (d) All of the above. The use of drugs is as old as the history of man. In the United States special periods have had special drug abuse problems. During the Civil War opium was used medically, and since its addictive properties were not clearly understood, many wounded soldiers became addicted. Following the Civil War, the practice of opium smoking became popular on the West Coast and spread to many urban areas.
   Throughout the century, there were periodic "drug scares" created by the use of cocaine at the turn of the century, heroin in the 1920s, marijuana in the 1930s, and heroin again in the 1950s. The 1960s saw a social explosion of drug use of all kinds from LSD to heroin and marijuana.

2. (e) All of the above. Drug abuse is found in all age groups. The recent focus on use of drugs by young people has been out of proportion.

3. (b) Through their friends. With the exception of alcohol, which is usually first used at home, most drug users are introduced to drugs by friends.

4. (b) Alcohol. Estimates show that about 9 million Americans are alcoholic persons.

5. (b) Marijuana. In the past marijuana has been legally classified as a narcotic, but it isn't now. Marijuana's psychopharmacological effects are similar to stimulants, sedatives, or hallucinogens, and its actual effects depend on dose, frequency of use, set (personality and expectation of the user), setting (environ-

ment), and other factors. Morphine and heroin are legally and pharmacologically classified as narcotics. Methadone is a synthetic narcotic.

6. (c) Mescaline. All are stimulants except mescaline, which is a hallucinogen with effects similar to LSD.

7. (d) MPA. MPA is not an acronym for any known drug. MDA, LSD, and STP are all hallucinogens with similar effects. MDA (Mellow Drug of America) and STP (Serenity, Tranquility, Peace) are street drugs.

8. (c) Peyote. Physical dependence on mescaline (the active ingredient of the peyote cactus) or many other hallucinogens has not been verified.

9. (a) Inhalants. Sniffing aerosols, glue, or other volatile substances can result in immediate death, although experts disagree on explanations for the rapidity of death. Although "mainlining" heroin can result in immediate death, most experimentation with heroin includes sniffing or skin-popping (injecting it under the skin but not in a vein).

10. (d) Different for each person. Although the time it takes for a person to become physically dependent on heroin may vary, we know that repeated use of heroin ultimately causes physical dependence, and people can become physically dependent after as few as three or four uses.

11. (a) Lysergic acid diethylamide. Street drug analyses indicate that lysergic acid diethylamide (LSD) is often a major ingredient of street "mescaline," although it varies from city to city. Street

mescaline may also contain psilocybin, amphetamines, phencyclidine (PCP),* or other contaminants, but none of the drugs listed in (b), (c), or (d) have been reported. Street mescaline is rarely pure mescaline and often contains no mescaline at all.

12. (d) All of the above. In particular, in the case of illicit drug use, nonsterile equipment (b) is a serious hazard often overlooked by the drug user.

13. (b) Relieve discomfort. When a person stops taking a drug that he is physically dependent on, he develops physical withdrawal symptoms (such as muscle spasms, vomiting, sweating, insomnia, etc.). Taking the drug relieves the discomfort of onset of withdrawal symptoms.

14. (d) Psilocybin. Psilocybin is a hallucinogen which has no accepted medical use. All of the other drugs have at various times been used to treat narcotic addiction. When heroin was introduced in 1898, some people thought it had possibilities for treatment of "morphinism." Methadone, cyclazocine, and naloxone are used currently to block the "high" from use of heroin.

15. (e) All of the above. All have been used successfully to treat drug abusers, and many of the methods have been used in combination.

___

*PCP, or phencyclidine, which has gained popularity on the street, is an animal tranquilizer. However, because of its different effects at different dose levels, PCP cannot be accurately placed in the "standard" stimulant, depressant, or hallucinogenic categories, although it acts pharmacologically like both a hallucinogen and a central nervous system stimulant.

DUCTLESS GLANDS   Glands which secrete their products directly into the bloodstream, instead of through ducts into the other organs or to the exterior of the body, are known as ductless or endocrine glands (see ENDOCRINE SYSTEM).

GLANDS

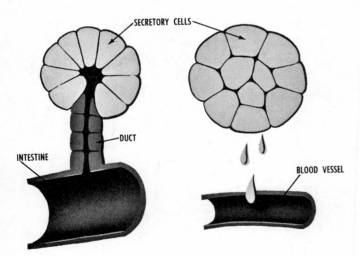

Exocrine glands (with ducts) empty into intestines or onto the skin.

Endocrine glands (ductless) empty directly into the blood stream.

DUMPING SYNDROME   After the surgical removal for any reason of all or part of the stomach, a group of symptoms known as the dumping syndrome sometimes occurs. The symptoms arise from two different mechanisms. In the first or immediate dumping syndrome the patient is aware of pain, distention, and sometimes nausea and vomiting immediately after eating. These symptoms occur as a result of the decrease in storage space due to the removal of a portion of the stomach; the ingested food then distends the first part of the intestine, causing the pain and vomiting.

In the second and more serious type of dumping syndrome, the symptoms occur usually about one-half hour to an hour after eating; therefore its name, the delayed dumping syndrome. In both cases, the symptoms are abdominal pain, palpitation, occasionally nausea and vomiting, and (in severe cases) actual loss of consciousness. The cause of these distressing symptoms is not entirely known or understood, but the presumption is that there are large fluid-shifts from the bloodstream into the small intestine, causing changes in the

206

delicate balance of fluid in and out of the vascular system. It is also thought that the sudden entrance of large amounts of food into the small intestine causes the pancreas to secrete larger amounts of insulin and other enzymes than would occur if food were released periodically, as it is in a normal stomach. This distressing condition is one of the reasons why removal of stomach tissue should be very carefully considered for conditions like peptic ulcers, which usually respond to other, less drastic, forms of treatment. The treatment for the dumping syndrome consists of avoiding consumption of large amounts of food at any one time. Small frequent feedings of bland food are consequently recommended.

DUODENUM   Literally duodenum means twelve fingerbreadths and refers to approximately the first twelve inches of the small intestine. It is joined at the stomach by the pylorus, curves around the head of the pancreas, and extends to the left upper portion of the abdomen where it joins the second portion of the small intestine (the jejunum). The bile from the gallbladder empties into the duodenum via the common bile duct. The pancreatic juices likewise empty into it to aid in the further breakdown of food.

The most common disorder of the duodenum is peptic ulcer. Interestingly, cancer of the duodenum—and indeed of the entire small intestine—is an extremely rare condition. Because of the constant irritation of the surface cells, this is an unexpected finding. Much investigative work is being carried out in an attempt to find out why this particular tissue in the body is almost immune to the ravages of cancer.

DWARFISM, PITUITARY   Failure of the peanut-sized pituitary gland at the base of the skull to secrete growth hormone before the age of maturity results in dwarfism. Pituitary dwarfs retain their

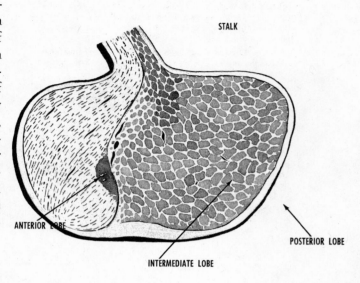

THE PITUITARY GLAND
(THE MASTER ENDOCRINE GLAND)

STALK

ANTERIOR LOBE

INTERMEDIATE LOBE

POSTERIOR LOBE

The anterior lobe produces at least six chemicals (hormones). These exert control over the other endocrine glands and the body in general. The posterior lobe secretes two hormones which control urine output and uterine muscular contractions. The function of the intermediate lobe is not certain.

childlike body proportions and do not undergo the normal prepuberal growth spurt. Because sexual maturation is absent or incomplete, older pituitary dwarfs may be considered by untrained individuals to be simply small children. Growth retardation is often apparent in early childhood; on the other hand, slow growth may continue into the mid-twenties, with eventual heights of four to four and one-half feet.

When failure to develop into adulthood becomes evident, the pituitary origin of the problem is suspected. If the entire pituitary gland is nonfunctional, as may occur with certain congenital anomalies and tumors, the child will also have signs of deficiency of thyroid and adrenal secretion. In about half the cases of pituitary dwarfism, the cause cannot be found. Intelligence is usually normal unless there is an associated thyroid deficiency or abnormality of the brain, either of which by itself would produce lack of mental development. (Emotional immaturity is often present because dwarfed children continue to be treated by adults as though they were younger.)

Because our knowledge of growth hormone is still incomplete, it is often not possible to make an accurate diagnosis of pituitary dwarfism at an early age. Until the age of one or two years, the child may appear to be as fully developed as other children. When concern about growth is brought to the attention of the physician, he must consider such things as family background, nutrition, and the presence of other congenital or hereditary diseases which limit growth and the function of other glands—particularly the thyroid. There is no specific laboratory test for diagnosing pituitary dwarfism, although X-ray of the skull will frequently reveal developmental defects or tumors in the region of the pituitary gland.

Treatment. The treatment of pituitary dwarfism will undoubtedly undergo revolutionary changes in the next few years. At present, administration of human growth hormone, which must be extracted from pituitary glands obtained at autopsy, is available for a very few patients in medical centers. For those individuals who have associated deficiencies in other endocrine glands, it is possible to obtain maturation and some degree of growth by treatment with thyroid substance, adrenal hormones, and—at the proper age—with male or female sex hormones. It is very important that persons having daily contact with those afflicted with pituitary dwarfism should be aware of the nature of their problem so they may be handled in accord with their age, and not with their height. This applies especially to parents and other relatives, teachers, social workers, schoolmates, and playmates. With proper care dwarfed individuals will have a normal life expectancy.

DYSENTERY   Dysentery, a more serious type of diarrhea, is the passage of very loose and watery, often bloody, stools seen in an intestinal infection due to a variety of bacteria. The disease is more often contracted in foreign countries, especially in warmer climates.

Symptoms. Dysentery is usually accompanied by fever and extreme prostration, the patient becoming rapidly dehydrated and going in a state of shock; the onset of the symptoms is rather rapid. Epidemics may occur, and on a lesser scale, whole families may suffer simultaneously after drinking from a common, contaminated source, such as a well. In carefully traced epidemics, one person will be found as the source of infection. This person may have no knowledge that he is a carrier (his system being immune to the effects of the germ), but his stools nevertheless contain the bacteria. Several germs are involved in dysentery, their identification depending upon their effect on different sugars when they are incubated: these include the typhoid, paratyphoid, *Salmonella,* and *Shigella.* In spite of good sanitation, these germs are still to be found sporadically in the United States and, of course, are rampant in tropical and low-income areas. Travelers learn not to drink unboiled water in those countries and are usually immunized against this disease before going abroad.

Treatment. Treatment for dysentery depends on the severity of the symptoms, but if the patient is severely ill he should be hospitalized, since intravenous fluids and perhaps blood may be needed. Usually a sample is taken of the stool and a drug or two started immediately; once the germ is identified, the most effective antibiotic is continued. Results are often dramatic within twenty-four to forty-eight hours if the patient has not been dehydrated or is not too seriously sick.

DYSMENORRHEA   Very few "female

troubles" can be as distressing to the patient, and occasionally to the doctor, as dysmenorrhea—severe, sometimes incapacitating, pain accompanying the monthly menstrual flow. It occurs predominately in younger women (late teens to late twenties) and improves or disappears after childbearing. It is much more common among better-educated, middle- and upper-class women, this latter fact lending support to those who believe that psychological factors are the primary cause, or at least account for the vast majority of the cases. Whether the cause is anatomical, hormonal, or psychosomatic, the fact remains that dysmenorrhea is a very painful experience for the patient. Its monthly recurrence may tremendously affect the personality of its sufferers.

Symptoms. Symptoms vary from an acute, colicky type of lower-abdominal (pelvic) pain lasting for the first one or two days of the menstrual flow, to milder but steadier pelvic soreness, not infrequently affecting the patient's thighs, knees, and legs. The patient may also complain of sensations of heaviness and fullness in the lower abdomen, with mild or moderate nausea and (occasionally) vomiting. Headaches, nervousness, and a general feeling of being "unwell" may be a part of the total picture. Part or all of these symptoms usually disappear one or two days after the beginning of menstrual flow.

Treatment. Such a complex and poorly understood entity as dysmenorrhea requires a carefully planned and individually suited program for its relief. Sympathetic understanding and cooperation between physician and patient are a prerequisite for the treatment. Relatively mild analgesics (aspirin or equivalents) will suffice for the milder cases. Stronger analgesics (narcotics) may be required for a day or two in more severe cases, and for uncooperative patients. Mild sedatives (in addition to the analgesics) will make it easier for the patient to withstand moderate dis-

comfort. Quite successful also are diuretic drugs given for two to three days before the onset of menstruation; they help relieve the sensation of heaviness and fullness of the lower abdomen, while nausea and vomiting is usually much improved or disappears. In some persistent cases, dilatation of the mouth of the womb and scraping of the uterus (D&C) may help temporarily or permanently.

In very resistant cases, temporary interruption of the menstrual periods by the use of hormones will definitely rid the patient of her symptoms, and quite often she will not require further treatment after her periods are allowed to occur normally. In any event, the majority of patients will benefit from a more natural cure in the form of marriage and childbearing.

DYSPAREUNIA   Pain experienced by the female during intercourse, dyspareunia may be caused by a variety of conditions. Often the male is responsible, either because of an excessively large penis, or because of ignorance of the act of proper sexual relations. In the female, the most common causes are: (1) infection of the vagina or the adjoining structures; (2) an extremely narrow or tight hymen, or too small a vagina (atrophic vagina being a relatively common cause of dyspareunia in postmenopausal women); (3) congenital anomalies of the vagina; (4) abnormal placement of the womb, so that it is turned backwards and sits on top of the birth-canal; (5) abnormal placement of the ovaries or infection of the tubes; or (6) psychosomatic factors—alone, or in coexistence with one or more of the above.

Treatment. Treatment depends on the cause. Infections should be treated; congenital anomalies, acquired malpositions, or tumors should be corrected surgically; a tight hymen must be cut or stretched; and atrophic vaginas of older women can be treated with hormones. Younger, inexperienced couples should be intelligently instructed about the physiological methods of intercourse and the usefulness of lubricants. Psychosomatic factors should be eliminated through careful analysis and psychotherapy. The overall prognosis is very good, and the majority of patients can be helped through specialized professional care.

DYSPEPSIA   See INDIGESTION

DYSTOCIA   This term applies to difficulties in labor and delivery. The most common causes are large babies or small pelvic-size of the mother, inability of the pregnant uterus to contract normally, pelvic tumors, etc. Treatment will depend on the cause of dystocia. Quite often caesarean section is required.

EAR   The ear and hearing mechanism is one of the most remarkable sense organs in the animal world. Its complexity is exceeded only by the human brain; its tiny mechanism is as fine and sensitive as the best of our miniscule man-made electrical-mechanical wonders.

There is a natural division of the ear into three parts. The first is the one we see: the outer ear. In some lower animals the outermost ear (pinna or auricle) still has the function of picking up sounds and is even able to turn so as to perform this function more efficiently. The best that man can do is wiggle his ears, and most of us can not even do that. The outer ear of man serves almost no hearing function. We are concerned about it mostly for cosmetic purposes and for hooking on eyeglasses.

From the outer ear and extending inward is a canal (the external auditory canal) a little over an inch long, which is lined by skin. This canal is supported at its outer third by cartilage and at its inner two-thirds by bone. The outermost skin of the canal has hair follicles and special glands which produce wax (cerumen). The innermost skin of the canal is very thin, tightly bound to the underlying bone, and devoid of hair and glands. The outer ear,

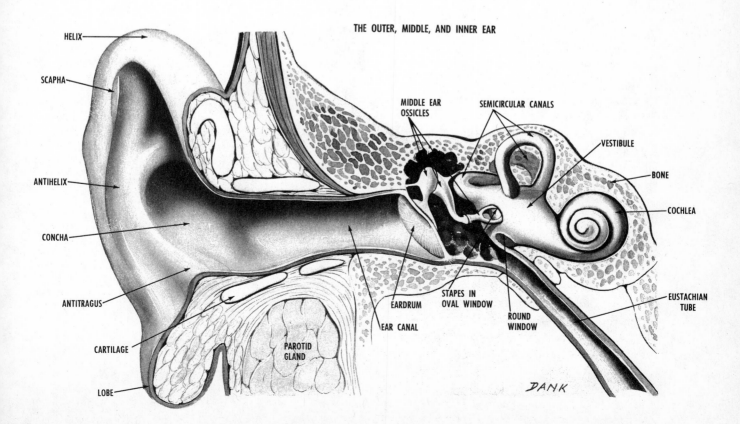

THE OUTER, MIDDLE, AND INNER EAR

HELIX — SCAPHA — ANTIHELIX — CONCHA — ANTITRAGUS — CARTILAGE — LOBE — MIDDLE EAR OSSICLES — SEMICIRCULAR CANALS — VESTIBULE — BONE — COCHLEA — EARDRUM — EAR CANAL — STAPES IN OVAL WINDOW — ROUND WINDOW — EUSTACHIAN TUBE — PAROTID GLAND — DANK

then, is composed of the pinna and the external auditory canal.

Separating the external from the middle ear is the eardrum (tympanic membrane or drumhead), an exceedingly thin membrane composed of five layers. The eardrum is about three-quarters the size of a dime, with a thickness of 1/250 of an inch.

Embedded in the fibrous layer of the vibrating eardrum is part of the first of the three bones of the middle ear. Shaped roughly like a hammer, this first bone has its handle attached to the eardrum and the head articulated with the second bone, which approximates an anvil in design. The anvil, in turn, has a delicate connection with the smallest bone in the human body, the last of the three bones of the middle ear, which fits into the "oval window" or *fenestra ovalis*. (This smallest bone is shaped very much like a stirrup, so the three bones are sometimes called the hammer, anvil, and stirrup. Their more sophisticated Latin names are the *malleus*, *incus*, and *stapes*, and it is these which we shall use in the text.) The stapes is flexibly bound to the oval window by an oval ligament.

The inner ear begins just below the oval window with a two-fluid system and is housed deep in the temporal bone in a special casing of extremely dense bone. The delicate organs of balance (the semi-circular canals) and of hearing (the cochlea) are housed in this special casing and share fluid systems in common. Although they are known by different names, the general mechanical construction of both are similar.

The chief pathway of sound traveling through the hearing mechanism is: into outer ear—ear canal—tympanic membrane—malleus—incus—stapes—stapes-footplate (which in its virbrations sets the outer fluid in motion)—basilar membrane of the organ of Corti (in the cochlea)—inner fluid—haircells of the organ of Corti

cochlear nerve—nuclei of the cochlea—lower brain-centers—higher brain-centers (where sound is recognized, associated, and interpreted).

There is a small tube indirectly associated with hearing which extends from the middle ear to the back of the throat at the level of the nose, called the Eustachian tube. This tube is ordinarily kept closed by muscles at the throat and is opened during yawning and swallowing, thereby keeping the air pressure on the middle ear side of the eardrum equal to that on the outer (atmospheric) side. The ear and hearing mechanisms are enormously complex, and this is a very simplified version; however, sufficient information has been given to understand the more common problems of hearing loss. (See also HEARING LOSS; HEARING TESTS; HEARING AIDS.)

EARDRUM, PERFORATION OF THE

The main mechanism of the middle ear depends upon the relatively large area of the eardrum acting via the three middle-ear bones (ossicles) on the relatively small area of the stapes-footplate. This mechanism is called "the sound-pressure transformer." The eardrum is an extremely important part of the sound-pressure transformer because it provides a seventeen to one increase in pressure at the stapes footplate. A perforation of the eardrum lowers this ratio (among other factors), thus causing hearing loss. Keeping water out of a normal ear is a good idea, but keeping water out of an ear with a perforated eardrum is an absolute necessity—and that means no swimming.

Treatment. There are several methods of closing eardrum perforations. If no infection or damage exists other than the hole in the eardrum, any hearing loss caused by the perforation can be remedied if the eardrum is repaired. Because a perforated eardrum more easily allows infection to enter the middle ear, it is wise to see an ear specialist about any eardrum perforation. Home remedies such as oils, Merthiolate®, and water irrigations are definitely contraindicated.

The patient should place a clean piece of cotton in the ear, take aspirin for pain, keep the ear dry, and plan to consult a physician soon. From office-treatment to major surgical procedures in the hospital, hearing loss through drum perforation can be repaired in a high percentage of cases. If there are no other defects except the perforated eardrum itself, the chances of successful therapy are over 90 per cent.

EAR, INFECTION OF THE MIDDLE

Infection of the middle ear is called otitis media. This should not be confused with serous otitis media, which (see page 377) does not refer to an *infected* middle ear. Usually the infection results from an upper respiratory infection and affects the middle ear via the Eustachian tube. The symptoms of otitis media are pain in the ear, hearing loss, and fullness in the ear during, or following, an upper respiratory infection.

Treatment. The treatment may be myringotomy with antibiotics or antibiotics alone. (The usual "cold," however, is caused by a virus, not by bacteria. If however, the bacteria *have* gained a foothold, it can be safely assumed that the virus has prepared the way. To put it another way, antibiotics are not in the least effective against the viruses causing colds, and it is only when bacterial invasion has been added that they are indicated. The patient demanding antibiotics for the common cold is therefore foolish and is trying to get the doctor to do something against his better judgment which will not help, and on the other hand may harm, the patient. Only a physician is in a position to decide what medication to use.) In otitis media as in other ear diseases, it is wise to avoid putting anything in the ear unless prescribed by a physician. If the ear begins to drain, this indicates the drum has

broken, providing a natural myringotomy. If this happens, clean cotton may be used in the ear to catch the drainage. The cotton should be very clean and be changed often; washing the hands before and after changing the cotton is a good idea. The doctor should be consulted *as soon as possible.*

Acute extension of a middle ear infection into the air spaces of the mastoid bone (acute mastoiditis) is now relatively uncommon because of the advances in medicine. Chronic mastoiditis is a different condition, however, and is often associated with chronically closed Eustachian tube (or cholesteatoma). Surgery for this kind of mastoid problem is still relatively frequent.

EAR, SOME COMMON DISEASES OF THE EXTERNAL

The skin of the external ear is subject to the same diseases as skin in other locations of the body. The very thin skin closely bound to the sculptured cartilage of the pinna is most subject to deforming injury. The skin of the ear canal is most subject to chronic inflammation and infections because of the tendency toward retention of moisture.

The pinna is the most frequent site of frostbite. Common signs are loss of skin sensation, color changes from flesh to yellow-white, and hardening of the ear. When these occur, the entire body should be warmed and a physician seen at once. Heat or massage should not be applied to the frostbitten ear. In later stages of frostbite the ear becomes painful and swollen, and blisters (blebs) occur on the skin. Protection against infection and prevention of permanent shut-off of blood vessels may prevent gangrene. Neglect of the condition by the frostbitten patient can result in gangrene and loss of the ear.

Injury to the ear can cause blood to accumulate under the skin, forming a hematoma (literally blood-tumor). The blood should be evacuated and protection against

212

infection secured. Consolidation of the hematoma can produce the "cauliflower ear." Like most ear problems, this is not amenable to home therapy, and a doctor should be seen.

Perichondritis is an infection of the lining between the skin and the cartilage of the outer ear. It can occur after injury, hematoma, frostbite, burns, or other damage. The ear becomes very thick and dusky red in color. This condition must be vigorously treated with antibiotics. Abscesses must be evacuated. Other modalities such as ultraviolet light may be recommended by the physician.

The skin behind the lobule of the ear has many sebaceous glands. When obstruction of a gland occurs, a cyst (called a sebaceous cyst) may form. This happens frequently behind the ear or earlobe. Surgical excision is the treatment of choice.

Keloids are an accumulation of scar tissue from any damage to the ear. They frequently occur after the earlobe is pierced for earrings. Surgical incision, sometimes followed by small amounts of X-ray, may prevent recurrence.

A localized form of external otitis, furuncles are really just pustules which can cause severe pain and tenderness of the ear. If treatment is started early, the infection can be corrected with local application of medication; later, incision and drainage may be necessary.

Lop-ear or protruding ear is a condition which can often be corrected by surgery. The purpose of surgery for a protruding ear is purely cosmetic. The ear cartilages are usually too soft to operate upon satisfactorily under the age of four, but after this age results are satisfying. The operation is called otoplasty.

EAR, TUMORS OF THE Tumors of the ear are not common. There are three kinds of cancer of the outer ear and three of the middle ear. There is also one benign (but dangerous) tumor of the inner ear. Hearing loss, sores that do not heal, bleeding from the ear, inability to move some facial muscles, and constant discharge from the ear are among symptoms of both benign and malignant conditions. The diagnosis must be made by your physician.

EATING PROBLEMS Problems with food usually develop because of insufficient knowledge on the mother's part, or because of emotional tensions that are brought to the table. The most common complaint is that the child (usually aged two to four years) will not eat.

It is possible that the "non-eating" child is sick or anemic and needs medicine or a tonic; in most cases, however, difficulties stem from the fact that the mother's idea of what the child should eat and the child's idea of what he will eat are two different things. The mother is used to the big appetite that the child had when he was four months old (and gaining two to three pounds in a month), but the child is now growing—and eating—less.

Treatment. If the child is healthy, happy, and up-and-around, he is obviously not starving, and the mother must stop worrying and pushing the food down his throat unless she wants a neurotic child. The best way to feed the two-to-four-year-old is to put small amounts of food (amounts he will be sure to eat) in front of him on a saucer; then if he wants more, he will ask for it. This is a far better situation than having the mother continually pleading with the child to eat.

The types of foods are important. In infancy milk was the baby's most important food. After one year of age it is probably the least important and, like all white foods, is merely a "bonus" of extra calories after the basic meat and fruit (vegetables if the child wants them) are consumed.

Too many mothers have been falsely led to believe that if the child at least drinks his milk he will be all right, even if nothing else is eaten. This is a fallacy. Milk lacks iron, is often highly constipating, and some people are allergic to it, suffering embarrassing amounts of gas and stomach cramps. This is not to say milk should be neglected or avoided, however. Since it is a major source of calcium, it should unquestionably be part of the diet of all children.

Children in the two-to-four group do not chew easily, so they are apt to prefer ground meat. Frankfurters, hamburgers, and soft-cooked chicken are about the only flesh-foods that small children will eat willingly. Fruits and vegetables have the same nutritional elements in them, and are therefore quite interchangeable. Bread and dairy products round out the diet. Since vitamins are found in all these foods, supplements are not usually necessary.

Sometimes it is best for the child to have only one meal a day. Although a child can be taught most of the good and bad eating habits of the parents, there is very little truth to the rule that if the parents like or dislike a specific food, the child will also dislike or like it. It is simply not so. The best rule is: keep mealtimes simple and keep them pleasant.

ECLAMPSIA   See Toxemias of Pregnancy

ECZEMA   In eczema the affected skin is red, scaly, itchy, and often "weepy," and the child with this problem is unable to leave the area alone. The usual locations of the eruption are the cheeks, the inner areas of the elbows, and the backs of the knees, but it can be found on any part of the body. In most cases the condition is caused by allergy to some kind of food and will disappear when the food is withdrawn from the diet. When it occurs in a very small baby, a milk-substitute has to be found (soybean, goat's milk, etc.). In older children and in teenagers the condition is sometimes assumed to be related to a sensitizing food. The more common offenders include milk, wheat, eggs, chocolate, citrus, pork, nuts, fish, corn, and vitamins.

Chronic eczema (neurodermatitis) is the name applied when the condition drags on for months or years; this may not disappear even with a strict elimination diet. The skin becomes thickened, remains scaly, but red only during acute flare-ups. Such flare-ups may be triggered by emotion, certain foods, contact with some irritants (soap, wool, etc.).

Treatment. Various ointments, especially those containing cortisone, will give temporary relief; but until the offending agent is removed the problem will recur. Many eczematous lesions become infected, so an antibiotic ointment may be necessary to help clear the condition.

Antihistaminics given internally, and external use of coal tar and cortisone ointments, as well as oil baths, will mollify the problem of chronic eczema, but nothing really cures it. (See also Infantile Eczema; Allergic Skin Diseases; Atopic Dermatitis; Contact Dermatitis.)

EDEMA   Edema is the presence of excessive amounts of fluid in the tissues, between the cells of the body, or in the various body cavities, and whatever the form it takes, it may cause the symptoms of congestive heart-failure. It may be present in the legs or arms, the pleural cavities, the liver and spleen, the lungs, or the brain. Indeed, accumulations of fluid may appear simultaneously in any combination of the body reservoirs.

No matter what the primary cause of the circulatory weakness happens to be, circulation inefficiency can cause accumulation of edema fluid. Often as much as six quarts can accumulate in the body before edema becomes noticeable to the patient, in the form of swollen ankles or fingers. The condition itself may be a sign of primary congestive heart-failure, but also may be a secondary result of kidney disease, nutritional disorder, or any of a number of other conditions.

In all cases of edema there is usually a rise of pressure in the veins bringing blood back to the heart. For various reasons, fluid has failed to escape from the tissue reservoirs and makes its way into the capillaries which return it, via the veins, to the heart. There is passive venous congestion, or crowding, and this makes for very inefficient pick-up of tissue fluid into the venous circulation.

The edema (or dropsy) of circulatory failure may be due solely to inability of the right side of the heart to move blood efficiently (right heart-failure). Edema in right heart-failure occurs throughout the body, but because there is an inefficient flow of blood from the right ventricle to the lungs, the pulmonary vessels and tissue spaces in the lung itself do not usually show congestion and edema in the early phases of this condition.

More commonly, perhaps, edema is caused by failure of the *left* side of the heart to empty blood efficiently from the lungs. In this case lung edema will be almost immediate. This burden will cause gradual failure of the right side of the heart as well, so that total heart (pancardiac) failure can be present, together with failing circulation to and from the lungs.

As soon as deposits of fluid begin to accumulate abnormally in various tissue spaces, a number of unusual changes in the body's fluid-handling methods begin to appear. For some reason, when circulation is inefficient the kidneys fail to excrete sodium in the usual amount. Excess sodium thereupon accumulates in the body and will attract and hold water in an effort to prevent the body fluids from becoming "too salty."

EJACULATION   The forceful discharge of semen (sperm) from the urethra opening at the tip of the penis is known as ejaculation. This process is rhythmic and begins at the base of the penis, where the ejaculatory duct enters on each side mixing the sperm with the secretion of the prostate gland.

EKG   EKG usually refer to the written record that comes from the electrocardiograph machine.

ELECTRA COMPLEX   Sigmund Freud defined the Electra complex as an unhealthy emotional attachment of a daughter toward her father, in which the daughter was unable to adjust to men of her own age because of a morbid attachment to the father. According to psychoanalytic theory, each young girl's ideal conception of the opposite sex is based on the relationship with her father. Normally, she is able to break away from her over-idealized father-image and make a normal adjustment to some younger man; when the father fixation is unduly strong, however, the girl may never be able to break away from her father's influence, thus making satisfactory adjustment to a man of her own age impossible. Fathers would be wise to discourage undue dependence by daughters, who should be encouraged to make their own decisions in becoming acquainted with many young men.

ELECTROCARDIOGRAPHY   The individual muscle fibers are stimulated to contract by electrical-voltage changes at the junction of the nerve and contracting fiber. To insure rhythmic pumping motion of the chambers, the impulse for contracture begins in healthy subjects at the pacemaker in the wall of the right auricle. The electrical current (excitation wave) moves along the muscle fibers themselves, and is conducted specifically by a system much like a telegraph cable. This special tissue, the bundle of His (beginning at the atrioventricular node), takes the electrical wave from the auricles into the ventricles, which ordinarily contract after auricular contracture has concluded. The bundle of His fibers take the wave of excitation to the tip of the ventricles and thence, after dividing into left and right branches, to all the fibers of the ventricular chambers.

Impulse transmission is very rapid along the bundle and its branches but relatively slow as it spreads out in the muscle, gradually passing to all the fibers in the contracting chamber.

In the relaxed, resting state, the heart-muscle fiber is charged positively on the surface. In this state, the muscle cell or fiber is said to be polarized. (The sodium ion at the surface is apparently a major influence in maintaining this positive surface charge.) When the muscle fiber contracts, the sodium ion moves within the cell membrane, and the surface charge turns negative. The muscle fiber is now said to be depolarized.

Experimentally, metal contact-points can be wired to the heart surface and led to a galvanometer, so that the spread of positive-to-negative potential can be traced as the muscle wave of contracture moves from its point of origin to the last heart fiber contracting in that beat. The resulting device is known as an electrocardiograph (EKG or ECG). Abnormal electrocardiogram tracings are present in most of the disease states that affect the heart.

In practice, the wired contacts do not actually touch the heart; the patient's body conducts the current, small though it is, the wires (or leads) being fastened to the arms and legs, or even along the wall of the chest over the heart. In these locations they provide a good tracing of the electrical activity within the heart.

Individual waves on the cardiographic tracing are called the P,Q,R,S, and T waves for reference. The P wave is the one which occurs at the beginning of the contraction of the auricles. The next wave, the QRS complex, occurs during contraction of the ventricles, and consists of three parts, above and below the zero line. The Q component comes as the impulse produces electrical changes in the fibers of the wall between the ventricles; the R and S components occur as the impulse spreads throughout the ventricles and out onto the heart surface, which is the last to tense. The T wave is recorded as the electrical charge along the conduction system begins to reverse polarity in the recovery, or relaxation, phase of the heartbeat.

In practical use, the electrocardiographic tracing is most useful both in the diagnosis and the observation of clinical progress of most heart patients. The machine is readily available, and little or no discomfort is experienced by the patient as the record is being made.

ELECTROENCEPHALOGRAM   An electroencephalogram is a graphic record of the electrical activity recorded from the surface of the brain by electrodes placed on the scalp. The electroencephalogram is a valuable diagnostic aid in a number of neurologic disorders. Perhaps the most important application of electroencephalography is in the diagnosis and improved understanding of convulsive seizures (epilepsy), since abnormal electrical wave patterns occur during convulsive attacks. Also, in more than half the patients with epilepsy, abnormal activity is recorded on the electroencephalogram between attacks. Localized brain disorders may be associated with abnormal electrical patterns on the electroencephalogram; hence, these are sometimes a valuable laboratory aid in diagnosis.

ELEMENTS (MINERALS)   Of the more than one hundred chemical elements now recognized, fourteen appear to be essential for human nutrition. These minerals (a preferred term) are widely distributed in foods, and under conditions of health there is little danger of a dietary deficiency developing. In certain disease states, however, abnormalities of mineral-nutrition do occur. Like vitamins, with which many are connected, minerals have important bodily functions.

The essential minerals are sodium, potassium, chlorine, calcium, phosphorus, sulfur, magnesium, iron, copper, iodine, manganese, cobalt, zinc, and molybdenum. (Several are discussed in separate entries under their own names.)

ELEPHANTIASIS This is a condition most often seen in the legs, which are markedly enlarged due to excessive subcutaneous (beneath the skin) fluid and thickening of the tissues. There is obliteration of normal ankle and calf contours, giving the impression of elephant legs. The fundamental cause is blockage of the flow of lymph. In temperate and colder regions the disfigurement is usually due to a developmental defect present at birth. However, elephantiasis may be seen after multiple attacks of erysipelas, and in other chronic infections involving the lymphatics.

EMBOLISM Circulatory disease is frequently caused or complicated by embolism, the formation of a foreign body (embolus) such as a blood clot or a cluster of bacteria. After a fracture of bone, a fragment of fatty material may escape from the bone marrow into a vein and form a fat embolus. A laceration of a vein in the neck as made, for example, by a penetrating piece of glass at the time of an automobile accident, will sometimes permit air to enter the circulation and produce an air embolus. Many small gas emboli form in the bloodstream when a deep sea diver is lifted to the surface rapidly; gas that was held in the body fluids by the high underwater pressure suddenly bubbles free (diver's bends).

Within the heart, any disease area tends to be roughened, and blood may form clots in those surfaces that are not smooth, especially if for any reason there is a slowing of the circulation. In heart disease both roughened intima and slowed circulation are frequently present, especially in association with diseased valve leaflets.

If the embolus forms in the right side of the heart it may fragment and particles of it pass to the pulmonary artery branches: pulmonary embolus. If the clot is formed in and breaks away from the left side of the heart, it can move through the arterial system to any organ of the body: the brain, kidney, or intestine, for example. The embolus can cause serious changes in the organ in which it lodges: even death will result if the vital area of the brain is so involved and deprived of blood supply.

Perhaps most embolization originates in the veins, at points far distant from the heart. Thus, an inflammatory state of the leg veins called thrombophlebitis can produce clots of blood within the veins. Fragments may break away and drift in the moving blood into the right auricle of the heart, skip through the tricuspid valves into the right ventricle, and then push into the pulmonary artery. When the clot reaches a small branch of the pulmonary artery in one of the lungs, it firmly lodges and obstructs blood flow in that particular branch of the vessel. This produces death of the lung tissue supplied by the vessel, the destroyed portion of the lung being a pulmonary infarction.

While a small pulmonary infarct generally produces very little in the way of symptoms (chest pain, blood-tinged sputum), a large pulmonary infarct may even cause the death of a patient.

EMOTIONS Feelings and emotions constitute the affective life of a person and are regarded as one of the three major components of psychic life, the other two being cognition (Reason) and volition. Feelings and emotions are biologically more primitive than intellect, appearing earlier, both in the history of the race and the development of a person.

The basic feelings are pleasure-pain, excitement-relaxation, and like-dislike. Feelings and emotions may be understood as primitive evaluatory reactions which underlie intuition. The basic emotions are fear, anger, and love. All emotions involve a fusion of physiological and psychological components, and are true psychosomatic reactions. Every emotion involves not only a mental state, but also a physiological pattern; both are integrated and coordinated in a unified emotional experience.

In order to understand each emotion, it is necessary to understand not only the primitive, instinctive, conscious component, but also the physical changes occurring simultaneously. When one is angry, the

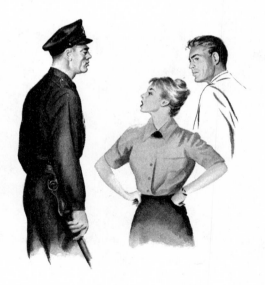

heart beats faster, blood pressure goes up, blood is distributed to the body musculature, the face becomes flushed, and the adrenal glands pour extra adrenalin into the bloodstream—all these changes being physical preparation for fighting. Anger is thus a biologic emergency-state. If one becomes angry often enough, he may remain in a constant state of biologic preparedness, associated with high blood

pressure (hypertension) and other unhealthy circulatory changes.

In contrast, fear is associated with an entirely different pattern of physical changes. A person may suddenly become pale, start to tremble and shake, feel general weakness, and even empty bladder and bowels involuntarily. There may be feelings of dizziness, fast or irregular pulse, abdominal faintness or quivering, and generalized muscular trembling. In chronic neurotic states, these fear symptoms may persist indefinitely, to the point of disabling the person.

Under the influence of love, a person feels happy and at ease. He may experience feelings of pleasurable excitement and tension, but ordinarily these do not interfere with his work. The person in love tends to be friendly, uncritical, and at peace with the world. His vital functions proceed normally and harmoniously.

The negative emotions of fear and anger are associated with disruptive physiological changes which can seriously interfere with healthy living. It is desirable to have a healthy and active emotional life, but excessive emotionalism almost inevitably results in a wide variety of psychosomatic symptoms and physiological disorders both in the person himself and in those who must react to him. The term neurotic refers to nonorganic disorders of emotional origin, and upset emotions are found in all neurotic disorders. Emotions provide the powerhouse of mental life and are healthy as long as they are kept under control, but can be associated with all kinds of symptom formations if they get out of control. It is therefore important for the individual to understand what his emotions are and, also, how to control and modify them.

EMOTIONS IN ALLERGY   Emotional disturbances can influence the course of an allergic disorder and, conversely, allergic problems can cause emotional disturbances. There are, however, only a few allergic-type diseases in which emotional problems are a true cause of the disorder (psychogenic urticaria, some cases of migraine headaches, and pseudoallergy). In general, psychosomatic states are a secondary factor, as emotional upsets will intensify and even trigger an allergic attack.

Psychological problems frequently arise where chronic allergic states are involved. For instance, there are overprotective mothers who go to extremes in taking care of an allergic child with asthma or eczema. In this situation the family life revolves entirely around a self-centered, selfish child. The rest of the family become irritable and unhappy. The suddenness of asthmatic attacks keeps both the family and the sick person continually worried and anxious, and fear of suffocating often converts a mild asthmatic attack into a severe one.

Fully as bad as the overprotective mother is her direct opposite: the indifferent careless parent who neglects the basic cares of her allergic offspring. This maternal rejection leads to severe psychological problems.

At school, teachers must contend with the sniffing, itching, coughing, restless, overactive, sensitive, and chronically ill child. Their reactions to the allergic child will in part affect the child's emotional response to his illness.

Persons with allergic rhinitis, with their constant noisy breathing and sniffing, constitute an annoyance to the people around them. This soon becomes obvious to afflicted individuals, who then tend to avoid human contact and keep to themselves.

Individuals with atopic dermatitis who are constantly scratching and reveal an unattractive eczema also avoid public exposure and try to lead a solitary, self-pitying type of existence. The emotional status of such people is affected by discomfort, sleeplessness, disfigurement, and the chronic quality of their skin disorders.

Allergic headaches may be accompanied by mental symptoms (confusion and personality changes) due to edema of the brain. Some migraine headaches of nonallergic origin are psychogenic; individuals suffering from these are usually perfectionists, tense, and have very rigid personalities.

There is a true allergy of the nervous system with such symptoms as overactivity, restlessness, clumsiness, irritability, insomnia, sluggishness or depression, unusual behavor, inability to concentrate and nervous tics or paleness, dark circles under the eyes, stuffy nose, swollen eyelids, excessive saliva, heavy sweating, abdominal pains, headaches, and bed-wetting. Before considering allergy, a physician should rule out all other possible causes when confronted with such an array of symptoms.

Certain cases of chronic hives (psychogenic urticaria) occur as a response to emotional conflict. These are most common in middle-aged women and older children. The wheals usually develop with a burning sensation.

When a person escapes reality and responsibilities by laying the blame for an unpleasant situation onto an allergy, he is said to have a pseudoallergy. This type of individual can have all the classic symptoms of any truly allergic disorder.

Emotional disturbances may be symptoms of treatment-reaction, since such states as drowsiness, irrational behavior, hysteria, confusion, impotence, and nervous movements can be caused by the medications being used in treating the allergic patient. (See ALLERGIC CORYZA; ALLERGIC REACTIONS IN CHILDREN; ASTHMA; ALLERGIES, DIAGNOSIS OF; HEADACHES; HIVES.)

EMPHYSEMA This word is derived from the Greek and means to inflate. It designates a variety of states in which overinflation occurs in any part of the body. In common usage, emphysema refers to a condition in which the smallest lung sacs (alveoli) become overdistended and lose their normal structure, and in which progressive "trapping" of air in the lung takes place. An additional important characteristic of the disease is the development of severe obstruction to airflow; at the present time it is not clear whether this obstruction precedes or follows the anatomical destruction. Emphysema is a disease much more prevalent in men than in women (ten to one ratio).

Overdistention of the lung may be purely a functional change without significant disease implications, as many otherwise healthy elderly individuals exhibit this feature. Pure emphysema (also called chronic pulmonary emphysema, or obstructive or hypertrophic pulmonary emphysema) is a disease in which overinflation is accompanied by anatomical destruction of lung-tissue, leading to the formation of small or large cavities called bulla; these become functionless, and in turn encroach upon and impair the function of still-normal lung areas. (See Obstructive Lung Disease.)

The cause, or causes, of emphysema are unknown. Commonly-held theories link the condition to chronic bronchitis, which almost invariably antecedes it. It is believed that emphysema is the final result of the sustained irritation to the bronchial tubes which follows in the wake of excessive smoking, air pollution, or repeated episodes of respiratory infection or allergic asthma. The common factor in all these conditions is the development of obstruction to airflow; this may be intermittent and reversible at the beginning (bronchoconstriction) but is eventually superseded by excessive mucous secretions which progressively narrow the bronchial passageway. With progression of the disease, air is allowed to flow in but is partially trapped on its way out, leading to formation of larger and larger air sacs. More respiratory pressure must then be exerted to promote airflow. This, in turn, further contributes to closing down the already narrowed and unsupported bronchial tubes.

Symptoms. Chronic pulmonary emphysema is a disease of insidious and progressive nature. A typical case might be a male in his late fifties who has been a heavy smoker for more than thirty years. He will have had a chronic sputum-productive cough for many years—one which was always dismissed as a "cigarette cough." For the past ten to fifteen years he has given up certain physical efforts which produce uncomfortable breathing (dyspnea), such as fast walking, running to catch a bus, or climbing more than two flights of stairs.

Because of the gradual development of this incapacitation, the typical patient often disregards it and does not volunteer such information until specifically questioned. At some point a respiratory infection develops and the patient becomes acutely ill and overcome by severe shortness of breath which clearly prevents him from performing his common daily activities. Cough and expectoration increase. The chest acquires a barrel shape, the shoulders are thrown forward and the patient gasps for breath. Usually the lips become bluish and the fingernails "clubbed" (similar in shape to drumsticks). Breathing ceases to be an effortless, unconscious mechanism and becomes a struggle.

The respiratory muscles have to perform a tremendous amount of work to get enough oxygen into the lungs and to transfer it to the blood in order to provide for the metabolic needs of the body; here, more oxygen is also required. This creates the following paradox: reduced lung function provides less than the necessary amount of oxygen, which is avidly "fought for" by both the body and the very respiratory muscles whose own need of oxygen is abnormally increased because of excess labor in moving an overdistended and inefficient chest.

Since breathing must continue, the respiratory muscles have "priority" on the available oxygen. Next in line for use of oxygen are the important organs of circulation and digestion, the brain, etc. Thus, very little is left in the end for use by the skeletal muscles and such activities as walking, for example, have to be severely curtailed. Effective expectoration of sputum is impaired, and mucus "plugs" create more bronchial obstruction. The stage is set for the development of repeated episodes of bronchial infection which acutely reduce the already chronically impaired breathing capacity. Curtailment of breathing capacity (particularly in acute emphysema) throws a burden onto the heart, which is forced to strain itself to maintain circulation through the lungs. Thus, heart-failure or pulmonary heart disease is a common complication in the advanced stages of chronic pulmonary emphysema.

Treatment. At present, treatment is mostly symptomatic and directed toward obtaining "bronchial cleansing." In essence, it is the treatment of chronic bronchitis. During its early stages, effective regimes may considerably delay the otherwise expected downward course of emphysema. Breathing exercises and abdominal belts are useful in reeducating the breathing pattern and can ease the work of the respiratory muscles. Slight degrees of physical activity (below the point of marked discomfort) are to be encouraged under a progressive program of rehabilitation. At the beginning of such a program, oxygen may be added to lengthen the training periods. Chronic use of oxygen at the patient's home has to be watched carefully, because in certain patients it may induce severe respiratory depression—the so-called "carbon dioxide narcosis syndrome." Symptoms of heart-failure are treated with digitalis and other drugs (diuretics) designed to promote urinary output and prevent fluid accumulation in the body.

ENCEPHALITIS   Encephalitis is an inflammatory reaction of the brain, usually involving both the cerebral hemispheres and the brainstem. It is frequently associated with inflammation of the meninges, and is then referred to as meningoencephalitis. A wide variety of disorders produce encephalitis, including various infections and intoxications. Infections, in turn, may be due to viruses, rickettsiae, fungi, and a few bacteria such as the bacilli which produce tuberculosis. Some forms

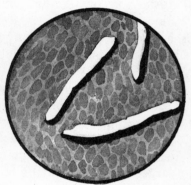

TUBERCLE BACILLI

of encephalitis occur in epidemics and others occur sporadically. Birds are the reservoir of the virus of equine encephalitis, which is transmitted by mosquitoes to horses and man and occasionally results in epidemics of encephalitis. Other viral diseases produce similar epidemic spread. Rarely, encephalitis is also a complication of measles, chickenpox, and mumps, as well as vaccination against rabies and smallpox. Encephalitis may also occur with lead poisoning.

Symptoms. The patient is either drowsy or stuporous. The neck may be stiff and there may be headache and fever. Localized weakness, visual disturbances, disorders of speech and swallowing may be present. The patient may be irritable. In extreme cases, loss of consciousness and convulsions may indicate early demise. Examination of the cerebrospinal fluid usually reveals a slight increase in the number of white blood cells. The organism responsible for some types of encephalitis can be cultured from the cerebrospinal fluid. In other types of infections, studies of the blood serum during the acute and convalescent phases of the illness may determine the cause. Skin lesions associated with some of these infections may be characteristic.

Treatment. Specific antibiotic and chemical agents are used in the treatment of rickettsial infections such as Rocky Mountain spotted fever, tuberculous meningoencephalitis, and cryptococci meningoencephalitis. No specific drugs are available for the treatment of virus infections producing encephalitis. The patient with severe encephalitis requires constant nursing care and attention, with careful check of blood pressure and respiration. If there is severe difficulty in swallowing, the patient may require an opening into the windpipe (tracheotomy). If the patient is unable to breathe adequately because of weakness of the respiratory muscles, respiratory aids are required. Intravenous fluids are often needed to prevent dehydration in patients who are stuporous or who vomit frequently. Physical therapy and, subsequently, occupational therapy are essential for those who develop motor weakness or paralysis.

ENDOCARDITIS   The endocardium is the smooth and glistening membrane that covers the entire inner surface of the heart walls and valves. Invasion of an area of the endocardium by bacterial organisms is called bacterial endocarditis.

When "blood-poisoning" is present from peritonitis, childbirth fever, or from an overwhelming infection due to almost any type of bacteria, the heart may be infected secondarily to the disease. The acute bacterial endocarditis that may be present in any case of "blood-poisoning"

is not primarily an affliction of the heart, and is rarely discussed in association with the circulatory diseases.

Subacute bacterial endocarditis is a distinct heart disease. It is due to bacteria of rather low toxicity that have colonized an area of the inner heart surface which has usually already been damaged by rheumatic fever or congenital deformity. This damage focuses a harsh stream of blood on a small bit of surface within the heart and causes the formation of a surface erosion that is vulnerable to bacterial implantation.

The organism involved is usually the so-called "non-hemolytic streptococcus" that can ordinarily be found in the mouth of even healthy subjects. A tooth extraction or sore throat may cause escape of these bacteria into the bloodstream where they freely travel to the heart and may attach themselves to endocardial spots roughened by stress changes or prior disease.

Symptoms. The symptoms of subacute bacterial endocarditis are usually those of a low grade fever and weakness. If these occur in a rheumatic patient or one with congenital heart disease, subacute bacterial endocarditis (SBE) must always be suspected. Diagnosis is based on a specimen of blood which shows the offending organism. The blood sedimentation rate is elevated, and anemia is often present as a complication.

Treatment. Vigorous antibiotic therapy and bed rest have brought down the mortality-rate to a figure below 30 per cent in the active phase of the infection. Those who recover usually show marked damage to the valves that were involved in the process.

Adequate surgical correction of congenital heart defects will prevent bacterial endocarditis. Sometimes the only indication for surgery in a patient with no symptoms related to congenital deformity may be the prevention of bacterial endocarditis.

ENDOCRINE ADENOMATOSIS This condition exists when tumors arise simultaneously in several endocrine organs. Although rare, it is important for the physician to recognize. Tumors may be seen at one and the same time in the parathyroid, the pancreas, and the pituitary, each of which produces its own characteristic effects which mingle with the effects of the tumors in the other glands. This complexity makes the entire disease-picture exceedingly difficult to diagnose.

ENDOCRINE SYSTEM The group of glands which secrete their products directly into the bloodstream are known collectively as the endocrine (ductless glands) system. The glands are to a great extent interrelated, the thyroid, adrenal glands, and sex glands being dependent for their normal functioning on secretion of the pituitary gland. It is for this reason that the pituitary is known as the "master" or controlling gland. The function of the pituitary gland is in turn regulated by a "feedback" mechanism which permits the pituitary to turn off its supply of hormones when they are not needed. Thus we may speak of a pituitary-thyroid or pituitary-adrenal axis which keeps the gland secretions in balance. Evidence that the endocrine glands operate as an interrelated system is also seen in the development of multiple tumors of various endocrine glands.

ENDOMETRIOSIS This is characteristically known as the "disease of the career girl," because it occurs predominantly in white women with a good educational background, gainfully employed, who have never been pregnant. It affects women in their middle or late twenties, but may begin as early as the late teens; it disappears after the menopause. The disease is due to the presence of endometrial tissue in areas other than the cavity of the womb.

During menstruation this "out-of-place" (ectopic) tissue undergoes the same changes as the normal endometrium, growing, becoming congested, and causing severe pain. The mechanism through which this endometrial tissue becomes ectopic is still an unsettled problem. It becomes commonly implanted on the ovaries, tubes, ligaments of the womb, top of the vagina, and occasionally in such unusual places as the rectum, lungs, etc.

Symptoms. Depending on the organ involved and the extent of the lesions, endometriosis is marked by severe pain at, or just before, the onset of the menstrual flow. Acute intermittent cramps in the lower abdomen, or a constant "achy" feeling in the pelvis with dyspareunia, nervousness, and irritability are common.

Temporary or permanent changes in the personality of the patient may take place because of the repeated, accurately scheduled, and thus anticipated painful experience. The ovaries are sometimes involved in extensive endometriosis, resulting in sterility and therefore the loss of the only natural way of treatment of endometriosis: pregnancy. If the bladder is involved, the patient may experience burning on urination during menstrual periods, while involvement of the rectum will result in difficulties of defecation and occasional rectal bleeding. Involvement of the lungs (very rare) may result in "spitting of blood" during the menstrual period.

Treatment. Surgery has been very commonly used in the past for the treatment of endometriosis, but is today almost entirely replaced with hormone therapy. The purpose is to prevent the ovary from ovulating and the uterus from menstruating; in this way, the ectopic endometrial tissue remains dormant, not undergoing the monthly cyclic changes. When hormone therapy is continued for at least six months, most of the patients obtain permanent, or at least prolonged relief. Pregnancy accomplishes the same end by a natural

THE ENDOCRINE GLANDS

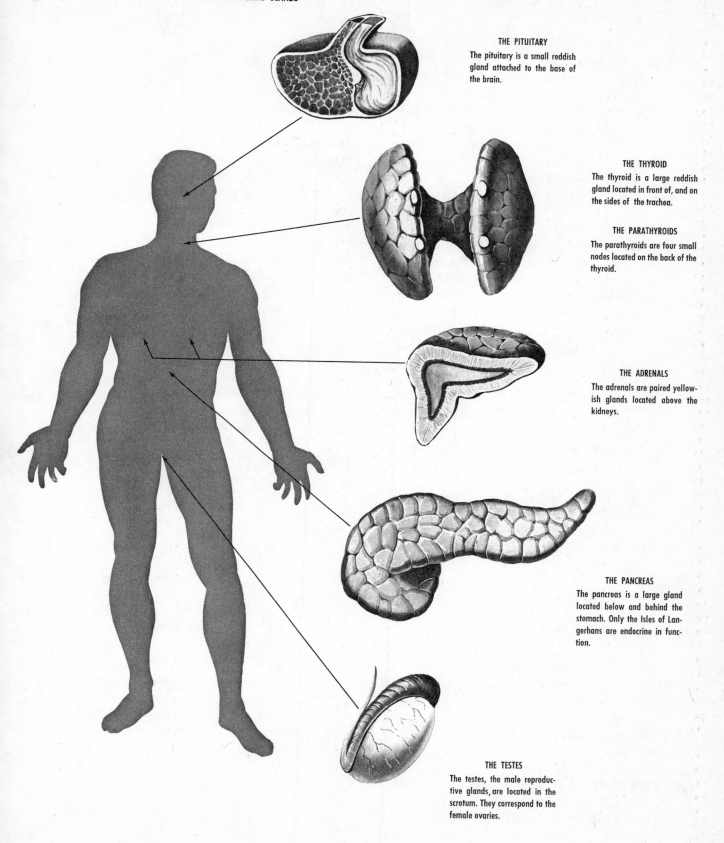

THE PITUITARY
The pituitary is a small reddish gland attached to the base of the brain.

THE THYROID
The thyroid is a large reddish gland located in front of, and on the sides of the trachea.

THE PARATHYROIDS
The parathyroids are four small nodes located on the back of the thyroid.

THE ADRENALS
The adrenals are paired yellowish glands located above the kidneys.

THE PANCREAS
The pancreas is a large gland located below and behind the stomach. Only the Isles of Langerhans are endocrine in function.

THE TESTES
The testes, the male reproductive glands, are located in the scrotum. They correspond to the female ovaries.

process. Some patients (about 20 per cent) may need to take more than one course of treatment, while others are better candidates for surgery. The hormones used for treatment of endometriosis are combinations of estrogen and progestrone-like drugs, taken daily by mouth. The prognosis is generally good, and some of the patients may become pregnant.

ENDOMETRITIS   Endometritis is an acute or chronic infection of the endometrium. The most common type of acute endometritis occurs three to four days after childbirth and is characterized by lower-abdominal pain, fever, and bloody foul-smelling vaginal discharge. The infection responds to treatment with antibiotics, and the prognosis is good.

ENDOMETRIUM   The tissue lining the inside of the womb, the endometrium is under the constant influence of the ovarian hormones during the reproductive life of a woman. It undergoes hypertrophy (growth) and is eventually shed, together with blood, in the form of menstrual flow. If pregnancy occurs, the endometrium serves for the implantation of the afterbirth (placenta) and the nourishment of the fetus.

ENGAGEMENT, OBSTETRICAL   In obstetrics, engagement of the baby's head means the descent of the head into the true bony pelvis of the mother. It occurs much more commonly in mothers carrying their first baby, and may take place several weeks before term. The mother feels the change, observing that her "womb has dropped," about the beginning of the ninth month.

ENTERITIS   Enteritis is an inflammation of the lining of any portion of the small intestine. Probably the commonest form of enteritis encountered is that which is commonly called intestinal flu. (The

influenza virus has nothing to do with the cause of this disorder.) This condition is often caused by several different types of viruses and is characterized by a rapid onset of cramping, abdominal pain, and diarrhea. The symptoms usually are short-lived and within twenty-four to forty-eight hours recovery is more or less complete. If the diarrhea is intense, and if vomiting also occurs, severe dehydration and shock may ensue—particularly in elderly people and in young infants. Other causes of enteritis are overindulgence in laxatives, excessive alcoholic intake, and food-poisoning. Typhoid fever and cholera produce severe bacterial forms of acute enteritis. It has been estimated that until modern times, enteritis or dysentery probably killed more soldiers than the wounds of battle. In the United States, modern, sanitary facilities make outbreaks of typhoid and other bacillary dysenteries rather rare, but sporadic cases continue to occur.

EPIDIDYMIS   This structure lies adjacent to the testis and is a collecting duct for the sperm. It is frequently the site of infection which may be acute or chronic. The most common chronic infection of this structure is tuberculosis.

EPILEPSY   Epilepsy is not a single disease, but a general term for symptoms of convulsive disorders. Epilepsy must therefore be understood as a symptom which may occur in any of a number of brain diseases. Scientific experiments show that the brain produces rhythmic electrical potentials, necessary for normal function. In normal persons, during the waking state these brain waves occur at the rate of 9 to 14 per second and are known as alpha rhythms. In sleep or under conditions of coma, the rhythms slow down to 3 to 6 per second and are known as delta waves. Apparently underlying all convulsive disorders is an abnormality of the electric potentials or waves produced in the normal brain. In such disorders therefore occur out-of-step waves (cerebral dysrhythmias) now recognized medically as indicative of epilepsy. Diagnosis of epilepsy, and location of the brain-areas producing abnormal rhythms, can now be positively made with b r a i n - w a v e (electroencephalographic) equipment available at most modern hospitals.

Symptoms. It was formerly thought that different forms of epilepsy could be diagnosed by the types of seizure involved. Three main patterns of epilepsy have been identified classically. In grand mal seizures, the person suddenly loses consciousness, falls to the ground in a convulsive seizure involving contraction and relaxation of all muscle groups. Frequently the epileptic bites his tongue or injures himself in other ways, for example, by falling against hot or hard objects. The seizure usually terminates spontaneously within a few minutes, following which there is gradual recovery of consciousness and reorientation. (Some grand mal epileptics report a warning aura—such as unusual visceral sensation—which gives warning of an impending seizure.)

Petit mal seizures usually involve a limited convulsive movement or temporary alteration of consciousness, but the patient does not lose consciousness completely or show generalized convulsion. The convulsive movement or alteration of consciousness may be so slight in petit mal epilepsy that only the patient himself or someone well acquainted with him knows that it has occurred. As in grand mal epilepsy, a petit mal diagnosis can be confirmed by brain-wave analysis (encephalography).

Psychomotor epilepsy involves involuntary alterations of conscious mental life, usually without any overt convulsive disorder. The pattern consists of a period of uncontrolled and unpremeditated behavior; the person may perform senseless or atypical actions without knowing why.

In medical circles the term epilepsy has largely been replaced by the designations convulsive disorder or cerebral dysrhythmia.

Treatment. Great advances have been made in chemotherapy of epilepsy, and it is entirely probable that future research will show the abnormal physical and chemical disorders underlying all convulsive conditions. The first step in treatment is to positively identify the cerebral dysrhythmia by means of brain-wave study. After abnormal cerebral rhythms have been found a large number of very effective drugs are available to control all types of convulsive symptoms.

It is absolutely essential for the epileptic to admit that he has a convulsive disorder. He must accept certain limitations on his life pattern; never engaging, for example, in any activity—driving, swimming, climbing in high places—where the onset of convulsions might be dangerous to himself or others. (See also CONVULSIONS.)

EPISIOTOMY The cutting of the tissues between the vagina and the rectum during delivery, episiotomy facilitates the passage of the baby. This procedure is advisable in every delivery because, in addition to allowing the baby to be born without too much squeezing through the birth canal, it protects against irregular tearing and overstretching of the vagina.

ERYSIPELAS Also known as "St. Anthony's Fire," erysipelas is a bacterial (streptococcus) infection of the skin manifested as well-outlined, red, swollen lesions, with fever and generalized malaise.

The cause is a blood-destroying (hemolytic) variety of streptococcus; its route of entry into the skin is not precisely known. Furthermore, since the advent of antibiotics the disease is seldom seen. When it comes to the attention of the physician today it is most often in aged persons who suffer chronic, debilitating disorders.

Symptoms. At first, there are chills, fever, and perhaps vomiting. Within forty-eight hours, one or more skin lesions appear which are shiny, raised, and well out-lined. In severe instances blisters of varying sizes may form. Although there are itching and burning, these are seldom extreme. The lesions tend to spread, and complications may ensue such as involvement of the kidneys and pneumonia.

Treatment. Among the most effective antibiotics are erythromycin and penicillin. Local relief is effected by packs soaked in cold magnesium sulfate. Aspirin, codeine, and other analgesic agents may be prescribed. The prognosis is excellent.

EROSION   The term "erosion" may refer to two very different health problems.

Erosion may refer to the wedge-shaped loss of the hard substance of a tooth, usually on the surfaces of teeth next to the lips and cheeks near the gum line. The eroded area is usually highly polished, and the condition is believed to be caused by a combination of mechanical and chemical (acid) factors. Severe cases of erosion must be restored by filling.

Erosion may also refer to an ulcerous condition of the cervix (the outer neck of the uterus). Cervical erosion occurs when cells covering the outer portion of the cervix are lost and substituted for by cells that are usually found in the interior portion of the cervix. Cervical erosion may cause bleeding or produce a vaginal discharge. The condition is most common among pregnant women. Other than the increased possibility of infection, cervical erosion is not considered a problem causing serious complication—especially if treated early, usually by cauterizing the affected area.

ERYTHEMA   Erythema is skin redness due to blushing, emotional stress, exposure to sun, X-ray, and ultraviolet emanations, drugs, certain diseases (particularly of the skin), and local injury.

ESOPHAGUS AND ESOPHAGITIS
The esophagus is a muscular tube leading from the back of the throat down through the chest cavity and an opening in the diaphragm and ending in the stomach. The first third of the esophagus contains muscles that are under voluntary control; swallowing is initiated in this region. In the other two-thirds, automatic reflexes take over to push the food into the stomach. The lining of the lower portion of the esophagus has some of the same cells that are found in the stomach, secreting enzymes and acid.

Occasionally the muscles of the esophagus will go into spasm, and it is thought that this is one cause of the familiar symptoms of heartburn. Often a case of esophagitis causes pain and discomfort that resembles other health problems. Caustic poisons such as lye or commercial acids, when swallowed, can cause severe inflammation and scarring of the esophagus so that surgery may be necessary to widen the passage. Diverticuli (balloon-like projections from the wall of the esophagus) are sometimes seen and can cause burning pain and difficulty in swallowing.

ESSENTIAL HYPERTENSION   High blood pressure, or essential hypertension, causes a high percentage of all heart disease. It may be found in persons of all social and economic levels.

Most cases of essential hypertension come in middle-aged persons, or those past middle age. Men and women share the disease equally. There seems to be a strong tendency for cases to run in families although what—if any—factor causes the individual to develop this type of blood pressure disability has not yet been discovered.

The physical disability caused by essential hypertension may slowly progress for many years; or it may occasionally advance to complete disability in a few months or years, and even lead to an early death. In spite of widespread research in many directions, little real information has been obtained about the true cause of the disorder and exactly why it leads to progressively destructive changes in the blood supply of the heart vessels and of the heart muscle as well.

There are, of course, many theories. Heredity, emotional stress, hormonal imbalance, and specific substances released abnormally by tissues diseased in a peculiar way are known at times to cause high pressures in the artery system. However, no clear-cut single cause of essential hypertension is yet known.

Even in normally healthy people blood pressure will rise when the individual is under emotional stress. Physical exertion, lifting, and almost any circumstance in which an extra demand for blood is made by the tissues, can also cause an elevation in artery pressures. But as soon as the stress and urgent tissue demands for replenishment of substances or oxygen are over, blood pressure ordinarily falls back to normal in a short period of time. When there is hypertensive heart disease, however, no matter whether the patient is resting or exerting himself, blood pressure stays at levels very much higher than in unaffected persons.

Symptoms. There are few, if any, symptoms directly caused by high blood pressure. Most patients, indeed, feel very well, and typically many of them seem to thrive at a high level of energy and activity at home, in social life, or in business. As a group, these patients seem to be content with themselves and with life. They prefer not to complain about anything, and often the diagnosis comes only after a routine employment or insurance examination.

Headaches and dizzy spells may express circulatory fatigue in persons with essential hypertension, but are perhaps complained of more by persons with normal blood pressure readings. If the structures of the heart or blood vessels, or the lung circulation, have been damaged by excessive pressures over a period of time, short breathing, pain in the chest, or cramping legs may be noticeable—especially on severe exertion. These are symptoms of the tissue changes caused by high blood pressure, and can, once they occur, indicate the need for close medical attention.

High blood pressure is never diagnosed as a disease-condition on the basis of a single blood-pressure reading. Repeated examinations must continue to show high readings if essential hypertension is to be diagnosed. As an indication of disease, systolic pressure readings should be consistently above 150 or 160 millimeters of mercury, and the diastolic pressures usually above 90 or 95 millimeters.

Treatment. A large percentage of patients kept under modern drug therapy may expect to lead nearly normal lives, and have a good life expectancy. Neglect of medical care, however, may lead to disaster.

ESTROGENS Hormones produced by the ovaries, the estrogens are responsible for the development of female sex characteristics (development of breasts, general female contour of the body) and the preparation of the uterus for the monthly menstrual flow. Cessation of estrogen-production results in the female climacteric or "change of life." Natural and synthetic estrogens are commercially available and are used for the treatment of various abnormalities caused by estrogen deficiencies.

EUNUCHOIDISM A male who has been castrated is referred to as a eunuch. When castration is accomplished before growth has been completed, the individual may become excessively tall because the androgens, which normally cause bone-growth to stop, are absent; or he may develop effeminate characteristics and become excessively fat. Many years ago it was a practice of rulers in the Far-Eastern countries to castrate slaves who were placed in charge of harems. Today eunuchs are seen only when there is congenital absence of the testes or failure of testicular development due to an endocrine disturbance.

EUSTACHIAN TUBE, BLOCKAGE OF THE   The function of the Eustachian tube is maintenance of equal pressure on both sides of the eardrum. If the Eustachian tube becomes blocked, this function is unfulfilled. In this case the oxygen in the middle ear is rapidly absorbed; the eardrum is pushed inward by the greater atmospheric pressure outside; and the delicate mucosal lining of the middle ear fills with a watery substance instead of air. The result is hearing loss. This condition is known by several names: serous otitis media, secretory otitis media, tubotympanitis, hydrotympanum, and others.

Treatment. The methods of treatment are directed at relieving the tubal blockage and evacuating the middle ear fluid. This may be accomplished by the procedure called myringotomy, an incision through the eardrum. The myringotomy must be performed carefully, under adequate lighting, with special instruments in the safe area of the eardrum. Suction may be used to aspirate the middle-ear fluid. The incision heals rapidly, usually in one day. This procedure may be done under general anesthesia for children; local anesthesia or even none will suffice for adults, and probably no anesthesia at all is safest for infants.

The hearing loss is relieved by myringotomy, but in order to avoid recurrence the doctor must also treat the underlying cause: the blocked Eustachian tube. Tub-

al obstruction may be due to a swelling around the throat (pharyngeal) end of the tube resulting from allergy or from upper respiratory infection (such as a cold). Occlusion may also be due to adenoids, tumor and, rarely, malocclusion of the teeth.

Fluid loss in the middle ear is the most common cause of hearing loss in children. The factors responsible are usually adenoids and allergy. If allergy is the problem, desensitization and myringotomy may prove successful. If the condition is a long-standing one, with need for long-term allergy management, an indwelling polyethylene tube is sometimes placed through the eardrum to promote drainage and to prevent the eardrum from closing too quickly; this method makes repeated myringotomies unnecessary. When the adenoids are responsible, their removal (and, if indicated, removal of the tonsils) together with the myringotomy should prove successful in relieving the hearing loss.

Medication, alone or in conjunction with opening the eardrum, is often sufficient for treating serous otitis media due to a cold. The danger of a negligent attitude is that after a long period of time the fluid in the middle ear tends to thicken and coalesce, causing possible adhesions. The adhesions then bind the ossicles, preventing their proper vibration and causing hearing loss. This type of hearing loss responds poorly to surgery. Therefore, neglect of the fluid in the middle ear can, in a small percentage of cases, lead to more or less permanent hearing loss. Thus, it pays to care for the ears promptly.

EXISTENTIAL PSYCHIATRY   This is a new movement in psychiatry, involving application of forms of existentialism to problems of mental illness. Existentialism is concerned with the meanings of being and living. Psychiatrists are meeting increasingly large numbers of patients who complain of a newly-recognized pattern which existential psychiatrists call the noögenic neurosis: doubts that life has any meaning, and despair about existence in general. A leading existential psychiatrist attributes this condition to an existential vacuum, caused by Man's loss of primitive security-in-instinct and loss of certain traditional values of the kind which governed life in earlier times. Modern man has lost his traditional belief in religion and established authority and has found nothing to replace them, so that he is left bankrupt, in a spiritual vacuum. Existentialism is concerned with the search for life meanings and reasons for being. When faced with patients who complain that life no longer seems to have meaning, the existential psychiatrist attempts to teach more solid values to live by.

A major concern of existential psychiatrists is self-actualization, or helping the patient to become what he can become. Many persons become thwarted and feel stalemated by internal and external factors which block personal growth. (Psychologists believe that there are many psychic conflicts which can act as blocks and that personal growth tends to resume if negative factors are removed.) An important part of the problem consists in helping people to see themselves more positively and hopefully, so that their lives open up in new directions. Anything which stimulates positive growth-resources tends to result in genuine self-actualization.

EXTRADURAL HEMATOMA
An extradural hematoma is a collection of blood between the outer coverings of the brain and the skull due to a tear in an artery which runs just beneath the temporal bone of the skull. Extradural hematomas are due to direct blows to the skull.

Symptoms. Usually the individual will develop a headache, vomiting, and drowsiness within a few hours after head injury. A bruise in one temporal area may be noted and weakness of the arm and leg on the opposite side of the body from the blow subsequently develops. The patient may rapidly become comatose and develop irregular breathing and convulsions.

Treatment. The patient should be hospitalized immediately and surgical removal of the hematoma carried out as soon as possible. Recovery is usually rapid and complete if treatment is prompt. Late treatment may result in partial recovery with residual weakness or speech disorder. If there has been a delay, and if severe damage to the brainstem has occurred, death may result in spite of surgical therapy.

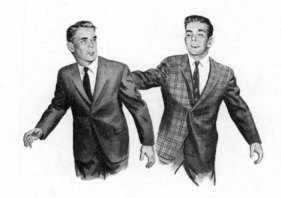

EXTROVERSION — INTROVERSION
The famous Austrian psychologist Carl G. Jung was the first to construct a psychological scheme based upon the outgoing or inward-looking nature of a person's whole approach to life. Extroversion is defined as the trait of being basically outgoing, interested in the outer world, and liking others. Introversion involves an inward-looking, sensitive, withdrawn, shy approach to life. At first it was believed the two types represented opposite and distinct forms of personality; later research has shown that pure forms of either are rare. Most people represent a balance of outgoing and introverted traits. An individual may be extroverted in social situations in which he feels at ease and introverted where he feels insecure. Except in

extreme degrees, introversion and extroversion are both normal traits, apparently determined by inherited or constitutional factors.

The extremely introverted child may have some difficulty adjusting socially, because of shyness and self-consciousness. It does no good to force such a child to socialize; this may make the child more anxious and insecure. Best is the application of gentle but firm pressure on the child to relate to other children, providing opportunities for easy social relationships, yet not making the child feel conspicuous by calling attention to his shyness.

It should be clearly understood that both extroverts and introverts can succeed well in life, each in his own way. Much harm can be done by trying to force a child to be something he is not. The extroverted child usually has an easier time developing socially because of his outgoing interest in other people, but most introverts are able to make compensatory adjustments for getting ahead socially. This is a problem which each child must be allowed to work out in his own way.

EYE, ARTIFICIAL After injury or disease it is sometimes necessary to remove the eyeball. A stump remains containing muscles and blood vessels. Over this may be placed a shell, usually of plastic, containing a disc which matches the remaining eye in color and appearance. Many artificial eyes do not have the full range of movement of the normal eye, and those wearing one should move their head rather than the eye to look to the side. Infection may be introduced into the socket by the fingers; the hands must therefore be scrupulously clean before touching the artificial eye to replace it. If one eye has been lost, it is wise to wear shatterproof lenses to protect the remaining one.

EYE, BLOWS TO THE The eyes are well protected by the bony structure surrounding them, and large blunt objects usually damage only the eyelids. A "black eye" consists of blood beneath the thin skin of the eyelids and is usually associated with swelling. If vision is normal, it is usually of minor import. During the first twenty-four hours, cold or iced compresses applied for ten minutes every hour will limit swelling. After twenty-four hours, hot compresses may be used. (See EYE, HYGIENE OF.)

A blow to the eyeball itself may cause severe injury. If the vision is decreased, if the pupil is not round, or if there is blood in front of the colored iris, medical care is indicated.

EYE, BURNS OF THE Chemical burns of the conjunctiva and cornea are best treated by immediate irrigation with water. No time should be wasted in seeking the appropriate neutralizing solution, but rather the eye should be copiously irrigated as soon as possible with clear water. The most effective method is to plunge the entire face into a container of water and then open the eyes under water.

Acid burns are quickly neutralized by the tissues and the immediate injury is usually the full extent of the damage; alkali burns, however, become worse as time goes by. Medical care should be sought as soon as possible after a chemical burn has been irrigated thoroughly.

Heat burns of the eye usually involve only the eyelids because the eyeball is fairly well protected from injuries by quick closure of the lids. Burns from cigarettes or matches require medical care. Washing the eye as described under chemical burns may remove foreign particles. Bandaging or closing both eyes will then prevent the globe from moving and will minimize pain.

Burns of the eyelid may be extremely serious and if severe enough to cause blisters (second degree) must have medical care. Salves and lotions should not be applied except under medical direction.

Ultraviolet rays from arc welding, from reflections of sunlight off sand or snow, or from a sun lamp may cause extreme eye irritation. Like sunburn, the effect adds up and, usually during the night following exposure, the eyes burn and water and feel filled with sand. The irritation is so extreme that it may be nearly impossible to open the eyes. If the individual recalls exposure to ultraviolet rays, the diagnosis is usually simple, since there are few conditions which cause such discomfort in both eyes. The condition persists for from twelve to twenty-four hours. Bandaging of both eyes; rest in a quiet, darkened room; and sedation are usually all that is required. Medicines which anesthetize the eyeballs give comfort but delay healing, and should be used only under medical direction.

EYE, CHAMBERS OF THE

The eye contains three chambers which interconnect with one another. The front chamber is in front of the iris and behind the cornea. It contains a clear, slightly salty fluid which continually drains out of the eye through a channel at the junction of the cornea and sclera. Obstruction of this channel causes increase in pressure in the eye known as glaucoma.

A very small chamber, the posterior chamber, is located behind the iris and in front of the supporting fibers of the lens. It is important because this is where the ciliary body secretes the nutrient material for the lens, which has no blood supply of its own to feed it. The fluid secreted by the ciliary body flows through the pupil into the anterior chamber.

The largest chamber of the eye is the vitreous cavity containing a clear, gelatin-like material in which are suspended very few cells but much water.

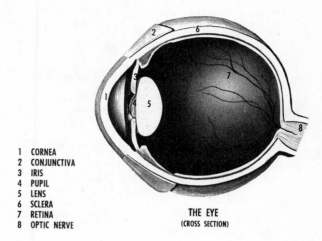

1 CORNEA
2 CONJUNCTIVA
3 IRIS
4 PUPIL
5 LENS
6 SCLERA
7 RETINA
8 OPTIC NERVE

THE EYE
(CROSS SECTION)

EYE, DRY

This occurs because of decreased tear secretion which may follow scarring of the lining of the lids, or occurs as part of a disease complex which includes decreased salivary secretion and rheumatoid arthritis. The eyes are dry and feel sandy, and are constantly irritated. It is frequently impossible to swallow a tablet without water. Diagnosis is made by measuring tear-formation. Treatment is by instillation of artificial tears.

EYE, FOREIGN BODIES IN THE

Dirt and cinders may be blown into the eye and cause a typical foreign-body sensation. Nearly always it feels as though the material is beneath the outer portion of the upper lid. There is watering of the eye but no disturbance of vision. The foreign body is usually lodged on the transparent tissue of the cornea or on the inside surface of the upper lid. If the foreign body is on the cornea, it may sometimes be washed out of the eye by placing the face in a basin of clean water and opening the eye under water. If this is not effective, the foreign particle may have to be gently lifted off the globe by a physician. Rubbing the eyelids is not helpful.

Foreign bodies on the lid are removed after first turning back the lid. A cotton-tipped applicator or the corner of a clean handerchief should be available before doing this, and a good light should be used. (The individual must look downward or the upper lid cannot be turned.) The lashes are grasped and the lid drawn gently away from the globe to break the suction. With a match held against the lid at the level of the fold in the skin about one-quarter of an inch above the margin, the lid may be folded back on itself. A cinder will frequently be at about the middle of the reddish exposed surface. The lower lid may be turned by placing the thumb against the skin surface and pressing gently inward.

Foreign bodies within the eye are extremely serious inasmuch as they damage the eye upon entering, may introduce infection, and may dissolve within the eye, causing further injury. Large objects are likely to destroy the eye. Most objects retained within the eye are small. Usually, but not always, the pupil is no longer round after the injury.

If the foreign object is wood or similar material, it may carry bacteria and cause an abscess to form in the eye. Small metallic foreign bodies frequently are sterilized by heat and are less likely to cause infection. Vision is frequently much reduced and a cataract may form.

X-rays indicate metallic objects within the eye but frequently fail to show wood, plastics, and glass. Iron and nickel foreign bodies may be removed by a surgeon with a magnet, but other metals and material are not magnetic. Some materials such as glass and some plastics are well tolerated by the tissues and need not be removed, while others are quickly covered by scar tissue and cause no harm. Some metals such as copper cause much damage, hence every effort must be made to remove them. In household accidents, the tool that may have been the source of the injury should be made available to the surgeon so he can learn its composition.

EYE, HYGIENE OF THE   The eyes are remarkably organized to provide vision with a minimum of care. They arise as an outgrowth of the brain and, like the brain, are designed for—and cannot be injured by—use.

Every individual should assure himself from time to time that his vision is unchanged, by testing each eye separately for both near and distant vision, and then checking side vision (see VISION, MEASUREMENT OF). Eye examinations are particularly important: (1) during the third year of life; (2) in the first, fourth, and ninth grades; and (3) at about age eighteen. After the age of forty to forty-five, examination every one or two years is desirable.

Poor lighting, excessive use of the eyes for close work, wrong glasses, or the need for glasses may give rise to burning and discomfort of the eyes, sometimes associated with headaches. The headaches are never severe and are always relieved by discontinuing the task at hand. If not relieved, the headaches are not caused by the eyes. The factors cited cause no permanent change but only discomfort. Excessive blinking, which occurs particularly in children, is seldom serious and usually disappears if attention is not directed to it.

It should not be necessary to use eyewashes at any time, unless prescribed for a definite disease. If an eyecup is used, it should be sterilized in boiling water and allowed to cool immediately prior to use. If one feels an eyewash is necessary, a satisfactory one can be made by dissolving a teaspoon of table salt in a pint of water, boiling for ten minutes, and then storing in a sterilized bottle. Old medications should be discarded. Inasmuch as the symptoms of many different eye diseases are the same, medicines should not be used by other family members.

The wearing of tinted and colored glasses is a personal preference and is rarely indicated for eye disease. The colored lenses provided by industry for protection in certain occupations should not be used outside of work as they frequently reduce vision excessively or interfere with the color vision necessary to recognizing traffic signals. A neutral gray or a greenish tint is the preferred color for sunglasses. Reddish tints may interfere with recognizing the red of traffic lights. All colored and tinted lenses interfere with night vision and should never be used at night. Individuals with normal eyes do not require colored lenses indoors.

The use of safety lenses made of plastic or hardened glass is preferable not only in industry and home workshops, but for general use. They should be worn even by those with normal vision in school laboratories and when working at home. Tools should be discarded if there is any danger of metal breaking off.

Hot or cold compresses may relieve tired, swollen eyelids. A washcloth wrung out in running hot or cold water, and then applied to the lids for ten minutes, relieves many nonspecific conditions. It is not necessary to add any medicine to the water.

EYE, INJURIES OF THE

Prompt and appropriate care of injuries of the eye may prevent much disability and may even be instrumental in making major corrective surgery unnecessary. If vision is to be saved, many steps cannot be delayed until medical care is available. (See also EYES, BLOWS TO THE; EYE, BURNS OF THE; EYE, FOREIGN BODIES IN THE; EYE, SCRATCHES OF THE.)

EYE, ITS PARTS AND FUNCTION

The eye is a hollow organ about one inch in diameter. It contains light-sensitive tissue, the retina, which is connected to the brain by nerve fibers in the optic nerve. It is protected by bone on all sides except at the front, and rests in a tissue hammock, surrounded by fat. Its movements arise from the action of six muscles.

In front, the eyelids keep the eye moist and protect it from external irritants and excessive light. So as to transmit light, the optical portions of the eye are transparent. The cornea and the crystalline lens both act as lenses to form images of external objects upon the retina. The pupil acts as a diaphragm to control the amount of light entering the eye and to reduce such blurring of the image as would be created by stray light entering a large opening.

EYELIDS

The front surface of the eye is covered by the eyelids—upper and lower curtains of skin, muscle, glands, mucous membrane, and a cartilage-like material. The eyelids serve to distribute fluid over the surface of the globe by periodic blinking and to protect the eye from external irritants and excessive light.

The skin covering the eyelids is extremely thin and is thrown into numerous folds to permit lid movements. It can stretch enormously following injury or when inflamed. Because of the thinness of the lids, blood vessels beneath the skin may be seen, sometimes as a dark blue line and at other times as a diffuse bluish discoloration of the entire lid. The conjunctiva is the mucous membrane lining the lid; it is continuous from the lid margin to the junction of the white (sclera) and the transparent portion (cornea) of the eye.

The lids contain voluntary and involuntary muscles which function in opening and closing. The muscle mainly responsible for closing is the obicularis oculi, a circular muscle in the upper and lower lid; this muscle holds the lids in close contact with the globe. The upper lid opens by means of the levator muscle which arises from the area surrounding the stem, or apex, of the orbit. Involuntary muscles in the lid elevate the upper and lower eyelid and give "tone" to the tissue.

Stability is provided in the lid by a

modified plate of dense tissue, the tarsus, which extends along the lid margin and deep into the lid. It contains glands producing an oily secretion which prevents the tears from overflowing.

The lid margins meet tightly to prevent fluids and irritating material from entering the eye. These margins each contain two layers of eyelashes and oil and sweat glands which may become infected to cause styes.

EYELIDS, BAGGY

The skin of the lids is so thin that it swells easily. Some persons inherit a tendency for the lids to be full; in others, there is a break in the deep tissues so that fat from the orbit protrudes into the lids. Long-time swelling of the lids may also produce laxness of the skin, with an unsightly appearance. These are cosmetic blemishes only. If severe, the individual may wish surgical correction.

EYELIDS, DROOPING (BLEPHARO-PTOSIS)

If the upper lids are too heavy because of scarring or tumors, or if there is weakness in the muscles which elevate them, they will droop. If marked enough, the lids cover the pupil and interfere with vision. Sometimes, because of misdirected nerves, the drooping disappears when the mouth is opened.

Symptoms. These arise only because of mechanical interference with vision, and a cosmetic defect.

Treatment. This depends upon the cause. If slight, no treatment is recommended; while if severe, the condition must be corrected surgically. Occasionally a "crutch" can be attached to a spectacle lens and support the lid.

Ptosis (drooping) usually occurs as a birth-defect and may involve one or both eyes. Later in life it occurs because of disease of the nerves, particularly strokes, mysthenia gravis, and muscular dystrophies.

EYELIDS, FUSED

Fusing of eyelids may occur as two clinical entities: ankyloblepharon and symblepharon. In ankyloblepharon the borders of the eyelids have grown together, partially or completely. In symblepharon the eyelid partially or completely adheres to the eyeball. Both conditions result from old inflammatory disorders, injury, or burn. Sometimes infants are born with either defect.

EYELIDS, INFLAMMATION OF THE

The exposed position of the skin of the eyelids makes them particularly subject to irritations and infection. Marked swelling may occur after insect bites and is best treated by cold compresses. Skin allergies from nail polish, perfumes, colored soaps, medicines, and the like may particularly affect the lids, sometimes only on one side when the irritant is carried to the lids by the fingers of a right- or left-handed individual. The condition recurs until the offending agent is removed.

Inflammations of the lid margin (blepharitis) causes an unsightly redness with fine, powdery scales on the lashes. The condition is frequently associated with dandruff of the scalp. There may be chronic irritation from bacterial infection, smoke, chemical fumes, or repeated rubbing. Treatment must be directed toward eliminating the cause.

EYELIDS, TURNED-IN (ENTROPION)

This condition, a turning-in of the lid margin, is caused by scarring of the inside or by continuous squeezing of the lids.

Symptoms. The turned-in lashes irritate the eyeball and cause redness and discomfort.

Treatment. Relief can sometimes be obtained by drawing the outer portion of the lid downward by means of adhesive tape; but if severe and persistent, surgery is required.

EYELIDS, TURNED-OUT (ECTROPION)

Turning-out of the lid margin is caused by scarring of the skin of the lids, and by paralysis or excessive contraction of the muscle closing the lids.

Symptoms. Irritation and tearing are produced by exposure of the inner lining of the lid.

Treatment. Surgical correction is indicated.

EYELIDS, TWITCHING OF THE

The delicate muscles of the lid may spontaneously contract. The condition is annoying but not serious, and is due to fatigue. Adequate rest is the only effective treatment.

EYE, OPTICAL DEFECTS OF THE

Rays of light entering the eye are bent by the transparent cornea, next by the lens; they then come to a focus. If the length of the eye is proportionate to the bending, the rays come to a focus at the back of the eye on the retina and a clear image is formed. If the degree of bending is not proportionate to the length of the eye, the focus is either in front of the retina or would be behind it if it were not stopped by the retina. Such a disproportion causes an error of refraction. Minor errors arise as a variation in growth and cannot be modified by such external influences as eyedrops, diet, lenses, exercises, or use of the eyes. (See also APHAKIA; ASTIGMATISM; FARSIGHTEDNESS; NEARSIGHTEDNESS; PRESBYOPIA.)

EYE, SCRATCHES OF THE

Scratches of the eyelid are generally not serious and require only cleanliness and treatment similar to that given for such injuries elsewhere in the body. Scratches of the surface of the eyeball are extremely painful. Inasmuch as they may become infected, prompt medical care is advisable. Some comfort may be obtained by closing or bandaging both eyes.

Cuts or lacerations of the eyelids vary in severity, but even apparently minor injuries may produce concealed damage. Cuts that parallel the lid margin may bleed profusely but, if there is no deeper damage, usually heal well, with the scar concealed in skin folds. Cuts at right angles to the lid margins usually gape widely and require skilled repair to avoid notching the lid.

Cuts of the eyeball are always extremely serious and require prompt and expert care. They are recognized by the protrusion of iris through the surface of the eye (so that the pupil is not round), or by the brownish tissue gaping through the cut. Both eyes should be bandaged and the individual should be moved on a stretcher. Examination of the eye should be avoided until surgical facilities are available. Even with expert care the damage may be so severe that vision cannot be saved.

Sympathetic ophthalmia is an inflammation of both eyes that follows a deep laceration of one. It requires at least fourteen days after the injury for this condition to develop, and will not happen if the injured eye is removed before that time. After the disease has been established, removal of the injured eye is not helpful, and it is probably best to retain it, since it may still be the better eye after the inflammation clears. The disease is now uncommon and responds fairly well to cortisone-like drugs.

EYE, TUMORS OF THE

Because of the ease with which they can invade the deeper structures of the head, if neglected, skin tumors are somewhat more serious in the eyelids than those elsewhere in the body. The most common new growth of the lid is a basal-cell cancer which usually occurs in the aged among those who are exposed to sun and wind. It is generally

236

about one-fourth of an inch in diameter, and has heaped-up sides with a depression in the center. It is treated either with surgery or by X-ray.

The most common malignant tumor in infants and young children is the retinoblastoma. It arises in the retina and is transmitted as a dominant hereditary characteristic to the children of survivors. It may occur in either one or both eyes, usually before the age of one year. It is usually first noticed when there is a white mass visible through the pupil. Such an eye must be removed as quickly as possible. Exact examination is required to detect early tumors in the remaining eye, which occur in about 25 per cent of cases. If a tumor is present, the second eye is treated with X-rays, anti-cancer medicines, and sometimes by an intense light directed through the pupil to coagulate the tumor. If the tumor continues to progress, it is necessary to remove the eye. Otherwise the tumor spreads by direct continuation into the brain and through the body via the bloodstream.

The most common eye tumor in adults is malignant melanoma, which arises in the blood-vessel coat of the eye—the choroid. The first symptoms arise because of loss of function in the adjacent retina with a resultant "island" of blindness. As the tumor grows, the island increases in size; later the eye becomes hard (secondary glaucoma), inflamed, red, and painful. The tumor spreads via the bloodstream to other parts of the body. Treatment for malignant melanoma is removal of the eye; if this is done while the tumor is relatively small, there is a good likelihood that malignancy has not spread to other parts of the body, hence that lasting cure can be achieved.

FACIAL NERVES The paired facial (or seventh cranial) nerves supply motor function to the muscles of the face and also carry sensory impulses of taste from the front two-thirds of the tongue to the brainstem. These nerves may be damaged by injury, infection, or neuritis.

FACIAL PARALYSIS (BELL'S PALSY) Bell's palsy, or facial paralysis, is a sudden palsy of the muscles of one side of the face, probably due to a neuritis of the facial nerve.

Symptoms. The muscles of one side of the face become weak or paralyzed without previous warning or illness. The eyelids may not close completely, and it may be difficult to use the lower portion of the face to smile and to chew food. Taste sensation may be lost on the side of the tongue on which the facial paralysis occurs.

Treatment. Most patients with Bell's palsy recover function of facial muscles. Recovery may be complete within a few weeks, or it may occur slowly and partially over a period of six to twelve months. No specific drug is uniformly effective in producing early recovery, although cortisone has been recommended. If function does not return after two years, plastic surgical repair may be required to obtain cosmetic improvement.

FALLOPIAN TUBES Approximately four inches in length, the fallopian tubes extend on each side of the uterus and serve to connect the cavity of the womb with the two ovaries. The tubes are necessary for transporting the egg from the ovaries to the uterus, and fertilization of the egg by a spermatozoan usually takes place in one of them. If both tubes are obstructed, fertilization is impossible. Tying of the tubes (tubal ligation) is a simple and popular method for surgical sterilization; it is successful in preventing pregnancy in approximately 99 per cent of the cases. (For infections of the tubes, see SALPINGITIS.)

FALSE PREGNANCY (PSEUDOCYESIS)

Occasionally, women who are overanxious to become pregnant stop menstruating, their abdomen becomes larger, they gain weight, their breasts become tender, and they experience morning sickness. This is termed false pregnancy, and may advance to such extremes as to create impressions of fetal movement or even establishment of false labor pains at nine months. Naturally this is a purely psychosomatic syndrome; when, after careful physical and endocrinological examination, the woman is assured that she is not pregnant, all the previously-mentioned symptoms disappear and the patient begins to menstruate normally.

FARSIGHTEDNESS (HYPEROPIA)

In this condition light rays from a distant object strike the retina before coming to a focus so that a blurred image is formed. The condition arises because there is either too little bending of light rays or too short an eyeball. It is extremely common and is usually compensated for by a change in the shape of the lens (accommodation) which increases its focusing power.

Symptoms. Minor degrees of farsightedness cause no symptoms, and both near and far vision are good because of the adjustment by accommodation. If there is a marked degree of farsightedness, accommodation may adjust the eye so that distant objects are seen clearly but the additional accommodation required for close work causes eyestrain or blurring of vision. Inasmuch as accommodation becomes less with age, an older eye cannot compensate as well for farsightedness as a youthful eye.

Treatment. Farsightedness is corrected by means of convex (magnifying) lenses. Considerable judgment is required to learn if symptoms arise because of the farsightedness, what should be the power of the lens required, and whether glasses should be worn constantly or only occasionally.

FATS

Fats are an important part of the everyday diet. They are more than twice as rich in potential energy as are carbohydrates or proteins, nine calories being released for each gram of the average type of fat processed by the body (metabolized). In other words, fats contain a large amount of energy in a small volume.

A meal high in fat tends to have a more prolonged effect on the sensation of "fullness"; fats also add to the palatability of food and serve as a vehicle for fat-soluble vitamins. Food energy not immediately utilized is stored in the form of fat within the body as a "reservoir" for future use. As tissue, fat serves as a protective cushion for certain organs and helps insulate the body against temperature changes.

On the basis of certain physical and chemical properties, the group of substances known as fats may be classified as follows:

1. Neutral fats (triglycerides), which make up the greater part of the fats in the diet and are typical of fat in animal tissue such as meat. Triglycerides are composed of the simple chemical glycerol, attached to which are three fatty acids. The latter are simple, long chains of carbon atoms, perhaps eighteen to twenty-one atoms long, with an "acid" chemical configuration at one end.
2. Waxes, which include the esters (fatty acids connected onto another substance) of cholesterol and vitamins A and D
3. Phospholipids (containing phosphoric acid), present in all cells and particularly concentrated in certain portions of the central nervous system
4. Glycolipids or cerebrosides, fatty

material containing carbohydrate, found in the white matter of the brain

5. Steroids, including cholesterol, certain hormones, vitamin D, and bile acids

Fatty acids have been also classified on the basis of saturation. When the bonds between the carbon atoms, which are arranged in a long chain, are each covered with a hydrogen atom, the fatty acid is said to be a saturated fatty acid. Some of the more important fatty acids are partially unsaturated; that is, they have some bonds between the carbons which do not have hydrogen molecules attached. Three of the unsaturated fatty acids (linoleic, linolenic, and arachidonic) apparently cannot be synthesized by animals and man, and have been termed essential.

Foods of relatively high fat content include milk, cream, butter, egg yolks, fish liver, other meats (especially pork), and vegetable oils of various types. Margarine is manufactured from vegetable oils that have been saturated (hydrogenated) in order to make melting less likely at room-temperature.

The average American daily diet contains about 100 grams of fat which supply about one-third of the total caloric intake. Perhaps two-thirds of the fats come from animal sources: meat, milk, eggs, dairy products, etc. The remainder come from vegetable materials. The precise role of fat in the diet with relation to heart attacks (atherosclerosis and coronary disease) is still being closely studied.

FEEDING (FROM BIRTH TO ONE YEAR OF AGE)

Milk is the most essential food for the baby in his first year of life. The adage that "breast milk is best milk" is a sound guide; but today (mostly for artificial and insufficient reasons) most babies are not breast-fed.

If breast milk is not available, suitably diluted cow's milk usually does very

well. (Four parts of whole milk should be mixed with one part of water; or two parts of evaporated milk with three parts of water.) Various prepared formulas are also readily available. The ones most commonly used are either in powder or in liquid ready-to-use form; both kinds are wholly satisfactory.

To gain weight and receive enough fluid, a baby up to three months of age should receive a minimum of two ounces of any standard milk for every pound of weight each twenty-four hours. Thus a seven-pound baby should get more than fourteen ounces of milk in a twenty-four hour period of time: this might be given on a schedule of three ounces five times a day. Most babies will gain one to three pounds of weight per month on this feeding for the first six months, depending on how large a person the infant will ultimately be as an adult. Ideally, the baby should be weighed and checked monthly.

The big controversy in infant feeding arises over the optimum time for introducing solid foods. If a baby consumes only milk in the first year, he will develop an iron-deficiency anemia because the iron received from the mother must be distributed through a body three times the size it was a year previously. To avoid this nutritional lack, solid foods (cereal, fruit, vegetable, and meat), which almost all contain iron, are started in the first six months of life. Variety is not important; the idea is to add a few minerals to the diet and get the baby used to the spoon.

The more common allergy-producing foods (egg, citrus, green vegetables, chocolate, peaches, pork, and wheat) are usually not offered until after a child's first birthday. One new food is usually added every four to eight weeks, beginning with rice, then adding strained pears, applesauce, and mashed banana. Strained yellow vegetables and strained meat are next introduced in small amounts at about six to eight months of life. A good general rule is to offer the milk first, before the solids, in the first six months of life because milk is the most important food during that rapid growth period; after the sixth month, give the solids first and let the baby decide (depending on rate of growth) how much milk he should have after eating his solids.

An average six-months-old baby takes about two ounces of solids, with or without cereal, at each of the three feedings a day. At eight months he is taking about four ounces three times a day and anywhere from two to eight ounces of milk afterwards (depending on whether he will be five feet or six-and-a-half feet tall when he grows up). At ten months the infant is usually getting about eight ounces of solids three times a day; this may still be strained foods, although many babies early refuse to be fed by others, insisting on table-foods. The infant is usually not adept at handling the spoon, so "finger-food" is usually served (chunks of bananas, boiled carrots, beans, potatoes, bits of ground meats, spaghetti, zwieback, cheese—anything that can be stuck together). From six months on, solids are more important than milk, and meat and fruit are probably the most important of the solids.

Vitamins are essential throughout life and a supplement of these is usually given in the first year. Once the diet is well balanced and the baby is no longer growing so fast, he probably gets enough from his food. Vitamin D, however, is often given in the winter, and fluoride (to inhibit cavity-formation) should be given if the water supply is deficient.

FEVER   Fever is elevation of the body temperature above normal. Rectal temperature, which is the more accurate, usually varies between 98.0° F. to 98.5° F. in the morning, and 98.5° F. and 99.0° F. in the evening; the highest acceptable normal temperature rectally would probably be no more than 99.5° F. A temperature-swing of more than 1.5 degrees during the day is also abnormal (98.0° in the A.M. and 99.5° in the P.M). Many people erroneously subtract a degree after taking a rectal temperature. The rectal temperature indicated is accurate and is always more reliable than temperatures registered at the mouth or armpit.

No one really knows why the temperature rises with disease, particularly with infection, but it is assumed that bacteria, viruses, or their toxic products irritate the temperature-regulating center in the brain. Some feel that fever is beneficial in that it helps kill the invading organisms, but this has not been proven.

Children are especially prone to high fevers, some temperatures having risen to 107° F. with no apparent damage. Fevers which rise high and rapidly may, however, produce convulsions; these are frightening; but although they seem to do no particular damage, swift action is always called for.

Treatment. Aspirin is the best immediate remedy for fever in a child. As a rule, one grain of aspirin for every ten pounds of body weight is safe to give over a long period of time. If the fever is reduced—at least temporarily—and the patient feels better within an hour and a half, the disease causing the fever is quite possibly not very serious; a day or two may be allowed to go by without seeking medical help.

A comfortable hot bath at only about 96° F. is useful in combating fever in that it serves to bring the hot blood to the skin surface where heat is radiated away. Sponging the skin with a wet washcloth and allowing the water to exaporate will further help to reduce the fever. A method used under careful medical supervision in cases of very high fever with delirium and dehydration is an enema of lukewarm water allowed to run into and out of the rectum in order to cool the body inside, where it is the hottest, and give the patient a "drink of water," since the colon effectively absorbs fluids. If attempted by the layman, however, this "tap water enema" may be dangerous to infants, leading to water intoxication, coma and even death. It should therefore *not* be encouraged as a home remedy for infants. However, a mild variation—namely, a small cool enema — might give relief to an older child or adult. With some fever-associated convulsions it may be necessary to give sedatives by injection to alleviate the spasms. The most important point, of course, is to call the doctor to ascertain the cause of fever, which in children is often obscure. Among these causes are infectious diseases, ear infections, or urinary infections.

FIBRILLATION   An auricle is said to be in fibrillation when its orderly, regular rate is replaced by rapid trembling of heart muscle and ineffective contractions of that chamber. Auricular fibrillation occurs when an irritable focal point causes electrical discharges at a rate of 500 or more per minute, in contrast to the normal and efficient 78 or 80 beats per minute, and produces irregular and ineffective muscular twitching in the auricle instead of a coordinated pulsation. Blood moves into the ventricle without the mechanical assistance of auricular contractions, and only a small portion of the hundreds of electrical impulses are transmitted to the ventricle; in fact, the ventricular rate in untreated auricular fibrillation usually lies between 120 and 200 per minute.

In ventricular fibrillation, the purposeful contraction of the muscular chamber is replaced by chaotic twitching in groups of muscle fibers; the forward flow of blood comes to a halt. Death will occur in a matter of minutes unless artificial maintenance of the circulation be provided until defibrillation can be attempted with the electronic defibrillator.

FIBROCYSTIC DISEASE   This is a congenital, hereditary condition which is manifested by chronic bronchitis; persistent, large and very smelly stools; and growth failure—all with variable degrees of severity in different cases. In some the stool symptoms border on diarrhea and the lungs are affected only minimally. In others it may be just the reverse; the bronchitis is so bad that multiple abscesses and scar tissue form in the lungs, causing backpressure in the right side of the heart, heart-failure, and even death.

The condition is not too difficult to diagnose if it is thought of. A sample of the sweat is analyzed to determine the salt concentration; in fibrocystic disease this is usually high, and patients therefore do poorly in hot climates.

Treatment. Treatment can only be directed toward maintaining good nutrition (with digestive enzymes) and keeping the chronic bronchitis under control with antibiotics.

FIBROIDS (FIBROMYOMATA OF THE WOMB)   These benign tumors are more prevalent between the ages of thirty-five and fifty. They are usually multiple tumors, quite firm, and their growth is slow —especially after the menopause, when they practically cease growing. Fibroids vary from marble-size to huge tumors weighing up to fifty pounds. The cause of these nonmalignant growths is unknown, although there has been definite association between their development and high levels of estrogenic hormones.

Symptoms. The symptoms of fibroids depend on their location and size. If they are located inside or very close to the cavity of the womb, they cause abnormal vaginal bleeding as well as infertility. When located at the outside surface, they may not be noticed until they grow very large; a feeling of fullness and heaviness in the lower abdomen and constant backache may then occur because of their size. Very often fibroids press the top of the bladder and cause difficulties in urination, kidney infections, etc.

About 1 per cent of fibroids may change into malignant tumors. Fibroids may also be responsible for infertility, or for abortion if pregnancy occurs. Often such tumors, growing from a small cord, (pedicle) become twisted and inflamed, and severe abdominal pain follows. If fibroids are present during a full-term pregnancy, they may cause difficulties in labor and delivery.

Treatment. Treatment of fibroids will depend on the symptoms. Fibroid tumors located very close to the cavity of the womb and producing bleeding will have to be removed, usually by removing the whole womb; if they are outside the womb and the patient is young, able, and willing to have children, then the tumors only are removed and the womb is left intact. Truly large tumors are usually removed together with the uterus.

Fibroid tumors in patients who have passed the menopause are removed only if they are too large and cause pressure difficulties; or if they cause bleeding, regardless of their size. In general, the choice will have to be left to the gynecologist who, during the operation, will use his best judgment in deciding whether the womb can be saved for a useful purpose, or whether everything should be removed. The patient should always be prepared to face the fact that childbearing may become impossible for her.

FIXATION, DEVELOPMENTAL Studies have shown that young people normally pass through a series of developmental stages in more or less orderly patterns. The child's sex interests, for example, are first directed towards sensations from his or her own body (autoeroticism), then toward experiences with the same sex (homoeroticism), and finally (after puberty) towards relationships with the opposite sex. Freud was first to emphasize that

developmental fixations may occur in which the person becomes "frozen" on one level, failing to mature towards higher levels. Developmental fixation has been suggested as one cause of homosexuality, the child becoming fixated on objects of the same sex, and failing to develop normal opposite-sex interests. Similarly, fixations may occur in eating or elimination habits, so that the person fails to mature beyond infantile levels because of emotional conflicts. Many adults show arrested emotional maturation caused by childhood fixations which impeded normal development.

FLATFOOT Flatfoot is a layman's term used to describe a loss of height in the longitudinal arch of the foot. In rare cases it may be due to abnormality of the bone, but is usually due to ligament or muscular weakness. Flatfeet are rarely painful in childhood, and most adults with flatfeet are able to lead active lives without any pain or discomfort. If foot discomfort develops, it may be relieved by appropriate shoe modifications such as heel wedges and pads and, if the foot is mobile, by an arch-support.

Some orthopedists feel that children with painless flatfeet should nevertheless be treated by means of shoe modifications and exercises in an attempt to strengthen their weak feet. The patient is taught consciously to try to flex his toes as he walks and to walk with his feet pointing directly forward, vigorously resisting the tendency of his feet to turn outward.

FLATULENCE (GAS) Excessive gas may accumulate in either the stomach or the intestine. An excess in the stomach may be expelled by belching, while collections of intestinal gas are relieved by the passage of flatus.

Gas in the stomach is the result of swallowing air, usually while eating or drinking; the ingestion of large quantities of carbonated beverages will likewise cause stomach gas. If excessive, the swallowed air can cause symptoms of pressure, fullness, and occasionally heartburn. Some individuals attempting to relieve this pressure by belching can cause further discomfort by swallowing more air.

Intestinal gas also results mostly from swallowed air, forced through the tract by peristalsis. Putrefaction of intestinal contents by bacterial action produces the rest. As is well known, certain foods such as beans, tomatoes, and other raw vegetables tend to cause excessive amounts of intestinal gas. Flatulence in this region can cause the same symptoms of fullness, abdominal cramping, and general distress as stomach gas. Gas-pains after abdominal surgery can be extremely distressing and must often be relieved by the use of a rectal tube. (This accumulation of gas is caused by a temporary paralysis of the intestinal tract so that the patient is unable to pass flatus voluntarily.)

FLEA BITES   The common flea (*Pulex irritans*) and the flea endemic to cats and dogs (*Ctenocephalus canis*) cause hive-like lesions in groups of two or three, arranged in a line or arc, with a tiny central puncture point. Any area of the body can be affected, and the eruption is accompanied by considerable itching. There appears to be variable susceptibility in responsiveness to the bite of a flea, and the diagnosis cannot be ruled out in the absence of similar lesions in other persons residing in the household of the affected member.

Treatment. Eradication of the fleas by fumigation, and de-fleaing the domestic animal are essential to a cure. It must be remembered, however, that if a dog or a cat is the source of the infection, the animal should not be removed lest the fleas attack the human being for nourishment in the absence of the prime host. The animal can be treated by a variety of household measures. For the existing bites, soothing lotion (calamine) and orally administered antihistaminic drugs, both for the relief of itching and allaying of the swelling, are effective. If the insects cannot be readily eradicated, the use of locally applied insect repellants may be necessary for persons highly reactive to the flea-venom.

FLUORIDE (FLUORIDATION)   A fluoride is a compound of the element fluorine with another element (such as sodium or tin) which in solution "disassociates" to liberate the fluoride ion. When incorporated into the teeth in one manner or another in proper trace amounts, this ion tends to reduce the incidence of dental caries.

There are two methods of administering fluorides: (1) topical application (directly to the teeth); and (2) ingestion through the digestive tract. Topical application is best accomplished by particular procedures utilized by the dentist, although another method is the regular use of fluoridated dentifrice. (Topical application implies that the teeth have already erupted into the mouth and are accessible.) Ingestion of fluorides may be accomplished by including them in drinking water or taking them in prescribed liquid or tablet form. This ingestion of fluoride is most beneficial during the actual formation of the tooth.

The exact mechanism of the action of fluoride in increasing the resistance of teeth to dental caries is still unknown. However, the fact remains that in our lifetime few methods of disease control have been more completely researched or thoroughly proved than fluoridation. The opposition to the inclusion of fluorides in drinking water cannot help but make one think of the opposition that once existed to any mass preventive measures, such as inoculation for smallpox and diphtheria.

In order effectively to reduce the incidence of dental caries, it is known that the fluoride compound must be in solution and actually deposited within the tooth in the form of the fluoride ion. This is accomplished much more thoroughly and readily when the ion is deposited in the tooth during its actual formation, although once a tooth has formed and erupted into the oral cavity, fluoride may be deposited into the teeth by means of topical application by the dentist. An ideal situation would be one in which the pregnant mother ingested fluoride compound in proper amounts; the child received fluoride by ingestion during the ages in which teeth were forming (up to twelve to fifteen years); and periodic topical applications were made by the dentist.

The effectiveness of fluoridation varies with the individual, and is directly related to many other factors, such as diet, heredity, dental caries-susceptibility, habits, arrangement of teeth, and oral hygiene. Fluoridation should therefore not be considered a panacea. It does not reduce the need for the competent advice of a dentist.

FOLIC ACID
Folic acid (also known as pteroylglutamic acid or folacin) is a member of the vitamin B complex. It is best known for its effect on the bone marrow, and it plays an essential role in the normal development of the red blood cell.

In the absence of adequate amounts of folic acid, a certain type of anemia may occur, identified by the presence of large cells (macrocytosis) and characteristic changes in the bone marrow (megaloblastic anemia). This type of anemia may be present in pregnancy and in infancy. Folic acid deficiency may also occur at times in diseases of abnormal intestinal absorption found particularly in tropical countries.

Folic acid is closely related to vitamin B_{12} in that both play a role in the normal maturation and development of the red cells. Folic acid is present in foods in both free and combined (conjugated) forms. It appears that folic acid is converted in the body to folinic acid, also known as citrovor-

um factor, which may be the more active form. (There is some evidence that ascorbic acid [vitamin C] assists in the conversion of folic acid to folinic acid.)

The best dietary sources for folic acid appear to be liver, green leafy vegetables, kidney, muscle meat, and whole-wheat cereals. The average diet probably contains under 0.5 mg. of folic acid compounds a day. Folic acid is also synthesized by intestinal bacteria, and this may be an important source of supply in man.

Certain drugs act against leukemia—a so-called "blood cancer"—by serving as antagonists of folic acid. When these folic acid antagonists are administered, symptoms of folic acid deficiency may be produced, including a red, inflamed tongue, diarrhea, and anemia.

FOOD ALLERGY
There is probably no food grown or processed to which someone is not allergic. To complicate the picture further, an allergic response to some foods may not be due to the food itself. There are today multiple food additives to which the individual may also be allergic: coloring agents, acids, alkalis, antioxidants, bleaches, maturing agents, flavors, emulsifiers, preservatives, stabilizers, thickeners, and nutritional supplements.

Food allergy may start at any age but most commonly first appears in infancy. The reaction to the food may occur immediately or be delayed for up to twelve hours after eating. Even if an individual is allergic to a certain food, exposure to it does not always cause a reaction; there seem to be external factors that control this. Infection, frequent consumption of the food, eating a great deal of it at one time, cold weather, emotional tension, and a general lowered physical resistance seem to increase the reaction to the offending food. Symptoms in a food-sensitive person can be provoked by eating the food, smelling it, or receiving blood from a donor who has eaten the suspicious food a few hours earlier. The most common foods to which people are allergic are cow's milk, wheat, eggs, sea food, chocolate, strawberries, and citrus fruits.

Symptoms. Food allergy in infants will manifest itself as colic, excessive "spitting up," chronic diarrhea, eczema, and a stuffy, runny nose. Some unexplained deaths in infancy may also be due to severe food allergy. It has been reported that some hypersensitive infants have gone into shock after eating milk and eggs. A positive skin test to egg white in a very young asthmatic child usually is a bad sign, indicating a severe course ahead.

Food allergy in children usually causes diarrhea, eczema, or hives. In adults the common symptoms are hives, diarrhea, rhinitis, headache, and asthma. Other symptoms reportedly attributable to food allergy in some cases are: hand dermatitis, ulcerative colitis, indigestion, abdominal pain, earaches, inflammation of the mouth, canker sores, excessive sweating, bad breath, constipation, frequency of urination, bed-wetting, contact dermatitis, conjunctivitis, personality changes, and so forth. An aromatic oil in coffee has been held responsible for the allergic symptoms of migraine, asthma, indigestion, malaise, rhinitis, and hives in those who drink the brew.

Diagnosis of food allergy is made by a careful and complete history. A "food diary" is helpful in recording the foods eaten and any reactions that may have developed. An elimination diet instituted by removing suspicious foods may help pin down the cause or causes of the difficulty. Skin tests may be used but have to be interpreted very carefully, as they are not too reliable in food allergy.

Treatment. Treatment consists of simple avoidance of the offending foodstuff. This is difficult and will require a great deal of label-reading—especially if a common food such as eggs, milk, corn, or wheat is involved. Special "allergy-free" recipes

are available so that the remaining permissible foods can be prepared in an appetizing and attractive manner.

In the case of the potentially allergic child, one should delay introducing eggs, wheat, fish, corn, cocoa, and cow's milk into the diet. The nursery should be kept free of feathers, kapok, and wool. One should avoid unnecessary injections of horse-serum medications as well as antibiotics. A pregnant woman from an allergic family should cut down on eggs, nuts, fish, and spices during her confinement so as to reduce the possibility of sensitizing the unborn child.

FOOD POISONING (BOTULISM) Botulism is a serious form of acute poisoning following the ingestion of food containing a toxin produced by the bacterium *Clostridium botulinum*. The disease is almost always caused by the eating of improperly preserved food, usually a home-canned product. The toxin produced by the bacteria may be found in such foods as string beans, corn, spinach, olives, beets, seafood, pork products, and beef. Cooking food at a temperature of at least 176° F. for thirty minutes before eating is a safeguard against botulism.

Symptoms. Symptoms develop within a day or two after eating contaminated food. The patient feels weak and tired and develops such visual disturbances as double vision, followed by difficulty in speaking and swallowing. The muscles of the extremities and trunk become weak; however, the mental faculties remain clear. There is no significant fever, and blood and urine tests are normal.

Mortality in botulism may be as high as 65 per cent. Most fatalities occur between the second and ninth day and result from respiratory paralysis or bronchial pneumonia. Recovery is slow in those who survive.

It may be difficult to diagnose a single case of botulism, but the simultaneous occurrence of several cases following consumption of the same meal makes the diagnosis more likely. Bacteriologic tests often indicate the guilty organism.

Prevention depends on proper home canning and adequate heating of food before serving. Food showing any evidence of spoilage should be discarded.

Treatment. Treatment usually requires hospitalization. Antiserum may be used, particularly in those who were exposed to contaminated food, but who have not yet developed symptoms of poisoning. For those with active botulism, treatment is largely supportive; that is, sedation, fluids by vein, antibiotics for respiratory infection, and so forth.

FOOT PROBLEMS, ADULT Most commonplace adult foot complaints are either due to, or aggravated by, poorly fitting shoes; painful bunions and hammertoes are almost exclusively related to pressure from tight shoes. Improper length is rarely a problem in shoe fit. Improper width and abnormal tapering of the toe box cause most of the difficulties. It is impossible to fit an ellipsoid foot into pointed shoes. Either the foot will deform the shoe or the shoe will deform the foot. Properly fitting shoes should be firm about the heel and amply wide in the toe area.

The fit of a shoe is best checked in the upright position. There should be half an inch of room in front of the big toe, and enough room at the level of the bases of the toes for the foot to be able to move

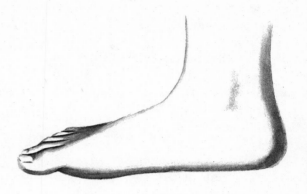

FALLEN ARCH
(FLAT FOOT)

ever so slightly inside the shoe. Any shoe that causes pain is improper and should not be worn.

Shoe modifications (such as arches, insoles, metatarsal pads, and wedges) are helpful in the relief of pain due to static orthopedic deformities. To achieve best results, professional examination and prescription is advised. If improperly selected, commercially available appliances may increase rather than relieve the painful symptoms.

FORCEPS These are several types of long, spoon-like obstetrical instruments, made of stainless steel or aluminum and used for the extraction of the baby's head from the patient's birth canal. When used under the proper circumstances and by experienced obstetricians, forceps deliveries are much safer than the spontaneous type. The patient is usually given some type of

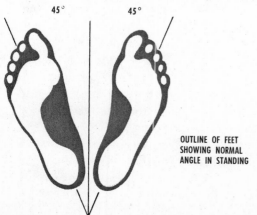

OUTLINE OF FEET
SHOWING NORMAL
ANGLE IN STANDING

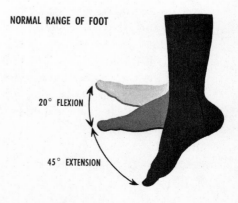

NORMAL RANGE OF FOOT

20° FLEXION

45° EXTENSION

satisfactory anesthetic, and the baby's head is delivered with forceps, under the physician's control; in this way the baby as well as the mother are less liable to be injured by very rapid delivery. The slight marks left on the baby's face and scalp disappear very promptly.

FOREIGN BODIES, INSERTION OF

If children find a hole, they love to put something into it. All the openings of the body have been subjected to this maltreatment with various effects.

The nose is probably the most accessible site and many objects have been inserted into it. If a child insists on repeating this activity, it may mean that he has a nasal allergy and is trying to scratch the lining. Most of the objects put into the nose are harmless and will soon ride out on the extra mucus secreted and/or be ejected by a healthy sneeze.

A very effective and safe way to dislodge an object from the nose is for an adult to make mouth-to-mouth contact with the child and to blow suddenly and powerfully, while holding the unaffected nostril closed with a handkerchief. The object will be blown out of the nose into the handkerchief (or onto the blower's cheek).

The nose is not the only body orifice into which the child may insert foreign bodies, however. Stopped-up ears will usually have to be washed out with a syringe and lukewarm water. An object left in the vagina will, after only a few days, begin to produce a very disagreeable and "dead" odor; special lights and instruments, and occasionally an anesthetic, will sometimes be necessary for surgical removal of the object inserted here.

When an object is successfully swallowed, it will usually pass through the entire tract, for the most narrow segment is from the throat to the stomach. Sometimes it will not pass the exit from the stomach (pylorus) but if it reaches the stomach it is assumed the object will continue on through. Occasionally, however, an oblong or irregular-shaped object must be "teased" through the anal opening.

X-rays of the intestines are not necessary unless symptoms of pain and vomiting occur. *Note:* An object in the lungs will make itself known by cough and wheeze; this needs immediate very special, skilled medical attention.

FORESKIN   See PENIS

FRACTURES   A fracture is a break in the structure of a bone. The two general types are simple (or closed) and compound (or open) fractures. A closed fracture is one in which the bone is broken but the overlying skin remains intact. An open fracture, on the other hand, is an injury severe enough not only to break the bone but also damage the overlying soft tissues and lacerate the skin. An open fracture is far more serious both because it is the result of a more violent injury and because of the danger of contamination of the bone-ends through the skin laceration. Every attempt should be made to minimize further damage and contamination of the injured limb while in transit to the hospital. It should be supported by a splint or a roll of newspaper or magazines, and if there are any lacerations, dry sterile dressings should be applied.

Fractures heal slowly in comparison with soft-tissue injuries. While a skin laceration will be well healed in about ten days, a finger fracture may require one month to heal, and a large bone such as a shin-bone (tibia) four to six months. Bones require not only ample time for healing, but also proper adjustment (reduction) to restore correct position and sufficient immobilization to maintain it through the long healing period.

Closed (non-operative) reduction is chosen whenever possible. Traction is employed to "unwedge" (disimpact) the fracture and regain length; the fractured limb is then manipulated so as to correct any deformation that may have developed. After clinical and X-ray examination have revealed satisfactory position, a plaster of Paris cast is applied to retain the reduced fracture until bony healing occurs. In some situations closed reduction is unsatisfactory and open reduction is required. With the fracture site directly visible, the orthopedic surgeon may employ various nails, plates, and screws to aid in the retention of the fracture after reduction has been achieved.

It is very important that the patient be as active as possible while the fracture is healing. Joint stiffness from disuse is one of the most troublesome fracture complications, and is to a large degree avoidable. With a fractured wrist, for example, the fingers and shoulders are free and should be vigorously exercised even while the forearm and wrist are immobilized. The shoulder should be put through a full range of active motion by swinging it freely like a pendulum, and the fingers exercised by squeezing a bar of soap or a mass of clay. (See also FIRST AID AND EMERGENCIES.)

FRECKLES Almost universally prevalent, and resulting from a simple dominant inherited characteristic, freckles are both elicited and made more prominent by exposure to sunlight. In identical twins, freckling will appear in identical distribution and intensity. Except when this condition is very intense and is part of a very rare disease of photosensitization (xeroderma pigmentosum), there are no indications for altering the process. For cosmetic purposes, however, bleaching applications, notably ointments containing monobenzyl ether of hydroquinone, can be effective but are attended with some risk of producing allergic dermatitis.

FREUD, SIGMUND Freud is now

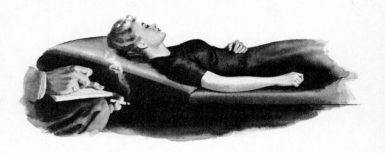

recognized as one of the most creative thinkers of all time, undoubtedly the major influence on developments in modern psychological and psychiatric science. Born in 1856, he studied medicine and showed an early interest in neurological and psychological disorders. While still studying in Paris under Charcot, he made the startling observation that seemingly physical disorders might be caused by psychological conflicts. Freud's greatest contribution was his theory of an unconscious mental life, in which ideas or impulses incompatible with the conscience (superego) are thrust back (repressed) into the unconscious—from which they can gain expression only in disguised form, such as formation of symptoms, humor, or mistakes.

Before Freud, no attempt had been made to comprehend the symbolic meanings of the (apparently) incoherent and irrational ravings of the mentally disordered. Freud was the first to attempt to differentiate between the manifest and latent meanings of behavior. (Manifest signifies the obvious or apparent meaning of behavior, latent referring to its unconscious significance.) He first discovered the possible significance of latent meanings in his study of dreams, where he was able to show that—though apparently meaningless—dreams might actually be interpreted in terms of unconscious complexes. Freud applied this same method to the understanding of latent or unconscious motivation in many other types of psychological phenomena: neurotic symptoms, origins of wit and humor, and the small distresses (psychopathology) of everyday life.

Early in his investigations, Freud became convinced that unconscious sex-conflicts were a major factor in causing mental disorders. His development of the theory of psychoanalysis involved intensive study of the various stages of psychosexual development through which everyone passes. He gave special emphasis to disorders resulting from unhealthy resolutions of the Oedipus complex, which involves unconscious love of the male child for his mother (with corresponding hostility towards the father), or, conversely, the Electra complex if the child is a girl.

Psychoanalysis may be seen as an attempt to understand the psychology of unconscious complexes and their symbolic representations. An important offshoot of psychoanalysis has been the development of projective psychologies, which involve methods for discovering the unconscious significance of obvious behavior. Freud's greatest contribution was perhaps his insistence on understanding and studying the emotional-impulsive determiners of mental life. Though Freud died in 1939, many years of intensive research will be needed to determine the validity of many of his theories.

One of Freud's major contributions was his invention of an entirely new school of psychology: the topological psychology of the unconscious. This theory pictures mental life as dominated by the dynamic conflict of powerful forces, both instinctive and acquired. Freud termed the innate, instinctive, unlearned drives and energies the id—conceived to include socially unacceptable expressions of sex, hate, life- and death-instincts. Opposing the forces of the id (instinct), Freud postulated the ego (the "I"), incorporating all the training imposed by society. That part of the ego involving concepts of right-and-wrong was designated by Freud as the superego (the censor or conscience).

Freud postulated continuous conflict between the forces of the id seeking expression, and repressive control exerted by the superego. He explained certain mental disorders as occurring when the superego was no longer strong enough to repress impulses from the id, the imbalance gaining expression through symptom-formation. "Psychoanalysis" comprises methods devised by Freud for the investigation of unconscious conflict, and the bringing of them into consciousness under conditions where they can effectively be controlled and turned into socially acceptable channels. The general validity of the Freudian theory of the unconscious has now gained wide acceptance, though specific applications have not been proved scientifically.

A cogent criticism of Freudian theory is that it places too much emphasis on the problems of psychosexual development to the exclusion of other factors known to influence behavior. Though psychosexual aberrations may underlie some types of mental disorder, these are only one of many potential causes. Historical evidence indicates that Freud was self-critical, modest, and self-effacing. He would have been the first to admit the limitations of his theories. Much of the controversy and criticism of psychoanalysis in recent years has arisen from efforts of his disciples to create an authoritarian and dogmatic psychoanalytic cult.

Even if many Freudian theories are eventually proved to be invalid, Freud's everlasting contribution will be that his discoveries opened up entire new areas for scientific investigation and forced a complete reappraisal of earlier theories.

FRIGIDITY, SEXUAL Sexual frigidity—indifference or aversion to sexual relations—among women is a complex psychiatric problem, and its many causes require intensive study. There are large innate differences in sexual excitability which exist on a constitutional basis. Studies in both lower animals and man have shown wide individual differences in sex drive; some cases of apparent frigidity may therefore be understood simply in terms of constitutional lack of sex drive.

Psychoanalytical theory, however, stresses the presence of emotional conflict and ambivalence as the major factor in most nonorganic frigidity. Of the three primitive emotions of fear, anger, and (sexual) love, fear and anger are biologically overriding because of their survival-value; they thus tend to inhibit the sex drive. Strong fear or strong anger, therefore, typically inhibit sexuality, so that sexual frigidity may occur in any situation where emotions of fear or anger predominate. This means that for optimum sex performance a woman should be free of internal conflict, anger, or fear.

Psychological studies universally indicate that sex behavior in human beings is learned, not instinctive. Adult performance is largely determined by sexual experience in early life. Where the child has been conditioned by unpleasant, frightening, or painful experiences with sex, frigidity may occur in later life. Psychoanalytic studies place special emphasis on sexual trauma (shocking experience) in which the child has been conditioned to respond to sex in unhealthy patterns. The victim of rape or sexual attack, for example, may subsequently show neurotic aversion to sex experiences.

Much also depends on early sex-attitudes. Many young girls are taught by older women that men are brutes, that sex is disgusting, and that menstruation and childbearing are curses which must be (unwillingly) borne. Such teachings tend to produce fear and revulsion concerning sex later in life. It is far more healthy for mothers to teach young girls that love can be beautiful; that men and women naturally complement each other; that menstruation is to be welcomed as an event indicating preparation for motherhood. More adequate sex education would undoubtedly prevent much of the frigidity now produced by ignorance and lack of proper training in sex roles. Persistent frigidity usually requires psychiatric treatment to discover its causes, and no young person should be too embarrassed to seek such help.

"FROG TEST"   One of the many animal tests for pregnancy, the "frog test" has been replaced by much simpler, cheaper laboratory tests of the immunological or chemical type. The most widely used are chemical tests performed on a small amount of urine placed on a slide. Unlike the animal tests, the chemical test takes only a few minutes.

FROSTBITE   See FIRST AID AND EMERGENCIES

FRUSTRATION TOLERANCE   Frustration tolerance is a psychiatric concept referring to a person's ability to tolerate normal amounts of frustration and thwarting without breaking down emotionally.

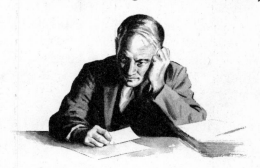

Psychoanalytic theory points out that many very young children develop feelings of "infantile omnipotence" during the first weeks and months of life when they are more or less pampered and spoiled, the parents attempting to satisfy all their needs. Freud explained this phenomenon by pointing out that the behavior of young or immature people is largely determined by the Pleasure-Pain principle, whereby the child seeks only pleasures and avoids pain. He also pointed out that as the child grows older he begins to face the Reality principle, the demands and limitations exerted by the culture in which he lives. Each person must therefore learn to balance the Pleasure-Pain principle against the demands of Reality.

Very young children develop rage reactions and have temper tantrums whenever thwarted and not allowed to have their own way. In the course of normal development the child learns, however, to accept and tolerate a certain amount of interference and thwarting of his needs. The degree to which any person learns to tolerate frustration without breaking down emotionally is termed the frustration tolerance.

One of the goals of education and conduct training is to teach the child to face increasingly difficult problems in life while remaining psychologically whole and in control of the situation. School systems, athletic programs, and military training programs provide tasks of progressively increasing difficulty which the child is trained to master by developing all types of self-control. The adult who displays temper tantrums or a break-down in emotional behavior lacks that frustration tolerance which can be acquired only through emotional retraining under psychiatric supervision.

FUNCTIONAL MENTAL DISORDER
See NEUROSIS

FUNGI   Of the thousands of varieties of fungi, a few are found on the cutaneous surface and cause no disease; even fewer produce infection of the skin (superficial mycosis) and of internal organs (deep mycosis). Fungi are the subject of many and diverse types of classification, according to their morphology, growth habits, and geographic distribution. In their ability to be provocative of disease, they can be

divided into three groups: (1) those capable of digesting skin keratin and using it for growth, and therefore capable of producing disease of destruction (ringworm of the hair and nails) or of allergic sensitization (ringworm of the groin and other skin sites); (2) those incapable of digesting keratin and therefore unable to infect, except very superficially (tinea versicolor, erythrasma); and (3) those capable of invading the skin and other organs and causing diseases the common feature of which is a fungating lesion or mass known as a granuloma (blastomycosis, sporotrichosis, histoplasmosis, coccidioidomycosis).

In addition to causing disease by invasion and growth, fungi are a common cause of allergic reactions of the respiratory tract, being responsible for a significant incidence of asthmatic attacks. The importance of fungi as a cause of disease depends to some degree on the geographic distribution of the organisms and their habits of growth, which are largely governed by climate, flora, geology, etc. However, the susceptibility (or resistance) of the individual host is undoubtedly the determining factor in the complexity of influences giving rise to disease.

THE GALLBLADDER AND LIVER

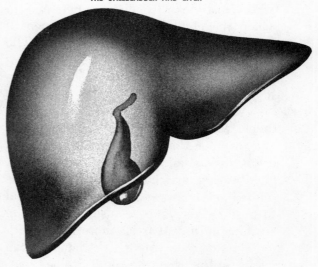

GALLBLADDER   This sack-like structure is primarily a reservoir for bile, which is produced by the liver. It is situated under the right lobe of the liver in the right-upper portion of the abdominal cavity. Bile helps in the digestion of fatty substances and is a thick liquid containing many salts. It is released from the gallbladder into the duodenum by the common bile duct. Removal of the gallbladder does not seem to be harmful in any way and digestion continues as before. Infections of the gallbladder are relatively common.

GALLSTONES   Gallstones are estimated to be present in 10 per cent of the population. Many individuals may have a gallbladder loaded with stones and yet never have symptoms. By contrast, others may have only a single gallstone which can cause agonizing pain and serious difficulties requiring extensive surgery. Acute attacks of biliary colic often occur in overweight, middle-aged women of light complexion, giving rise to the axiom that right-upper abdominal pain in a woman who is "fair, fat, and forty" is most likely due to gallstones. The causes of gallstones are not entirely known. Faulty metabolism of cholesterol (one of the substances in bile), chronic infection of the lining of the gallbladder, and partial obstruction of the bile duct are all thought to play a part.

Symptoms. Typically, a gallbladder attack will start as a cramping pain in the upper right portion of the abdomen, usually after a heavy meal. The pain then becomes more severe and often radiates into the back under the right shoulder blade. (This type of radiating pain is characteristic of gallbladder disease.) Nausea and vomiting are common, and the pain can become extremely severe.

Occasionally a stone will travel into the common bile duct and obstruct the flow of bile. If the obstruction continues, bile will back up through the liver and eventually stain the skin, causing jaundice; the characteristic color of this condition

is due to certain pigments that are found in bile. If the obstruction is severe, the stools may become very light since the normal brown color of feces is due to bile pigment. An attack of biliary colic usually subsides spontaneously in a few hours, only to make its presence felt at some later time.

Treatment. Surgical removal of the gallbladder and its stones is by far the most effective cure. Most authorities agree that when gallstones are found on routine X-ray examination, surgery is often indicated, as future likelihood of acute attacks is great. Other useful measures are reduction in weight and the avoidance of fats in the diet. Surgery is seldom indicated in patients whose gallbladders contain a single large stone where there is no danger of passage into the bile ducts and no associated infection. However, acute and chronic infections of the gallbladder are commonly associated with gallstones. These conditions are discussed under CHOLECYCYSTITIS.

GASTRIC JUICES   The lining of the stomach secretes a variable mixture of powerful digestive juices including hydrochloric acid; the enzymes pepsin, rennin, and lipase; and a thick, protective mucus. The secreting cells respond to stimuli initiated by the sight, smell, or thought of food, as well as by reacting to the presence of food in the alimentary canal.

GASTRITIS   Gastritis is an acute inflammation of the lining of the stomach. Usually of brief duration, it is sometimes sudden and violent. Several types of gastritis exist. One form may be caused by the ingestion of single substances, such as alcohol, creosote, sulfa drugs, antibiotics, iodine or bromine compounds, very hot foods, an allergy-producing food (such as milk, eggs, or fish when taken by hypersensitive individuals), and so forth. Another type may be caused by swallowing strong acids or caustics (iodine, arsenic, zinc, lead, etc.). Still a third type of gastritis is produced by infectious or toxic material and may be seen in patients with influenza, measles, scarlet fever, pneumonia, or diphtheria. (A rare form may be caused by such bacteria as the streptococcus or colon bacillus.)

Symptoms. In gastritis the lining of the stomach is intensely congested with small areas of hemorrhage, and there may actually be ulceration. Symptoms include loss of appetite, pressure sensation in the stomach area, headache, vomiting, and exhaustion. In milder cases these symptoms may subside within twenty-four to forty-eight hours. If the gastritis is due to a corrosive poison, there will be collapse, severe pain, and a rigid abdomen, and chills and fever will occur if the cause is toxic or infectious.

Treatment. In the more common form of gastritis, complete bed rest is necessary. Drugs that reduce the tendency to nausea are indicated, and analgesics or narcotics may be given for severe pain. (Morphine, however, is not to be given in the presence of nausea or vomiting.) No solid or semisolid food should be given for the first day or two. Water, bouillon with salt, hot tea and sugar, and thin soups may be given orally, although in some cases nourishment must be injected into the vein. Later, bland foods may be taken. These include buttered toast, soft-boiled eggs, cooked cereals, mashed potatoes, milk and cream, gelatin desserts, and so forth. This type of diet may be necessary for several weeks.

GASTRITIS, CHRONIC Chronic gastritis is a continual inflammation of the wall of the stomach. The cause is unknown, although some instances may be psychosomatic. Patients have a sensation of heartburn or fullness in the upper part of their abdomen, especially after the ingestion of food. Loss of appetite, nausea and vomit-

ing, or hemorrhages occur infrequently. An ulcer-like pain is present in many patients and loss of weight is common.

Treatment. When chronic gastritis is suspected, all stomach irritants such as alcohol, nicotine, spices, aspirin-related or iodine compounds, or harsh laxatives, should be avoided. A bland diet, such as is used for peptic ulcer, is recommended. Because of the nutritional limitation of foods in this diet, large amounts of vitamin B complex and vitamin C are added. In view of the fact that the disease is hard to distinguish from peptic ulcer or other more serious conditions of the gastrointestinal tract, the patient should be placed under a physician's care.

GASTROINTESTINAL DISORDERS The gastrointestinal system (or alimentary canal) can properly be considered a hollow tube with various bulges and attached glands, extending from mouth to anus. Its purpose is to prepare and extract fluid and nourishment from foodstuffs, to provide energy and building material for the body, and then to reject the resulting waste at the convenience of the host. This tube is lined with various types of cells which, in addition to other specific functions, protect the body in much the same way as does the skin. The canal should be considered not as an inner part of the body, but merely as another surface in contact with the outside environment.

The alimentary canal includes the mouth, the esophagus (or tube from throat to stomach), and stomach, the small intestine with its associated organs—the liver, gallbladder, and pancreas—the large intestine, the rectum, and the anus. This complicated apparatus is subject to many diseases and malfunctions both of its components individually and of the system as a whole. Disturbances of function may arise from infections, ingested food or poisons, injuries, tumors, lack of essential foods, and in many instances from so-called psychosomatic or "functional" difficulties.

In our society a vast amount of attention is given to affairs of the alimentary canal. The infant is urged to eat; the adult is urged not to eat after the previous lessons have been too well learned; the teenager fears halitosis (a term coined by an advertising man for the promotion of a certain now-famous mouthwash); and nearly everyone is at least occasionally preoccupied with "regularity" or lack of it. It is no wonder that an estimated 30 per cent of patients with gastrointestinal complaints are found to have no demonstrable disease to account for their symptoms. Conversely, very real and often serious disorders such as peptic ulcers, ulcerative colitis, and even cirrhosis of the liver may have at least partial psychologic origins.

GENITAL HYGIENE   The uncircumsized penis should be cleansed periodically by completely pulling back the foreskin (prepuce) and washing the secretion known as smegma from the glans penis and the indented area behind it. In the female, the region of the clitoris should likewise be cleansed by washing, with the "small lips" (labia minora) spread apart. A mild douche powder may be used if there is heavy discharge. (Frequent douching or douching with strong substances should be avoided as it may injure the delicate membranes of the vagina.)

GEOGRAPHIC TONGUE   Frequently noted and thought to be of no importance is the changing appearance of the tongue due to temporary loss of papillae (tongue ridges) in areas of varying size and shape. The areas containing normal papillae seem to be enlarged and give the impression of being the mountain ridges of a basrelief map. Changes in the sites of involvement result in new configurations of the "ridges" and "valleys." There are usually no associated symptoms, and there is no significance to either the change in appearance or the persistence of the condition. Geographic tongue exists as a medical oddity.

Geriatrics

GERIATRICS   Geriatrics is the branch of medicine that deals specifically with the health problems of elderly people. Many geriatric physicians explain that as specialists they are particularly concerned with health problems that directly or indirectly involve the physiological complications of the aging process. Their clients are generally more than seventy-five years of age because younger people usually have health problems not linked specifically to aging. Geriatric doctors do not expressly seek to prolong life, but rather strive to give the elderly a quality of health as free of discomfort and disability as possible.

Geriatric medical research explores areas of study such as the determination of "normal" physiological change due to age—as apart from illness not directly related to aging. Researchers also attempt to discover the best approaches in the treatment of chronic illness associated with advanced age, as well as finding the most beneficial methods of care to give individuals confined to hospitals, nursing homes, and private homes. Research that deals with the health problems of the elderly in holistic terms, including the role of regular exercise, proper nutrition, and the psychological needs of the elderly, is also an important area of scientific investigation.

In addition, geriatric physicians emphasize the point that individuals age at different rates and that the different organs of the body age independently of each other. In terms of living a healthy life and possessing a "well body," someone of seventy-five years of age who follows a regular regimen of exercise, has proper diet and hygiene, and a satisfactory sleep routine could conceivably be "fitter" than a much younger person with poor personal health habits. Too, one should not assume elderly people who have difficulty walking or standing, seeing or hearing, necessarily have impaired intellectual faculties as well.

It is true, however, that as people reach an advanced age they become more susceptible to a wide range of illnesses. Of the elderly living in hospitals or nursing homes, a large majority suffer from more than one major chronic illness. The three most common causes of death for people over age sixty-five are heart disease, cancer, and stroke. Too, the risk of injury due to accident increases with age.

Every day about 4000 citizens are added to the number of Americans over the age of sixty-five. In 1980, Americans over age sixty-five comprised almost 13 percent of the population and accounted for more than 30 percent of all health care expenditures.

The Aging Process. With the biological process of aging, certain changes in body metabolism and physiology are to be expected. Various vital organs undergo alterations that can be considered "normal" within the context of advancing age. These changes characteristic of aging may become aggra-

Major causes of death among the elderly population, 1977:

Cause	Rate per 100,000 population
Aged 65 to 74 years	
Heart disease	1,250
Cancer	792
Stroke	260
Diabetes mellitus	66
Accidents	62
Pneumonia	57
Cirrhosis of the liver	43
Aged 75 and more	
Heart disease	4,106
Stroke	1,309
Cancer	1,308
Pneumonia	342
Arteriosclerosis	266
Accidents	170
Diabetes millitus	157
Emphysema	69

vated, however, and then contribute to associated complaints, injury, and illness.

The Skin. As a person ages changes occur in the skin. The ability of the skin to respond to temperature changes decreases, as does sensitivity to pain. Sweat glands tend to degenerate, which decreases the body's capacity to regulate body temperature via evaporation. These changes of the skin raise the probability of the elderly to succumb to burn accidents and heat prostration.

The Heart. The aging process has especially significant influence upon the physiology of the heart. The heart muscle loses its former contracting strength, heart valves have increased calcification, and the ability of the heart to function in situations of stress (e.g. accident, shock, surgery, excessive physical exertion) may greatly diminish.

Cardiac complications associated with these changes in an aging heart include endocarditis, heart murmurs, abnormal heart rhythm, and heart blockages.

The Brain. The brain characteristically loses weight and loses brain cells in certain areas of the brain. Blood vessels of the brain become more susceptible to athersclerosis and the efficiency of nerve signals, as expressed in reaction speed, decreases.

Complications of the aging brain may produce confusion, loss of memory, senile dementia (including Alzheimer's disease) and depression. It is important to note, however, that the changes the brain undergoes in the course of normal aging do not, of themselves, indicate an inevitable loss of intellectual capacity. Some studies have shown that verbal proficiency, as measured in IQ testing, may increase in later life.

Digestive Tract. The organs of the digestive tract change with advancing age. There is a probability of decreased hydrochloric acid production, decreased awareness of thirst, decreased moving ability of the large intestine, and diminished calcium absorption. Complications can lead to chronic constipation, dehydration, and osteoporosis.

Renal System. Aging usually means a decrease in the holding capacity of the bladder, a decrease in the size of the kidneys, less efficient filtration, and decreased blood flow through the kidneys. Complications commonly encountered include increased frequency of urination, lack of bladder control, and heightened drug sensitivity, especially for drugs expelled primarily through the renal system.

Bones and Muscles. Advancing age usually causes decreased stature, bone weight, and elasticity, as well as decreased muscle size and strength. Osteoporosis (bone degeneration due to lack of calcium absorption), fractures caused by falls, and muscle fatigue are associated complications.

Vision. Advanced age normally brings with it increased lens density, a lessening of the ability to discriminate light intensities, and alterations of the aqueous humor. Complications include cataracts and glaucoma.

Intellect. Impairment of the intellect or mental confusion should not be considered a natural characteristic of the aging process. Of people more than seventy-five years of age only 25 percent manifest discernible states of mental confusion. Often such conditions in elderly people are caused by factors only indirectly associated with advanced age, such as drug side effects, certain types of infections, dietary deficiencies, and anemia. Abnormal emotional behavior, or sudden personality changes, may also be induced by medications, poor diet, and other factors not considered a part of the overall aging process. Most of these disorders are reversible when a correct diagnosis is made, which leads to proper treatment.

When a brain disorder first occurs it may be diagnosed as acute organic brain syndrome (OBS), and various treatments are possible to reverse its effects. However, when a disorder is prolonged and brain damage or degeneration is not affected by treatment, the condition may then be termed chronic brain syndrome (CBS). At this stage the disorder and its associated effects, such as confusion, loss of time and space orientation, etc., is virtually irreversible. One such brain disorder is Alzheimer's disease.

Alzheimer's disease is a particular problem among the elderly. This condition is initially characterized by mental impairments such as mood changes, memory lapses, and time and spatial disorientation. As the disease progresses the individual may become irascible, increasingly confused, suffer attacks of anxiety, and become restless to the extent of wandering at night. Efforts at meaningful communication are often futile. The late phase of Alzheimer's disease may include severe apathy, total lack of bowel control, and lack of reaction to sensory stimuli. Postmortem brain examination usually reveals loss of brain weight and fewer brain neurons plus, for reasons not yet understood, high concentrations of aluminum. Because it is a chronic, irreversible disorder that requires long term medical care, some authorities consider Alzheimer's disease to be America's most costly illness. It is the chief reason for the six billion dollars annually spent on the care of patients with adult dementia.

Medical care for the elderly who suffer chronic illness or disability can be obtained in hospitals, nursing homes, and private homes. Usually factors such as the nature of the illness, the type of medical care required, and the long term cost of care determine which environment is chosen. Between 20 and 30 percent of all elderly people will spend some portion of their lives in a type of nursing home facility.

Nursing Home. There are different classes of nursing homes based upon the level of medical attention provided. Nursing homes that are designated "skilled nursing" facilities are obligated by federal regulation to provide their clients rehabilitation, pharmaceutical, radiological, laboratory, and dietetic services, in addition to providing social activites. There are about 7000 skilled nursing facilities in the United States.

Nursing homes designated "intermediate care" facilities are to accommodate clients with less severe disability or illness than those in a skilled nursing facility. This type of institution is state-licensed to provide regular medical services to its clients.

The type of facility that usually provides only room and board, and possibly recreational activities, is designated a "domiciliary" facility. Its clients usually should not require constant medical care apart from periodic checkups or self-administered medication.

Trying to locate the particular nursing facility that provides the best possible care for its clients can be made easier by considering the following points:

1. Be sure that the nursing home and the nursing home administrator have state-issued licenses. Do not be afraid to ask to see these certificates if they are not openly displayed. Be sure, too, that these licenses are up-to-date. Do not use a home that cannot produce these documents for your inspection.

Also, find out whether the institution is certified by the Joint Commission on Accreditation of Hospitals. This is a nongovernment organization that inspects and judges the care given in hospitals and nursing homes.

2. Consider the interests and desires of the prospective client. Does he or she prefer a rural or an urban environment? Does the nursing facility offer interesting recreational and social activities? Is there a lawn, park, or garden area open to the home's residents?

3. What professional medical staff is a permanent part of the nursing home's health care personnel? Is a geriatric physician or nurse a member of the staff? If needed, are rehabilitation and special dietetic programs available?

Better nursing homes require each new client to have a complete physical examination in order to assess the client's individual medical care needs. Questions concerning emergency arrangements with nearby hospitals and provisions for pharmaceutical needs should also be asked.

4. Be sure that the nursing home has been inspected, and complies with, state and federal fire safety codes. Avoid homes that have not been inspected within a year. Also, notice whether the home's furnishings were designed to minimize the risk of accidents. Do the hallways have hand railings? Do the toilets and bathrooms have support bars?

5. Is the home clean? Be sure to notice whether common areas such as dining rooms, hallways, activity rooms, and lounge areas are cleaned regularly.

6. What are the costs? Are there any charges that are separated from the basic monthly rate, such as laundry service or telephone access? Find out what exactly is provided for the amount charged. Discover if the prospective client is entitled to Medicare or Medicaid benefits. Always take the time to compare the costs and services of several nursing homes. Do not use a home that is not eligible to participate in federal, state, or private financial assistance programs.

Alternatives to Nursing Facilities. For many elderly people the peace of mind gained by living in familiar surroundings or among relatives, cannot be obtained in any other environment. Often arrangements that meet health care needs using available financial resources can be made to allow the elderly to live in their own homes, eliminating the need for institutionalized care. When elderly people can deal with their everyday needs in their own homes, or in the homes of relatives—with the help of family, visiting health care professionals and aides, and community social service personnel—much can be done to maintain their senses of self-worth and independence.

If older family members are capable of living in their own homes, or in the homes of their relatives—and elect to do so—various

measures can be taken to lessen the risk of accidents. Hand rails for steps, stairs, and on walls near bathtubs and toilets can be installed. Ramps can be added to outside entrances to facilitate entry.

A list of telephone numbers, perhaps in large print, can be located near the telephone. This list should include the phone numbers of physicians, nurses, and friends that the elderly individual may need or want to contact.

Medicines not in current use should be kept in a secured cabinet since geriatric patients may become forgetful. Family members can help make sure that medications are taken as prescribed. Family members can also be alert for danger signals specific to their elderly relative's particular health problems.

Preventive Measures. There are some simple measures that can be taken to improve general health. Regular health examination with a physician is important. Also, following the instructions in health care, resulting from this consultation, is necessary. Follow the doctor's orders.

Regular, moderate exercise helps to maintain good digestion, circulation of blood, and strengthens the heart. But care should be used not to produce strain and exhaustion, and exercise should be discontinued before one is tired. Adequate rest is also essential. Research shows that most elderly persons who sleep eight to ten hours have fewer health problems than those who sleep less.

A well-balanced diet is the key to maintaining good health. Many older persons, due to specific medical problems, are on restricted diets. For health reasons they should eliminate salt, sugar, fats, and caffeine products from their daily menu. This may result in a lack of interest in tasteless foods. But it is of the utmost importance that good nutritional foods be eaten to maintain health and energy levels. Digestion and elimination affect the overall health picture. A properly planned diet of

MEDICAL ASSISTANCE

Medicare

This health insurance program is designed to serve everyone over 65 years of age and disabled persons under 65 years of age who:

(1) have been entitled to receive Social Security disability benefits for a total of 24 months; or

(2) who need dialysis treatments or a kidney transplant because of permanent kidney failure.

The program is not based on income, but is available regardless of financial need. The Medicare program has two parts:

Part A: Hospital insurance at no cost that helps pay for care while in the hospital and for related health care services after leaving the hospital.

Part B: Voluntary medical insurance at a monthly premium that helps pay doctor bills and other approved medical services.

More information about Medicare is available from your local Social Security Office, or by writing to:

Health Care Financing Administration
Inquiries Branch
Rm. 1–N–4, East Lowrise Bldg.
Baltimore, MD 21235

Medicaid

Medicaid (Medical Assistance Programs) is a joint Federal/state program to provide physical and related health care services to persons with low incomes. Disabled persons may be eligible for Medicaid on the basis of their income.

Because eligibility is determined by your state program of public assistance (welfare) on the basis of broad Federal guidelines, there are geographic differences between eligibility requirements and types of services covered. Generally, persons may be eligible for Medicaid if they are receiving welfare or other public assistance benefits or Supplemental Security Income or are blind or disabled. Medicaid services are available in all states except Arizona.

Individuals with higher incomes may be eligible for Medicaid Supplemental Medical Care Assistance, or their children may be eligible if medical expenses exceed a given percentage of their annual income.

Each state establishes its own eligibility requirements for Medicaid.

Further information on Medicaid and assistance in applying is available from your local or state welfare or public assistance office.

If you cannot get information locally, write to:

Health Care Financing Administration
Inquiries Branch
Rm. 1–N–4, East Lowrise Bldg.
Baltimore, MD 21235

fresh fruit and vegetables, which contain fiber, improves both digestion and elimination, as does drinking six to eight glasses of water daily. Water flushes poison from the kidneys and bladder, helping to prevent problems in these vital organs.

Varieties of Financial Assistance for

Health Related Expenses. Government financial assistance programs that may offer help to the elderly include Medicare, Medicaid, Social Security, and food stamps.

Medicare is a program that shares medical costs with the individual. Application for Medicare assistance is through the local Social Security office. Because benefit eligibility requirements and specific guidelines governing the amounts of financial assistance given may vary as laws are changed, up-to-date information should be obtained from the nearest Social Security office.

Medicaid is a government program geared for those who fail to be eligible for Medicare or who do not have the funds necessary to pay the expenses Medicare does not cover. Administration of Medicaid is through state welfare agencies and these agencies should be contacted for the most current eligibility requirements.

Nongovernment health insurance programs and policies are also available. Blue Cross/Blue Shield and other companies offer policies that might be beneficial. Caution should be taken when considering the purchase of supplemental health insurance. Be sure the money spent obtains the most reliable and widest range of coverage possible.

The Problem of Boredom. Prolonged inactivity or boredom can lead to serious consequences, such as severe depression or alcoholism. If the older individual finds enjoyment in a hobby or other activity, members of the family can encourage its continuance. Many communities have agencies that involve older citizens in social service work. Often the years of experience and acquired skills an elderly person has can be of particular benefit to others—if the proper matching of human needs and resources is made. This is especially true of individuals who have led very active lives before retirement.

Older people have highly diversified interests, personalities, illnesses, and disabilities. Some improve in mind and body and acquire ambition and the ability to participate in family and community affairs to a greater degree than much younger people.

Facing Incurable Diseases. A large number of elderly patients have illnesses that are terminal. The majority of incurable diseases fall into two categories: cancer, and cardiac and circulatory disease. Many older people have specific desires concerning the use of medical techniques and equipment engaged only to prolong life temporarily. Some have "living wills" that instruct physicians not to employ sophisticated methods of treatment if the condition is irreversible.

The recent research and writings of Dr. Elisabeth Kübler-Ross and others have

---

Some organizations and agencies that deal with the health-related concerns of the elderly:

U.S. Administration on Aging
3303 C St. SW
HHS South
Washington, D.C. 20024

National Council on the Aging
Suite 504
1828 L St. NW
Washington, D.C. 20036

Center for the Study of Aging
 and Human Development
Duke University
Durham, NC 27710

Family Service Association of America
44 W. 23rd St.
New York, NY 10010

American Cancer Society
219 E. 42nd St.
New York, NY 10023

Andrus Gerontology Center
University of Southern California
Los Angeles, CA 90007

Gray Panthers
3635 Chestnut St.
Philadelphia, PA 19104

260

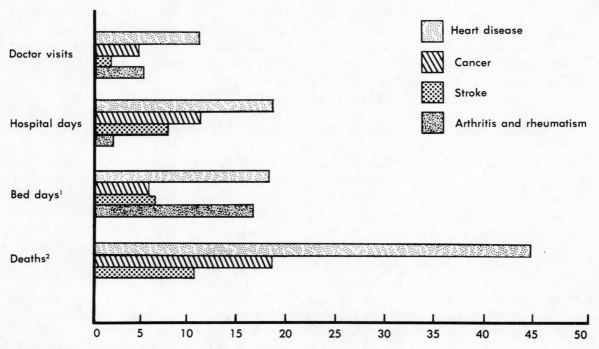

¹Average for 1979 and 1980.
²Provisional data.
SOURCE: National Center for Health Statistics: Division of Health Care Statistics, Division of Health Interview Statistics, and Division of Vital Statistics.

Burden of illness for persons 65 years of age and over, according to selected conditions: United States, 1980

increased the general public's awareness of the psychological and social needs of a dying person. Family members, medical professionals, and spiritual advisors can do much to make the terminally ill gain peace of mind about their condition.

Gerontology

GERONTOLOGY Gerontology is the scientific study of old age and the aging process, which includes the broadest range of biological, social, and psychological investigation.

Biological Theories of Aging. There are a number of theories that attempt to explain the aging process. Some of these theories take into account one or more of the following considerations:

1. The possibility that as the body ages there is a decrease in the amount of certain vitally essential substances within the cell.

2. The dysfunction and subsequent inoperation of vital organs is caused by the clogging of essential activities by waste products.

3. That there is a definite limitation on the cell division capacity of cells; thus, after this limitation is reached, cellular replace-

ment necessary to maintain life becomes impossible.

4. That there is a definite limit to the cumulative effect of repeated stress and strain; and that when this limit is achieved a deadly malfunction of intracellular activities or body metabolic regulation will occur.

Studies have also been conducted to explore how the biochemical mechanisms of growth might inhibit the aging process. By reducing the calories in the diet of young rats to that sufficient to sustain life but insufficient for growth, researchers have extended the life span of laboratory rats to more than twice the average length. However, the lack of proper nutrition early in life, aside from stunting growth, caused brain damage and other disorders.

Longevity Studies and Life Expectancy. In the United States the life expectancy at birth in the middle of the 19th century was a mere 39.4 years. By 1979, life expectancy at birth had risen to 73.7 years. Most of this increase was due to the falling infant mortality rates and in the improved treatment of childhood diseases. The more relevant statistic, in terms of the longevity of the elderly, is that in 1850 the life expectancy at age sixty was 16.3 additional years; in 1960, the additional life expectancy was a slight increase to 17.3 years. Some authorities estimate that even if deaths from diseases were totally eliminated, human life expectancy at birth still would not exceed 100 years due to the irreversible physiological deterioration of the body caused by the aging process.

Factors that contribute to a potentially long life include a rural living environment, marriage, a family history of longevity into the eighties and nineties, and maintaining moderate eating habits. There is also almost an eight-year difference between the life expectancy at birth of females compared to males.

A number of explanations for the disparity between the life expectancy of men and women have been offered. Many argue that men are more likely to have stressful careers that may induce health problems such as ulcers, high blood pressure, and heart disorders, which ultimately shorten life. Too, some psychologists maintain that cultural attitudes requiring boys and men to suppress emotions add stress to their lives, thus placing additional strain on their well-being.

Mortality figures for males and females sixty-five years of age and over show a disparity that has increased since 1950, when the age-adjusted mortality rate for males was 34 percent higher than females. By 1979, the difference between the sexes had risen to 69 percent. The difference is particularly evident in the mortality rate of cancer. Lung cancer alone had a mortality rate five times higher for men than women in 1979, largely due to the greater number of men who smoke cigarettes.

There is also reason to suspect that the female hormone estrogen may lower the risk of heart disease for women. The exact mechanisms involved, however, are not fully understood.

America's elderly: current and projected figures

Population of persons 65 and over	1975	2000	2030
Number in millions	22.4	31.8	55.0
Percent of total population	10.5	12.2	18.3
Population of persons 75 of age and over:			
Number in millions	8.5	14.3	23.2
Percent of total population	4.0	5.5	7.7

262

Living situation of men and women age 65 and over: (percentage figures)

Male	65–74 years	Over 75
With family	85.0	74.5
Alone	12.1	18.2
Institutionalized	2.9	7.4
Female		
With family	64.6	49.4
Alone	32.9	40.6
Institutionalized	2.5	10.0

Source: Bureau of the Census

Demography. About 4000 Americans join the ranks of citizens over sixty-five years of age each day. Projections indicate that if present trends continue, 18.3 percent of the general population will be elderly by the year 2030. The fastest growing subgroup is the portion of the elderly population over the age of seventy-five.

In the United States two-thirds of the elderly population live in urban areas. Only one-fifth live on farms or in a rural locale. California, Florida, and four other states contain about half of America's elderly.

Figures from 1976 reveal that a large majority of the elderly under age seventy-five live with their family. More than twice the number of elderly women than men live alone, due to the fact that more wives outlive their husbands. The number of elderly living in nursing homes or other health care facilities rises dramatically after age eighty. The average age of the institutionalized elderly is about eighty-two years.

The Elderly and Mental Health. Advancing age brings with it the need to adjust to change. Many older people must deal with problems such as decreased mobility, chronic illness, inactivity, isolation, and fixed income. Usually, the elderly can adapt to these conditions without becoming func-

tionally disabled by frustration, anxiety, or depression. However, at times the stress of adjusting to age-related change has a very negative effect upon the mental and physical health of the elderly.

Estimates suggest that between 13 and 15 percent of the population sixty-five and over have some form of functional mental health problem. The social isolation experienced by the elderly who live alone may be a factor in the development of late-life schizophrenia. The grief, depression, or melancholy that may occur after the deaths of spouses or peers may also lead to severe mental disorders, depending on the individual and his or her social and economic situation.

The physical health problems of the elderly may also contribute to a mental disorder. A sudden loss of mobility, unaccustomed pain, and the realization that their illness may be terminal may give rise to intense frustration or bouts of extreme depression or anxiety.

All too often elderly people who suffer some form of mental health disorder go untreated. Some authorities estimate that as much as 80 percent of the elderly who need mental health care are neglected. In some cases the consequence of this neglect is self-destruction. Of all suicides reported in the United States, about 25 percent are committed by persons sixty-five or over. Compared to other age groups, men over the age of seventy-five have the highest rate of suicide. Factors that might contribute to an emotional state leading to suicide include the trauma of forced retirement, physical disability, and social isolation. However, with proper treatment, many of the mental health problems of the elderly can be alleviated.

Community mental health centers provide many services, including inpatient, outpatient, partial hospitalization, and aftercare.

Mental Health Associations provide information about mental health resources available in the community.

For further information on mental health and mental illness, write to:

Public Inquiries, Room 11A21
National Clearinghouse for Mental
  Health Information
Division of Scientific and Public
  Information
National Institute of Mental Health
5600 Fishers Lane
Rockville, Maryland 20857

National Association for Mental Health
1800 North Kent Street
Arlington, VA 22209

Supplemental Security Income. Supplemental security income (SSI) makes monthly payments to aged, disabled, and blind people who have limited income and resources (assets).

To receive SSI payments on the basis of disability or blindness, you must meet the social security definition of "disabled" or "blind." But, you do not need any social security work credits to get SSI payments. People may be eligible for SSI even if they have never worked. And, people who get SSI checks can get social security checks, too, if they are eligible for both.

To be eligible for SSI, you must have limited income and resources, be a resident of the U.S. or Northern Mariana Islands,

and be either a U.S. citizen or a lawfully admitted immigrant.

Not all of your income and resources are counted in determining if you are eligible for SSI. Generally, the first $20 a month of unearned income and the first $65 a month in earnings are not counted. Income above these levels usually reduces the amount of the basic SSI payment. A home and the land adjacent to it are not counted. Personal effects or household goods, a car, and life insurance policies may not count, depending on their value. The Federal Government does not put liens on recipients' homes.

Rent Assistance. Low income families (including the handicapped) may be eligible for housing assistance payments from the U.S. Department of Housing and Urban Development (HUD). Payments by HUD are made directly to the owners of rental units to make up the difference between the HUD-approved rental amount and the amount the tenant is required to pay. Tenants pay between 25 and 30% of their adjusted income (gross income less certain deductions and exceptions). Rental assistance payments under this arrangement are not considered additional income to the tenant who is also eligible for Supplemental Security Income payments from the Social Security Administration.

For further information on rent assistance or other housing programs benefiting the elderly, write to:

U.S. Department of Housing & Urban
  Development
Washington, D.C. 20410

Income. The United States Department of Agriculture defines poverty as a restriction of income to cover only basic necessities. The poverty level is determined by multiplying by three the cost of groceries for a thirty-day period. Monthly income below this amount is considered to be poverty level. The individual income level for 1984 is $8,991 per year.

A special committee on aging has found

**Income sources for those 65 and over
(percent of total income)**

Source	Married couples	Non-married men	Non-married women
Social Security	33	41	47
Other pensions	18	21	14
Earnings	29	17	11
Assets	18	15	21
Other	2	6	7

that elderly minority persons are twice as likely to live at the poverty level as members of the elderly white population.

Income Sources. In most cases the sources of income for the elderly are limited. There are retirement benefits such as Social Security, public and private pensions. Some are eligible for veterans benefits or for Supplemental Security Income.

Assets of Aging. People tend to dwell on the liabilities that accompany the aging process. However, the elderly possess physical, mental, and emotional assets also.

Mental Assets. Mental confusion is not a part of normal aging. Learning tests have proven that though older people tend to learn more slowly, they also learn more thoroughly than younger students.

It is now known that memory is related to interests, and though older people may forget recent events, it is because many are only concerned with the past.

Older people also have an advantage when it comes to judgment, which depends upon experience as well as reason.

Emotional Assets. A person that is well-adjusted is not as self-conscious as he was in earlier years. He has more poise and self-control, and is generally more tolerant of others.

Feelings of insecurity, fear, and anxiety are damaging to older people's well-being. Irritability in some aged men and women is sometimes caused by an inability to sleep well. There may be a suspicious attitude toward anything new, many times due to a lack of self-confidence. However, older people who are emotionally secure do not generally respond in this way.

After middle age some persons are quite disturbed with thoughts of death. Sometimes it helps them to talk about this with friends or family members.

Physical Assets. The process of aging is generally uneven. In many persons some organs will be impaired and others still remain young. As people get older, they have an immunity to some diseases they have already had or to which they have been exposed. Often they have acquired some immunity to other infections as well.

Resources*

Action for Independent Maturity, 1909 K St., NW, Washington, DC 20049.
American Association of Homes for the Aging, 1050 17th St., NW, Washington, DC 20036.
American Association of Retired Persons, 215 Long Beach Blvd., Long Beach, CA 90801.
American Geriatrics Society, 10 Columbus Circle, New York, NY 10011.
American Health Care Association, 2500 15th St., NW, Washington, DC 20015.
American Physical Therapy Association, 1740 Broadway, New York, NY 10019.
American Red Cross, 17th and D Sts., NW, Washington, DC 20006.
Association of Rehabilitation Facilities, 5530 Wisconsin Ave., NW, Washington, DC 20015.
Center for the Study of Aging and Human Development, Duke University, Durham, NC 27710.
Elderhostel, 100 Boylston St., Suite 200, Boston, MA 02116.
Family Service Association of America, 44 W. 23rd St., New York, NY 10010.
Gerontological Society, 1 Dupont Circle, Washington, DC 20036.
National Council on the Aging, Suite 504, 1828 L St., NW, Washington, DC 20036.
National Council for Homemaker-Home Health Aide Services, 67 Irving Place, New York, NY 10003.
National Council of Senior Citizens, 1511 K St., NW, Room 202, Washington, DC 20005.
National Interfaith Coalition on Aging, Inc., P.O. Box 1986, Indianapolis, IN 46206.
U.S. Administration on Aging, 3303 C St., SW, HHS South, Washington, DC 20024. (Administers ten regional offices. Each state has its own Department, Office, or Commission on Aging, usually located in the state capital.)

---

*Excerpt from John Gillies, *A Guide to Caring For and Coping With Aging Parents,* (Nashville: Thomas Nelson, Inc., Publishers, 1981), pp. 207–208.

GIGANTISM   When a pituitary tumor of the eosinophil type develops before adolescence, it stimulates overgrowth in all body tissues. Because the growth of bone is not complete, such afflicted individuals grow to an excessive height. In addition, there occur some of the features described under ACROMEGALY.

GINGIVITIS   Inflammation of the soft tissue (gingiva) covering around the necks of the teeth is called gingivitis. It may be localized or generalized, depending upon the number of teeth involved. It may be caused by local irritation, overfunction of the related tooth, lack of stimulation to the tissues, the eruption of teeth, faulty restoration, viruses, bacteria, psychosomatic factors, and general body disturbances.

Symptoms. Gingivitis produces redness, swelling, tenderness, and possible bleeding of the gingival tissue.

Treatment. As with all diseases, primary treatment is removal of the cause. Generally the cause can be ascertained only by a dentist, but proper diet and oral hygiene are under the control of the patient. The vast majority of cases will respond to proper gingival stimulation, but untreated gingivitis may progress to more serious periodontal disease.

GLANDS   The term glands refers to organized collections of tissue which secrete substances showing chemical activity in the body. The two main types of glands are the exocrine and endocrine: exocrine glands (e.g., sweat, stomach, and salivary glands) secrete substances into the digestive tract, other body-tubes, or to the surface of the skin; endocrine glands are those which secrete their product directly into the bloodstream, and are hence often referred to as ductless glands. (The liver and pancreas are large glands which combine exocrine and endocrine functions in the same organ.)

GLANDULAR FEVER (INFECTIOUS MONONUCLEOSIS)   This is a contagious disease (not common in small children), manifested by fever, swollen glands, and general malaise. It is usually accompanied by a sore throat and there may be a headache and stiff neck, a measle-like rash, and/or jaundice. The majority of the patients have an enlarged spleen. Some complain of fatigue for weeks and months. The diagnosis is based on the finding of typical white cells in the blood and by the special Paul-Bunnell test. Since infectious mononucleosis is more likely to be found in young adults or in older children, it is commonly called "the kissing disease." It can, but should not, be confused with hepatitis.

Treatment. Recent studies have implicated a specific virus, the Epstein-Barr (E-B) virus, as the cause of the disease. There is no specific treatment, although cortisone drugs may be of symptomatic value. The patient should rest adequately; associated fatigue states are common.

GLARE   Any brightness within the field of vision that causes an unpleasant sensation or temporary blurring of vision is defined as glare. It cannot be measured scientifically and symptoms vary considerably in different persons. Particular sources of glare are reflections: from bright surfaces such as desk tops, automobile windshields and hoods, sand, and sky. Unshielded light sources may cause discomfort. Colored lenses may minimize symptoms, but a change in lighting conditions is more effective.

GLAUCOMA   This is an eye disease in which the pressure within the eye is so increased as to cause interference with vision. The severity of the increased pressure is not the same in every eye, and some individuals may tolerate for long periods a pressure which would rapidly blind another. A pressure of 24 mm. of mercury, as measured with a special instrument, is usually considered the maximum pressure compatible with continued health of the eye.

Glaucoma is divided into primary and secondary types. Primary glaucoma is in turn further divided into two sub-types: (1) simple glaucoma; and (2) angle-closure glaucoma.

GLAUCOMA, ANGLE-CLOSURE

This is an uncommon type (5 per cent of all primary glaucoma) in which the iris is too close to the cornea. The pressure in the eye is normal, but conditions which cause dilation of the pupil, (such as looking at movies, being in prolonged darkness, emotional disturbances, and the like) result in the iris touching the cornea and closing the area through which fluid exits from the eye.

Symptoms. An acute attack is ushered in with a dull, aching pain in one or both eyes, which gradually becomes more severe. There is marked loss of vision, sensitivity to light, watering of the eye, and extreme redness of the affected eye. The pupil is dilated, the eye is sensitive to the touch, the iris pattern appears muddy, and the individual appears severely ill.

Treatment. This is directed initially to lowering the pressure within the eye by means of local eye drops, injections behind the eye, and systemic medication. If the acute attack cannot be interrupted immediately, surgery must be performed. If the acute attack is stopped, surgery is indicated in the interval between attacks.

Most individuals with angle-closure glaucoma have mild transient attacks that do not damage the eye. The chief symptoms are mild dimness of vision and halos around lights. The attack is frequently corrected by sleep, during which the pupil is small and constricted. The predisposition to attacks of angle-closure glaucoma can be detected by careful examination of the position of the iris in respect to the cornea, sometimes by controlled dilation of the pupil.

Once diagnosed, angle-closure glaucoma should be corrected by surgical means. Even faithful use of medications designed to prevent acute attacks may be useless, while the disease *can* be cured with surgery.

GLAUCOMA, CONGENITAL

This is a secondary type of glaucoma which arises because of a developmental abnormality involving the outflow channels of the eye. Males are affected about twice as frequently as females.

Symptoms. Signs may be evident at birth or up to one year of age. The earliest sign is marked tearing of the eye with an associated sensitivity to light. The normally transparent cornea becomes hazy, and the pattern of the colored iris is seen with difficulty. The eye then enlarges and there is loss of vision.

Treatment. This is surgical and should be carried out as soon as the diagnosis is made.

GLAUCOMA, SECONDARY

Increased pressure of the eye occurs as a complication of a number of eye diseases. The main signs and symptoms are those of the primary disease. Treatment is usually directed toward the cause of the glaucoma rather than toward the increased pressure itself.

GLAUCOMA, SIMPLE

This is the most common type of primary glaucoma, and frequently causes severe visual damage without prominent symptoms. It arises because of an obstruction to the exit of fluid from the eye.

Symptoms. The eye has a normal appearance. There may be loss of focusing power for near objects and a development of farsightedness. Night vision may be poor. If there is a sudden increase in eye pressure, there may be blurring of vision and the appearance of halos around lights. This last symptom, however, is not as common in simple glaucoma as in the angle-closure type.

As the increased pressure continues, the optic nerve is injured and there is loss of side vision. Vision directly ahead (central vision) is usually preserved until a late stage. If the disease is detected and treated in time, optic-nerve changes are not likely to occur.

The condition is diagnosed by discovering increased pressure in the eye by means of an instrument applied directly to the eye. If optic-nerve damage is present, it may be evaluated by means of an instrument directing light through the pupil (ophthalmoscope). Measurement of side vision will indicate the degree of damage present.

Treatment. This is directed to maintaining the pressure within the eye at a normal level by means of drops in the eyes and sometimes tablets taken by mouth. Coffee is usually limited to no more than two cups daily, and drinking excessive amounts of fluid is discouraged. Usually the drops are used at regular intervals, and before and after a person has been in prolonged darkness, such as at the movies, which tends to dilate the pupil.

Medical treatment is preferred in simple glaucoma; but if the disease progresses despite adequate care, surgery is indicated. A variety of surgical procedures is used, to lower eye pressure either by establishment of drainage valves, or reduction of the flow of fluid through the eye.

GLOMERULUS   See NEPHRON

GLOSSITIS   Inflammatory conditions of the tongue may result from bacterial infections, yeast-like infections (thrush), and from certain nutritional deficiencies. Because of the rich blood supply to the tongue, bacterial infections are uncommon in otherwise healthy individuals. Rarely,

vitamin deficiencies can cause glossitis; specific replacement therapy will usually give dramatic results. Pernicious anemia may be accompanied by glossitis which is characterized by a disappearance of the taste buds and results in a smooth shiny tongue. Such glossitis may be the first symptom of this serious condition.

GLOSSOPHARYNGEAL NERVES   The two glossopharyngeal (or eleventh cranial) nerves carry sensory impulses such as pain and temperature from the throat and also taste sensation from the back one-third of the tongue. These nerves may be damaged by injury or infection.

GNAT BITES   See MOSQUITO BITES

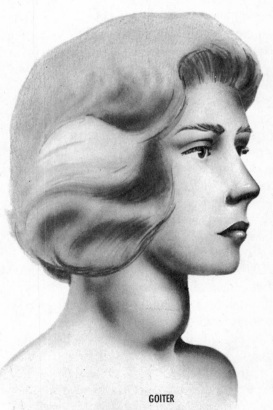

GOITER

A goiter is an enlargement of the thyroid body, causing a swelling in the front part of the neck.

GOITER   When the thyroid gland becomes enlarged for any reason, it is spoken of as a goiter. Various forms of goiter occur: the toxic goiter with hyperthyroidism; the non-toxic goiter present with iodine deficiency or due to congenital or hereditary disturbances; and swelling of the thyroid in various forms of thyroiditis. The treatment of goiter depends upon its cause. A toxic goiter is treated by surgery, or by administration of radioactive iodine or antithyroid drugs. Simple goiter, if due to iodine deficiency, is treatable by administration of iodine in the form of drops or iodized salt. Goiter which is due to congenital disorders is usually best treated by the administration of thyroid hormone.

GONADS   The gonads are the sex glands; in the female they are the ovaries, and in the male the testes.

The ovaries are located in the pelvic region of the abdominal cavity, one on each side of the uterus. They produce the eggs (ova) which travel along the fallopian tubes to the uterus. If fertilized by a male sperm-cell (spermatozoon), an egg is implanted in the uterine wall and grows to form the fetus. The ovaries are also the site of production of estrogen (female hormone) and progesterone (pregnancy hormone).

The testes lie in the male scrotum and produce spermatozoa, which fertilize the ovum in the female uterus.

GONORRHEA   This is the most common of the venereal diseases, both of the male and female. With the advent of antibiotics, incidence of gonorrhea has been greatly reduced, but it is by no means eradicated. The infection is due to the gonococcus, and is contacted almost exclusively through intercourse. It is one of the commonest causes of infertility, because if left untreated it obstructs the tubes (male epididymis and female fallopian tubes).

Symptoms. The symptoms of gonorrhea will depend on the organ involved. The first symptoms usually appear a week

after exposure, and consist of burning during urination, difficulty in emptying the bladder, and excessive discharge, with pus. In the male the testicles may become swollen and tender; in the female the same thing happens to the glands at the entrance to the birth canal (Bartholin's glands). If the infection spreads through the womb to the fallopian tubes and ovaries, the woman will complain of severe lower-abdominal pains and fever, and the whole picture will often be difficult to differentiate from acute appendicitis. Occasionally the joints can become involved, becoming warm, swollen, and tender (gonococcal arthritis).

Treatment. After proper diagnosis, treatment is relatively simple. Most cases can be cured with penicillin. It is important to find the original host of the infection and treat him or her, otherwise a cycle of reinfection is very likely to occur.

GOOSE FLESH (GOOSE PIMPLES) This common symptom of rapid and simultaneous elevation of myriads of tiny papules of the skin on sudden and extreme joy, sorrow, cold, or fright is the result of the contraction of muscle fibers (erectores pilorum) attached to the outer lining of the hair follicle just below the attachment of the sebaceous gland. The muscle extends from this point in a diagonal manner to an area just below the epidermal layer, at which point the "puckering" or goose pimple forms.

GOUT   Gout is a body-chemistry disturbance with recurrent attacks of acute arthritis which may become chronic and deforming. The disease has been known since ancient times and occurs predominantly in middle-aged males. The cause is unknown. It is obviously a disturbance in the processing of vital chemicals known as urate and purine. The protein materials found in the nuclei of cells (nucleoproteins) are the principal source of the body's uric acid; certain foods, such as organ meats (liver, kidney, and sweetbread) and sardines, are the source of purine in the diet. In gout, the serum uric level is elevated. Urate deposits, which eventually form small nodules called tophi, are a distinguishing feature. These nodules may be found in cartilage, certain parts of the bone, ligaments, and tendons.

Symptoms. In acute gout there is a sudden, sharp, severe pain, often at night, and not infrequently in the joint of the great toe. The joint becomes swollen and extremely tender. The skin is red, hot, and shiny. There may be fever and chills. Attacks may last for a few days or may persist, with intermissions, for several weeks.

Only after numerous attacks over a period of years in inadequately treated patients will there be permanent deformity. This can take the form of limited motion in many joints of the hands or feet, and sometimes in other joints.

A frequent and sometimes serious complication is kidney disease. This is usually related to urate stones that develop in this organ.

Treatment. A patient with acute gout responds rapidly to large doses of colchicine. Other forms of arthritis do not respond to this drug. Cortisone derivatives and Indocin® are also useful.

In recent years a new form of therapy appeared with the development of the drug allopurinol (Zyloprim®). Allopurinol reduces the body's manufacture of uric acid and thus acts on the fundamental mechanism behind the disease. It has to be taken several times per day on an indefinite basis in most patients.

GRANULOMA PYOGENICUM   A growth of proliferating blood vessels resulting from an infection in which the pus formation is minimal, the globular tumor mass of granuloma pyogenicum is characterized by bleeding on slight injury.

Because the blood vessels have little or no elasticity, the bleeding is difficult to control. The lesion is usually the size of a pea, intensely red and glistening, and occasionally crusted. Any part of the skin can be affected; the condition occurs most commonly on the face.

Treatment. The lesions can be readily destroyed by electrocautery. Only rarely does the lesion disappear without being deliberately destroyed. The persistent bleeding can be alarming; it can be controlled until treatment is available by applying pressure.

GRASS POLLEN   Grass pollen is produced in the late spring and during the summer. The common grasses causing "grass hay fever" are bluegrass, timothy, orchard, redtop, Bermuda, Johnson, sweet vernal, and rye.

The symptoms of pollen reaction (pollinosis) consist of red, teary eyes, stuffed and runny nose, and spasmodic sneezing.

GRAVES' DISEASE   When the thyroid gland becomes overactive and diffusely enlarged, the increased amounts of circulating thyroid hormone produce changes throughout the body. These changes, especially noticeable in the heart and circulatory system, are known as thyrotoxicosis, or Graves' disease (named after the man who described the changes many years ago). Chiefly affected are women between the ages of twenty and forty.

Symptoms. Characteristically, patients with Graves' disease appear highly nervous and overactive. They are quite apt to be emotional and excitable, and often complain of intolerance to heat. Weight loss is common, there is excessive perspiration, and a tremor is often noticeable. The eyes usually present a staring appearance and often bulge noticeably; indeed, eye symptoms may be the most prominent and serious feature of Graves' disease. Diagnosis is made by measuring the circulating blood iodine, and in more recent years by the use of the radioactive iodine-uptake test. (For many years the basal metabolic rate has been a standard test; this is usually elevated by 30 or 40 per cent when Graves' disease is present.)

Treatment. A number of so-called "antithyroid drugs" are available for temporary alleviation of this condition; however, they are rarely capable of producing a lasting cure. The two definitive forms of therapy are surgery and administration of radioactive iodine. Before surgery can be performed, it is necessary to bring thyroid overactivity under control by means of antithyroid drugs and iodine; radioactive iodine, on the other hand, is usually administered without prior preparation.

Because of the unpredictable nature of Graves' disease, it may be expected that about 15 per cent of the patients treated either by surgery or radioactive iodine will development permanent underactivity of the gland—hypothyroidism. This is easily treated by administration of thyroid hormone, however, and is a much less dangerous and formidable condition than is Graves' disease itself. In a few individuals the eye protrusion becomes worse after treatment of the thyroid condition. If the eyes become too irritated or swollen, surgical removal of a portion of the bony orbit may become necessary. Often, however, the protrusion will stabilize after several months and slowly recede.

GROUP THERAPY   Practical psychiatric experience indicates that a number of patients with similar problems may be treated in group-therapy sessions. The earliest experiments with group therapy started with the "Washingtonian Movement" (an early association of alcoholics to help themselves) and with Alcoholics Anonymous, where it was discovered that a large number of individuals could help one another in many ways. Group therapy works best with patients of roughly the same age, education, and clinical type, who presumably have lived through similar experiences. Members of a therapy group lose their embarrassment over being mentally ill in the course of talking with others who have the same problems and who are also learning how to solve them. Those just entering a therapy group are comforted by the acceptance and friendship of people who have "been through the mill" and know what it is all about.

If group therapy sessions are properly conducted, participants learn to be frank in discussing their problems, particularly things about which they have been oversensitive in the past. Frank group discussion encourages members to give their opinions and reactions in helping each other. Psychiatrically, group therapy is most effective and economical because it makes help available to a large number of people simultaneously.

GROWTH HORMONE   This product of the pituitary has been actively investigated in recent years and is now available in a few clinical centers for experimental administration to human beings. Unfortunately, when obtained from animals, it is not effective in humans. Its availability at the present time is therefore limited by the availability of human pituitary glands at autopsy.

GUILT   Feelings of guilt stem from self-hate and regret over transgression of the moral code. Every society tries to instill morality in children by rewarding good and punishing bad behavior, so that moral codes become second nature (are internalized) and operate as conscience (censor, superego). The whole question of Right-and-Wrong is complicated by great differences in standards between cultures. Some cultures (or parents) make a terrible fuss over relatively slight misbehavior, while others accept relatively serious transgressions without much punishment.

There is currently a great deal of scientific controversy over the role of punishment in instilling good behavior habits and over the whole question of sin and evil. Modern psychiatry takes the position that wrongdoing is always caused by mental ill-health rather than by sinfulness, and that problems of misbehavior should therefore be handled by healing methods rather than punishment. In the history of psychiatry there is little evidence that punishment has any beneficial effect in curing mental illness; on the contrary, only a healing attitude is capable of helping people understand the reason for their misbehavior. Modern psychiatry believes that feelings of guilt may frequently make a person more unhealthy. Instead of continuing to punish the self by continued guilt feelings, it is healthier for the patient to understand reasons for unhealthy behaviors and to try to correct them.

Psychiatrists try never to take a "laying down the law" (authoritarian) attitude towards misbehavior or to criticize the patient in any way for what he has done. Experience indicates that such attitudes simply create more conflict and do not contribute to constructive solutions; the psychiatrist must maintain an accepting attitude, no matter what the patient says or does.

GYNECOLOGY   This is the medical specialty concerned with the diagnosis and treatment, both medical and surgical, of diseases of the female genital organs. In recent years great progress in gynecology has been made through intensive research, mainly in the field of hormones, and the early detection and treatment of genital cancer.

Specialists practicing gynecology are called gynecologists; most of them—especially the younger ones—are given combined training in both gynecology and obstetrics.

HAIR, EXCESSIVE See HIRSUTISM

HAIR-LOSS   There are several types of loss of hair in addition to the oft-encountered male type of baldness and the distinctive hair loss of alopecia areata.

Hair can be lost by reason of chemical, physical, or mechanical damage; or as the result of infections having a unique affinity for hair involvement. Aside from singeing the hair by the application of very warm or hot instruments, hair can be so "softened" by chemical or physical agents designed to straighten, curl or color it that it can break off. Hair damaged in this manner is no different from hair that had been cut off. Regrowth will take place at the usual rate—providing no injury was sustained by the scalp.

Hair can also be broken off mechanically as the result of a habit mechanism not unlike that of fingernail-biting. This condition is called trichotillomania and can only be alleviated by the patient's being made aware of the condition and seeking help in breaking the habit. Cure of this condition is especially difficult in those patients in whom the eyelashes are the site of the pulling-out, the twisting, or the breaking-off. It is usually not necessary to probe the original cause of the habit which, as with fingernail-biting, has long ceased to matter. Breaking the habit can be accomplished with devices (greasing the hair to make it impossible to get a grip on it), rewards (in addition to the obvious one of improvement of appearance), and—rarely—threats (infection, deformity of hair regrowth).

Other apparent loss of hair is encountered in ringworm infection of the scalp, in which the hair shaft is invaded by the fungus and the hair breaks off and gives the appearance of bald spots. This is discussed elsewhere. Loss of hair in the secondary stage of syphilitic infection gives the scalp a "moth-eaten" appearance. This, too, is discussed elsewhere.

Probably even more common than baldness in men is the loss of hair in women, either as a result of pregnancy or in relationship to some change in endocrine activity. The hair-loss of pregnancy usually ceases after delivery, or after the menstrual cycle is reestablished. While it is usual for only a portion of the hair to regrow, there is sufficient regrowth to reassure the patient that she will not be bald even if the condition recurs with each pregnancy. The most distressing loss of hair is that which occurs in young women and appears not to be related to hair appliances like curlers, wave-set lotions, permanent waves, etc., and seems also not to be related to the metabolic rate, menstrual cycle, or other organic or psychic distress (except as a result of the loss of hair). In spite of the absence of findings of any significance in recent extensive investigations, there is a continuing impression that this type of hair loss is related to some malfunctioning of the endocrine glands. To this end, the patient is well-advised to seek help from the internist. Correcting even minor defects in the general health may possibly result in the cessation of the hair-loss, though not insure its regrowth.

HALITOSIS (MOUTH ODORS)

Unpleasant odors of the mouth may be due to a variety of causes: primarily, they arise from the decomposition of substances within the mouth which also create a bad taste. These decomposed products include both the dental tissues (teeth and gums) and accumulated food debris, and oral hygiene, properly practiced, is the best defense against the problem. Basic to such hygiene is the rapid removal of debris from the teeth and the furrows of the tongue by brushing. Furthermore, it is evident that certain foods possess a characteristic odor which influence the breath. This can be corrected by a scented mouthwash.

In some cases odors may be related to infected tonsils, severe cirrhosis of the liver, and systemic problems of the lungs or digestive tract. The uncontrolled diabetic may have a "fruity breath" and a person with kidney problems may retain urea, giving rise to "ammonia breath." In persistent breath problem, medical and dental examination is indicated.

HALLUCINATIONS

Hallucinations involve the projection of inner experiences into states of clear consciousness so vividly that the individual cannot distinguish them from the real world and believes they actually exist. Most common are auditory hallucinations, in which the person thinks he hears voices talking or giving him commands, which he then frequently feels compelled to obey. In visual hallucinations, the patient sees people or things which are not truly present. (More rarely, there may be olfactory or tactual hallucinations, in which the patient smells or feels things which have no real existence.)

Hallucinations must be interpreted as expressions of unconscious mental life, which the patient is unable to distinguish from real events. They occur particularly in schizophrenia, but are also encountered in other psychoses. The patient may state that God is talking to him, or that a deceased parent is reproving him. (A particular danger is that hallucinating patients may commit antisocial acts while under the impression that they are carrying out the commands of God.) There are no specific treatments for hallucinations except the general methods directed towards removal of causes of underlying psychotic disorder.

HANGNAIL

Resulting from an injury (tear) of the skin around the nail which affects the nail fold, a hangnail almost always causes infection at the site of the injury. When not induced by the biting of nails, these lesions are caused by an irritation from the irregular shedding of the cuticle or by repeated injury sustained in active use of the fingers or toes.

Treatment. To prevent further irritation from friction of the torn epidermis or cuticle, the torn skin should be cut as close to its attachment to normal skin as possible, and an antibiotic ointment should be applied. To prevent frequent recurrences, the cuticle should be kept soft and pliable with the application of simple lubricants like vaseline or lanolin.

HARELIP   This congenital anomaly is obvious at birth, a slit or gap being present from the nostril to the mouth on one or both sides of the upper lip. It is usually associated with a cleft palate. If the gum and palate are cleft, the baby has trouble creating any suction; the surgeon therefore tries to correct the lip as early in life as possible. Modern surgical techniques have been so perfected that some of these defects defy detection.

HAY FEVER   Hay fever is a very poor term for a disorder which involves neither hay allergy nor increased temperature. The disease is now more properly called pollinosis. It is more commonly found in individuals with an allergic background.

There are three types: tree hay fever, which occurs in the spring and early summer; grass hay fever, which occurs in the late spring and summer; and weed hay fever, which starts during the late summer and continues until the frost. The symptoms are due to an allergy to the pollen of one or more plants. The severity of the complaint depends on the amount of pollen present in the air.

Symptoms. The eyes become itchy, red, swollen, tearful, and begin to burn; the throat becomes swollen, with attendant itching and burning; and the nose itches, burns and feels full. There is a watery-to-thick nasal discharge, together with sudden attacks of severe sneezing. The sinus cavities may swell and become full of fluid. (These symptoms are seasonal, depending on the type of pollen to which the individual is allergic.) Nasal polyps, sinusitis, and asthma are the most common complications.

Diagnosis is made on the basis of a history of seasonal complaints plus positive skin tests. A smear made from the nasal membranes shows an abundance of a certain type of cell (eosinophil).

Treatment. Treatment consists of hyposensitization, nasal sprays for temporary relief, antihistamines, ephedrine, epinephrine, masks and nasal filters, installation of air conditioning, and—if necessary—change of climate during the pollen season.

HEADACHE   Headache is a very common symptom that occurs at some time in all individuals and has many different causes. Constant generalized headaches occurring periodically are frequently related to emotional stress, while headaches that throb on one side are characteristic of migraine. Headaches occur in association with a wide variety of systemic diseases. Acute fever (due to many causes) is frequently accompanied by headache, and infections of the ears and mastoids are also associated with local head-pain. Sinusitis, too, is a common cause of headache.

Less commonly, neurologic disorders such as meningitis, encephalitis, brain tumor, disease of cerebral blood vessels, or head injury may also produce headaches of varying severity.

Headache is usually characterized by the dilation (enlargement) of the blood vessels in the head. This dilation exerts pressure upon the nerves that surround the blood vessels, thereby producing the pain of headache.

The most common type of headache is the tension headache. This may be caused by the tightening of the muscles of the back of the neck and the scalp. Prolonged neck strain, for example, during long distance driving may induce tension headache. Emotional stress that causes the neck and scalp muscles to tighten involuntarily is responsible for most tension headaches.

Headache associated with fever is

usually generalized and present on both sides of the head, whereas ear and mastoid infections and migraine frequently produce intense one-sided headache. Localized frontal head-pain occurs with frontal sinusitis; with maxillary sinusitis, pain over the cheek is common. Headache caused by neurologic disorders may be either one-sided or generalized.

Treatment. Because headache is a symptom of various health disorders, identifying the underlying cause is important in determining treatment. If headache is associated with acute infection, drug therapy focused at the infection should eliminate headache. Dealing successfully with the causes of emotional stress can remove tension headaches. Minor headache pain often responds to treatment with aspirin, or other non-aspirin analgesics. With severe or chronic headaches, it is important that careful examination is done to determine the cause of the headache. Persistent headache that does not respond to aspirin or a non-aspirin analgesic (such as acetominophen) should be reported to a physician.

HEADACHES, ALLERGIC

Headaches may be due to an allergic reaction to a food, drink, or inhalant, or may be a secondary manifestation associated with an allergy. If unrelated to allergy, headaches may be due to emotional stress, various infectious diseases, tumors, or exposure to noxious fumes.

The primary allergic headache is caused by a hypersensitivity to a food (e.g., milk, chocolate, grains) or an inhalant (e.g., molds, dust). The headache pain is probably due to dilation of the blood vessels of the brain, which occurs upon exposure to the substance causing the allergy. Allergy symptoms such as dizziness, vision impairment, abdominal pain, nausea, and vomiting may accompany headache. Migraine headache, with its throbbing, recurrent one-sided pain, may be induced by sensitivity to certain foods and drugs.

Allergic rhinitis and sinusitis in which there is swelling, infection, and pressure will produce secondary allergic headache. In such a circumstance the headache is usually over the forehead or on the top of the head.

Treatment of allergic headaches consists of finding the cause of the allergy and removing it. Headache pain can be alleviated with antihistamines, analgesics such as aspirin, vasoconstrictors, and whenever possible, desensitization to the allergy-inducing substances.

HEADACHES, MIGRAINE

Migraine headache is an intensely painful type of headache that may last several days and temporarily incapacitate its victim. A migraine attack may bring with it dizziness, chills, and sensitivity to light.

What exactly causes migraine headache is not completely known. A variety of factors that predispose individuals to migraine are known, however. Researchers have discovered a genetic disposition for migraine, as well as a connection to hormonal imbalance. Also twice as many women as men have migraine. Quite a number of migraine victims have personalities that may be characterized as compulsive, tending to be perfectionists with high standards set for themselves and not prone to communicating their anxieties to others.

A migraine attack is an excruciating experience. It may begin with flashes of light or other impairment of vision. The pain is almost always on one side of the head and can be accompanied by nausea, vomiting, and soreness of the scalp. Migraine, like many types of headache, involves painful dilation of cerebral blood vessels but is not caused by organic problems. For many sufferers migraine attacks can be induced by abrupt temperature and air pressure changes and by an allergic reaction to certain foods or drugs.

Treatment. Migraine may be relieved by vasoconstricting drugs, such as dihydroergotamine. Methysergide maleate is sometimes prescribed in the attempt to decrease the frequency of migraine episodes in very severe cases. Throbbing, suddenly recurrent headache may also be associated with elevated blood pressure, for which the treatment is reduction of blood pressure by use of drugs and by training of the individual to be emotionally calm. Some migraine victims benefit from warm baths and bed rest.

A large percentage of migraine attacks, as well as lesser types of headaches, have psychogenic causes, such as emotional conflicts, psychological instability, and intense anxiety. Two forms of headache characteristically occur in association with emotional instability. These are "belt-like" headaches in the region of the temples, with the sufferer complaining of a constricting sensation around the skull, and occipital headaches involving a dull ache in the muscles at the back of the head and neck. Psychogenic headaches should be treated with psychotherapy directed at discovery and removal of the causes of emotional conflict.

HEAD INJURY (TRAUMA)   It is possible for a sharp blow on the head to cause hearing loss either because of dislocations of the ossicles, or because of fracture of the temporal bone which extends through the cochlea.

HEARING AIDS   The proper way to get a hearing aid is as follows: (1) Go to an ear, nose, and throat specialist. If his diagnosis is a nerve-loss, a hearing aid will perhaps help. (2) Ask the doctor to recommend a place where it is possible to get a "Hearing Aid Evaluation." This is a long series of special hearing tests to determine what type of hearing aid will best help. Doctors' offices are usually not equipped to give such tests, but hospital, university, and otology centers are so equipped; these centers are usually located in or near big cities. The tests may take half a day and cost approximately twenty-five dollars. For those thinking of a hearing aid, the evaluation test is the best investment which can be made. From the results of these tests the examiners (who are experts in the testing of hearing but usually are not M.D.'s) can tell whether or not a patient will be benefited by an aid, what type he should get, and when and how to use it.

Aids are expensive, and the constant replacement of batteries makes them even more so over the years. It therefore pays to see a doctor to determine whether medication or surgery can help; it pays to get a Hearing Aid Evaluation to find out whether or not a mechanical aid will help, and if so, what type is needed. Merely walking into a store and picking up a hearing aid is a poor way of choosing—even if a thirty-day trial offer goes with it.

HEARING LOSS   Hearing loss can result from abnormal conditions affecting any one of the three parts of the ear: outer, middle, or inner. If the outer or middle ear is responsible, the hearing loss is said to be conductive and is very often reparable by the use of medication or surgery. When the inner ear, cochlear nerve, or central connections are at fault, the hearing loss is nonconductive and is called neurosensory or perceptive. Only two kinds of nonconductive hearing loss respond to medical repair: labyrinthine hydrops (Ménières disease) and psychological hearing loss. (See CONDUCTIVE HEARING LOSS; NONCONDUCTIVE HEARING LOSS.)

HEARING TESTS   In order to give the reader a more thorough understanding of procedure in the otologist's office, a brief word about the audiogram is included.

An audiogram is a report plotted on a graph, describing the hearing. There are many special tests which can be performed to give the otologist information about different factors in the hearing mechanism;

the basic data recorded by means of the audiometer, however, are the air- and bone-conduction curves.

The audiometer itself is an electronic machine giving off controllable sounds of varying intensity (loudness) and frequency (pitch). These sounds are applied to the outer ear, and the patient indicates when he hears the sound. The audiometrist records this information on a specially prepared graph, this constituting an air-conduction audiogram. When the sounds are channeled to the patient by means of a bone-conductor, most commonly placed on the mastoid bone in back of the pinna, the resulting graph is called a bone-conduction audiogram. The doctor often uses various tuningfork tests to verify the audiogram.

Heart

ADRENERGIC BLOCKING AGENTS Drugs which block the normal response of an organ or tissue to nerve impulses transmitted by the adrenergic nervous system (more or less the same as the sympathetic nervous system). Blocking adrenergic nerves to the heart and blood vessels tends to decrease heart rate and the vigor of heart contraction and to suppress the constriction of blood vessels. Adrenergic blocking agents are often used to treat angina pectoris (since by reducing heart work they reduce its need for oxygen). Some are also used to treat arrhythmias and to control high blood pressure, especially when it is accompanied by a hyperactive heart.

There are two classes of these drugs, alpha- and beta-adrenergic blocking agents. Both can be used in cardiovascular disorders, although beta-adrenergic blocking agents are used more often; of these, propranolol is the most common.

ANEURISM A ballooning-out of the wall of a vein, an artery or the heart due to weakening of the wall by disease, traumatic injury or an abnormality present at birth. (See ANEURISM.)

ANGINA PECTORIS An episode of chest pain due to a temporary discrepancy between the supply and demand of oxygen to the heart. (See ANGINA PECTORIS.)

HEART AND BLOOD VESSEL X-RAYS (ANGIOCARDIOGRAPHY) Machines have been designed to take a series of X-ray pictures at intervals of much less than one second; as the heart beats, the changes taking place in its size and shape can be filmed throughout the cycle of contraction (systole) and relaxation (diastole). Study of the precise movements of the heart's outline can lead to important conclusions about its anatomical structure and the efficiency of each chamber in performing the work of the pumping blood.

Angiocardiography is an X-ray study of the movement of blood through the heart and vessels. When a fluid that throws a shadow onto the film (contrast material) is injected into the blood, its passage through the heart, lungs, and blood vessels can be recorded on rapidly-taken X-ray films, or even on motion-picture film that can later be observed in normal or even slow motion. By means of this procedure, the actual pumping can be observed: first the blood enters the receiving chamber of the heart (right auricle) which lies within the right portion of the heart shadow. Next it moves into the pumping chamber (right ventricle) and is then dispersed in the lungs. A moment later, the contrasting material is seen collecting in the left auricle, moving to the left ventricle, then being pumped out of the heart into the aortic system of arteries.

Selective angiocardiograms are usually made during heart catheterization. After pressures have been taken in the heart chambers and samples of blood withdrawn for oxygen saturation percentage, contrast material is then introduced through the same catheter and X-rays taken as it moves through the heart and vessels.

Narrowing of any chambers can be recorded with great accuracy on these X-ray films and the records kept for future reference and comparison. Valve efficiency also is demonstrated well; if any valve happens to be "leaking," the location and quantity of the backward flow can be seen clearly. Any vessel abnormalities, unusual openings between chambers or vessels, can be observed as well.

Angiocardiography can often furnish a good anatomical presentation of the heart in action when other diagnostic procedures may fail to uncover the precise nature of early disease changes or very small birth defects. In addition, if surgical correction is made, the angiocardiogram can be repeated after operation to demonstrate the improved circulation.

A technique of injecting contrast material into the aorta near the coronary arteries will make the arteries of the heart visible on motion-picture film. Abnormal vessels, narrow points in the coronary artery, and inborn (congenital) defects can be studied by coronary motion-picture angiograms.

From these studies, surgical correction of diseased coronary vessels can be planned

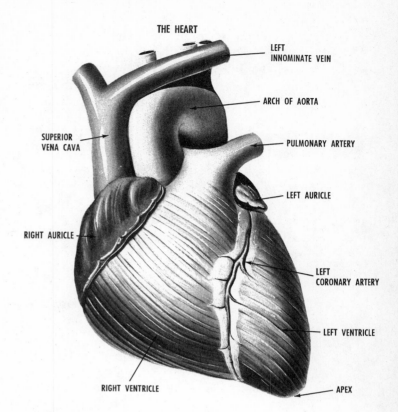

THE HEART

LEFT INNOMINATE VEIN

ARCH OF AORTA

SUPERIOR VENA CAVA

PULMONARY ARTERY

LEFT AURICLE

RIGHT AURICLE

LEFT CORONARY ARTERY

LEFT VENTRICLE

RIGHT VENTRICLE

APEX

and then achieved. Each year, more and more patients are having circulation restored to the heart-muscle by surgically relieving the obstructions or abnormal vessel-attachments as shown in film studies of this important type.

"HEART ATTACKS" The term heart attack has no exact meaning in medical practice. Sudden chest pain, sudden weakness or breathlessness, a sudden blackout, or even sudden death is referred to as a heart attack by many laymen.

Sudden chest pain comes with angina pectoris, coronary insufficiency, aneurism, and pulmonary infarction, but it may also appear in pleurisy and in disorders completely unrelated to the heart.

Palpitations may indicate heart disease, or on the other hand may be expressions of fear.

Sudden unconsciousness may appear in heart disease, but also in cerebrovascular accidents, diabetes, or shock from any cause.

What is often suspected as a heart attack may eventually prove to be an episode completely unrelated to malfunctions of the heart: asthma, epilepsy, gallstone, intercostal neuritis, slipped cervical disc, or even an anxiety state. Until a diagnosis of heart disease is made by the physician, needless anxiety should be held in check, especially by the patient's family and friends.

HEARTBEAT, IRREGULAR (ARRHYTHMIA)

In most persons of all ages, the heart beats at regularly timed intervals, even though the rate can vary from slow to fast. However, if the heart- or pulsebeats are not regular, a disorder—an arrhythmia—or cardiac rhythm may exist.

A disturbance in rhythm can come on and leave quickly, or it can be more or less permanent. The heart may show an occasional irregular beat or a total irregularity (as happens when each beat seems independent of all others, and each interval between beats of different length). Beats may even come in groups of fast, then slow, pulsations: an "irregular irregularity."

Arrhythmias may have no real significance. Simple ones may be caused by extraordinary stress, strange foods, drugs, or even intense excitement. These may be quite a nuisance to the patient, but often cause more embarrassment than real disability.

A serious arrhythmia, however, can cause a profound drop in blood pressure. The patient may become pale, breathless, and weak, or even fall into a state of shock or coma. Occasionally, a patient is quite unaware that he has a heart-rhythm disorder. There may be times, however, when he notices a strange beating in his chest, a "flippity-flop" sensation of fluttering under the ribs somewhere, or a feeling that he is about to "pass out."

Ordinarily, no pain whatever is experienced with a rhythm disorder. If pain is present, it usually means that heart disease may be the primary cause of the irregular heartbeat. All arrhythmias should be called to the attention of a physician, for sometimes a serious crisis may thus be averted.

HEARTBURN

This commonly used term describes a sensation of burning and pressure under the lower portion of the breastbone. It results from distension of the lower portion of the esophagus or from the presence of regurgitated stomach-contents in the area. Heartburn does not necessarily result from the presence of stomach acid, as persons with no acid-production may experience this symptom. Simple measures such as change in position, or the drinking of a small amount of milk or antacid mixture will most often relieve this condition.

HEART (CARDIAC) DISEASE

Heart disease can be the result of tissue changes primarily in the heart itself. Good examples are the congenital heart malformations which, if not correctable by surgery, often lead to death in infancy.

On the other hand, heart disease severe enough to result in a death of cardiac origin can come from disease entirely separate from the heart: failing kidneys can sometimes affect the heart so severely that it develops changes incompatible with life; while some tumors of the body may produce severe high blood pressure, with death eventually resulting from a heart that fails in the end because of the hypertensive changes produced in it.

Some heart diseases show changes in the heart not too different from those found in tissues elsewhere. Thus, changes typical of rheumatic heart disease occur in the lungs, in some of the joints, and in other areas as well. Poisons and drugs that affect the heart will usually also cause disease of the kidneys and liver. High blood pressure is as much an arterial as a heart disorder, and coronary artery disease may be only one manifestation of wide-spread atherosclerosis.

Each variety of heart disease occurs in a characteristic age group, and involves special tissue changes. Symptoms and tissue alterations may be limited to the heart alone or to the entire heart and blood-vessel system, but occasionally other organs, such as the brain, joints, liver, and spleen, are typically involved in the structural changes brought about by the heart disorder. The patient may even complain bitterly about symptoms in parts of the body completely unrelated to the region of the heart itself.

Important causes of heart disease might include congenital structural defects, rheumatic carditis, syphilitic heart disease, hypertensive (high blood pressure) heart disease, arteriosclerotic heart disease, and bacterial endocarditis. The less common causes of heart disease may include thyroid disease, heart tumors, heart injuries, diphtheria carditis, beriberi, and other nutritional heart disorders, and functional heart disease.

Treatment. Diagnosis and management of heart disease must include studies not only of the heart and the efficiency of its functional operation, but also the operational state of the lungs and the demands or requirements of the entire body: whether it requires a higher-than-normal cardiac output and therefore places an abnormal work-load on the heart.

HEART (CARDIAC) EMERGENCIES
Patients with acute cardiac conditions are urged as soon as practicable to enter a hospital where constant observation and care may prevent a sudden unnecessary complication, or even death. With efficient drugs and special equipment, adverse changes in blood pressure, heart output, lung blockage, heart-rate and -rhythm, and cyanosis can in many instances be effectively met and overcome.

Symptoms. Serious emergencies in heart disease come with hemorrhage, shock, and respiratory distress. Although palpitations, cardiac pain, and coma are distressing to all concerned—a source of great anxiety for patient and family alike— they are less serious in their implications.

Treatment. The patient must be reassured and not allowed to panic, for anxiety will increase his distress. He should be permitted to sit up, lie down, go to a window, and do what is most comfortable for him until professional help arrives.

A patient in an acute attack probably should not be transported from his place of employment or his home until the advice of a physician can be obtained on when and how to do so. If unconscious, the patient should be given nothing by mouth, and the head should be turned to one side in case of vomiting. Clothing should be loosened. Chest pain may be relieved slightly with an ice pack. Emergency oxygen may be ordered, when facilities are available, if a physician cannot be contacted immediately. Ordinarily medication should not be given, unless it be a dose of drug previously prescribed for use in just such a catastrophe.

Acute distress experienced in heart-function can require emergency care from the doctor more often than with any other organ in the body. Prompt use of drugs, oxygen, and electrical stimulation when indicated, will save lives that can otherwise be lost. Even convalescent time is shortened by prompt use of established methods in cardiology; indeed, serious complications of a failing heart can often be prevented by use of quickly-administered accurate treatment. Acute disorders of the heart usually indicate the need for hospital observation and care, if all available medical knowledge is going to be used and contribute to the ultimate welfare of the patient.

It thus becomes evident that there is almost no place for simple home remedies

280

in the care of a true cardiac emergency.

HEART (CARDIAC) PAIN The heart is almost devoid of nerves that carry sensations, so that a great many diseases of the heart are completely painless. There are however, two important sources of pain in the heart structures:

1. Pericardial Pain. Some of the sac (pericardium) that encloses the heart chambers is supplied by the same nerve that goes to the diaphragm—the phrenic nerve. Acute inflammation in the pericardium can therefore result in sharp "pleurisy" pains. If the pericardium is irritated by injury or stretched by blood or by fluid trapped within its membranes, a dull, painful ache may be felt over the heart, sometimes spreading to the tip of the shoulderblade.

2. Coronary-artery Pain. Ordinarily, the sympathetic nerves do not carry pain (or even cause it in the conscious mind). There are however, a number of exceptions to this rule, one of which involves the nerve endings that lace themselves about the arteries of the heart (the coronary arteries). These nerves can be stimulated to produce painful alarm signals when there is deficiency of oxygen for tissue activity in the area supplied by a coronary artery. Painful stimuli travel to the upper sympathetic chain in the left (or at times the right) chest and in some way escape into nearby sensory nerves. The result is real, often excruciating, pain characteristically felt behind the breastbone and down the left arm into one or more fingers. Because the cause of the pain is apparently indirect in its production, a great variability in its location, character, and intensity is noticed from one patient to the next.

True heart (or coronary-artery) pain almost always indicates a serious failure of the artery to supply an adequate flow of refreshed blood to the active heart-muscle fibers. This deficit state (myocardial ischemia) can usually be traced to narrowing of the coronary artery's diameter by at least one focal point of partial obstruction.

HEART CATHETERIZATION A catheter is a piece of special tubing that can be introduced into the body to drain out samples of fluid. A rather long section of plastic tubing less than one-sixteenth inch in diameter can be inserted into an arm vein. When this slender tube is pushed inside the vein, it travels with the blood returning to the heart, reaching the right auricle, right ventricle and then the pulmonary artery and lung vessels. This exploration of the vessels is called right-heart catheterization.

Because the plastic catheter is visible on the X-ray (fluoroscopic) screen, the doctor can observe the path the catheter takes, and serious defects may be studied visually. Thus, the catheter may pass through a defect in the septum that divides the right from the left chambers of the heart, and thereby give pictorial proof of the presence and location of that defect. Then too, any narrow points in the pulmonary valve or vessel may prevent the catheter from passing out of the right ventricle into the pulmonary artery, and may be revealed.

Because the catheter is an open tube, pressure at its tip can be measured. Structural deformities can cause abnormal pressures in the right auricle, right ventricle, and even in the pulmonary circulation: pressure measurements therefore serve a useful purpose in diagnosis and can indicate any unusual strain or work load from which the heart may be suffering.

Defects, or windows between the right and left chambers and vessels, are almost always birth defects. As blood flows through the heart, some of it can move abnormally through these openings, shunting from the high-pressure side of the low-pressure area. The exact position of the catheter tip will indicate the region of the defect; if the pressure changes vary greatly from normal, a serious abnormality may be presumed.

Samples of blood are taken in the right auricle, right ventricle, and pulmonary artery. Oxygen saturation is then measured. Before passing through the lungs, 65 per cent saturation may be taken as average, whereas fully saturated blood (97 per cent oxygen-laden) circulates in the left heart system. Therefore as the catheter tip passes through the right heart, oxygen saturations higher than usual can indicate an abnormal passageway from one side of the heart to the other; elevations far above 65 per cent will be noted when the catheter tip happens to lie close to the abnormal interchamber connection. The amount of leakage through the defect can be estimated by the amount of saturated blood that moves into the unsaturated portion.

In selective angiocardiograms, contrast material that is visible on X-ray film is injected through the catheter; it will outline the structures in the area of the catheter tip. Repeated small injections can be made and observed on the fluoroscopic screen, so that, for example, exact details of any anatomic changes in that region of the heart can be photographed. Minute variations in the structure and efficiency of valve leaflets can be studied very nicely by this procedure.

Dyes are sometimes injected through the catheter and their concentration in systemic blood can be estimated by photoelectric methods, usually sensed by means of a tiny electronic device attached to the ear. Shunts of blood from right to left can be demonstrated by this method because the time interval between injection and earlobe arrival is shortened when the lung circulation is partially by-passed.

When disease changes are present in the mitral or aortic valves, left-heart catheterization may be helpful. This can be done by passing a catheter inserted in an artery of the body back to the heart and then through the aortic valve leaflets. Pressure and oxygen studies can be done as in right-heart catheterization, and selective angiocardiography carried out. Estimation of rheumatic fever damage to the mitral and aortic valves must be made by left-heart catheterization.

HEART DISEASE, EXERCISE AND

Not long ago, rest was the keystone of treatment in heart disease. The modern trend is to encourage some form of activity or physiotherapy as soon as it is reasonably safe to do so. Recovery from heart disease or a heart attack can be speeded by gradual measures that will include both supervised exercise and occupational rehabilitation. With careful use, the working heart is strengthened and can even facilitate the development of new blood vessels within the heart muscle.

HEART-FAILURE

Heart-failure is usually defined as that stage of heart disease at which, even while the patient is resting, the heart can no longer fill the needs of the tissues for refreshed blood. The symptoms of excessive heart work no longer disappear after rest; fatigue, heart pain, and even attacks of shortness of breath often follow a pattern unique for a particular patient; and the established pattern of their appearance from day to day can rarely be eliminated by enforced rest periods alone.

Symptoms. When the heart is unable to keep up a fresh supply of blood to the tissues, fatigue (muscular weakness) is almost always present. During muscular activity almost all the output of refreshed blood from the heart is diverted from organs to the working muscles. When the output of the heart is unable to increase on demand, as in severe heart disease, even the slightest muscular effort may be hard for the patient to endure.

Often an individual finds himself easily fatigued. This of itself, however, is not often a sign of heart disease. Almost every person will have periods of emotional stress

282

which, even with a healthy heart and blood vessels, will cause useless muscle tension and so deplete the nutritional reserves of muscle fibers. Emotional tension, therefore, and not heart disease is probably the most common cause for the tendency to fatigue.

Everyone may experience breathlessness on effort. As a symptom of heart disease, however, shortness of breath is caused by inability of the heart to move blood through the lungs and into the tissues to keep pace with body demands as these change from minute to minute. Acute distress in breathing, along with a sense of suffocation, may compel the patient to sit down and rest or lie down in a propped-up position.

Fainting is sometimes a symptom of the failing heart, especially when it is produced by either moderate or very little exertion; it is thought to be due to temporary lack of fresh blood circulated to the brain.

Heart-failure of very serious degree causes very poor kidney function, with a low daily output of urine and accumulation of sodium and fluid in the tissue reservoirs; visible swelling of the feet and ankles may indicate the possibility of this complication. Excessive fluid in the lung tissues may result in a chronic cough, sometimes producing phlegm that is streaked with dark flecks of blood. An abdominal swelling may indicate that excessive fluid has accumulated in the peritoneal reservoir.

Treatment. Satisfactory treatment of heart failure depends upon strict adherence to the doctor's orders. First of all, the cause of failure must be remedied, if possible. A toxic goiter or anemia, for example, can be treated successfully so that heart failure, if caused by either disease, will be completely relieved, if there is a good response to that specific treatment. Structural defects and abnormal vessels may be corrected by surgery and thereby relieve the burdened heart.

If failure occurs during the last months of pregnancy, it may respond well to medical treatment, but when present in the first few months, termination of the pregnancy may need consideration to prevent disaster to both mother and unborn child.

Physical rest is important in treatment, the patient usually being nursed in a half-sitting position. Often an armchair is more convenient than a special bed, for this position itself can relieve congestion in the veins near the heart and reduce heart work to a minimum. Breathing is improved by a somewhat upright position and swelling may drift to the lower legs where it will do the least harm to an overburdened heart.

Drugs in the digitalis group act directly on the failing heart muscle, increasing the strength of its contraction and thereby speeding the evacuation of blood from engorged veins leading to the heart and in addition, improve the heart's output so that a greater volume of blood will flow to the kidneys, brain, and other vital organs that have been deprived of an adequate circulation.

A low sodium diet can bring about the removal of excessive body fluid because the sodium already present within the body will "pull water through the kidneys" as it passes through them. Low sodium diets are not difficult for the patient to follow, especially when salt substitutes replace the usual table salt.

A group of useful drugs that enhance kidney action (diuretics) are very effective as an aid in the removal of fluid trapped in the body by circulatory failure. They may be administered for many weeks without the occurrence of harmful side-effects. Once in a while, small skin incisions will be needed to provide an escape route for very swollen legs, especially when conservative treatment has not been effective in removal of this "dropsy" (edema) fluid. Drainage, produced through the skin incisions can continue for days with sometimes the fortuitous escape of many quarts of fluid. Fluid that has accumulated in the chest or abdominal cavities may need to be removed by needle puncture.

HEART MURMURS As blood passes through the healthy heart, characteristic sounds are made as the heart valves open by the tensed—and resonating—muscle walls of the heart chamber; and again by the resonant vibrations of the heart valves as they close at the end of muscle contracture (systole).

If there are abnormal surfaces along the valve margins, and especially if these surface changes prevent normal closure of the valve leaflets, murmurs or noises are made by the blood as it rushes past the abnormal surface irregularities or leaks back through misshapen valve leaflets that fail to close completely.

Any defects, inborn or acquired, may be potential causes of murmurs of varying intensity, pitch, and quality. Murmurs recur with each cycle of the heartbeat, and are generally classified as systolic murmurs if they are heard during active contracture of the ventricles, or diastolic if they come during the phase of ventricular relaxation.

Careful study of the murmur, listening to it many times and in a great many areas over the heart, is rewarding to the physician. He can gather an accurate impression of the disorder that causes the murmur, inasmuch as specific changes in the heart chambers or valves tend to produce murmurs that are quite typical. What they

sound like, how intense they are, where best heard, and the exact time in the heart cycle when they appear all contribute to the unique character of the various heart murmurs, hence to diagnosis of their underlying causes.

HEART MUSCLE The myocardium, the heart muscle, differs from muscle of the skeletal system in many ways. It has the ability to contract rhythmically both with and without external stimulation, and can do so continuously for long intervals of time with no evidence of fatigue. In the adult, the heart muscle weighs about one pound and provides the pumping pressure to move nearly five hundred gallons of blood through the vascular system every day of a person's life.

HEART SOUNDS When listening through the stethoscope, one can ordinarily hear two heart sounds in adults; these are known as the first and second sounds. In children, a soft third sound is often audible, and under unusual conditions fourth (auricular) sound may occur just before the first.

The first and second sounds are the usual ones to be concerned with. The first is caused by closure of the ventricular (mitral and tricuspid) valves and is audible at the beginning of ventricular contractions (systole). The second sound, in contrast, is due to closure of the aortic and pulmonary valves and is heard just at the beginning of ventricular relaxation (diastole).

HEAT, COLD, AND LIGHT ALLERGY
See PHYSICAL ALLERGIES

HEMOPHILIA Years ago any abnormal bleeding in a child was inaccurately called hemophilia. The true hemophiliac is a

male who has acquired his bleeding trait through the mother's side of the family.

Symptoms. The hemophilic boy bruises easily; blood may be passed in his urine from insignificant back injury, or a wrenched knee-joint may fill up with blood and result in a crippling deformity. Dental extraction produces prolonged bleeding.

Treatment. For years, transfusions of fresh blood or plasma were the mainstay of treatment. More recently an essential clotting factor (Factor VIII, AHF-antihemophilic factor) has been isolated. In relatively small amounts it corrects the clotting deficiency of hemophilia.

HEMORRHAGE, SUBARACHNOID

Subarachnoid hemorrhage is a bleeding into the spaces between the inner coverings of the brain. Brain injury from external violence is the most common cause. Spontaneous subarachnoid hemorrhage occurs as a result of the rupture of a weakening (aneurysm) in a cerebral artery, or of a vascular malformation. In one-third of cases the cause of bleeding is not found.

Symptoms. Severe headache is usually followed by drowsiness and stiff neck. Vomiting, double vision, weakness of one arm and leg, and other signs of neurologic deficit may develop, particularly if there is associated intracerebral bleeding. The patient may become comatose and show irregular respiration. The cerebrospinal fluid is bloody.

Treatment. Subarachnoid hemorrhage associated with head injury may result in severe complications. Spontaneous subarachnoid hemorrhage is of the greatest importance due to the threat posed by the leaking arterial aneurysm. (The blood in the subarachnoid space itself is absorbed within two to three weeks.) Approximately one-third of patients die after the first episode of spontaneous subarachnoid hemorrhage. Among survivers of the initial attack, the aneurysm may bleed again within a few weeks or months, with an increasing mortality rate. Surgical treatment is recommended for selected cases of aneurysm with rupture. This, however, is a major operative procedure and is associated with a high mortality rate. The aneurysm is located by X-ray studies made immediately after injecting oil which is opaque to X-rays into the cerebral circulation. An opening into the skull is then made to expose the aneurysm, to place clips on it, and to prevent it from rebleeding. Hospital care is required for every patient with subarachnoid hemorrhage. Intravenous fluids are frequently needed. If there is difficulty in swallowing, suction is necessary to maintain adequate aeration of the lungs.

HEMORRHOIDS (PILES)

Hemorrhoids are swellings of the veins in the lower rectum and anus. If they protrude through the anal opening (sphincter) they are external. If they are confined to the anal canal they are internal. Hemorrhoids are seldom painful unless the blood becomes clotted in these swollen areas. Hemorrhoids have been called "a disease of upright posture," as they are seldom noted in four-footed creatures. They may result from constipation, pregnancy, rectal infections, an enlarged prostate gland, severe obesity, or lack of exercise. Rarely, the appearance of hemorrhoids may signify an obstruction of the normal blood flow from the intestinal tract to the liver via the portal vein, such as seen in cirrhosis of the liver.

Symptoms. Internal hemorrhoids may cause itching, a feeling of fullness in the rectum, and pain if they become filled with clotted blood. Frequently the first sign of internal hemorrhoids will be bright-red blood from the rectum coating the stool. The bleeding is quite often painless. External hemorrhoids can be felt as small grape-like protrusions from the anus. They often contain clotted blood and can be extremely painful. Because of the pain associated with the passage of a bowel movement, the patient is likely to neglect his normal bowel habits, causing further hardening of the stool and thus making passage even more difficult. It cannot be assumed that all bright-red painless bleeding from the rectum is due to hemorrhoids, because painless tumors or polyps may also bleed even though hemorrhoids are known to be present. Examination is essential in these cases.

Treatment. The treatment of hemorrhoids may be very satisfactorily accomplished by such simple measures as sitz baths and anesthetic ointments. The avoidance of constipation and of the consequent straining at stool is most important in eradicating this condition. Severe pain and bleeding or chronic recurrence are indications for surgical removal.

HEMOTHORAX

HEMOTHORAX Collection of blood in the chest (pleural) space is referred to as hemothorox. This may vary in degree from very small amounts to a massive collection. The condition represents one form of internal bleeding. Hemopneumothorax is a combination of air and blood in the same location.

There are four principal causes of hemothorax: (1) pleural inflammation, either localized primarily in the pleura or most commonly following a lung inflammation such as pneumonia or pulmonary infarct; (2) rupture of a blood vessel following or as a sequel to chest-wall injury of a rib or other penetrating chest wound; (3) tumors which in their progressive course invade and erode blood vessels; (4) as a complication of a partial pneumothorax (air in the pleura) due to rupture of an adhesion-band.

Symptoms. If the collection of blood is small the condition may go undetected in the course of the primary disease, or may be manifested only by mild pain. With increased amounts, the fluid compresses the lung and breathlessness and bluish discoloration (cyanosis) become prominent. Massive collections, beside producing the above, give rise to rapid heartbeat, pallor, drop in blood pressure, and shock (internal hemorrhage).

Treatment. Cases of small hemo-

thorax do not ordinarily require specific treatment other than that for the primary cause. When large, the blood should be evacuated by the same procedures described in the treatment of pleurisy.

HEPATITIS The commonly seen infections of the liver are caused by viruses. Infectious hepatitis or catarrhal jaundice is the result of ingesting food or water contaminated by fecal material containing the virus.

Serum hepatitis is caused by a virus which gains access to the body through injections. Contamination of needles, syringes, tubing, ampoules, or the injected material itself may be present. To combat this hazard great care is taken by pharmaceutical manufacturers to produce absolutely sterile injectable medications. Blood and plasma may contain the virus, and the patient who is given several transfusions is thereby increasingly exposed to the risk of hepatitis. Improved methods of processing blood and plasma have greatly diminished this risk. The grossly unsterile techniques of drug addicts using homemade syringes and needles (or discarded hypodermic needles) is a troublesome source of serum hepatitis.

Symptoms. The symptoms of the two types are similar, as is the treatment. The incubation period in serum hepatitis is usually longer, and the infection may not be apparent until three to six months after introduction of the offending material.

The symptoms in both forms of hepatitis often begin abruptly and include loss of appetite, nausea and vomiting, fever, and tenderness over the liver area. Often the taste for tobacco is lost. Jaundice usually becomes evident in four to five days and is due to an inability of the diseased liver to handle the pigment from the broken-down red blood cells. In epidemics of infectious hepatitis, however, jaundice may not be noticeable. Recovery is usually uneventful after six to eight weeks of illness. Relapses are common

286

and are often due to too quick a resumption of activity. In a small percentage of cases severe liver damage may occur and treatment is difficult. Therapy is non-specific and bed rest is mandatory. The diet should be rich in protein, carbohydrates, and vitamins. Proper nutrition is often difficult because of continued nausea. Rarely, after severe cases of hepatitis, the liver may become cirrhotic.

HEREDITY Heredity is the endowment of offspring by parents (beginning with the fertilized egg) with physical and psychical characters. Reproduction never results in an exact replica of either progenitor although there may be a remarkable resemblance. Variation in offspring actually opposes heredity. The germ cells arising from sexual reproduction bear certain substances which account for inheritance. Of paramount importance are the carriers of hereditary factors, the chromosomes. Recent research indicates that there are 46 in each human cell, except in the mature sperm and ovum in which there are 23 in each. Thus, a child inherits 23 chromosomes from each parent. The chromosomes carry genes which are hereditary factors.

Neither natural science, nor anthropology, nor medicine, nor any other division of science has ever fully explained how a single fertilized egg can develop into an organism with billions of differentiated cells, with the capacity to reproduce itself, and with an almost endless number of functions, complex organs, and feelings. Molecular biologists seem to have the answer in the cellular substances DNA (desoxyribonucleic acid) and RNA (ribonucleic acid).

DNA and RNA are found in every living cell, animal and vegetable. In brief, DNA transmits orders from cell to cell (through its "executive officer" and "roving ambassador," RNA), and from one generation to another. We have reason to

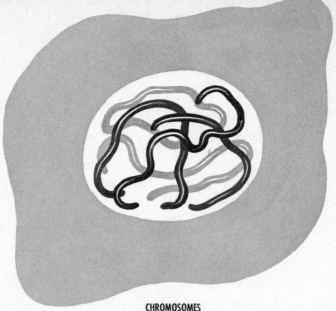

CHROMOSOMES

Chromosomes are small, dark-staining, and more or less rod-shaped bodies which appear in the nucleus of a cell at the time of cell division. They are supposed to be made up of genes. The number of chromosomes in any species is usually constant.

believe that DNA is responsible for life's processes, life's origin, life's evolution, and life's future on this planet. That DNA can split in two on its own implies that this force is behind the beginning of life, its differentiation, and its very origin. Furthermore, DNA builds proteins in the cells, and without amino acids (derivatives of proteins) life is not possible. The endless permutations that DNA undergoes in its fissuring explains inheritance; the unusual and even recessive combinations in DNA particles that can suddenly pop up in one generation (never seen before or existing in generations before) strips the mystery from the "sport" which geneticists have never been able to explain in their otherwise set theory of mutation.

In psychiatry, there is no proof that mental illness or retardation can be inherited or that they are familial in nature. Nevertheless certain types of mental retardation are known to be inheritable, for example, amaurotic family idiocy (Tay-Sachs disease). It is also true that an inherited constitutional predisposition does appear to play a role in some mental afflictions, but the emergence of a psychosis or a psychoneurosis in a given individual is determined by many factors. It has also

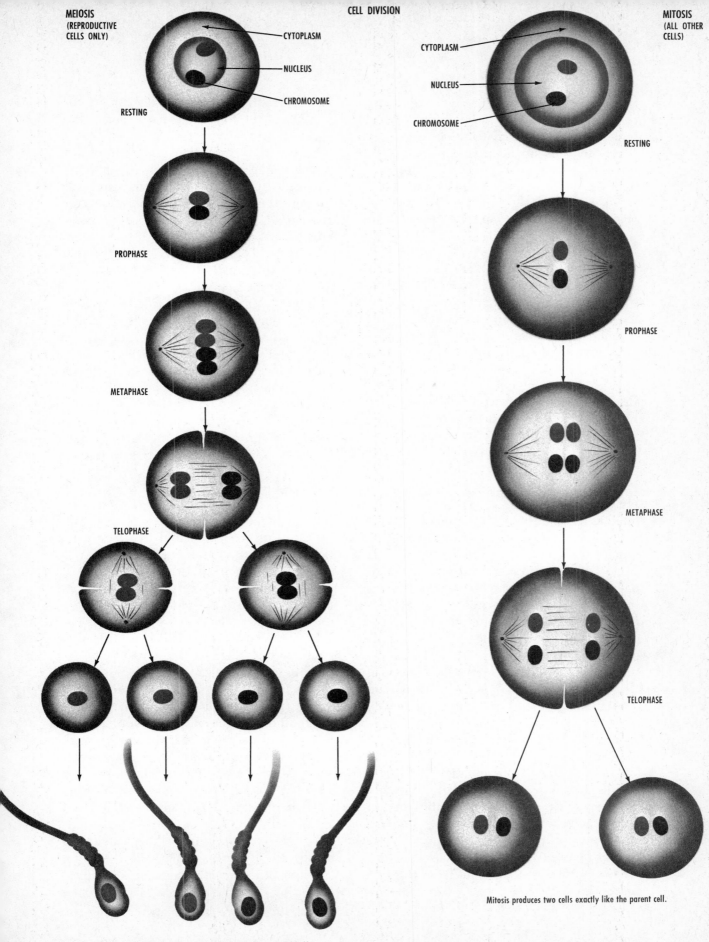

MEIOSIS
(REPRODUCTIVE
CELLS ONLY)

CELL DIVISION

MITOSIS
(ALL OTHER
CELLS)

CYTOPLASM

NUCLEUS

CHROMOSOME

CYTOPLASM

NUCLEUS

CHROMOSOME

RESTING

RESTING

PROPHASE

PROPHASE

METAPHASE

METAPHASE

TELOPHASE

TELOPHASE

Meiosis produces four cells, each containing one-half
the chromosomes of the parent cell.

Mitosis produces two cells exactly like the parent cell.

been shown that a predisposition to epilepsy is inheritable, since normal children of epileptic parents may produce epileptic brain rhythms in electroencephalographic tracings.

HERMAPHRODITISM   This very interesting condition is named after the Greek god Hermes, and the Greek goddess Aphrodite. In mythology, their child Hermaphroditos possessed the traits of both sexes, and the name has been applied to conditions which represent male and female features in the same individual. True hermaphrodites have one or more testicles and one or more ovaries. The individual may have the physical appearance of a male or female, depending on the predominance of the ovary or the testis. Often the true hermaphrodite will appear to be a completely normal female who is found at surgery to have testes in the groin region. (See also ADRENOGENITAL SYNDROME.)

HERNIA   A hernia or rupture is defined as the abnormal protrusion of a loop of the intestine or of some part of an internal organ through an abnormal opening of the cavity which contains it. In the gastrointestinal system, the commonly seen hernias include hiatus hernia—protrusion of a portion of the stomach through the hole in the diaphragm through which the esophagus passes; ventral hernia—protrusion of intestinal loops through a defect in the midline of the abdominal wall; and inguinal and femoral hernia—loops of intestine which pass through the inguinal canal into the scrotum or (in females) through the femoral canal into the upper thigh.

A hiatus (diaphragmatic) hernia is usually the result of a congenitally large hole (or hiatus) in the diaphragmatic muscle which allows a portion of the stomach actually to protrude into the chest cavity; rarely, severe injury to the abdomen may force a portion of the stomach up through the hiatus.

A ventral hernia may occur in the midline of the abdomen, particularly after repeated pregnancies. This is due to the relaxation and separation of the muscles of the abdomen and can be quite distressing. Occasionally a ventral hernia may protrude through the site of a former incision in the abdomen. This is known as an incisional hernia.

Inguinal hernias are of two major types: indirect and direct. The indirect type refers to the protrusion of a loop of intestine through the inguinal canal which leads from the abdominal cavity into the scrotum. (Normally the entrance to this canal closes over shortly after birth.) A direct inguinal hernia, on the other hand, does not travel through the length of the inguinal canal, but pushes into it at some distance beyond its origin. If the loop of intestine which herniates through the abnormal opening becomes kinked (strangulated), serious consequences may follow unless the hernia is quickly reduced: because of blockage to intestinal flow, a bowel obstruction is present, the flow of blood becomes impaired, and there is actual tissue-destruction. This type of strangulated hernia is a surgical emergency. In many instances, however, the defect is relatively large so that the loop of intestine is easily pushed back up into place, either manually or by a truss. Inguinal hernias may result from excessive straining or lifting, but a preexisting weakened inguinal canal is usually necessary for producing a hernia in this manner.

A femoral hernia is the protrusion of a loop of intestine (usually in women) into the femoral canal—the potential space through which the large blood vessels and nerves leave the pelvis and go into the upper leg. This type of hernia may likewise be relatively benign, producing no symptoms, but occasionally here also surgery is required.

In a certain percentage of newborn babies there is protrusion of a loop of intestine at the navel, causing an umbilical hernia. This may be rather frightening to the

THE NERVOUS SYSTEM

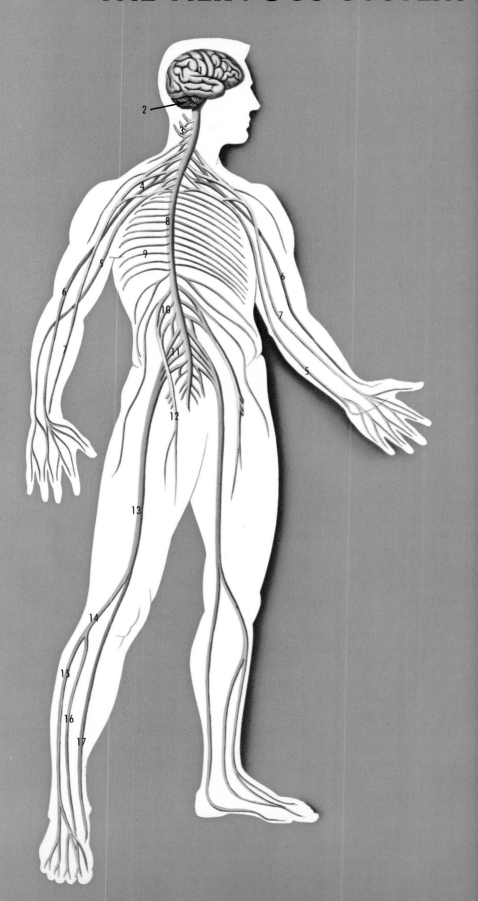

THE MAJOR NERVES

1　CEREBRUM
2　CEREBELLUM
3　CERVICAL PLEXUS
4　BRACHIAL PLEXUS
5　ULNAR
6　RADIAL
7　MEDIAN
8　SPINAL CORD
9　INTERCOSTAL
10　LUMBAR PLEXUS
11　LUMBO-SACRAL PLEXUS
12　FEMORAL
13　SCIATIC
14　COMMON PERONEAL
15　SUPERFICIAL PERONEAL
16　DEEP PERONEAL
17　TIBIAL

ILLUSTRATED BY

LEONARD D. DANK

ST. LUKE'S HOSPITAL
NEW YORK CITY

PARTS OF THE NERVOUS SYSTEM

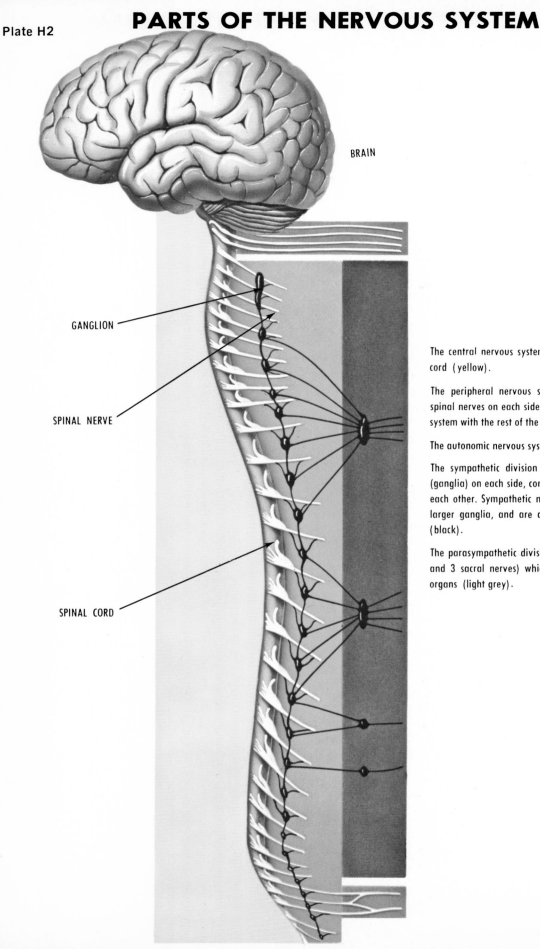

BRAIN

GANGLION

SPINAL NERVE

SPINAL CORD

The central nervous system consists of the brain and spinal cord (yellow).

The peripheral nervous system consists of a series of 31 spinal nerves on each side which connect the central nervous system with the rest of the body (blue).

The autonomic nervous system has two subdivisions:

The sympathetic division consists of a series of 25 nodes (ganglia) on each side, connected to the spinal nerves and to each other. Sympathetic nerves leave the ganglia, travel to larger ganglia, and are distributed to the internal organs (black).

The parasympathetic division consists of 7 nerves (4 cranial and 3 sacral nerves) which are distributed to the internal organs (light grey).

ANATOMY OF THE CENTRAL NERVOUS SYSTEM

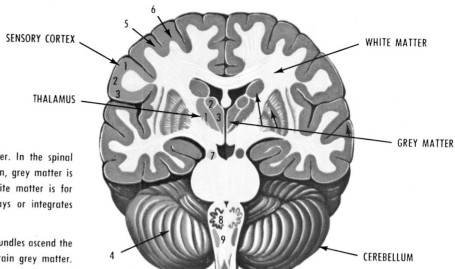

SENSORY CORTEX

WHITE MATTER

THALAMUS

GREY MATTER

CEREBELLUM

CROSS SECTION OF BRAIN

Nervous tissue is composed of grey and white matter. In the spinal cord, grey matter is within white matter. In the brain, grey matter is both over and within white matter. In general, white matter is for transportation of impulses, grey matter either relays or integrates these impulses.

White matter is arranged into fiber bundles. Sensory bundles ascend the cord, traverse the brain white matter, and end in brain grey matter. These bundles and their terminations in the brain are in tones of red and numbered 1-4. Motor bundles begin in brain grey matter, travel down brain white matter, and descend the cord. These bundles and their brain origins are in tones of blue and numbered 5-9. Not only does each bundle occupy a specific location in both brain and cord, it also carries a specific type of impulse. For example, pain-sensation impulses from most of the body ascend the lateral spinothalamic bundle, travel to the thalamus, and are relayed to the sensory cortex. Note that the right cord bundles are linked with the left side of the brain.

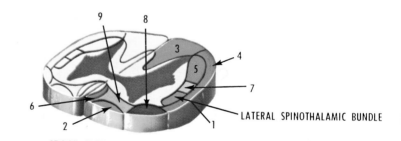

LATERAL SPINOTHALAMIC BUNDLE

CROSS SECTION OF SPINAL CORD

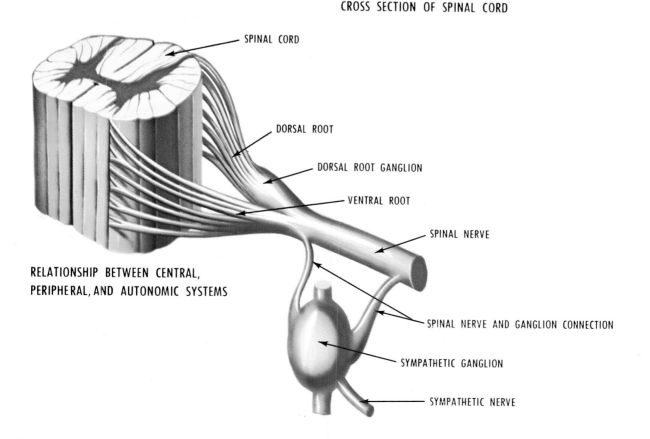

SPINAL CORD

DORSAL ROOT

DORSAL ROOT GANGLION

VENTRAL ROOT

SPINAL NERVE

RELATIONSHIP BETWEEN CENTRAL, PERIPHERAL, AND AUTONOMIC SYSTEMS

SPINAL NERVE AND GANGLION CONNECTION

SYMPATHETIC GANGLION

SYMPATHETIC NERVE

THE NEURON—LOCATION AND ANATOMY

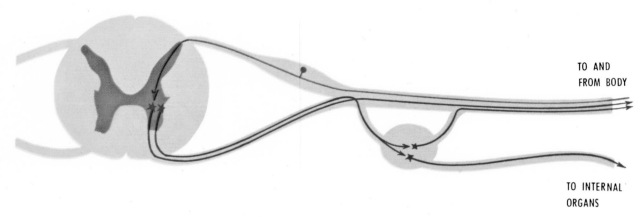

TO AND
FROM BODY

TO INTERNAL
ORGANS

The neuron is the basic impulse-carrying cell of all parts of the nervous system. Excluding specialized brain neurons, there are two types. Sensory neurons (red) bring sensation impulses to the spinal cord grey matter. They synapse with motor neurons carrying command or action impulses to the muscles and glands of the body and internal organs.

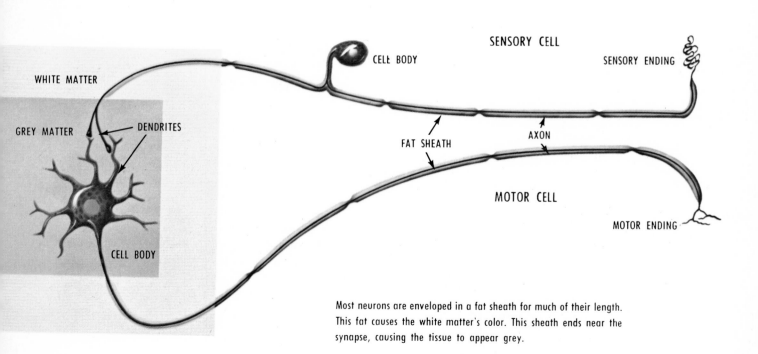

WHITE MATTER

GREY MATTER — DENDRITES

CELL BODY

CELL BODY

SENSORY CELL

SENSORY ENDING

FAT SHEATH

AXON

MOTOR CELL

MOTOR ENDING

Most neurons are enveloped in a fat sheath for much of their length. This fat causes the white matter's color. This sheath ends near the synapse, causing the tissue to appear grey.

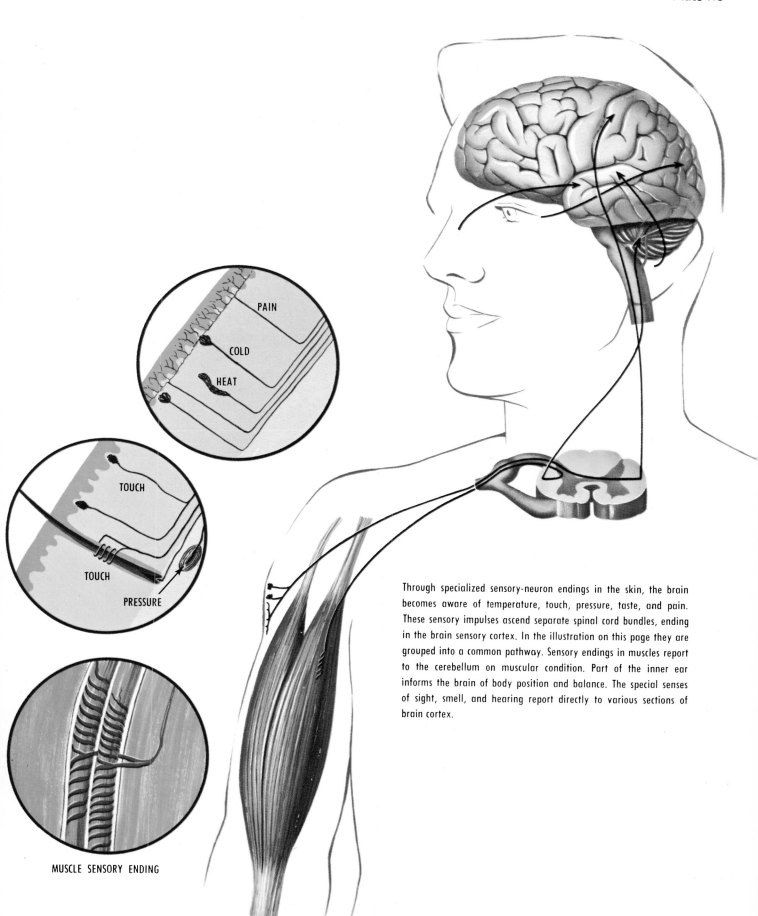

PAIN

COLD

HEAT

TOUCH

TOUCH

PRESSURE

MUSCLE SENSORY ENDING

Through specialized sensory-neuron endings in the skin, the brain becomes aware of temperature, touch, pressure, taste, and pain. These sensory impulses ascend separate spinal cord bundles, ending in the brain sensory cortex. In the illustration on this page they are grouped into a common pathway. Sensory endings in muscles report to the cerebellum on muscular condition. Part of the inner ear informs the brain of body position and balance. The special senses of sight, smell, and hearing report directly to various sections of brain cortex.

CONTACT WITH THE MUSCLES

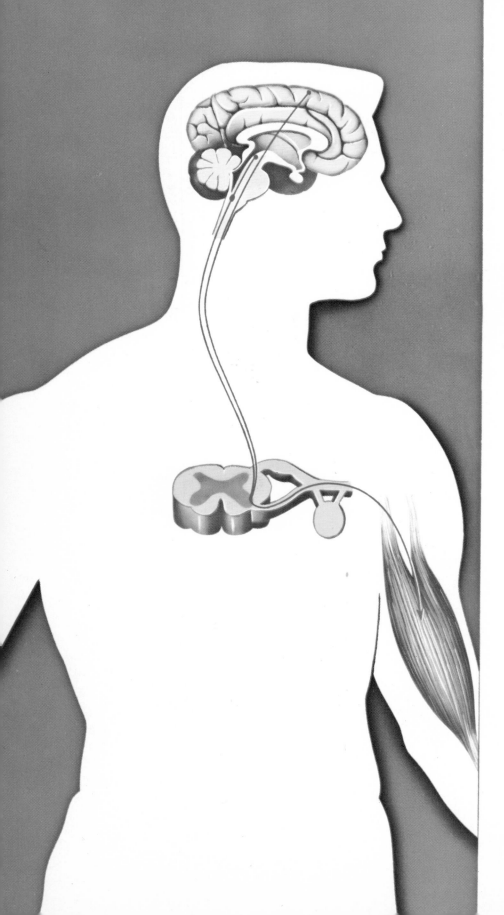

In response to the vast amount of information collected by the body, the brain directs innumerable movements. Motor impulses originating either in the brain grey motor cortex, or in other muscle coordinating brain centers, descend the spinal cord. The impulses travel out a spinal nerve to the muscle. A complicated voluntary movement may involve several hundred motor neurons.

The autonomic nervous system controls the internal activities. Each organ (the stomach is used as an example) receives a nerve supply from the parasympathetic division (light blue) which takes a direct route independent of the spinal cord. Each organ also receives a sympathetic nerve supply (dark blue) which descends the spinal cord, exits into a ganglion, and travels a sympathetic nerve to the organ. Sensory nerves (black) travel to the lower, nonconscious portions of the brain, where autonomic regulatory centers are located. In response to sensory information regarding the stomach's muscle and gland activity, a speed-up impulse is sent via the parasympathetic nerve, or a slow-down impulse via the sympathetic nerve. Thus each organ is maintained in delicate balance. Occasionally, unusual pain or discomfort will cause sensory impulses (dotted black) to register in the conscious mind.

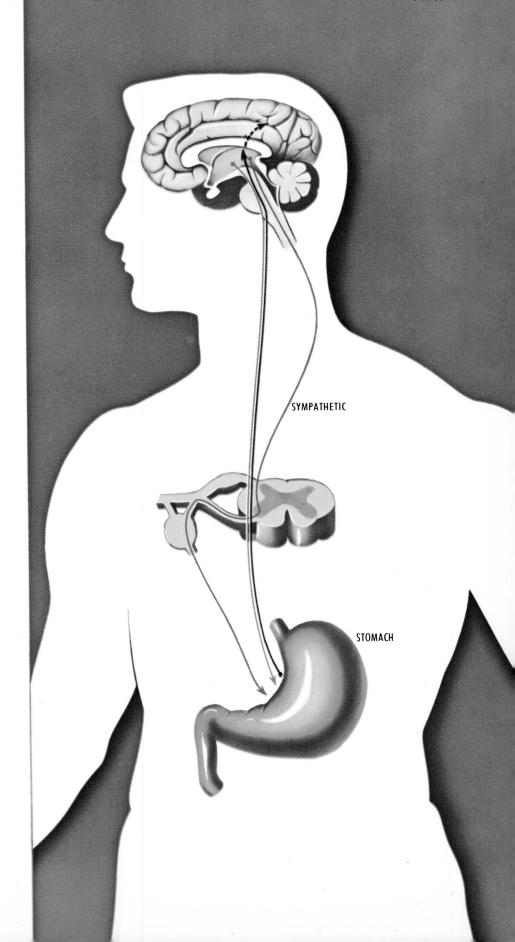

SYMPATHETIC

STOMACH

REFLEX ACTIVITIES OF SPINAL CORD

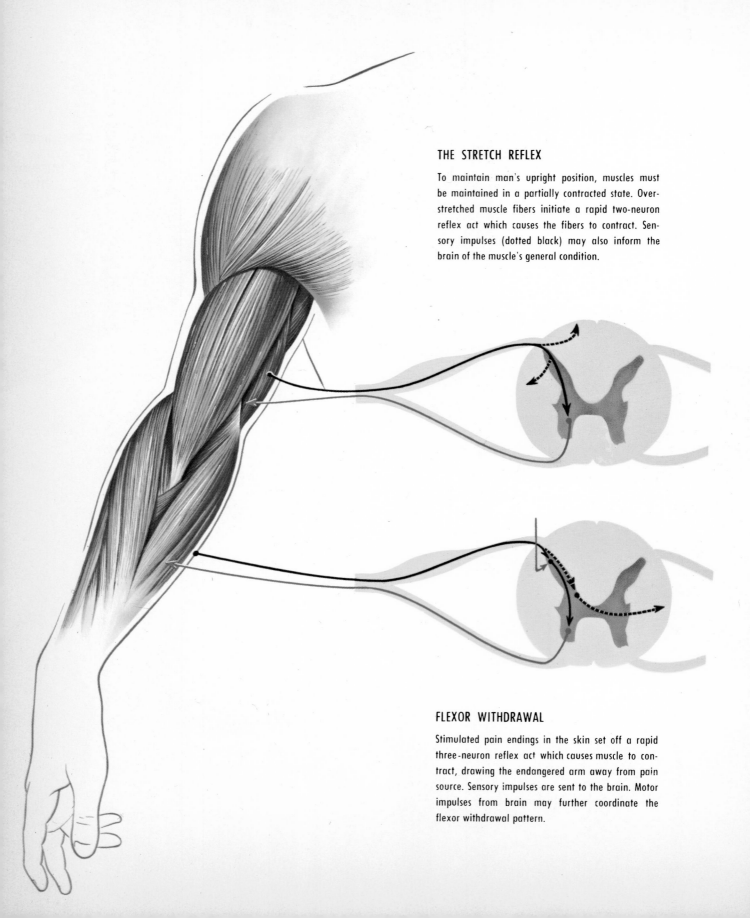

THE STRETCH REFLEX

To maintain man's upright position, muscles must be maintained in a partially contracted state. Over-stretched muscle fibers initiate a rapid two-neuron reflex act which causes the fibers to contract. Sensory impulses (dotted black) may also inform the brain of the muscle's general condition.

FLEXOR WITHDRAWAL

Stimulated pain endings in the skin set off a rapid three-neuron reflex act which causes muscle to contract, drawing the endangered arm away from pain source. Sensory impulses are sent to the brain. Motor impulses from brain may further coordinate the flexor withdrawal pattern.

parents, but such hernias almost always disappear after one or two years and seldom require surgical repair. However, if surgery is required for a large hernia, the baby will take only about two to four weeks to recover.

HERPES SIMPLEX   Of the more than seventy herpes viruses identified, five are known to infect humans. Of these five, herpes simplex Type I and herpes simplex Type II are the most common.

Herpes simplex Type I produces cold sores and fever blisters, usually on the lips or on the mouth. On rare occasions Type I can erupt in the genital area. The disease can be transmitted by direct contact with active lesions. (See also COLD SORES.)

Herpes simplex Type II causes genital herpes, perhaps the fastest spreading sexually transmitted disease in the United States. It is highly contagious whenever the characteristic blisters appear. The first instance of Type II, accompanied by burning and itching sensations, may last as long as a month.

The first symptoms of Type II would occur about six days after contact with an infected person. Prior to the appearance of the blisters, the individual may have fever, headache, or a generalized discomfort.

Often Type II infections occur again; for some individuals repeated attacks of the active phase have been reported. Usually the severity of the recurrence lessens over time, but they may continue for years at sporadic intervals.

Women with herpes simplex Type II antibodies have a much greater risk of developing cervical cancer. Pregnant women with Type II risk miscarriage, early delivery, and possible birth defects, especially if the baby is exposed to the virus during birth. Delivery by caesarean section may be recommended to reduce the risk of infecting the baby.

It is possible for the herpes virus to spread into the bloodstream and infect other organs in certain individuals, such as cancer patients or persons with kidney, lung, or blood diseases. These people have difficulty in fighting most infections.

There is no cure as yet for Type II herpes, although testing for vaccines is now underway. Some relief from symptoms can be obtained with medications such as Domeboro and Zovirax. Sexual contact during the active phase of Type II should be avoided.

Current information about herpes can be obtained by sending a self-addressed, stamped envelope to Herpes Resource Center, Box 100, Palo Alto, CA, 94302.

HICCUP (HICCOUGH)   This is an involuntary spasm of the diaphragm during its inspiratory (inhale-phase) contraction which is checked suddenly by the closure of the voice box (larynx). It is often caused by fast eating. It usually repeats itself for several minutes and disappears spontaneously, or by simple measures such as holding the breath, drinking cold water, or pulling the tongue out firmly. Sometimes, eating granulated sugar will stop it.

Persistent hiccup is of medical significance because of its underlying cause, which may be an irritation of the gastrointestinal tract, the pleura, lung, heart, central nervous system, or of the diaphragm itself. In such cases it is postulated that an abnormal nerve-reflex mechanism is at fault, persistently stimulating the diaphragmatic motor-nerve pathways. Contact a physician if the condition is prolonged.

Treatment. Treatment for this condition should be aimed at controlling the basic underlying cause. In addition, the following measures are occasionally effective: rebreathing into a paper bag; gastric lavage; breathing a mixture of 10 per cent carbon dioxide in oxygen, or injecting antinausea drugs such as chlorpromazine. If all fails, one may have to resort to surgical interruption or temporary paralyzation of the phrenic nerve in the neck.

HIGH BLOOD PRESSURE If blood pressure (measured in millimeters of mercury) remains above 150 to 160 in systole, or 90 to 95 millimeters in diastole, even after a period of rest, high blood pressure as a disease entity can be suspected. To prove that a state of high blood pressure exists as an abnormality, the doctor will take a series of pressure readings at various times during the day, after simple exercise tests, or following the administration of certain drugs. If high readings are constantly present, a state of hypertension (high blood pressure) may be said to exist. If present, it may represent a specific disease entity (essential hypertension) or be an indication of a disorder in one of the body organs, such as the kidneys or adrenal glands.

HIGH-RESIDUE DIET This type of diet is indicated in constipation due to lack of muscle tone (atonic constipation). The intestinal muscles are stimulated by bulky foods that are high in cellulose-content—basically fruits and vegetables. In addition, at least six to eight glasses of water per day should be drunk.

HIP DEFORMITIES IN CHILDHOOD Any child who walks with a limp or states that he has a pain in the hip or knee should be suspected of having disease of the hips and needs immediate medical attention. Likewise, any infant who has limited motion of one hip or who cries when his legs are spread in diapering should also be suspected of having hip involvement.

HIRSUTISM Excessive growth of hair on the face (and other areas) of women is not infrequently first seen in early adult life, but is an almost universal occurrence in women of middle age. Both the time of onset and the distribution of facial hair growth are governed to some degree by an inheritance factor. Other factors, including endocrine activity and metabolic imbalances, may be of significance in some patients but are not capable of being determined in the light of our present knowledge.

Symptoms. Dark, relatively stiff hairs may be confined to the upper lip, the chin, the anterior chest or the breasts; or they may be present in all or in several of these areas. More rarely, the forearms and the thighs are the sites of excessive hair growth. The appearance of a diffuse growth of fine, light-colored "down," usually on the cheeks, is not necessarily a forerunner of a growth of real hair, the color and texture of this hair almost always remaining unaltered. Hair is rarely found in the ears of women, usual as it is in the ears of men.

Treatment. Permanent removal of hair can be accomplished by electrolysis or by electrocautery. Both processes are tedious and seemingly endless, requiring repeated treatment; but both are finally effective. Temporary removal with depilatories is a practical procedure for excessive hair of the extremities. Removal with wax applications or with tweezers affords longer periods of relief because removing the hair with its root prolongs the time before reappearance of the hair at the surface of the skin. With both these methods it is necessary for the hair to be long enough to permit its being clutched without injuring the skin.

While the eradication of unwanted hair is feasible, if difficult, the prevention of additional hair growth already destined to appear is not possible. The commonly held view that pulling out, or otherwise removing, hair induces further growth probably stems from the fact that early appearance of hair is the first evidence of the likelihood of more growth; and the removal of this first growth is erroneously cited as the cause of later-appearing hair.

It is impractical to attempt removal

of the fuzz type of downy hair except under extraordinary circumstances. Wax depilation is probably the most useful for this purpose.

Bleaching of excessive hair growth is most often used for the forearms, legs, and upper lip. Usually no problems are encountered except in people who have an allergic sensitivity to the bleaches and dyes.

HISTOPLASMOSIS Caused by the *Histoplasma capsulatum*, this deep mycotic infection usually results from inhalation of the spores, which reside in the soil and have been found most frequently in the Mississippi and Ohio River valleys. The infection varies from a disease with practically no symptoms to overwhelming infection, and the condition is often difficult to differentiate from tuberculosis. Active infection is probably the result of a general depletion of immunity as is evidenced by the high susceptibility of infants to the progressive form of the disease.

Symptoms. Aside from the skin involvement in the overwhelming progressive form, primary infection of the skin is rare and usually self-limiting. The red, nodular lesions of the skin occur more frequently on the penis, around the mouth, and on the buccal mucous membranes.

Bed rest and supportive measures are useful, and may alone be curative. For more serious cases a drug called amphotericin B is given in intravenous solution.

HIVES (URTICARIA) This common eruption consisting of raised, reddened lesions often surrounded by a halo of unelevated redness, occurs at all ages and represents an allergic reaction of the "immediate" type. While a period of about ten days (but often more) is required for an allergy to develop the first time a patient shows evidence of having become allergic to a substance, the succeeding attacks will occur in from only a few minutes to several hours after exposure to the causative substance.

Symptoms. The eruption is usually generalized in distribution but may be confined to particular parts. Thus, only the arms and legs may be involved; or the eyelids, lips or face; or only portions of the body exposed to the sun (photoallergy). Each lesion goes through a cycle of redness, swelling, surrounding pink halo (flare), and gradual fading. The presence of lesions in different stages of development, and often joining with each other, gives the appearance of blotchiness. This eruption is accompanied by much itching, and when the palms and soles or the lips or eyelids are intensely swollen there may be pain and burning sensation.

Depending on the type of hives and the nature of the causative agent, the eruption can be of short duration or last for many months; and it can occur as a single attack or be a recurrent disease.

Hives can occasionally be of such large size as to warrant the designation giant hives (angioneurotic edema). The lesions can reach the size of a lemon and completely involve areas like an eyelid or the lip. This type of lesion is not usually present over the entire skin but can nevertheless be of more serious nature than the eruption of more usual size. Not only does the involved part become distorted and incapable of function, but there is also not infrequent association of swelling of the throat and larynx with impairment of breathing. Neither the causes nor the treatment differ from the more usual type of hives; only the need for early, effective treatment is more immediate.

Still another type of hives is papular urticaria, seen mostly in young children. This disease tends to recur seasonally, usually in the spring. The eruption, which is usually confined to the outer sides of the arms and legs, consists of small, hard papules of a shot-like consistency, slightly reddened and usually scratched. Often the scars and discolorations of lesions of previous attacks are mixed with the current ones. A very high percentage of cases of papular urticaria is caused by an allergy to insects, accounting for the seasonal occurrence. Treatment is the same as for hives of other appearance and causation, except that the use of insect repellents is effective in prevention. It should also be noted that, almost without exception, this type of reaction is seen in children only, and spontaneous cure even in severe and prolonged cases is the rule.

The most common cause of hives is medication taken by mouth or administered by injection. Contrary to general belief, drugs of such ordinary usage as to be considered household remedies, no matter how frequently taken previously or in what dosage, can at any time in the patient's use of them cause an attack of hives which will be followed by like attacks each time the drug is taken thereafter. Some drugs are more likely to produce this type of allergic reaction, and it is necessary for this reason for patients with known previous reactions (hives) to be especially cautious not only in taking new remedies, but also in the use of previously tried remedies with a high incidence of allergic responses. Excretion of drugs is variable and the hives persist for as long as the drug remains in the body. It is obviously urgent to determine the cause of the eruption as quickly as possible in order to discontinue the taking of the offending agent.

Older than drugs, of course, among the known causes of hives is food. While patients often indict unusual foods as causative of an attack, neither the uncommonness, the "spiciness," nor any other taste-related characteristic of the food is a factor in its being constituted as an allergenic cause of hives. Why a person becomes allergic at one particular exposure to a food and remains allergic to that food from then on is not yet known. There is neither a common factor among the causative allergens nor among the persons affected.

Hives can also be caused by physical agents, such as light (including ultraviolet rays), heat, cold, stroking, and physical pressure of varying intensities. As in hives of other causation, the reason for the sudden onset is unknown.

Substances foreign to the body, as for instance serum from another animal species (horse serum) or from an incompatible human source (serum or blood), can cause hives without additional systemic involvement or can produce a more inclusive reaction, serum sickness. These instances are usually readily recognized because of the immediately preceding administration (but sometimes as long as ten days earlier) of the causative material.

The cases not included in the previously mentioned possible causes comprise a large number variously considered attributable to chronic infection (teeth, tonsils, appendix, gallbladder), noninfectious diseases (leukemia, liver disease), pregnancy, emotional stress, animal dander, plants, fungi, etc.

Treatment. Removal and future avoidance of the causative substance is essential for cure. In patients in whom it is not possible to determine the cause (and in all cases before specific treatment was available) alleviation of this eruption results either from unknowing removal of the allergen or from a spontaneous immunization, the mechanism of which is also unknown.

The antihistaminic drugs and the cortisones are the most effective remedies, though each may be more effective than another in different circumstances. Local remedies include cold compresses and lotions. Administration of adrenalin, heretofore a frequently used remedy, is now reserved for relief of great swelling interfering with function (eyes, mouth, hands, and feet), and is followed by the previously-mentioned antihistaminics and cortisone drugs.

HOARSENESS   Hoarseness is a heavy,

rough, or harsh quality of the voice, usually lower in pitch than a person's normal voice. The most frequent causes of hoarseness are: tumors, inflammation, trauma, scars, paralysis and foreign bodies. (See TUMORS OF THE LARYNX; LARYNGITIS; LARYNX, INJURIES OF THE, AND FOREIGN BODIES; VOCAL CORDS, PARALYSIS OF THE.)

HODGKIN'S DISEASE

Hodgkin's disease is a progressive, often fatal disease marked by increasing enlargement of lymph nodes and often of the liver and the spleen, with terminal anemia, fever, and profound weakness. The cause is unknown.

Symptoms. Generally, the patient first notices a single lymph node that is enlarged. This may be in the neck, armpit, groin, or anywhere else in the body. This can be the sole complaint for months. He may suffer pruritus (severe itching) that is resistant to local treatment. The lymph node involvement slowly but steadily progresses to involve other nodes; at first they are separate, but with time they "mat" together. Sometimes enlargement of the spleen and liver is the only sign. When bones are implicated there is pain and disability with compression, and even fracture, of a vertebra. Lesions within the spinal column press on the cord and cause various neurologic signs, palsies, paralyses, etc. Invasion of the lung may produce a clinical picture closely resembling pneumonia. Large nodules pressing: (1) on the superior vena cava (one of the body's largest veins, located in the chest cavity) will result in edema (collection of serum) and cyanosis (bluishness) of the neck and face; (2) on the bronchial tubes, in infection and shortness of breath; (3) on nerves in the neck, in a constricted pupil of the eye of the same side, the orbit itself receding into its bony cavity, and there will be alterations in flushing and perspiration on that side of the face; (4) on spinal nerves as they emerge from the cord, in neuritic

pains; (5) on bile ducts, in jaundice; and (6) on the inferior vena cava, in edema of the legs ("dropsy").

As time goes on, the pruritus may worsen. There is often an increase in the white blood cells (leukocytosis), progressive weakness, and fever. Drinking of alcoholic beverages may cause pain in one or more of the lesions. Herpes zoster ("shingles") frequently occurs. This is an acute infection of the central nervous system characterized by blebs of the skin, pain, and perhaps itching of the involved area.

Early, the blood smear may show an increase in the lymphocyte count. Eosinophils (another variety of blood cells) are sometimes markedly increased in number. Anemia is usually present. It is difficult to specify the length of life after onset. It varies, with intensive treatment, from five to twenty or more years.

Treatment. Therapy includes radiation treatment and antineoplastic ("against new growth") agents, such as nitrogen mustard (mechlorethamine), triethylenemelamine (TEM), or chlorambucil. Adrenocortical therapy is also used.

HOMOSEXUALITY, SEX INVERSION

In this century great psychiatric progress has been made in understanding the causes and methods for dealing with homosexuality—sexual preference for a person of the same sex—an area in which superstition and misunderstanding have done much to confuse scientific study of sex deviations.

Prior to the studies of Freud, homosexuality was considered a form of degeneracy which was subjected to severe punishment. Freud's studies of psychosexual development showed that almost all young people normally pass through a period of interest in members of their own sex, and that such interest should be considered morbid homosexuality only when a person, on becoming an adult, sought sexual outlet with the same sex. Thus, because of the influence of psychoanalytic studies, homosexuality has come to be regarded as a variant of normal development rather than as a separate mental disorder.

In actual practice, modern societies tend to leave homosexuals to their own devices so long as their activities do not become socially obnoxious or dangerous to the morals of the young. Scientific studies (such as the Kinsey report) show a high incidence of homosexual activity among both sexes. Although much of this might consist of mutual masturbation or minor petting practices among teen-agers, the Kinsey report helped to dilute the connotations of severe abnormality to at least some homosexual behavior.

Symptoms. A distinction should be made between the confirmed homosexual who shows no interest whatsoever in the opposite sex and otherwise-normal persons who have occasional homosexual feelings. It is entirely normal for an individual to feel sexually attracted by a person of the same sex; such feelings alone should not cause panic unless they are acted out in such ways as to interfere with relations with the opposite sex (heterosexuality). Studies of men in army or prison situations, where there is no possibility of contact with the opposite sex, indicate that many normal men and women have transient attachments to persons of their own sex which are broken off when normal heterosexual opportunities again return. Probably no man is 100 per cent masculine, nor any woman 100 per cent feminine; rather, everyone represents some combination of masculinity and femininity in such ratios as 90-10, 70-30, 50-50, etc. Some people are optionally (facultatively) homosexual; that is, attracted to both sexes and without a firm preference for either.

Homosexual tendencies may be either latent or manifest, depending on whether they are unconscious and unexpressed, or conscious and overt. Psychiatric experience indicates that many normal people have latent homosexual tendencies which may never be expressed in action unless the person is subjected to some form of sexual attack or seduction.

The causes of homosexuality have not been exactly established and are very complex. In a small number of cases there appears to be a physical basis, the person having many secondary sexual characteristics of the opposite sex. In other instances homosexual attack or seduction in early life may undoubtedly be a predisposing cause, particularly if occurring during crucial periods of psychosexual development. Another possible factor is failure of the child to achieve a healthy identification with the parent of the same sex. In boys, for example, it is desirable for the father to set a healthy pattern for masculine identification, so that the son early learns normal male sex roles.

Treatment. Homosexuality constitutes a difficult therapeutic problem, usually requiring intensive psychoanalytic treatment. This has been estimated to produce "cures" in about one-fourth of such patients. Others may show varying states of improvement including restoration of potency with members of the opposite sex, capacity for heterosexual marriage with occasional lapses, etc. Decreasing automatic disapproval of the homosexual, increasing militancy of the so-called gay groups, and more open discussion of the problem are evidences of change toward less punitive attitudes in society at large.

HORMONES A hormone is a substance of complex chemical composition secreted by an endocrine gland directly into the bloodstream, traveling to organs and tissues where it stimulates chemical reactions. Glands which secrete hormones are the pituitary, thyroid, adrenals, male and female sex glands, and the parathyroid. (Hormones are also secreted by the stomach, liver, and kidney, but these are not as well understood.) Hormones are used in the treatment of deficiencies of the glands which normally manufacture them. Certain hormones have been synthesized in the laboratory; most important of these are cortisone, thyroxine, and sex hormones. Thyroid, cortisone, and sex hormones may be given by mouth. Insulin and ACTH are examples of hormones which must be given by injection.

HOUSE-DUST ALLERGY   House dust is a conglomeration of many materials. It contains small amounts of kapok, cotton lint, feathers, wool, fragments of paper, orrisroot, silk, molds, tobacco, insects, pyrethrum, animal danders, flaxseed, and glue. It is found all over the house but mainly in mattresses, box springs, pillows, toys, upholstered furniture, comforters, heavy drapery, rugs, stored clothing, and in heating systems. The older the furnishings the more potent the house dust.

House-dust sensitivity is more common in people who have a family history of allergy. In springtime, housecleaning will bring on symptoms. In the fall, the use of a furnace that has been standing idle for several months will precipitate attacks—one reason why house-dust difficulties are more common in the colder northern climates.

Symptoms.   Nasal congestion, spasmodic sneezing, postnasal drip, wheezing (asthma), and headaches are common symptoms of house-dust sensitivity.

Treatment.   Reducing the dust exposure, decreasing clinical sensitivity, and relieving symptoms are the basic means of therapy.

Dust-control is difficult but very necessary—especially in the case of the highly allergic individual. There should be no upholstered furniture; no rugs and rug pads; no pillows containing kapok, down, or feathers; no stuffed toys; no heavy draperies; no comforters or quilts; no stored clothing in the bedroom; no dry sweeping;

and no animals in the home. The mattress and box spring should be covered with special covers. Furniture should be cleaned with oiled cloths. If possible, steam-heating units should be used rather than hot-air furnaces. If this is not possible, then all parts of the furnace system should be thoroughly cleaned (and not by the house-dust allergic person!) before turning the heat on for the winter season. Use commercially available dust-sealers on furniture and rugs. Wherever possible, use linoleum floor coverings. Bedcovers may be of cotton or rayon. Pillows should be made of Dacron or foam rubber. A filter mask should be worn when the house is being cleaned. An electrostatic precipitator or room water-filter will lower the dust-content in the circulating air.

The usual method of reducing clinical sensitivity is by hyposensitization, employing the perennial method. Some doctors hyposensitize by using the house-dust extract in special dilutions mixed with glycerin, then placed under the tongue and allowed to dissolve there.

The individual symptoms may be relieved by using the appropriate medications (Antihistamines, mild, nasal decongestants, analgesics).

HUNGER, UNUSUAL   Hunger is a complicated sensation that has physiological as well as psychological origins. True hunger should not be confused with appetite, as appetite may continue long after hunger pangs have been satisfied by the first few mouthfuls of food. Hunger pangs result from actual contractions of the stomach, causing disagreeable sensations in the upper abdomen when expected food is not forthcoming.

The level of circulating blood-sugar (controlled by insulin from the pancreas) is thought to be important in the regulation of hunger sensations. Thus, pancreatic disturbances may cause unusual hunger if excessive amounts of insulin are being secreted. Where the food that is actually digested and absorbed is inadequate, continued hunger may result. At times of increased need for foods, such as during the heavy growth-periods of teenagers, hunger is also prominent. Because of the intimate psychological relationships between hunger and appetite, however, there are many instances of chronic disease when hunger is strangely not present. Persistent unusual hunger in an individual who is consuming adequate amounts of food should lead one to suspect the possibility of intestinal parasites, such as tape worms—which are not as uncommon as generally believed.

HUNTINGTON'S CHOREA   Huntington's chorea is a familial disorder occurring during adult life, and is associated with involuntary movements and mental deterioration.

Symptoms. Involuntary movements of the face, arms, and legs are noted, usually between twenty and forty years of age; these gradually increase in severity. The patient has difficulty in writing and in performing other precise movements of the hands. The gait has a dancing quality. Together with these involuntary movements, or subsequent to them, the patient undergoes intellectual changes: his ability to remember recent and remote events, his ability to calculate, and similar intellectual capacities decline. Subsequently psychotic behavior may require institutional care.

Treatment. The course of Huntington's chorea is progressively downhill over a period of years and ends fatally. No therapy is yet available to prevent intellectual deterioration.

HYDATIDIFORM MOLE   This is a disease of early pregnancy in which the fetus undergoes degeneration and takes the form and appearance of a bunch of vesicles (grape-like structures) which are eventually aborted. The disease is much more common in people of Asian origin. It becomes dangerous only when it changes to its malignant form, chorionepithelioma; this occurs in approximately 7 to 8 per cent of the cases.

Symptoms. The womb is usually much larger than in a normal pregnancy. The patient's blood pressure rises quite rapidly, and there are severe headaches, nausea and vomiting. The patient looks puffy, and eventually bleeding starts through the birth-canal. Labor pains usually follow, the bleeding becomes worse, and the patient may notice pieces of grape-like tissue filled with fluid coming out of the vagina.

Treatment. Treatment of hydatidiform mole consists of complete evacuation of the womb, followed by thorough scraping. The patient should be checked for at least a year, with special tests to make sure that the mole does not change to a malignant chorionepithelioma. (More than one scraping of the womb may be required, and blood transfusions may be necessary.) When tests are negative on three successive occasions, the patient may be considered cured, and another pregnancy can be permitted without fear that the same thing may happen again (at least with no more chance than in any other pregnancy). In certain cases, removal of the womb (hysterectomy) will be indicated; this will depend on the patient's age and the number of children she already has, as well as on pathological examination of the mole.

HYDRAMNIOS   This term refers to the production of excessive amounts of amniotic fluid ("baby's water") during pregnancy. The patient's abdomen will look huge, distended, and shiny; her weight will increase rapidly; and there may be swelling of the ankles and high blood pressure. What is more significant, and a real cause for concern, is the fact that hydramnios is usually associated with sever-

congenital malformations of the baby.

HYDROCELE   A collection of fluid in the small sac which partially surrounds the testicle is known as a hydrocele. It may be either congenital or acquired. (When acquired, it is often the result of infection or injury.) Hydrocele causes swelling of the scrotum and is easily treated by puncture of the sac with a needle and withdrawal of the fluid into a syringe. It often recurs, however, and may require surgical removal of the sac.

HYMEN   This anatomical structure of the female consists of a membranous formation located at the entrance of the birth canal (vagina). Its location and (usually) delicate consistency have made this organ so notorious a proof of virginity that many otherwise-harmonious marriages have been doomed to failure, especially in more conservative and less informed societies, if the bride's hymen is found missing. The ironic fact is that intact state of the hymen is far from being a reliable evidence of virginity. Its size and structure may vary from a very thin and fragile membrane which easily tears upon first intercourse, to a very thick and ring-like structure which occasionally remains intact even after delivery. (The majority of hymens, however, do rupture after normal sexual relations.) It is even possible for the hymen to rupture as a result of accidents (falls, traumas in that area, etc.). Occasionally the hymen is completely closed (imperforate hymen), so that, when the menstrual flow of the female first begins, it has no way to escape, accumulates in the vagina, and causes discomfort. The cure is simple: incision of the hymen.

HYPERACIDITY   The overproduction of gastric acid by the specialized glands in the lining of the stomach results in hyperacidity. The term refers to gastric acid only, and has nothing to do with the delicate acid-base balance of the blood and other body fluids. The consumption of acid-containing foods and liquids contributes very little to gastric acidity, as the acids contained in fruits and vegetables are extremely weak when compared with the hydrochloric acid manufactured by the stomach. Acid secretion is initiated by the ingestion of food, as well as by nervous impulses from the brain. This latter mechanism is the usual cause of hyperacidity and emotional stress is therefore a powerful contributing factor. Prolonged hyperacidity may cause gastritis and in many cases is a direct cause of a peptic (gastric or duodenal) ulcer.

HYPERINSULISM (OVERPRODUCTION OF INSULIN)   This very rare, very interesting condition is due to a tumor of the islets of Langerhans in the pancreas. Fortunately, it is usually amenable to surgical treatment by removal of the islet-cell tumor.

Some persons chronically secrete excessive amounts of insulin, so that their blood-sugar is kept low (hypoglycemia) when they are not eating, and the result is an almost constant state of nervous irritability, chronic headache, and fatigue. It is important to distinguish this condition from psychoneurotic states, which will not respond nearly as satisfactorily to the diet therapy discussed under HYPOGLYCEMIA.

HYPERPARATHYROIDISM   Excessive parathyroid secretion (hyperparathyroidism) may be produced by generalized enlargement of all the parathyroid glands, or by a growth in one of them.

Symptoms. The most indicative finding in hyperparathyroidism is an elevated level of calcium in the bloodstream. It is this hypercalcemia which is the cause of the other symptoms of the condition. The increased level of calcium in the blood

298

produces a high level of calcium in the urine. When the calcium becomes too concentrated in the urine, it precipitates in the small tubules of the kidney or in the larger collecting ducts. Stones form and may cause severe pain or destruction of kidney tissue. When there is widespread calcification of the kidneys much of their function is lost and the patient develops kidney failure (uremia) often resulting in death. In hyperparathyroidism it is also common to experience abdominal pain due to ulcers of the stomach and upper intestine.

Treatment. The only known treatment for hyperparathyroidism is surgical removal of the enlarged glands. The operation is delicate but carries little risk in the hands of a skilled surgeon.

HYPERPLASTIC RHINITIS After repeated nasal infections or recurrent sinusitis, sometimes at puberty, and temporarily during pregnancy or the menses, the nasal mucosa becomes thickened. It is swollen, secretes mucus excessively, and after a time shows thickening of the bone and bony lining (periosteum). These changes in the structure of the nose cause symptoms of nasal blockage and thick, sticky discharge. Difficult to treat, hyperplastic rhinitis requires finding and successfully treating underlying causative factors for its control.

HYPERTENSION With each heartbeat, blood is thrust into the elastic artery system under pressure and, propelled by this pressure, is delivered to the capillaries and the tissues. If there is a persistent elevation of the blood pressure, arterial hypertension is present. (When pressure is taken in the arm at the level of, or above the elbow, the upper normal limits for systole and disastole may be as much as 160/90 as measured in millimeters of mercury.) If, after screening for the usual causes of secondary hypertension, the cause of elevated pressure cannot be found, the patient is said to have high blood pressure of unknown cause: essential hypertension. (Secondary hypertension is that which results from a derangement other than that of the heart or blood vessels—as from some of the primary diseases of the kidneys or adrenal glands.)

HYPNOSIS; SUGGESTION Suggestibility underlies a wide range of phenomena including autosuggestion (self-hypnosis), hypnosis, posthypnotic suggestion, and similar trance states. It involves the establishment of a dominance-submission relationship in which the submitting (suggestible) member accepts and responds uncritically to suggestions or directions.

Suggestion-effects can occur in all degrees of strength, from the casual influence of one person by another during conversation, to the deepest levels of hypnosis. Psychologically, it comprises a process of communication in which one person attempts by use of stimuli—usually verbal or symbolic in nature, but exclusive of argument or direct command—to induce an idea, feeling, decision, or action in another by circumventing the latter's critical and intellectual powers. The procedure consists basically in presentation of stimuli which build up or release attitudes, or heighten the release of responses—all with a minimum of reflective thinking on the part of the person to whom the suggestions are given.

Suggestion-effects and hypnotism have been known and practiced ever since the earliest days of tribal communities. They have been used by religious healers in all ages, from the primitive witch-doctors to the modern, faith-healing cultist. Hypnotism was first studied scientifically by Mesmer, who believed that suggestion-effects were caused by passage of a current ("animal magnetism") from one person to another. Later experiments proved that there was no such current and that the effects were due purely to psychological dominance of one person over another. There are countless methods for securing suggestion-effects and hypnosis, including fixation of the subject's eyes on a bright object held just above eye-level; giving of suggestions in a low, monotonous voice; or use of other paraphernalia which the subject has been led to believe can control him mentally. Once a subject has been hypnotized successfully, it becomes easier and easier to produce the hypnotic state with minimal stimuli.

Medical specialists have done extensive investigation of the possibility of using suggestion and hypnotism for such therapeutic purposes as pain removal. Hypnosis has been widely used during minor surgery, childbirth, and the extraction of teeth, to suggest to the patient that he will feel no pain. Such methods are effective only with subjects who are able to enter deep stages of hypnosis. There is currently considerable controversy over the value of hypnosis in psychiatric practice, and its most valuable use today is confined to the uncovering of unconscious material which had been repressed or forgotten.

Use of hypnosis for symptom-removal has been less successful, and is now generally discredited. It had been hoped that both mental and physical symptoms could be eliminated by giving hypnotic suggestions that they would disappear. Experience has shown that only those symptoms caused by suggestion can be made to disappear through suggestion. In some cases where a symptom has been caused to vanish by hypnosis, it has been found that another symptom quickly appears to take its place.

Posthypnotic suggestion involves a method for continuing the effects of suggestion after the hypnotic trance has been terminated. It was learned that, while hypnotized, patients could be instructed to carry out tasks after the trance was ended. Under the influence of such posthypnotic suggestion, the subject carries out instructions automatically, often without conscious awareness of their source. Posthypnotic suggestions have been utilized for purposes of symptom-removal by suggesting, under hypnosis, that the person no longer experience the symptom on awakening. Unfortunately, this method has proved effective only with minor symptoms caused by suggestion effects; it is totally ineffective with symptoms determined by organic causes. Posthypnotic suggestion effects can have little influence on deep emotional conflicts which underlie many psychoneurotic disorders.

Hypnosis has also been used to produce automatic writing, for the study of unconscious conflicts. While under hypnosis, the subject is given a pen and instructed to write either about anything which comes to mind, or on some particular topic. The person is told not to censor his material but to attempt to recover forgotten memories. Under hypnosis many persons can remember events which are completely beyond their recall while conscious; this seems to be evidence in support of the psychoanalytic contention that nothing in life is ever completely forgotten.

HYPOCHONDRIASIS Excessive preoccupation with one's own health and fears concerning undiscovered diseases are very common neurotic symptoms. In hypochondriacs, unconscious anxiety and emotional conflict produce psychosomatic symptoms and fears of illness. A vicious circle develops in which increasing emotional instability stimulates increasing physical disturbances, resulting in psychosomatic symptoms about which the person becomes extremely worried and anxious.

Symptoms. Hypochondriacs typically go from physician to physician, searching for someone who can discover the cause for their emotionally upsetting symptoms; they frequently undergo all sorts of unnecessary medical or even surgical treatment in an attempt to cure nonexistent physical diseases. The hypochondriac examines himself constantly to discover if any new symptoms have appeared and is usually rewarded by finding something new to worry about. If one symptom is cured, it is usually replaced by another which the hypochondriac builds up out of all proportion to actual seriousness.

HYPOGLOSSAL NERVES   The two hypoglossal (or twelfth cranial) nerves innervate the tongue. If one of these nerves is damaged, the tongue becomes wrinkled and wasted on that side. When the tongue is protruded from the mouth, it deviates to the weak side. If both hypoglossal nerves are affected, the tongue becomes wasted on both sides and its function is lost.

HYSTERECTOMY

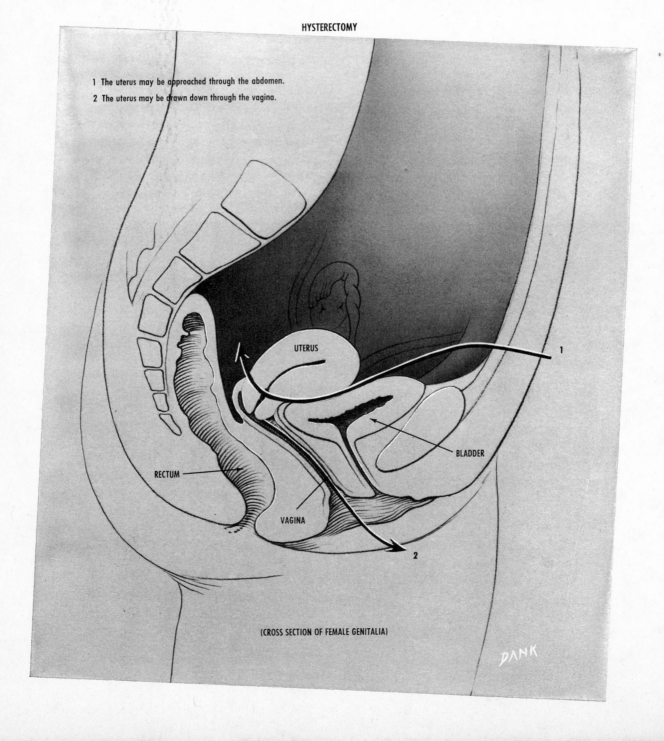

1 The uterus may be approached through the abdomen.

2 The uterus may be drawn down through the vagina.

UTERUS

BLADDER

RECTUM

VAGINA

1

2

(CROSS SECTION OF FEMALE GENITALIA)

DANK

HYPOGLYCEMIA   Hypoglycemia, which occurs when blood sugar level falls too low, is caused by too much insulin in the system. In diabetics this may be due to an overdose of insulin, too little to eat, strenuous activity, or not eating after insulin has been administered. Sugar or glucose should be given immediately if the afflicted individual is conscious and capable of swallowing. If the individual is unconscious, immediate medical attention is required.

Many people who are not diabetic suffer from mild to severe forms of hypoglycemia. Symptoms can include trembling, cold sweating, headache, feeling of faintness, fatigue, and anxiety. A sugar-tolerance test can measure the extent of the condition; a prescribed amount of glucose is taken by the patient on an empty stomach followed by analysis of blood sugar levels at stated intervals.

The prudent hypoglycemic strives to maintain a steady blood sugar level through a high protein diet. He or she eats a "good" breakfast immediately upon arising, does not skip meals or go too long between meals, if necessary having supplemental snacks such as nuts, cheese, or milk during the day and at bedtime. Discreet use of sweets may possibly be included in the diet if taken in conjunction with the necessary protein.

HYPOPARATHYROIDISM   When the parathyroid glands are absent or inactive, a condition ensues known as tetany. This is characterized by spasms of the muscles in various parts of the body, numbness of the fingers, and (sometimes) convulsions.

Although this condition may occur spontaneously, it is more frequently seen in patients who inadvertently have had their parathyroids removed in an operation for removal of the thyroid gland.

Diagnosis is made by measurement of calcium and phosphorus levels in the blood, and by the presence of clinical signs of irritability of the muscles.

Treatment. This condition does not yield to treatment by replacement of the absent hormone (parathormone). In fact, no effective preparation is available for long-term use. It is fortunate, however, that the symptoms may be well controlled by administration of calcium and vitamin D.

HYPOPITUITARISM   See SIMMONDS' DISEASE

HYPOTENSION   Hypotension, or low blood pressure, is compatible with old age. It rarely causes symptoms directly, but patients with consistently low blood pressure readings seem to complain of fatigue more than would be expected.

HYSTERECTOMY   The removal of the womb (uterus), hysterectomy may be done either through the abdomen (abdominal hysterectomy) or through the vagina (vaginal hysterectomy). Whenever the womb is enlarged or there is indication for removal of the ovaries, or when exploration of the abdomen is indicated, the abdominal route is preferred. On the other hand, when the womb is small—and especially when repair of the birth canal and the bladder is indicated—the vaginal approach is much more practical. In addition to avoiding a scar on the abdomen, a vaginal hysterectomy makes postoperative recovery of the patient faster and more comfortable.

HYSTERIA   See CONVERSION REACTION

HYSTEROGRAM (HYSTEROSALPINGOGRAM)   This is an X-ray picture of the womb and tubes, after injection into the uterus of a liquid impenetrable to X-rays. The purpose is to demonstrate whether the tubes are open or obstructed, and whether the cavity of the uterus is normal or deformed because of congenital malformations or acquired abnormalities (usually fibroid tumors).

ICHTHYOSIS   Ranging from mild, generalized dryness of the skin to severe fish-scale-patterned peeling, ichthyosis is first noted in infancy and early childhood. Not infrequently, there is some spontaneous improvement during and after adolescence. It is almost always congenital and tends to be more common in some families.

Symptoms. More prominent on the outer sides of the extremities, ichthyosis also involves the face and trunk; on the palms there is a thickening which results in exaggeration of the "lines." The upper arms and thighs often are also the site of plugging of the follicles and give the appearance and the feeling of a nutmeg grater. The condition is much less apparent and less inconveniencing in the summer months, largely because of the increase in sweating of the otherwise reduced number or the usually reduced activity of the sweat glands.

Treatment. Maintaining a comfortable environment may be difficult, but avoiding extremes of cold and of humidity is necessary, at least in the more severe cases. Bathing should be kept to a minimum; and water softeners or bath oils should be used in hard-water areas. Ordinary cold creams, liniments (lime water and olive oil combined), and mild peeling ointments are helpful. Medication with thyroid extract and vitamin A is occasionally indicated.

IDENTIFICATION CARDS Because of the severe reactions that can occur when one is exposed to a substance to which one is strongly allergic, it has been recommended that allergic individuals carry identification cards. Such cards would give the person's name and address, and supply information on blood-type, dates of vaccination, and all immunization procedures. Any previous or known drug, serum, extract, or vaccine reaction would be listed in a special space on the card. Such a card would be invaluable in emergencies when the patient's medical background is unknown. This card could save lives.

ILEITIS, REGIONAL (TERMINAL ILEITIS) The cause of this inflammatory condition which usually affects the final eight to twelve inches of the ileum (final portion of the small intestine) is not known. It is most frequently seen in young males but may affect all ages of both sexes. In the commonly-seen form of the disease there is diarrhea, cramping, abdominal pain, loss of weight, and a continued low fever. Occasionally the onset may be abrupt, with localized pain in the right-lower abdomen, and differentiation from acute appendicitis may be determined only at surgery. Many cases subside spontaneously; chronic cases, however, usually progress steadily and surgery may eventually be necessary. Because of the extensive involvement of the lining of the intestine, there is interference with the absorption of certain foods—particularly fats and certain vitamins. Diagnosis can usually be made in chronic cases on the basis of the patient's history and X-ray examination of the intestinal tract. This condition must be differentiated from functional gastrointestinal disorders, ulcerative colitis, sprue, and tumors. Rarely, tuberculosis of the intestines may cause similar symptoms.

ILEOSTOMY AND COLOSTOMY In cases where extensive portions of the large intestine or rectum have been surgically removed, the construction of an artificial anus may be necessary. This is accomplished by suturing the cut end of the bowel to an opening in the abdominal wall. The resulting opening is called an ileostomy or colostomy, depending upon whether the ileum or the colon has been brought up to the abdominal wall. An ileostomy, because of the fluid nature of the contents of the small intestine, is likely to require somewhat more care and the use of a bag held in place by various mechanical devices is often required; however, after training and experience, the individual with an ileostomy can carry on a completely normal life without fear of embarrassment. Most patients with a colostomy, because of the more normal consistency of the contained stool, are usually able to train themselves to have relatively normal bowel movements at predictable intervals and do not require any particular attachments to cover their abdominal opening.

There are thousands of patients with ileostomies and colostomies who lead perfectly normal lives. There are, in fact, formal societies of patients with such operations in most large cities throughout the country. Regular meetings are scheduled to which patients with recently acquired ileostomies or colostomies are invited. Much self-confidence is obtained through such organizations and the care and use of altered eliminatory apparatus becomes much less formidable.

ILEUM AND ILEITIS   See SMALL INTESTINE

IMMUNIZATIONS   The practice of giving live or dead material to a person in an effort to create an immunity or resistance to a particular disease is common today. Dead bacteria are given in shots to ward off whooping cough; toxoids are given to help the body resist diphtheria and tetanus; dead viruses "teach" the body to fight off poliomyelitis and measles; and finally, live viruses are used to build an immunity against smallpox, poliomyelitis, and measles. Special immunizations against rabies, mumps, Rocky Mountain spotted fever, and cholera are available, but are used only in unusual situations.

Diphtheria, whooping cough, and lock jaw (tetanus) shots are now universally given as a combined "DPT shot" beginning at one to three months of life; three of these are used, at monthly intervals. Simultaneously, or following soon thereafter, the poliomyelitis vaccines (live and/or dead) are given—and before the baby is eight to ten months old, the smallpox vaccination. Measles vaccine is given anytime after the tenth month.

A booster shot of the DPT is usually given in the second year, again at age five before school, and approximately every three to five years subsequently.

A number of recent studies show that the immunity conferred by tetanus immunization lasts longer than had been supposed. The immunity titers run high for 5 to 10 years and are easily boosted by another shot over this interval if the need arises. In 1971 the Public Health Service, taking note of findings that the need for routine smallpox vaccination for travelers appeared obsolescent because of the disappearance of the disease in modern countries, modified the every-three-years rule. Proof of vaccination on reentry to the United States is now needed only if the traveler returns from a country where smallpox has been reported in previous weeks.

There are still many ignorant, misinformed, or bigoted people who deny their children the benefit of these vaccines despite the overwhelming evidence that they suppress diseases. These people feel that they are better off getting immunity "the natural way"—which may or may not work. A child may die in the process, and countless other people are needlessly exposed.

IMPACTED TOOTH (IMPACTION)
A tooth which fails to erupt normally, and which does not assume its intended position in the dental arch, may be considered to be partially or completely impacted. A partially impacted tooth is visible, to various degrees, in the oral cavity, whereas a completely impacted tooth is not visible, and its position can only be ascertained by radiographs (photographs de-

pending upon X-rays instead of light). The completely impacted tooth may be covered only by the soft tissue of the mouth (mucosa), or it may be completely imbedded in the jawbone.

IMPETIGO   Common in childhood, but not unusual in adult life, this infectious and contagious disease is caused by bacilli (streptococci and staphylococci). It is characterized by pinhead to bean-size crusting and occasionally oozing lesions. The crusts are the color of honey, crumble easily, and can be removed with slight friction. Since the crusts themselves contain the infecting organisms, they carry the infection to surrounding areas directly and to remote areas by contact with clothes or by contact with other skin areas. The disease cannot be contracted except by direct contact with the affected part. No perceptible injury to the skin is necessary to initiate the eruption, and uncleanliness is not the cause except to the degree that washing with soap and water tends to remove, or alter the vitality of, possibly causative organisms.

In infants this disease not only has a different appearance, but also a different course. The lesions appear as blisters which often become very large before breaking; the patient is acutely ill even if no general symptoms are apparent. Early antibiotic therapy, usually by injection, is urgent and usually effective.

When the disease affects a hairy portion of the body (beard, armpits, groin), deeper infection of the hair follicles may occur together with the superficial crusting lesions, and may constitute a source of reinfection.

An impetigo-like eruption may be present as a complication of many other skin diseases, usually as a result of scratching, and appears as a diffuse crusting rather than discrete, sharply defined lesion.

Another variant of this disease occurs in the skin at the site of other draining infections; in pustular drainage of a middle-ear infection; on the eyelids and surrounding skin from "pinkeye"; or around a draining surgical wound. This condition is known as infectious eczematoid dermatitis. The yellowish crust forms in the area exposed to the infected draining exudate as a result of an allergic response to the bacteria. Curing the pre-existing infection and usual treatment with antibiotics for the skin involvement are both necessary for cure.

Treatment. Because the crusts of impetigo are the site of growth of the causative bacteria, and also because the crusts are so easily removed, wherever possible they should be removed and the remaining glistening, reddened area covered with an antibiotic ointment (bacitracin, neosporin). The crusts are formed again very quickly; it is therefore necessary to remove them repeatedly. An effective regime is to apply the ointment every two hours during the day, wiping off the crust before each application. Washing with soap and water should not be excessive lest the skin be irritated and further infection induced. In extensive cases it may be necessary to administer the antibiotics systemically, but local treatment will have to be carried out in addition. Other than the blistering impetigo of infancy, all other eruptions, whether primary or a secondary complication of other skin affliction, require the same basic treatment.

In children it is well to cut the nails short and apply the antibiotic ointment to the fingertips so that they are protected from spreading the infection. Patients should be instructed to use their own towels. Contaminated clothes should be boiled or dry-cleaned.

IMPOTENCE   Inability of the man to complete the sexual act satisfactorily is called impotence; the analogous situation in the female is spoken of as frigidity. Impotence may be caused by diseases and injuries which produce damage to the testicles. On the other hand, damage to the nerves which supply the male sex organs results in inability to achieve penile erections.

Impotence due to lack of sufficient male hormone in otherwise normal males is extremely rare. The most common cause of impotence is psychological. It is likewise the most difficult type to treat. Another common cause of impotence is diabetes. Injuries to the brain and spinal cord are less common causes.

INCISORS The incisors (literally cutters) are eight chisel-shaped front teeth, four in either arch, which are present in both the permanent and the deciduous sets of teeth. Those located nearest the middle of the face are termed the central incisors and those adjacent to these are the two lateral incisors.

INCONTINENCE When the sphincter muscle which closes the urethra is weak, torn, or damaged by disease there is an intermittent or constant flow of urine from the bladder. This is much more common in women than in men, and is prone to occur in aged people who are confined to their beds and have lost some of their faculties. In women it is commonly due to the damage of childbirth, and in men frequently occurs after surgery on the prostate gland. Treatment of incontinence is that of the disorder which causes it. Often the use of dilators will afford a good measure of relief.

INCONTINENCE (IN THE FEMALE) Involuntary loss of urine is a condition which can be classified as stress incontinence, in which the patient leaks urine with minimal stress, such as coughing, laughing, or sneezing; and urge incontinence, in which the patient suddenly feels that she must void immediately or she will lose urine. The cause of stress incontinence is an anatomical defect of the bladder and urethra, often brought about by repeated vaginal deliveries. It is corrected by surgery with generally good results. The cause of urge incontinence is infection, and requires medical treatment.

INCUBATOR Used for the maintenance of life in premature infants or those who are congenitally debilitated or severely ill, an incubator is a small glass-enclosed chamber with mechanical means for the control of oxygen supply, temperature, and humidity.

INDIGESTION Indigestion (also known as dyspepsia) is an indefinite term that is used differently by various writers. Because it is so nonspecific, it is really not useful.

The most common interpretation of the term is as a group of symptoms, including nausea, heartburn, upper abdominal pain, belching, passage of gas, a sense of fullness, and a feeling of distention.

Symptoms. Although the symptoms may be caused by organic disease of the digestive tract, they are more commonly produced by eating too much or too rapidly, inadequate chewing of the food (sometimes due to poor dentures), eating during emotional upsets or mental strain, and the swallowing of large amounts of air. Indigestion may also be produced by poorly cooked foods; those with high fat content; and—for some people—by specific items of diet, such as cucumbers, radishes, and gas-forming vegetables (beans, cabbage, etc.). Chronic gallbladder disease and allergies to specific foods can also cause symptoms.

The symptoms seem to be due to an alteration in the activeness (motility) of the digestive tract. Instead of a normal, smooth, rhythmic wave of contraction down the tract pushing the food material onward, under conditions of nervousness,

306

anxiety, fear, depression, or pain, the muscles may be inhibited or, may go into spasm and not relax. Because similar symptoms may be associated with significant organic disease, any patient who has frequently recurring episodes of indigestion should see a physician.

Treatment. The patient should eat a balanced diet. Food should be thoroughly chewed without haste, and meals should be eaten, whenever possible, in a pleasant, quiet, relaxed environment. Foods should be properly cooked, prepared in an appetizing way, and eaten in moderate amounts. Smoking immediately before meals should be prohibited. Excitement should be avoided after a meal. A number of drugs are used for indigestion, most of these act on the psychological aspects of the digestive process, but others are used to relieve spasm, reduce gastric acidity, improve bowel function, and so forth.

INFANTILE ECZEMA   Eczema in the infant results from a variety of causes. Encountered in earliest infancy is seborrheic eczema with greasy scaling of the scalp (cradle cap) and red scaly plaques of the brows, the cheeks, shoulders, back, and chest, and the skin behind the ears. Soon after birth, too, the infant is subject to eczema from excessive moisture in the groin and in the armpits. This condition, often associated with the previously mentioned seborrheic dermatitis, constitutes a hazard to the infant because of the frequent presence of yeast infestation (monilia), a condition common also to the mouth and tongue of the infant (thrush). A third type of eczema in the infant is that of allergic contact dermatitis, caused most often by the application of "baby oil," powders, medication applied for a preexisting condition; or, in older children, from contact with toilet seats (plastic) or materials in toys or clothes (dyes, finishers). This condition is no different in infants and children from that of adults

except that the causative agents are unique for the age group. Still another group of patients, small in number, suffers from eczema induced by infectious organisms which cause an allergic rather than an infecting response. The most important of the infantile eczemas is that of atopic dermatitis in which the eruption is the beginning evidence of an allergic state and indicates that the patient may require medical management of this and related conditions for some time. Eruption of atopic dermatitis is not unlike that of seborrheic dermatitis in the infant, although there is a greater tendency for the lesions to appear on the arms and legs and, after a relatively short period of time, to be confined to the bends of the elbows and knees.

Treatment. Although treatment is somewhat modified in the infant and very young child, symptomatic relief is sought through the application of soothing lotions (calamine), water-softened baths (starch, oatmeal, salts), oral antihistaminic drugs (see under specific diseases). The infant's nails should be cut short to prevent damage from scratching. Restraints (splints) are usually not necessary and are indeed often irritating to the infant in his attempts at moving about in the crib. Socks sewn (not pinned!) to the shirt will deflect some of the trauma of scratching although considerable irritation can be encountered from the rubbing of the sock.

In connection with eczema in infancy and early childhood it is necessary to emphasize the warning that these patients may not be vaccinated against smallpox. Every small damage of the skin is vulnerable to the pox inoculation, no matter what care is taken to keep the site of intended vaccination covered. Accidental inoculation into many skin areas results in a general infection. Although this disease is much milder than smallpox, it can be very serious and can involve the eyes sufficiently to cause much damage. Not only should children suffering from eczema be protected from the inoculation of smallpox virus, but their siblings or other persons in contact with them should also be removed from the environment lest accidental vaccination occur.

INFANTILE PARALYSIS (POLIOMYELITIS) "Polio" is an acute virus disease characterized by fever, headache, stiff neck and back, and sore muscles, which often leads to paralysis. Until recently there were widespread epidemics of this disease, but thanks to the polio shots and drops the disease is now rarely seen.

The poliomyelitis virus invades the nervous system, killing the nerve cells that activate muscles. Once these cells are killed, no more messages are sent to the afflicted muscle so that it stops working, shrinks, and becomes useless (atrophies): hence the paralysis. When the virus involves the nerves leading to the throat and diaphragm muscles, the victim has bulbar polio. Here the "iron lung" is often needed, because these are the muscles which control breathing; and without an adequate supply of air into the lungs the patient will die.

Treatment. Since polio is virus-caused, there is no specific treatment once the disease is established. Aspirin and hot packs are useful in easing the severe pain of the muscle spasms, and after the acute attack is over (in two to three weeks) a great deal is accomplished by the use of various physiotherapy devices to encourage weak muscles to regain strength and to reeducate good muscles to do the work of those whose use is permanently lost. Some authorities feel that at least two years are required for complete recovery, since muscle-function may be returning all this time. Later, orthopedic surgery may help a great deal to substitute good muscles for bad, and to restore function.

The best treatment would be prevention. There are two methods of protection, the Salk vaccine and the Sabin vaccine. The Salk shots contain all three polio viruses which have been killed; a basic immunizing series consists of three monthly shots with a booster several months later. The Sabin vaccine is the live virus but it has been weakened to the extent that it will not produce the disease but still allow the body to develop protective antibodies, with three types administered separately at monthly intervals; it is given orally by dropper or on a sugar cube. It is best to administer a booster of the Sabin vaccine several months later.

Both vaccines are safe and highly effective. One or both methods should be begun in the first few months of life, but all ages should be immunized. The oral type lends itself better to mass or community wide immunization methods and is, of course, not painful as the shots are.

INFANTILISM Infantilism is an inhibition or blocking of emotional development, so that the child remains at, or regresses back to, infantile patterns of behavior; for example, when a young child passes through a very painful emotional experience, it is not unusual for him to regress to infantile eating, speech, motor, and toilet habits. The child may have to be toilet-trained and taught to take care of himself once more, until he feels emotionally secure enough to develop more mature habits. Regression to infantile behavior patterns typically indicates feelings of great insecurity on the part of the child, who is symbolically asking to be loved and nurtured like a baby again.

Infantile behavior patterns tend to be reinforced and perpetuated by maternal overprotection, in which the mother spoils and pampers the child, thereby encouraging it to become neurotically dependent. Every child must learn to tolerate pain and adversity without breaking down emotionally, crying, or showing other infantile

308

patterns; children develop their personality resources and become emotionally independent only by resolutely facing and solving difficult problems of life.

Infantile regressions often occur when a new child is born into a family, partially displacing older children from parental attention and affection which they have been accustomed to receive. Such older children may regress back to infantile behavior in an attempt to regain the attentions which they have lost.

INFARCTION   See CORONARY OCCLUSION.

INFECTION   Infection is a disease process that is due to a specific organism, such as a germ, virus or fungus. The term is sometimes erroneously used to indicate invasion of the body by organisms of higher orders, such as worms, which is called infestation. A disease may be both infectious and contagious, such as gonorrhea. Infection also means the communication of disease from one part of the body to another; this is autoinfection. Thus, disease from diseased tonsils may spread through the bloodstream to joints and produce inflammatory arthritis.

INFESTATION   Infestation is the invasion of the body by organisms higher in order than germs, viruses, fungi, and similar organisms. The most common type of infestation is that by worms.

INFLUENZA   Also called the flu, grippe, catarrhal fever, this condition is a specific infectious disease of man. Acute and self-limiting in its course, the disease occurs in epidemic attacks which have sometimes acquired pandemic proportions. While epidemics recur at frequent intervals, the pandemics do so only every twenty to thirty years—the most recent having taken place in 1957 ("Asian" Influenza).

The disease is a viral infection. The first influenza virus (at present called Influenza A virus) was isolated in 1933; this was followed by the discovery of Influenza B in 1940 and C in 1949. (The three viruses have characteristics in common, but important differences do exist—particularly the fact that infection by one type of virus does not confer immunity against infection by another.) Each of these viruses can be further subdivided into strains.

Although epidemics tend to appear in the winter months, they may also occur in the summer and tend to show some cyclic tendency; thus, Influenza A occurs at about two to three year intervals and B at four to five year intervals. Occasionally both epidemics may run concurrently. Infection is transmitted through droplets and all persons are susceptible regardless of age, sex, or race.

Symptoms. Symptoms may vary widely in severity and duration. The incubation period is short (one to two days) and the onset is abruptly announced by fever, chills, headache, lassitude, and diffuse pains, particularly in the back and limbs. Respiratory symptoms are similar to those of a "cold" or upper respiratory infection, but are characteristically of much lesser magnitude than in these conditions; on the other hand, the general symptom of being "sick all over" is more prominent. Patients are usually acutely ill for no more than three to five days, the fever then subsiding gradually over several more days. Most characteristic is the feeling of prostration which follows the acute symptoms and may prolong convalescence for several weeks, particularly in debilitated patients. The disease usually runs an uneventful course and complications are rare. When the epidemic is severe, fatalities have, however, occurred—mainly because of superimposed bacterial pneumonia, which affects especially individuals suffering from pulmonary or heart diseases.

Treatment. There is no specific treatment presently available. Supportive hygienic measures and alleviation of troublesome symptoms are the same as described for other respiratory infections. In debilitated persons, a careful watch should be kept for the development of pneumonia in order to institute early antibiotic treatment.

As regards prevention, the currently available vaccines contain a certain number of strains of both Influenza A and B virus. About two weeks after administration, some defense substances (antibodies) appear, but their level in the blood is insufficient for immunity; a booster dose should therefore be given after six weeks. The protection afforded is almost complete, but only against the specific strains used, and only for a period ranging from two to eight months. Thus, booster injections should usually be administered every year before the winter season.

INGROWING TOE-NAIL   Ingrowing toe-nail occurs almost exclusively in the great toe. It is usually due to poorly fitting footwear. In the early stages, the form of the nail is unaltered, but the soft parts of the pulp are crowded over on its edge, and careless trimming of the nail on the edge predisposes to inflammation and to ulceration. Later, the edge of the nail becomes folded under, and by pressure on the pulp, aggravates the condition.

If treatment is continued for a sufficient time, a cure usually may be produced by keeping the parts free from pressure and by separating the overhanging skin from the nail either by antiseptic cotton stuffed into the chink or by drawing the skin aside with adhesive tape, while the ulcer is treated with local antibiotic powder or ointment after cauterizing its base. The nail should be cut square across the top, and never trimmed down its sides. If a rapid cure is desired, it is best to surgically remove the skin on the side of the nail affected (on both sides if necessary) by splitting the nail down the center with strong scissors, and grasping the portion to be removed by forceps.

INJECTION TREATMENT   The injection treatment of allergies refers to those methods in which doctors attempt to decrease the allergic symptoms by injections of various concentrations of the allergenic substance. These methods are known as desensitization or, more properly, hyposensitization. One cannot completely eliminate the hypersensitive state, but one can decrease it to the point where no symptoms are manifested upon exposure.

Injections may be given during the season of greatest sensitivity (co-seasonal), before the season of most difficulty (preseasonal), or all year round (perennial). (See ALLERGIES, TREATMENT OF.)

INLAY   An inlay is a filling consisting of gold, porcelain, or other materials which is constructed primarily outside the mouth and is then cemented into the prepared tooth.

INOSITOL   Little is known of the role of inositol in the nutrition of animals or man. In chemical structure it is related to glucose. It is present in large amounts in the heart, brain, and musculature of man, and also in bacteria, plants, and grains. It has been administered, together with other agents, in the treatment of several conditions, including liver disease, but the results have not been conclusive.

"INSANITY" (MENTAL ILLNESS)   Until the relatively recent development of Freudian psychoanalytic theory and modern psychopathology, little was known about the causes or nature of mental states. One of the most unfortunate historical beliefs related mental disorder to witchcraft; many of the early forms of psychiatric treatment in fact consisted of types of punishment supposed to drive out evil spirits. It is only within the last fifty years that mental cases have been moved from prisons and into the healing atmosphere of hospitals.

With this revolution in psychiatric thinking there has occurred a change in terminology: lunatic, derived from a mistaken belief that a relationship existed between lunar phases and onset of mental symptoms; insane, from the Latin *insanus*, unhealthy; and crazy have been abandoned in modern psychiatry as not being properly descriptive.

The question has even been raised whether many mental disorders are in fact diseases at all, rather than learned patterns of disturbed social relationships. During the nineteenth century determined efforts were made to discover physical causes for mental disorders, but these studies were largely unsuccessful, save in the case of organic brain syndromes such as general paresis, caused by syphilis of the central nervous system. To the present, studies of so-called "functional" (nonorganic) disorders have failed to demonstrate any cellular changes to account for the abnormal processes. Research studies in the near future may succeed in demonstrating deranged physical processes underlying some forms of schizophrenia; there remain, nevertheless, many functional disorders for which no organic basis can be demonstrated. These latter must be regarded as disorders conditioned by disturbed social relationships. It has therefore become usual to speak of personality problems, psychosocial problems, personality maladjustment, and life problems, rather than using such obsolete terms as insanity, lunacy, or mental disease.

INSECT ALLERGIES Insects can affect certain persons in a variety of ways. Some will develop asthma or allergic rhinitis on inhaling the dust from the bodies of some insects (May fly, caddis fly, housefly, mushroom fly, aphid, moth, butterfly, beetle, water flea, silkworm). Certain moths and caterpillars can cause a blister-

ing eruption on contact with the sensitive person's skin.

Symptoms. The most common reactions are produced by bites and stings. Most insects will cause a local wheal or hive at the site of the sting. Bee, mosquito, and yellow-jacket stings have caused acute urticaria. The bites of fleas, mites, and mosquitoes have caused a condition known as papular urticaria, in which there are many small, itchy, raised spots that develop long after the responsible insect is gone. Severe anaphylaxis and death are not uncommon immediately following the sting of bees, hornets, wasps, and yellow jackets. Nausea, vomiting, and diarrhea may occur after a bee string. Although not actually an insect, the spider also has been involved. A brown-spider bite is followed by local inflammation, then ulceration and scarring. The black widow spider will cause agonizing cramps and (in children) some fatalities.

Treatment. The treatment of insect allergies consists of antihistamines, epinephrine, ephedrine, steroids, calcium, and drying antiseptic lotion. After a bee sting one should flick the stinger out, rather than pull it out. As a preventative method, 5 per cent DDT or Chlordane® should be sprayed in the environmental area. Insect repellants may be used on the skin and clothing. Hyposensitization to bee, wasp, yellow jacket, and hornet venom may be necessary. Hyposensitization to insect inhalant antigens may help those asthmatics with this allergy.

Emergency treatment for an insect sting consists of applying a tourniquet (if stung on an arm or leg) above the sting-area and applying cold packs to the site. The doctor will inject epinephrine, aminophylline, and cortisone, and will give oxygen.

INSECURITY Emotional insecurity is now recognized psychiatrically as an important cause of neurotic anxiety symptoms. A person may feel insecure or deprived concerning both material and psychological needs. Most obvious deprivations concern physical needs for food, shelter, and material possessions, and thus one may feel insecure if physical livelihood is threatened.

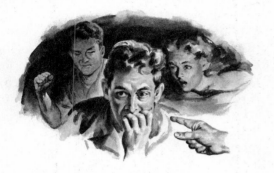

More subtle and important, however, are emotional insecurities relating to fears, threatening hostility, or loss of love. Psychoanalytic studies of early childhood indicate that each child must feel loved and wanted if he is to develop normal self-confidence and independence.

Another cause of feelings of insecurity is poor health or illness in early childhood which threaten existence. Children with delicate health tend to be insecure, fearful, and anxious. Lack of physical attractiveness, small size, or physical weakness or deformity may produce feelings of inferiority resulting in psychological insecurity.

INSOMNIA   Inability to go to sleep or easy arousal from sleep resulting in prolonged wakefulness are common symptoms of psychoneurotic states. The ability to sleep depends on progressive relaxation of all physical and mental activity; any exciting stimuli or states of emotional upset tend to interfere with normal sleep-inducing processes, resulting in wakefulness. Thus, anything which disturbs a person emotionally tends to excite him and keep him awake. Similarly, any exciting experience occurring just before bedtime tends to stimulate emotional excitement and prevent sleep.

There is no psychiatric evidence that insomnia is a cause of mental disorder; normal individuals can go without sleep for long periods with fatigue as the only undesirable effect. Worry over insomnia, rather than lack of sleep itself, stimulates neurotic emotional reactions.

Normal people vary greatly in the amount of sleep needed to control fatigue. The average person gets along well on eight hours of sleep. Older people require less sleep and can get along on as little as five or six hours if they nap or simply lie quietly, resting, once or twice during the day. Some people have learned that short naps of five or ten minutes every few hours can result in heightened mental acuity and ability to do with a minimum of sleep at night.

Treatment. The only effective treatment for insomnia is removal of the underlying causes of emotional conflict and instability. The insomniac should understand that natural sleep will occur with emotional tranquillity and relaxation. Intensive psychiatric treatment may be needed to discover the nature of unconscious emotional conflict causing prolonged insomnia.

The best way to handle insomnia on any particular night is for the sufferer to reassure himself that loss of sleep is annoying, but that nothing dangerous will happen because of it. People tending towards insomnia should make every effort not to become emotionally stimulated just before bedtime. It may help to become physically tired by taking a long walk just before bedtime, followed by a warm, relaxing bath.

Important in avoidance of insomnia is establishment of regular sleeping habits, rather than the taking of many short naps during the day on the grounds of chronic tiredness. People who are very tense and excitable should live in quiet neighborhoods and sleep in single beds. Those with insomnia should definitely avoid habit-forming sedatives; though temporary relief can be gained through use of many of these drugs, increasingly large doses are usually required with time. Toxic symptoms from over-sedation may result—a problem even more difficult to control than insomnia. The person who wishes to break addiction to habit-forming sedatives must accept a few nights of emotional anguish and nervous irritability until normal sleep habits reestablish themselves. If this cannot be achieved at home, hospitalization during the withdrawal treatment may be necessary.

INSULIN Insulin is a hormone necessary for the normal metabolism of sugar (carbohydrate). It is produced by "beta cells" present in a region of the pancreas known as the islets of Langerhans. Banting and Best, about forty years ago, first showed that the hormone (a protein) was necessary in metabolizing the sugars, glucose and dextrose. The disease diabetes mellitus is due to inadequate secretion of insulin, either in absolute amounts or relative to the body's needs. There is some evidence that many diabetics do indeed produce insulin, but that it is "bound," or in other ways ineffective.

Insulin consists of two long chains of amino acids linked together by sulfur-containing bridges, and the exact sequence of the constituent amino-acids has been determined. As a protein, insulin is digested if given by mouth and must therefore be injected. Insulin has been obtained from the pancreas in crystalline form; commercially, it is derived from both beef and pork sources.

A number of modifications of the insulin molecule have been made so that its action may be prolonged, thus avoiding the need for multiple daily injections. The physician today has a choice of several insulins, permitting him to adjust the dosage for the varying individual needs of his patients. Among the insulins now available are protamine zinc insulin, NPH (isophane), lente, semilente, ultralente, globin zinc, as well as unmodified "regular" insulin.

Every diabetic should be instructed in the proper technics of sterilization, injection, and storage of this life-saving drug.

The dosage must be tailored for the individual patient and will vary from time to time, depending on the patient's health, weight, age, the presence of pregnancy or infections, the type of diet, and exercise. The dosage schedule must be regulated by the physician because an overdose of insulin leads to hypoglycemia (insulin shock) and inadequate dosage results in poor diabetic control. In rare cases, allergy or resistance (the latter necessitating ever higher and excessive doses) has been reported.

When insulin is given to a diabetic it enhances the entry of glucose into tissue cells, enhances the burning (oxidation) of glucose to carbon dioxide and water; increases the storage of glucose as glycogen in the liver; promotes the formation of fatty acids from glucose; and is essential for normal protein metabolism. A deficiency or lack of insulin therefore results in many widespread metabolic defects.

Oral drugs have recently been introduced which are useful for some diabetics. They probably act by stimulating the diabetic pancreas to produce more insulin. However, not every diabetic responds to these agents, and in times of stress (such as after injury or during illness or surgery) insulin is the preferred agent.

INSULIN SHOCK Insulin shock refers to an abnormally high concentration of insulin in the blood. It frequently occurs when too much insulin is administered to a diabetic, or if too little food is taken with a regular dose of insulin. The excess insulin then lowers the blood sugar level and the symptoms of a severe hypoglycemic attack may result.

Symptoms. Insulin shock may be signaled by sudden weakness, tremors, and sweating. Vomiting is rare, although there may be some drooling from the mouth. Respiration and blood pressure are usually normal, and the pulse is full and bounding. The hands may tremble, and in the late stages convulsive seizures and unconsciousness may occur. In a typical case of hypoglycemia there will be no sugar in the urine. (All of the features mentioned above differ from those seen in diabetic coma, caused by ketoacidosis, a condition produced by insufficient insulin.)

Treatment. In a mild case of insulin shock, a carbohydrate such as sugar or candy may be given. A rapid improvement should result. In more serious cases it is preferable to administer a glucose solution by injection. This may be required if the individual is unconscious. Another possible treatment consists of the administration of glucagon, a hormone from the pancreas that raises blood sugar. This can be injected under the skin, in the same way as insulin.

It is important that the diabetic be taught to recognize the symptoms of insulin shock. Sugar or glucose may be carried at all times and taken if blurred vision or sudden weakness or dizziness occurs.

An identification card, stating that the patient has diabetes and takes insulin, will be helpful in case of an accident or a severe hypoglycemic reaction. Young people and children who are diabetic should be encouraged to wear a medical alert bracelet as they often do not carry identification.

INTELLIGENCE, NATURE OF

Theories concerning the nature of intelligence have recently undergone a revolutionary change and there is increasing recognition of the complexity of the problem of measuring human abilities. Earliest attempts to measure intelligence (around 1890) utilized memory tests since at that time intelligence was considered to be highly dependent upon memory. Within a short time it was discovered that memory comprises only a limited part of intelligence, and that memory tests cannot be used to predict intellectual level. The first modern intelligence test was devised shortly after 1900 by Alfred Binet, who designed age-scales consisting of intelligence test items suitable for children of different ages. The Stanford-Binet, an American revision of the original Binet scales, was the first formal test constructed of items arranged at different mental age levels and scored by an Intelligence Quotient (IQ). The Intelligence Quotient (IQ) is obtained by dividing the child's mental age in months by his chronological age. (See INTELLIGENCE QUOTIENT following this article.)

From the 1920's to the 1940's, the Stanford-Binet was the most widely used intelligence test in America, until the advent of the Wechsler intelligence scales for adults and children, developed after World War II. Both the Stanford-Binet and the Wechsler scales consisted of verbal and performance test items derived from practical experience concerning what children of different ages were able to do. Since both the Stanford-Binet and Wechsler scales resulted in one averaged IQ or mental ability score, it was believed that intelligence involved a single ability occurring in all persons to a greater or lesser degree. It was believed that this intelligence matured progressively from birth to about fourteen, paralleling the maturing of the cerebral cortex.

A new era was introduced after World War II with the invention of highly complex statistical methods for analyzing the correlations of scores on various types of intelligence tests. The new mathematical methods demonstrated that many different abilities are involved, rather than a single factor called intelligence. This newer system of classification recognizes general, group, and specific factors of intelligence. The general factor found in all measures of intelligence appears to be identical with the intelligence measured by the

Stanford-Binet and Wechsler scales. Among the group factors—less broad than the general factor, but still flexible enough to cover certain broad types of intelligence—are verbal, mathematical, memory, and mechanical factors. (The mathematical factor for example, involves the ability to handle numbers and other symbols in all kinds of mathematical applications.) In addition, there have been discovered a large number of specific intelligence factors involving very special abilities which are important in such things as musical or artistic performance.

This new concept of intelligence, recognizing that human intelligence depends upon a large number of abilities, has resulted in the construction of entirely new types of tests, measuring all the factors of ability which have been shown to exist. Thus, the whole field of intelligence measurement is far more complicated than formerly believed and requires much more extensive testing programs to measure all the newly discovered factors. The whole problem has become even more complicated since the discovery that actual performance is influenced by many other personality factors in addition to innate ability. Success in life, for example, is a product of emotional stability, level of motivation, levels of self-control, and many other specific psychosocial factors. An emotionally stable, highly motivated child of relatively low intelligence may actually perform better than a child of very high intelligence who is emotionally unstable and poorly motivated. So it is that many personality factors in addition to innate ability determine the actual level of performance.

INTELLIGENCE QUOTIENT (IQ) The IQ was devised to provide a standard method of comparing levels of intelligence among different groups of people at all age levels. It is obtained by dividing the person's mental age (as determined by his intelligence test scores) by his calendar (chronological) age expressed in months, then multiplying by 100. Thus, if a child has a determined mental age of 96 months, and his chronological age is also 96 months, his IQ is 100. The higher the mental age in relation to the chronological age, the higher the child's IQ.

Based on the distribution of IQ scores over the whole population, psychologists have developed an arbitrary system for classifying IQ levels as follows:

Classification	IQ Range
Idiot	0-20
Imbecile	20-50
Moron	50-70
Borderline intelligence	70-90
Normal	90-110
Superior and very superior	110-140
Near genius or genius	140-above

In recent years clinical psychologists have learned that the IQ should be evaluated with considerable caution in making predictions concerning a child's actual ability. Intelligence tests are highly weighted with items relating to verbal and symbol-handling abilities, so that children with high reading- and vocabulary-ability tend to get the best scores and may be overrated, while children lacking these abilities may be underrated. Though the IQ is one of the best predictors of academic success, it does not inevitably predict success in actual life situations. Clinical experience has shown that many people with very high IQ's have not been particularly successful in life, while many who are actually very successful never did well academically or on intelligence tests. Success in life is a most complex matter which is not necessarily predictable via intelligence tests.

School authorities sometimes place too much emphasis on IQ measurements when classifying children as to ability levels or predicting what they will do. Clinical psychologists have learned that success in later life may be more determined by a child's special abilities or talents, involving highly specific factors of intelligence, rather than by his average level of intelligence or IQ.

The whole field of intelligence testing is still in its infancy and many current tests are not valid for the purposes for which they are being used. They are often more valid for predicting what a child cannot do than what he can do. It is always necessary to test a child repeatedly in order to get a true estimate of his abilities, since he may not perform at his best on any one test. To get the most comprehensive measurement of a child's abilities, it is necessary to give dozens of tests measuring all known mental abilities in order to discover special talents on which later success may be based.

INTERTRIGO   This eruption occurs in areas of the body where one skin surface is in contact with an adjoining skin surface and causes a retention of sweat and moisture, affording opportunity for the skin to become macerated and for resident microorganisms to flourish. The most common areas are the under-surface of the breasts, the groin, and the armpits. In infants, the folds of the neck and the bends of the elbows and knees are often affected. These warm, moist sites are highly suitable for the growth of the causative organism, a yeast (*Monilia*), which is also the organism causing "thrush" in the infant.

Symptoms. The eruption is usually confined to the areas where skin "meets" skin and has an intensely red, moist, shiny and often dusky appearance, with a sharply demarcated border.

Treatment. Wherever possible, repeated drying of the area and avoidance of restricting and warming clothing are effective both in prevention and in implementing treatment. Drying lotions (calamine) carefully applied so that excessive amounts do not further macerate the skin may suffice in mild cases. In persistent or severe eruptions, specific antibiotic therapy (mycostatin) administered systemically or applied locally may be necessary. Solutions of Gentian Violet are also specific and effective and can be used when mycostatin is either unavailable or contra-indicated. The great inconvenience of purple staining on skin and clothes is a deterrent to the use of this otherwise excellent remedy.

INTRAOCULAR PRESSURE   The eyeball is hollow and in order for it not to collapse it must have an internal pressure in excess of the surrounding atmospheric pressure. Usually the pressure inside the eye is only slightly (10-20 mm. of mercury) above the atmospheric pressure. The pressure inside the eye arises from secretion of fluid, blood pressure, and a delicate control of the flow of fluid into and from the eye.

INVOLUTIONAL PSYCHOSIS   Involutional states occur during change of life (the climacteric), usually in the late forties in women and the late fifties in men. In women the menopause is associated with major changes both in endocrine status and in the whole plan of life, as child-bearing potential ends and age advances. The physical symptoms are less dramatic in men, but many experience progressive diminution of physical and mental vigor. In both sexes the change of life signals the end of youth and may be associated with states of melancholy.

Symptoms. Symptoms usually develop insidiously, often involving an exaggeration of prepsychotic habits of worry, peevishness, irritability, insomnia, and depression. These symptoms gradually worsen to psychotic levels of agitation and depression. The individual becomes preoccupied with feelings of unworthiness, guilt, delusions of sin, and concern over impending death. There may be blame for supposed unpardonable sins and unforgivable errors. Hallucinations are common, and many involutional patients feel that God has abandoned them and everybody is against them. Suicidal tendencies are also common as the person seeks to escape intolerable conflicts.

Involutional psychoses tend to be self-limited, about 40 per cent of cases recovering spontaneously.

Treatment. Because of the danger of suicide, involutional patients should always be hospitalized for at least an observation period, until depressive symptoms are well controlled. Twenty-four-hour nursing care is necessary to maintain nutritional status, as well as to provide constant supervision.

Electroshock therapy is rapidly effective in 80 to 90 per cent of involutional states. A course of fifteen to twenty shock treatments usually terminates the involutional state completely, and many patients show symptomatic recovery after only six or eight treatments. It is usually advisable for the patient to remain hospitalized for a week or two longer, until transient memory defects and the unnatural well-being (euphoria) resulting from electroshock treatment have leveled off.

Thanks to tranquilizers and psychic energizers, many involutional states can now be completely controlled without recourse to electroshock. However, it is safest to hospitalize potentially suicidal patients during chemotherapy because psychic energizer drugs frequently do not exert their full effects for two to three weeks, during which period it may be dangerous to leave the depressed patient unsupervised.

IODINE   The importance of the element iodine in human nutrition lies in the fact that it is necessary for the formation of thyroid hormone, which controls the rate of energy-production in the body. The human requirement for iodine is about 1 microgram per kilogram of body weight daily. The suggested daily amount, making allowance for physical activity, is 0.15 to 0.30 milligram; this amount can be supplied by the regular use of iodized salt.

Iodine is absorbed by the intestine and brought to the thyroid gland, which converts it into the active hormone. Various measurements of thyroid activity are based on iodine. Thus, one can measure the uptake of radioactive iodine by the thyroid gland. (This is increased in overactivity of the thyroid and decreased in underactivity.) In addition, the iodine in the blood, which is bound to protein and presumably represents circulating thyroid hormone, can be measured.

Iodine deficiency leads to the development of goiter, a swelling of the thyroid gland. Where the iodine content of the water and soil, and of foods grown therein, is low, the incidence of goiter is high. (However, it is important to note that goiter can be produced by factors other than iodine deficiency.) Where goiter is prevalent, cretinism, or congenital underactivity of the thyroid (hypothyroidism), is observed. Iodine is also essential for growth, normal fertility, and lactation.

Thyroid enlargement is also seen in normal situations during puberty and in pregnancy, during which time the need for iodine is increased.

Treatment. In the treatment of iodine deficiency, the mineral may be administered as an iodine solution (Lugol's solution), but the widespread use of iodized salt has greatly reduced prevalence of the typical iodine goiter seen in past generations.

IRIS, DISORDERS OF   Diseases, injuries, and abnormalities of the iris give rise to variations in its color, a loss of tissue substance, a distortion in shape of the pupil, and failure of the pupil to become smaller when bright light shines in the eye.

Absence of the whole iris (aniridia)

gives the eye a black appearance. It is associated with poor vision and frequently with treatment-resistant glaucoma.

The iris may change in color. Change of a brown iris to blue may occur because of an inflammation of unknown cause (heterochromic iritis) frequently associated with secondary glaucoma and cataract. A blue iris may become brown when a piece of metal containing iron is retained in the eye.

Blunt blows to the eye may tear the iris from its root and cause the appearance of two pupils—the normal central one and another at the edge. There is frequently blood in the anterior chamber between the iris behind and the cornea in front. If small, the rip in the iris is frequently not corrected.

Finally, in diabetes (and following closure of a retinal vein) new blood vessels may form on the iris surface and cause a glaucoma which is nearly impossible to control either medically or surgically. The disease usually involves only one eye and requires a microscope to diagnose accurately. (See also IRITIS.)

IRITIS   Inflammation of the iris may occur because of the same conditions that cause choroiditis and cyclitis.

Symptoms. The eye frequently becomes red and it aches. Vision is reduced and the iris pattern appears cloudy. The pupil at first is semidilated; later it adheres to the lens behind it and is irregular in shape.

Treatment. This is directed to dilation of the pupil by medication and treatment of the specific cause. Frequently cortisone-like eye-drops are used to minimize inflammation. Attacks tend to recur.

IRON   Iron, an essential element, is important chiefly because of its function in the blood. About two-thirds of the body's total amount of iron (four to five grams) is in heme, a compound which

when linked to the protein globin forms hemoglobin, the red pigment in red blood cells. Hemoglobin is responsible for carrying oxygen to the tissue cells and for removing waste carbon dioxide. When the body is deficient in iron, the amount of circulating hemoglobin is reduced and anemia results.

Some iron is found in certain enzymes. About 15 per cent of total iron is combined with a protein to form a storage compound known as ferritin.

The body tends to hold on to its store of iron; normal people excrete very little (about 1 milligram per day). Furthermore, most of the element released when red cells die is re-used. Under normal circumstances, little dietary iron (perhaps 10 per cent) is absorbed. However, when there is a need for iron, as in iron-deficiency anemia after a bleeding episode, the intestinal tract absorbs more iron from foods.

The recommended daily allowance for adults is 12 milligrams, with additional requirements during adolescence and pregnancy. This amount is generally supplied by a well-balanced diet. In many states of (iron-deficiency) anemia, iron is administered by mouth as ferrous sulfate and other iron-containing compounds.

Iron in excessive amounts may be toxic. For this reason medications containing iron should be kept out of reach of children.

IRON-DEFICIENCY ANEMIA IN PREGNANCY   This type of anemia is quite common in pregnancy because the baby takes up a large amount of iron from the mother's reserves in order to build up its own blood. It is therefore advisable that pregnant women, in addition to vitamin preparations, take iron pills regularly after the first three months of pregnancy. Today there are many preparations which combine iron and vitamins in one-a-day form and, if these do not suffice, supplementary iron pills must also be given. For the occasional patient who can not tolerate iron given by mouth, there are special iron solutions available by injection.

ISOMETRICS   See pages 319-22

ITCHING   Itching is not a disease but a symptom and is best described as the need to scratch to obtain relief. Itching can be elicited by a large number of substances and situations. Because so many skin conditions are accompanied by itching, it is not uncommon for a person afflicted with a skin disease to be astonished if there is none. The sensation can occur in the absence of any obvious change in the skin, as for instance in liver disease with no visible jaundice. The degree of itching and the extent of area responsive to itch stimuli vary greatly with the disease giving rise to the symptom and with the individual response of the patient. The pattern of itching is also variable. Thus patients with louse infestation produce long scratch marks of the torso; scabies infestation produces scratch marks of the papules only (and almost exclusively at night); patients with atopic dermatitis or with dermatitis herpetiformis rub the skin with the backs of the fingers and produce shiny nails (from the buffing). Itching can occur as a continuing low-grade symptom or as a crisis relieved only by gouging the skin (or by sedation). The severity of itching may far exceed the importance of the disease producing the symptom and may be the predominant factor in prognosis and treatment.

Preeminent among the several types of localized itching is that which occurs in the anus (pruritus ani), in the vulva of women (pruritus vulvae), and the scrotal sac of men. Although these conditions are extremely common, the cause is usually not known except in instances of recognizable diseases such as contact dermatitis, seborrheic dermatitis, moniliasis. Although often discouraging, treatment for relief of the itching should be pursued because continued scratching or rubbing of the site causes thickening (lichenification) which in itself produces itching.

Treatment. In addition to the specific therapy indicated for the causative disease, generalized itching is best controlled by tepid, water-softened (starch, Calgon®, oil) baths, oral antihistaminic drugs, soothing lotion or liniment (calamine), and cortisone remedies, both locally and systemically administered. When small areas are involved (eyelids, hand, foot) application of ice-cold water affords rapid relief. It should be mentioned that extremes of temperature afford relief from itching; and that it is apparent that cold applications are preferable since damage from excessive cold is less likely than damage from excessive heat (burn) in a patient already distressed and given to extremes in seeking relief. In blistering eruptions, opening the blisters under proper antisepsis affords some relief from itching. Persistent itching in the absence of a skin eruption should be investigated by the internist.

JAUNDICE   Jaundice results from the discoloration of tissues and body-fluids by bile pigment. There is a characteristic yellow color to the skin and mucous membranes. In dark-skinned individuals, the jaundice may not be readily apparent but is obvious in the white of the eyes. Occasionally, severe jaundice may cause a peculiar itching. This is usually seen in the obstructive type.

There are two major causes of jaundice: first is due to inability of the liver to dispose of the bile pigment which normally circulates in the blood—either because of increased formation of this pigment, or because of inability of the liver to secrete it into the bile (due to disease or liver-cell damage as seen in hepatitis), and the second results from a backing-up of the bile into the bloodstream due to

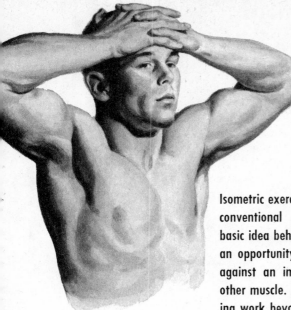

ISOMETRICS*

Isometric exercises are valuable supplements to conventional physical fitness programs. The basic idea behind isometrics is to give a muscle an opportunity to work by pushing or pulling against an immovable object or against another muscle. A muscle so engaged in performing work beyond the usual intensity will grow in strength. Research has indicated that one hard six-to-eight second isometric contraction per workout over a period of six months will produce a significant increase in the strength of a muscle.

In the exercises described in these pages, for each contraction maintain tension no more than eight seconds. Do little breathing during a contraction; breathe deeply between contractions. For the first few weeks exert only about one-half of what you think is your maximum force. If you experience pain, which indicates you are applying too much force, reduce the amount immediately. If pain continues, discontinue using the exercise for several weeks then try it again with less effort and if no pain occurs build up the effort gradually.

Starting position: Sit or stand, with interlaced fingers of hands on forehead.
Action: Forcibly exert a forward push of head while resisting equally hard with hands.

NECK

Starting position: Sit or stand, with palm of left hand on left side of head.
Action: Push with left hand while resisting with head and neck. Reverse using right hand on right side of head.

Starting position: Sit or stand, with interlaced fingers of hands behind head.
Action: Push head backward while exerting a forward pull with hands.

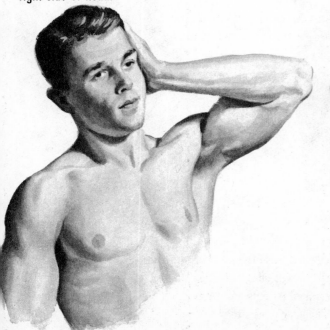

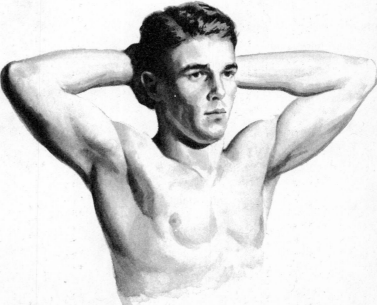

*Based on *Adult Physical Fitness* prepared by the President's Council on Physical Fitness.

320

UPPER BODY

Starting position: Stand, back to wall, hands at sides, palms toward wall.

Action: Press hands backward against wall, keeping arms straight.

Starting position: Stand, facing wall, hands at sides, palms toward wall.

Action: Press hands forward against wall, keeping arms straight.

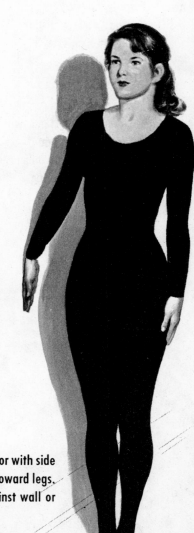

Starting position: Stand in doorway or with side against wall, arms at sides, palms toward legs.

Action: Press hand(s) outward against wall or doorframe, keeping arms straight.

ARMS AND CHEST

Starting position: Stand with feet comfortably spaced, knees slightly bent. Clasp hands, palms together, close to chest.

Action: Press hands together and hold.

Starting position: Stand with feet slightly apart, knees slightly bent. Grip fingers, arms close to chest.

Action: Pull hard and hold.

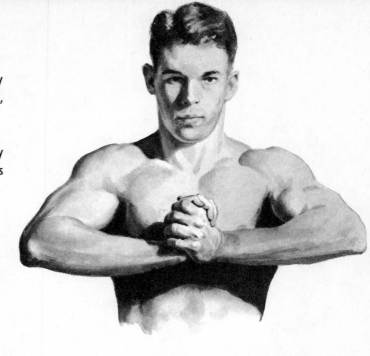

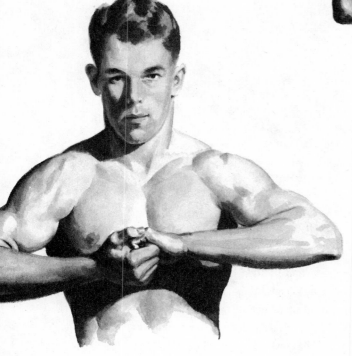

ARMS

Starting position: Stand with feet slightly apart. Flex right elbow, close to body, palm up. Place left hand over right.

Action: Forcibly attempt to curl right arm upward, while giving equally strong resistance with the left hand. Repeat with left arm.

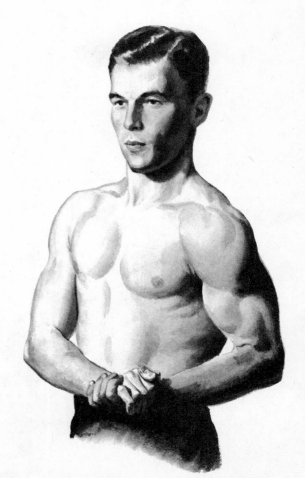

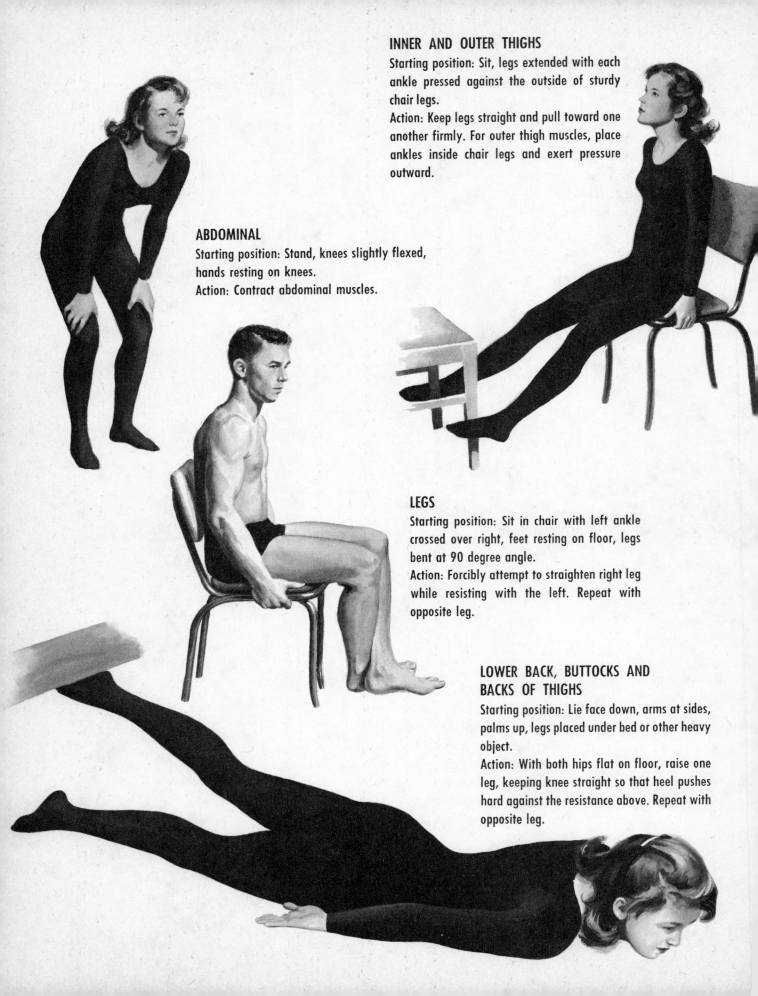

INNER AND OUTER THIGHS

Starting position: Sit, legs extended with each ankle pressed against the outside of sturdy chair legs.

Action: Keep legs straight and pull toward one another firmly. For outer thigh muscles, place ankles inside chair legs and exert pressure outward.

ABDOMINAL

Starting position: Stand, knees slightly flexed, hands resting on knees.

Action: Contract abdominal muscles.

LEGS

Starting position: Sit in chair with left ankle crossed over right, feet resting on floor, legs bent at 90 degree angle.

Action: Forcibly attempt to straighten right leg while resisting with the left. Repeat with opposite leg.

LOWER BACK, BUTTOCKS AND BACKS OF THIGHS

Starting position: Lie face down, arms at sides, palms up, legs placed under bed or other heavy object.

Action: With both hips flat on floor, raise one leg, keeping knee straight so that heel pushes hard against the resistance above. Repeat with opposite leg.

obstruction on the bile-collecting system (obstructive jaundice). The obstruction may occur in the small canals of the liver itself, or in the bile ducts. An impacted gallstone in the bile ducts or acute inflammation of the gallbladder are the two most common causes of this type of jaundice. Tumors in the region may also cause obstructive jaundice.

Treatment. Deep painless jaundice demands thorough investigation, as tumors are common causes. The bile-staining does not in itself cause any particular harm, and after the cause has been relieved the jaundice will gradually fade.

JAUNDICE OF THE NEWBORN

Half of all babies develop some yellow tinge to their skin during the first few days of life. This is due to as-yet faulty elimination of bilirubin, the breakdown-product of hemoglobin, or to put it more accurately, to the fact that the appropriate enzymes are not yet well enough developed in the newborn infant's liver to dispose of it.

What is occurring is this: Within the womb (in utero) the baby needs extra amounts of red blood cells and hemoglobin to carry the oxygen from the placenta (the organ connecting the child to the mother via the umbilical cord) to and through its body. As the fetus produces bilirubin, it crosses the placenta to the mother's bloodstream and is disposed of by the mother's liver. After birth, however, the mother's liver is no longer available; at the same time the infant needs fewer red cells and less hemoglobin. But the body mechanism for removing the hemoglobin (the liver) may still be too immature to function efficiently, and when this happens, the breakdown-product (bilirubin) may not be excreted fast enough. It is this accumulation of bilirubin in the body that may produce the symptoms of retention jaundice in the newborn infant.

In most hospitals, if a baby becomes jaundiced a blood test is taken to make sure that the level of bilirubin in the tissues does not rise above dangerous levels, since it is now known that if this does happen, irreversible damage to the nervous system may ensue, and the baby may develop cerebral palsy, or in extreme cases may die.

Jaundice, often coloring the skin a severe orange or pumpkin yellow, is found, together with anemia, in the disease erythroblastosis fetalis (Rh disease) which develops if the mother has Rh negative blood while the father is Rh positive. Retention jaundice and the jaundice of Rh disease are probably the most significant types found in the newborn. Since the term is applied to a whole class of liver disorders, however, there are many other ultimate causes possible. Thus, diagnosis of the underlying causative condition is essential in all cases of jaundice which, in a sense, is rather a symptom than a disease proper.

Treatment. Exchange-transfusion is the present treatment for Rh disease; the procedure is to transfuse normal blood into the baby's veins while its own original blood (containing the excess bilirubin) is removed.

Treatment of various other jaundices is directed to the underlying condition responsible, and must be undertaken by the physician.

JUVENILE WARTS (See also WARTS.)

The term juvenile refers to the size rather than the age of a certain type of warts. These warts, usually the size of the head of a pin, occur in groups and are found on the face and on the extremities. Because they often occur in such large numbers and in areas in which scarring would be cosmetically unacceptable, only the application of mild acids, oral medication or other non-destructive measures are suggested. Furthermore, the duration of this disorder, while very variable, is not lifelong, and the patient can be assured of the ultimate spontaneous disappearance of the warts.

KELOID This disease is the result of the depositing of an unusual form of connective-tissue fibers in areas of the skin which have been either accidentally or deliberately penetrated.

Symptoms. Firm nodules, pink in color, conforming to the site of disruption of skin and sometimes growing beyond it, appear at varying times after the injury and are accompanied by itching, burning, and sometimes pain. The nodules can become pale and occasionally even decrease in depth if not in extent after some time. Rarely does complete involution occur, and even then a marble-like disfigurement of the skin remains. The lesions have a tendency to occur in patients for varying periods of time (years) after even slight trauma (scratch). The condition also has a tendency to be more prevalent in some families, although no specific hereditary pattern has been noted. This condition can result in serious cosmetic disfigurement. Reports of malignant degeneration of the lesions are extremely rare. The disease is, however, one of great concern because of the distortion of the skin. Avoidance of all but essential surgery is a necessity of prevention.

Treatment. Repeated application of dry ice with minimal blistering, local injection of the cortisone drugs, and irradiation (radium, X-ray, Grenz ray) are among the available forms of treatment. In some instances it has been found useful to excise the involved area and administer X-ray immediately after surgery. The results of treatment vary considerably, and consideration should be given to the possibility of not treating lesions that do not constitute serious cosmetic problems.

KERATOSIS, SEBORRHEIC These

warty lesions begin to appear in middle age and usually increase in both size and number. There appears to be a familial tendency, though the lesions can be of limited number and occur in a single member of a large family.

Symptoms. The keratoses occur most commonly on the chest, face, and scalp. They first appear as small buff-colored or brown raised lesions covered with a greasy scaling and are sharply defined. They increase in diameter and in depth and often attain the size and shape of a walnut. The greasy scales peel off easily, leaving early lesions barely perceptible for a while. The large lesions often crack and bleed.

Although these lesions are almost always benign no matter what the size or duration, removal of seborrheic keratoses is necessary both for comfort and for esthetic reasons.

Treatment. Destruction of the lesions by electrocautery is both simple and effective. It is possible to destroy early lesions by repeated applications of several types of acid with little or no scarring. Surgical excision is usually not necessary.

KERATOSIS, SENILE Occurring most commonly in people past middle age, these lesions develop on areas of skin exposed to the sun (the face and back of the hand) and are often accompanied by other evidence of actinic change. They are precancerous, and if left untreated for a sufficient length of time undergo malignant degeneration. Because they so invariably do become cancerous, they are considered by some to be true cancers even in their earliest stage. Aging of the skin, whether because of occupational exposure to the sun as encountered by farmers and sailors, or because of inherited disease (xeroderma pigmentosum, hydroa aestivale), is an important factor in producing this condition in patients not otherwise aged.

Symptoms. The lesions are grayish black, small, sharply outlined flat papules, often covered with a dry tenacious scale. There is some reddening of the surrounding area which varies and gives the lesion a different appearance from time to time. Some early lesions remain undefined, red, scaly and unpigmented, making diagnosis more difficult. Even in a single area, the size of the lesions may vary greatly.

Treatment. Destruction by electrodesiccation is the treatment of choice. When removal of a lesion for biopsy study is indicated, surgical excision may be more practical. Repeated biopsy study is usually neither practical nor necessary when many such lesions are removed from a single area, but should be done when possible malignant degeneration is suspected.

KIDNEY   The kidneys are among the most important organs in the body; without them life is impossible for more than a few days. They are set deep and high within the abdomen, lying against the large muscles of the back on each side of the spine. They are shaped roughly like beans (hence the term kidney beans) and are normally about the size of a clenched fist.

The kidneys are essentially filters which remove poisonous substances from the blood and carefully regulate the amount of minerals, acids, and certain food substances in the bloodstream. For example, they keep the blood just slightly alkaline through their ability to transfer acid into the urine. They very efficiently prevent the collection of too much urea and other nitrogenous products in the body and carefully regulate the level of calcium, potassium, and sodium. They also permit the excretion of certain substances such as sugar only when its level is too high in the blood.

The actual filtering apparatus of the kidneys is known as the glomerulus. Blood is brought to this structure by an artery which divides from the abdominal aorta and breaks into many tiny branches. The first step in urine formation is the collection of a filtrate from the blood. This is then passed along a system of tubules which twist and turn through the inner portion of the kidney. During the passage of the blood-filtrate through the tubules, a good deal of water is extracted and substances which the body desires to dispose of are concentrated and eventually gathered in larger collecting ducts. The urine is next directed into a funnel-shaped structure (the kidney pelvis), from which it is passed down the ureters into the bladder, and from there through the urethra to the outside.

KIMMELSTIEL-WILSON SYNDROME
This syndrome is a type of kidney disease associated with diabetes mellitus. There is a characteristic abnormality seen in the filtering portion (glomerulus) of the kidney tubule when examined microscopically. The condition, when present, is usually found in individuals who have had diabetes for many years. Leakage of protein from the serum into the urine (proteinuria) is characteristic of this disease. There may be high blood pressure and distinctive blood-vessel disease in the retina as seen on ophthalmologic examination. Advanced cases may show an accumulation of nitrogen compounds in the blood (uremia). The disorder is also known as diabetic glomerulosclerosis.

KINSEY STUDIES   Alfred C. Kinsey, a zoologist, in collaboration with other researchers at the University of Indiana, did two pioneering studies in sexuality in the human male (1948) and female (1953). The studies established maximum male sexual performance at around age 18 and its age-related decline in the decades thereafter. The scholarly tone and detached attitude toward sexual behavior helped set the stage for the more intimate clinical studies of stimulation and orgasm made by William H. Masters and Virginia E. Johnson (1966).

KLEINFELTER'S SYNDROME This is a condition characterized by small testes and various degrees of eunuchoidism. In almost all cases spermatozoa are absent in the ejaculate, and there is some enlargement of the male breast. In recent years it has been discovered that men with this condition have a cell chromosome pattern similar to that seen in the female. In other respects most of them appear to be normally masculine.

KNOCK-KNEES These disorders in leg growth and development are rarely present at birth and usually are not manifest until the child walks. When either condition is mild, the child may be expected to outgrow it. If it is progressive, however, orthopedic attention is required. The child's diet should meanwhile be checked to make sure that he is receiving adequate milk and vitamin D, since these deformities are commonly seen in rickets, a disease due to vitamin D deficiency. Since these conditions are rarely painful in childhood, treatment is directed toward prevention of disability in adult life. Shoe wedges, manipulation and massage, and occasionally braces may be necessary to treat these deformities.

LABIA These are two pairs of folds of skin, one inside the other, at the entrance of the female birth canal (vagina). The inside pair (labia minora) is smaller than the outside pair (labia majora) and, unlike the latter, has no hair.

LABOR Active labor consists of regular contractions of the pregnant womb (uterus), which cause the mouth of the womb (cervix) to open wide and allow delivery of the baby. These contractions are felt by the mother as labor pains and should not be confused with the irregular, short, and slightly uncomfortable pains which the mother experiences for several weeks before term. These latter are known as Braxton-Hicks contractions and may be the cause of false labor; they are useful in preparing the cervix for active labor, but do not accomplish any dilatation of the cervix. When contractions are at regular intervals of fifteen minutes or less, and the mother starts to feel them as labor pains, then she enters the phase of true labor; the doctor should be notified and/or the patient taken to the hospital.

The duration of labor varies considerably, depending on the number of previous pregnancies and on the constitution of the individual patient. On the average, it lasts fifteen to eighteen hours in patients laboring on their first baby, and approximately six hours less in patients who have already had one or more children. For practical purposes, the entire length of labor is divided into three stages; namely:

The first stage of labor starts with the onset of regular uterine contractions and ends with the complete dilatation of the cervix. This covers about 90 per cent of the total length of labor. During the first stage, the labor pains become gradually stronger, longer, and closer together, and the patient requires drugs for relief. The patient may notice pink vaginal discharge, which is mucus from the mouth of the womb mixed with some blood. This is known as bloody show. The bag of waters (membranes) may or may not rupture during this stage.

The second stage covers the period between complete cervical dilatation and delivery of the baby. In patients having their first child, this stage lasts one to two hours; while in subsequent pregnancies it only lasts twenty to thirty minutes. During this stage the patient experiences a bearing-down sensation and she pushes voluntarily, using her abdominal muscles; this often results in precipitous uncontrolled delivery. When time allows, the patient should be given some form of anaesthesia, and the baby delivered under the control and with the help of the obstetrician.

The third stage of labor starts after the delivery of the baby and ends with the delivery of the afterbirth (placenta). This phase is approximately fifteen minutes in duration.

Under certain circumstances labor is induced artificially (induction of labor) for the benefit of the baby, the mother, or both. Induction of labor may occasionally be accomplished by the administration of enemas and castor oil, combined with stripping the membranes from the cervix. The only reliable means for induction of labor, however, are the so-called "oxytocic drugs"—hormones produced by the pituitary. When administered to the pregnant patient, these cause regular uterine contractions. These drugs are administered by continuous intravenous drip, diluted in large amounts of fluids. Intramuscular administration of oxytocic drugs should be avoided before the delivery of the baby.

In some instances labor starts normally, lasts for several hours, and—for a variety of reasons—may then slow down. (This is called uterine inertia.) In these cases the doctor will either resort to stimulation of labor with the same oxytocic drugs, or to caesarean section, depending on the individual case.

LACRIMAL GLAND   Tears are mainly formed by the lacrimal gland located in a depression in the front, upper, and outer portion of the bony orbit. Tears flow over the surface of the globe to the inner portion, where tiny openings are located in both the upper and lower lid. These openings lead to a duct which carries tears to the nose.

LACTATION   Lactation, the secretion of normal milk from the mother's breasts, starts two to three days after the delivery of the baby. At this time the mother notices her breasts becoming enlarged and

THE LACRIMAL APPARATUS

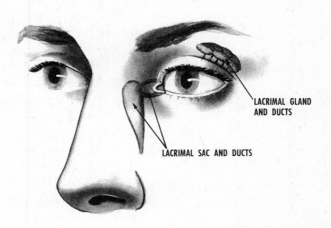

LACRIMAL GLAND AND DUCTS

LACRIMAL SAC AND DUCTS

The lacrimal gland secretes tears which are poured over the eyes through small ducts. The tears collect in the inner corner of the eye and pass through two small openings into the lacrimal ducts and into the lacrimal sac. The sac empties into the nose.

painful; milk may leak from the nipples.

Large amounts of nutritive substances and antibodies are secreted in the mother's milk. The diet of the lactating mother should therefore be improved in quality and quantity (about 1,000 more calories will be required in her daily diet). Drugs, alcohol, and other toxic substances are promptly secreted in the milk, and the mother should either avoid them or—if unable to do so—should stop nursing the baby.

Menstrual periods are usually absent for several months during lactation. Ovulation can occur however, and pregnancy may follow without a preceding menstrual flow; this creates difficulties in the recognition of early pregnancy, and not infrequently the mother becomes aware of a new pregnancy only when the baby starts moving. When this happens, nursing should be discontinued.

LARGE INTESTINE   The large intestine, or colon, is joined to the ileum (the final portion of the small intestine) at the cecum, a blind pouch to which the appendix is affixed. The colon is composed of four parts. The first portion, or ascending colon, originates in the lower right abdomen and rises along the right flank to just under the liver. The transverse colon crosses the upper part of the abdomen and makes a sharp turn downward, becoming the descending colon. Along the left flank, the descending colon dips into the pelvis and is then called the sigmoid (S-shaped) colon and ends at the rectum.

The main functions of the large intestine are storage of fecal material and the absorption of water. In this context it should be noted that the concept of intoxication due to poisons being absorbed through the wall of the colon has been amply disproved. Cleansing enemas are accordingly seldom required in the normal, healthy individual, and may in fact be harmful if resorted to frequently. The lining of the colon contains many mucus-secreting cells which aid in lubricating the fecal material and protecting the lining from excess roughage.

A condition called megacolon (large colon) is occasionally seen, in which the large intestine may attain a huge size due to a congenital defect in the nerve supply. Unlike the small intestine, the colon is relatively prone to tumors often arising from small polyps which may extend from the wall of the organ. Most authorities agree that polyps, whenever discovered, should be removed for this reason. Mucous colitis, or irritable colon, is a fairly common, annoying, but not serious condition which is discussed under COLITIS. Diverticulitis is another relatively common affliction of the colon and is described under a separate heading. Ulcerative colitis, a much more serious disease, requires early recognition and careful treatment. It is likewise discussed more fully in its own entry.

THE COLON

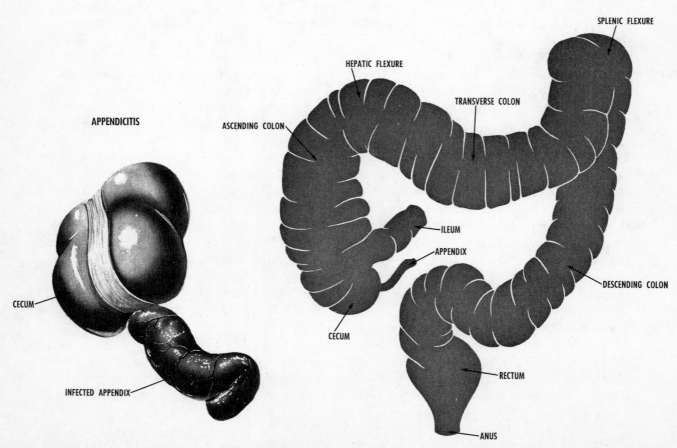

APPENDICITIS

CECUM

INFECTED APPENDIX

HEPATIC FLEXURE

SPLENIC FLEXURE

ASCENDING COLON

TRANSVERSE COLON

ILEUM

APPENDIX

CECUM

DESCENDING COLON

RECTUM

ANUS

LARYNGITIS   This common term may be defined as inflammation of the larynx (voice box), occurring most commonly as part of, and in the course of, upper-respiratory infections. It may be caused by bacteria, viruses, or an allergy. The main symptom is change of voice, ranging from hoarseness to severe degrees of incapacity to produce sounds. Breathing becomes more difficult and the obstruction may lead to sudden suffocation (asphyxia). The rest of the symptoms will depend on the other organs involved (nose, throat, glands). The laryngeal symptoms are more dramatic and develop faster than those in the other areas because of the relative smallness and unusual irritability of the larynx, especially in infants. The manifestations of diphtheric laryngitis are essentially similar to those caused by other bacteria or even viruses, and may be differentiated only by direct laryngeal examination and study of the secretions.

Another form of acute laryngitis is croup. This condition is due to an acute spasm of the laryngeal muscles. Its symptoms are the sudden onset of harsh, metallic cough (without warning or preceding symptoms, frequently at night) and alarming "rattling" sounds (stridor) during inhalation, accompanied by severe shortness of breath. The disease-picture is very dramatic, but can be quickly controlled by steam inhalations or induced vomiting, the patient being completely relieved the following morning. This should be clearly differentiated from the mild shortness of breath which is part of the symptomatology of common laryngitis, but which may progress (obstructive laryngeal dyspnea) to irreversible asphyxia and require an emergency operation.

Other forms of laryngitis are those chronic forms due to continued irritation (smoking, air pollutants) or caused by specific diseases such as tumors, tuberculosis, syphilis, or nerve diseases.

Treatment. In most cases common acute laryngitis requires only the hygienic measures described for other upper-respiratory infections. If the cause is bacterial, the proper antibiotic should be given. The important exception is diphtheria, which requires quick administration of diphtheria antitoxin if the patient has not been previously vaccinated. If a picture of breathing-difficulty (obstructive laryngeal dyspnea) begins to develop, regardless of cause (aside from the classical croup), an immediate tracheotomy should be performed (see TRACHEOTOMY).

LARYNGOSPASM   Laryngospasm, or spasms of the muscles of the larynx, occurs chiefly with the use of some kinds of anesthesia in the operating room (where it is readily taken care of) and in children between one and six years of age. In these latter cases the child typically awakens from a sound sleep with respiratory difficulty, although there is no immediate previous history of a cold or fever. Reassurance and deep regular breathing may relieve the problem. Breathing oxygen mixed with air may stop the attack. The inducing of vomiting has been used successfully for this problem, but is probably dangerous since there is a chance of sucking in vomited material.

LARYNX   The voice box, or larynx, is composed of cartilages held together by ligaments, muscles, and strong sheets of fibrous tissue. It can be felt in the front part of the neck. The most prominent bulge in the neck—approximately where the knot of a man's tie is—is the "Adam's-apple": the prominence of the thyroid cartilage of the larynx. Just below this is the only complete ring of the larynx, the cricoid cartilage. (Within the thyroid cartilage, near the Adam's-apple, is the attachment to the vocal cords.)

The real functions of the larynx are threefold: (1) as a sphincter—an organ of closure—to prevent fluids and food from entering the lungs; (2) as a rigid structure to permit and assure an open pathway for breathing; and (3) as a voice-producer. The intricate workings of the larynx are indeed wonderful; when not functioning well, however, the larynx gives rise to two recognizable and common symptoms: hoarseness and difficulty in breathing.

LARYNX, ABNORMALITIES OF THE
The most common problem under this category occurs in children under two years of age. The cartilages of the larynx —particularly the epigottis—are frequently very soft and flabby (laryngomalacia). These soft cartilages may be drawn inward on inhaling, thus producing difficulty in breathing. The child usually outgrows this problem by the age of two. Webs, cysts, and vascular rings are less common, but when found can often be relieved by surgery.

LARNYX, INJURIES OF THE, AND FOREIGN BODIES IN Trauma is a general term referring to injury. In its broad sense this can, for example, be injury from a cold or from tobacco. (Trauma can be caused by infections like the common cold.)

In a limited sense, trauma refers to an actual physical blow causing injury. This type of direct trauma to the larynx, and the resultant scar it can form, may be a cause of hoarseness. Direct blows to the larynx are dangerous and can break the cartilage. If the cricoid cartilage is broken, or if sufficient swelling and hemorrhage occur, respiration can be severely compromised, resulting in death.

Foreign matter sucked into the larynx can also obstruct the airway or produce swelling and hemorrhage. After an initial period of irritation and coughing, the foreign body may cause no further outward symptoms, but days or weeks later cause serious illness. Furthermore, suction of a foreign body into the lungs can cause

pneumonia or blockage of the main bronchus.

Treatment. Location of the foreign body by examination and X-rays, and removal by special instruments, is now performed by both ear-nose-and-throat specialists and by chest specialists. If a child is suspected of having inhaled foreign materials—anything from buttons to beans —he should be examined by a physician. The fact that the child has stopped coughing is no excuse for neglecting the possibility of retained foreign material.

LARYNX, TUMORS OF THE There are both benign and malignant (cancerous) tumors of the larynx; the vast majority manifest themselves through the symptom of hoarseness. Therapy for benign tumors consists of removal of these tumors and of voice-rest. Some benign tumors called papillomas are frequently multiple and tend to recur after removal, although not so readily once adolescence is past. One very common cause of hoarseness results from vocal nodules caused by vocal abuse. These nodules are not true tumors, but are called tumors for the sake of convenience. With proper use of the voice and removal of the tumor, the problem can be solved.

Malignant tumors, cancer, have only one early symptom: hoarseness. Pain is not an early manifestation.

The diagnosis can be made by your family physician or by an ear-nose-and-throat specialist. Mirror inspection of the larynx, viewed indirectly from the mouth, clearly reveals lesions of the vocal cords, but a small piece of tissue is necessary for absolute diagnosis. This is called a biopsy, and is most often taken with a special forceps through a long, hollow, lighted tube. Brief hospitalization is usually necessary for this procedure.

Treatment. Early cancer of the larynx is curable in a high percentage of people. In very early cancer of the vocal cords, radiation or surgery can cure in 85 per cent of cases. In view of the possibly dangerous nature of the symptom it is inexcusable for the patient to neglect hoarseness.

The position and/or size of tumors causing hoarseness may be such that airway obstruction also occurs. The loud objections to surgery on the part of some patients with cancer of the larynx who refuse surgery because they fear voice-loss are foolish; in most cases the size of the tumor and the swelling associated with it will eventually necessitate tracheotomy, and tumor-plus-tracheotomy will cause a loss of voice in any event. The patient will have lost valuable time and perhaps sacrificed his life for no good reason.

LEFT - ARM - AND - SHOULDER - PAIN

Left-arm-and-shoulder-pain is a common symptom of coronary artery disease. If the source of the pain is the heart, there is never any spot-tenderness of the shoulder or arm, for the pain only seems to reside in shoulder, arm, or fingers. Movement of the arm or shoulder neither augments, relieves, nor alters heart pain that happens to reflect itself in this area.

When there is an oxygen deficiency at endings of the sympathetic nerves of the coronary arteries, these nerves are aroused to send out pain impulses. The impulses are carried through to collecting stations (ganglia) near the upper five thoracic ribs, a few inches from the spine, and even to ganglia in the neck. From these ganglia, the impulses then escape by pathways near those used by the shoulder and left arm on their way into the spinal cord and thence to the brain.

Apparently this side-by-side position of the sympathetic pathways leading from the arteries of the heart and the peripheral nerve pathways leading from the arm and shoulder may have something to do with the fact that pain originating in the coronary vessels of the heart seems to originate in the arm and shoulder.

LENS   The lens of the eye is located behind the pupil and is held in position by fine fibers (the zonule) which are inserted into the ciliary body. The lens is transparent and, because of varying tension exerted by the zonule through connections with the ciliary body, varies in focusing power so that the normal eye forms clear images for objects located both near to and far from it (accommodation). The lens is formed by enclosure of a tissue which forms skin elsewhere in the body and is secondarily involved in some skin diseases. Like skin, it forms new layers throughout life, but unlike skin, it does not cast off the old ones; rather, these become concentrated in the center of the lens. These older fibers lose elasticity and their accumulation results in a gradual loss of focusing power (presbyopia), so that in about the forty-fifth year of life glasses may be necessary for clear close vision.

Sometimes, in cataracts, the loss of clearness of the hard fibers in the center of the lens results in a marked increase in total focusing ability, so that the eye becomes nearsighted and it is possible to read without glasses late in life. This "second sight" of the aged, however, is associated with decrease of vision for distance and is frequently not permanent.

LEPROSY   Known for over 2,000 years, leprosy is a disease of high incidence in the tropics, but is also present in many countries of the temperate zone. In the continental United States leprosy has been contracted occasionally in the southernmost states (Florida, Texas, Louisiana, and Southern California). Cases reported elsewhere in the United States have almost always been contracted in a tropical or sub-tropical area.

Commonly acquired in childhood and adolescence by natives of those areas of the world in which the disease is endemic, it is usually also acquired by adults whose childhood was spent in non-leprosy areas.

332

Both sexes are affected, though males appear to be more susceptible to the acute (lepromatous) type.

The mode of transmission of the causative organism, *Mycobacterium leprae* (Hansen's bacillus), is probably through the skin or mucous membranes of the nose or throat. What determines the acceptance of the disease by an exposed person, or the type of disease acquired, is not known. Classification of the disease is often difficult, many cases belonging to an indeterminate or borderline group. More concise are the lepromatous (acute, infectious) and tuberculoid (usually non-infectious, less actively progressive) types.

Symptoms. These vary greatly, depending on the type and stage of the disease. Thickening of the skin, either in the form of small nodules or large plaques, or as a diffuse generalized condition, is common to all forms of the disease—as is involvement of the mucous membrane and septum of the nose. Ulceration, especially of the mucous membranes, produces great deformity and interferes with function. Nerve involvement results in loss of sensation and loss of sweating of the area, and finally in actual atrophy and absorption of tissue (especially of the fingers and toes).

Treatment. The heretofore universally used chaulmoogra oil has been replaced with several drugs often used in combination (sulfones, para-aminosalicylate, streptomycin). The cortisone drugs are probably very effective in some types and stages of the disease, and are especially useful for at least temporary relief in the acute lesions of the eye and in the lesions based on an acute allergic response.

LEUKEMIA This distressing condition is a cancer of the white blood cells, and when found in children is almost universally fatal, the average length of life after onset being only six months. There are different forms of this disease, depending on the type of white cell involved.

Symptoms. The symptoms of leukemia are variable, but obvious to the pediatrician. The disease has been known occasionally to follow on the heels of a simple respiratory infection or bout of the flu. A blood test revealing abnormal types and numbers of white cells, and usually a severe anemia, directs the physician's attention to this disease. A specimen of the patient's bone marrow is obtained, usually by suction (needle aspiration), from which a more definitive diagnosis can be made.

The most difficult task for the doctor and the parents of the afflicted child is to decide how much treatment, testing, hospitalizing, and transfusion of blood should take place. Most authorities are of the opinion that the child should remain at home as much and as long as possible.

Treatment. At the present time the prognosis in leukemia is admittedly poor, but there has been some reason for encouragement because of recent progress in chemotherapy. Remissions are now more common, with the child able to lead a normal life; there is, in fact, an increasing number of children who, with treatment, live five years or longer. In addition to chemotherapy (which admittedly is more successful with adults than with children—the underlying principle being control of the growth-rate of white cells by means of various drugs) it is now believed that some forms of leukemia may be viral in origin, and if this is true, a vaccine becomes a possibility. There are even a few cases on record where massive blood transfusions (from a member of the same family with the same blood type) have produced apparent "cure"; but it is much too soon to tell whether the improvement is more than a temporary remission. All in all, while the eventual outcome of leukemia is today almost universally fatal, the medical profession believes that to prolong the patient's life is important because of the imminent possibility of new scientific discoveries, hence of new solutions. A further argument for treatment with drugs is that in the usual form of the disease, acute lymphocytic leukemia, these drugs sometimes do serve to make the patient more comfortable.

LEUKORRHEA   This condition represents excessive vaginal discharge, whitish or yellowish in color, and is due to infection of the vagina by trichomonas or monilia organisms. Treatment consists of vaginal or oral medications and vaginal douches. (See VAGINITIS.)

LICE   See PEDICULOSIS

LICHEN PLANUS   Lichen planus is of unknown causation but is thought to be related to stress, emotional crises, or worry. Lichen planus can occur as an acute, widely disseminated disease including lesions of the mucous membranes of the mouth and eyes; or it can appear gradually, persist, and become a thickened, horny and plaque-like condition usually of the shins. Occasionally drugs (most notably Atabrine®) produce this type of eruption.

Symptoms. The lesions consist of shiny, octagonal-shaped papules, purplish in color and with slightly depressed centers. They usually remain discrete, although they are often arranged in circles or parts of circles along a line of trauma (scratch or burn) and are most commonly found on the wrists, the flexor surfaces of the arms and legs, and the mucous membrane surfaces (mouth, eyelids, penis, vulva). Itching is both severe and persistent. Other forms of the disease include blistering, hyperpigmentation and atrophy. Although the incidence of recurrences is high, the disease constitutes no threat to the general health other than the unsightly appearance and the disability caused by the itching.

Treatment. The cortisone drugs are effective in some cases, and the older remedies (bismuth, arsenic) are worthy of trial in the absence of more specific therapy. Sedation, tranquilizers, relief from stress. and other supportive measures should be used. Local treatment consists of soothing lotions but they are of limited value except in the hypertrophic cases.

LIGAMENTS AND SPRAINS   The ligaments are bundles of tensile connective tissue specifically placed between adjacent bones. At the joints the ligaments are part of the joint capsule. The ligaments maintain the proper anatomical arrangement between the bones, acting in some instances as protective struts to limit unwanted motion and in others as guy-ropes transmitting force from one bony part to another.

A sprain is an injury to a limb in which ligaments and other soft tissues are torn. Marked pain and swelling are usually associated with it.

Treatment. The object of sprain-treatment is to control the distressing pain and swelling, and to allow the torn structures to heal precisely. The sprained limb should be put to rest, and an icebag applied locally in an attempt to prevent further swelling; an elastic compressive dressing may be applied to provide temporary support and to control the pain.

These home measures will in most cases be adequate treatment for minor sprains, but medical attention should be sought if pain and swelling persist for more than a few hours. A severe sprain may require taping, compression dressings, or plaster immobilization to allow adequate healing. Occasionally the tear of the ligaments may be sufficient to warrant surgical repair. Untreated sprains lead to unstable and weak joints which are then subject to repeated sprains from minor damage which would not be capable of injuring intact joints.

"LIGHTENING"   See ENGAGEMENT

LINGUAL TONSILLITIS   The part of Waldeyer's ring situated near the base of the tongue can become infected, although less frequently than the larger, deeper-set palatine tonsils. Treatment is similar to that for infections of the palatine tonsils.

LIVER   The largest organ in the body, the liver is situated mainly in the right-upper portion of the abdominal cavity, but does extend into the left upper quadrant as well. Because of the dome-like shape of the diaphragm (the muscular partition between the chest and the abdomen), the liver is normally protected by the lower ribs; in healthy individuals it is seldom felt on abdominal examination. The liver has many functions and is indispensible for life. Fortunately it has a great capacity of regeneration, and liver failure occurs only after an overwhelming infection or repeated injury. Among its more important functions are storage of digested food-products and energy; the manufacture of proteins; the storage of certain vitamins (the normal liver can store more than a year's supply of vitamin B_{12}); the production of bile from the breakdown products of the red blood cells; the manufacture of antibodies; and the detoxification of many harmful substances which may occasionally be present in the bloodstream. Its major functions are therefore storage, synthesis, and detoxification. The more common disorders of the liver include hepatitis, cirrhosis, and subsequent jaundice.

LIVER SPOTS   These flat, discrete and confluent lesions of excessive pigmentation occur most commonly in women, on the face, along the margin of the brow and on the cheek bones. They are sometimes so joined together as to seem to form a rim around the eyes. The eruption neither resembles the liver nor is it caused by diseases of the liver. The most usual condi-

tion alleged to precede this eruption is pregnancy. Many cases are also thought to be due to some functional ovarian disturbance, the exact nature of which is not known.

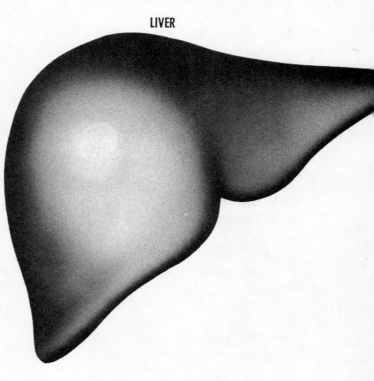

LIVER

   Treatment. Several types of local bleaching applications designed to interfere with the production of pigment or to alter already existing pigment are commercially available and may be of some benefit. Peeling of the affected sites with acid, or with blistering dry ice, or with abrasives like brush-planing, can be tried. Great care must be taken that the irritation from treatment does not in itself induce further hyperpigmentation and therefore worsen the condition.

LOBECTOMY   Lobectomy is surgical excision of a lung lobe. This procedure is indicated for destructive diseases, tumors, or chronically infected areas of the lung.

LOCHIA   This is a term applied to the vaginal discharge that follows delivery. For the first two to four days after delivery, the lochia are bloody, becoming pink for the next few days, and finally turning whitish.

LOCKJAW (TETANUS)   Lockjaw is a fatal disease caused by the toxin produced by bacteria introduced into the body through a break in the skin, usually a deep wound (like a nail-puncture). Although it is now rare, as compared with the early part of this century, it can still be fatal unless treated promptly and efficiently. It is relatively more frequent in children because they are more prone to puncture wounds. A newborn baby may acquire this disease if his umbilical cord is tied off with unsterile or dirty material.

Symptoms. Within a few days after tetanus germs have lodged in the body through a puncture wound, there appears some muscle stiffness, especially about the neck. Soon the patient cannot open his mouth, is apt to develop localized muscle spasms, and may then go into convulsions or coma.

Treatment. Treatment of lockjaw must be prevention. Once the active disease is contracted it is difficult to treat—in spite of antitoxin which neutralizes the toxin which produces the spasms. When treatment is started late, the death-rate is high.

It is simple to have basic tetanus shots in the first year of life; later on, all that is necessary at the time of a wound or cut is to give a "booster" of tetanus toxoid.

If a child has not been immunized, a doctor should always decide—even in minor injuries—whether antitoxin should be given.

LOW-BACK PAIN   Low-back pain is one of the most common complaints of mankind. It is probably related to man's erect posture since the four-legged animals rarely develop spinal difficulties. The terms lumbago and sciatica are commonly used to describe the clinical syndrome. Lumbago denotes pain localized to the low back area, and is increased by motion of the back; sciatica refers to acute pain in the back, radiating down the back of the leg along the distribution of the sciatic nerve.

Symptoms. A low-back syndrome may develop spontaneously or may follow an injury. The patient may state that his back "gave out" after he bent down to pick up a heavy object. Sciatic pain may or may not be present acutely. The patient describes difficulty in standing erect; his trunk is tilted forward and to the side; and he walks with a halting, painful gait. For many years this syndrome was labeled sacroiliac disease because of the pain localized over the sacroiliac joint, but there is now general agreement that the sacroiliac joint itself is rarely implicated.

Treatment. Mild acute low-back syndromes may be due to muscle sprain and will be relieved by a period of bed rest and a back support. The more severe cases are usually due to herniation of intervertebral discs, the discs sandwiched between adjacent spinal bones (vertebrae). In a severe injury, the retaining ligaments are disrupted and the disc material drops (prolapses) backward, pressing against a spinal nerve root.

Several weeks of complete bedrest on a firm mattress, with or without bed boards, is the usual treatment. When symptoms subside, the patient is slowly allowed to move, and a back brace or corset is prescribed to limit motion and provide some support to the weakened back. Certain rules are helpful for avoiding recurrence of back pain:

1. Never lift anything by bending forward at the hips only. Always bend the knees and lift from a squatting position.

2. Never sit up in bed with the legs

fully extended. Always get out of bed by rolling out sideways.

3. Never twist the trunk. Rather, maintain the trunk as a column and turn about at the hips.

The patient should lie down and rest whenever his back "gives out." Even when free of back symptoms, the low-back patient should sleep on a firm mattress and actively protect his back. Most low-back syndromes will be resolved under this regime. With massive disc protrusion and unabating neurological signs, surgery is occasionally required to relieve nerve-root pressure.

LOW BLOOD PRESSURE   See HYPO-TENSION

LOW-CHOLESTEROL DIET   Recent research has found the common form of heart attack (actually coronary atherosclerosis) highly prevalent among people who (among other things) eat a diet high in saturated fatty acids. Such a diet, rich in animal fat, such as fatty meats, is often associated with a high level of cholesterol in the blood serum. Because cholesterol is present in the injured portions of the damaged heart, it seems logical to attempt to lower its serum-level. This is done by reducing the "animal" or saturated fatty acids and by increasing the so-called "vegetable"—a poor term—or polyunsaturated fatty acids. There is some evidence that this will decrease serum cholesterol in many patients; however, it must be remembered that the long-term effect hoped for, a lessened likelihood of heart attack, still remains to be proved.

Lean cuts of meat, with visible fat removed and cooked (medium or well-done) by methods which drain off fat, are recommended. When a source of fat is needed in preparation of food, an oil such as corn-oil or safflower-oil, high in linoleic acid (an essential unsaturated fatty acid), is to be used. These oils may also serve as

a salad dressing. Frequent use should also be made of vegetables, nuts, and fruits.

A patient placed on a low-cholesterol diet will be told to avoid the following foods: butter, ordinary margarine and shortening, lard, sweet cream, sour cream, and foods containing the above in large amounts.

Also to be avoided are bacon, ham, pork, ice cream, sausage, frankfurters, luncheon meats, most salad dressings, brains, liver, kidney, sweetbreads, egg yolks, and all cheeses except dry cottage.

(Because fat, cheeses, and cream in any form should be omitted, macaroni, spaghetti, rice, or potatoes should be cooked without cheese, or fat-or-cream sauces.)

LOW-RESIDUE DIET   This is a diet used before and after surgery on the stomach and intestines in conditions of inflammation or irritation of the digestive (gastrointestinal) tract. The advantage of this diet is that it spares the digestive tract much work because it consists of small, frequent feedings that are easily digested and are low in residue.

Five meals a day are recommended—breakfast, midmorning snack, lunch, midafternoon snack, and supper. The patient should eat slowly and rest after each of the three main meals.

Foods to be avoided are: raw vegetables and raw fruits such as figs or raisins; whole wheat cereals and bread; pork; veal; spices; fried foods; excessively fat foods; rich desserts (pastries and pies); nuts; corn; beans; cabbage; onions; cucumbers; and rhubarb. Ice-cold liquids, such as soft drinks and iced tea or coffee, are not recommended.

Among the foods that are allowed are: weak coffee and tea; diluted orange juice (avoid iced drinks); and well-cooked cereals. Dairy products are recommended. Among desserts, one can select tapioca, rice pudding, spongecake or angel food cake, jello, custard (and similar dishes), marmalades, jellies, and cooked or canned fruits. Most meats, fish, and poultry may be eaten; these should be baked, broiled, boiled, or roasted—*not* fried. Consommé and creamed soups are also permissible.

LOW - SALT (LOW - SODIUM) DIETS

Salt is often restricted in the diet of many patients with high blood pressure (hypertension), congestive cardiac failure, certain forms of kidney disease, fluid in the abdomen (ascites), and in certain disorders (toxemia) of pregnancy. This is done because salt—the sodium portion of it—retains fluid in the body. A low-salt diet is therefore helpful in ridding the body of excess fluids and in lowering blood pressure. Drugs and other therapeutic measures are usually also recommended.

The average American diet contains from 5 to 10 grams of sodium a day (not all in the form of salt); but this varies considerably, depending on the foods consumed. In mild restriction (total sodium intake kept in the range of 2.5 to 4.5 grams per day), no salt is allowed at the table and is used sparingly, or not at all, in cooking. In moderate restriction (about 1 to 2.5 grams) no more than one-fourth of a teaspoon of salt may be used in preparation or at the table. In a strict diet (under 1 gram), all foods are prepared and eaten without salt.

The following dietetic recommendations are based on a strict low-salt ("salt-free") diet:

Basic list of low-sodium foods:

Beverages:
Coca Cola
Cocoa powder
Coffee
Fruit juices (except tomato)
Ginger ale
Tea

Seasoning Agents:
Allspice
Caraway
Cinnamon
Curry powder
Garlic
Mace
Mint leaves
Mustard powder
Nutmeg
Onions
Paprika
Pepper
Peppermint extract
Parsley
Sage
Thyme
Tumeric
Vanilla extract
Vinegar

Avoid onion salt, celery salt, and garlic salt. Also avoid all prepared sauces such as horse-radish, prepared mustard, Worcestershire sauce, and steak sauce.

Fats and Oils:
Beef drippings
Butter, unsalted
Olive oil
Crisco
Salad oil

Avoid bacon fats and other fats to which salt has been added.

Miscellaneous: (These foods are high in calories and should not be used if patient is overweight.)
Coconut, dry
Honey
Jam
Jelly
Marmalade
Peanuts, unsalted
Peanut butter, salt-free
Walnuts, unsalted
Sugar
Pure sugar candy (Life Savers, lemon drops, rock candy, peppermints)

The above-listed foods are extremely low in sodium and may be used if desired to flavor and add variety to the diet with-

338

out adding significantly to sodium intake. The use of herbs in cooking has always been advocated by the well-known good cooks; now when salt must be excluded from the diet, herb cookery becomes even more desirable. The addition of herbs and allowed condiments permits interesting flavors which compensate for the lack of salt. The use of a pressure cooker, too, enables the cook to preserve the natural flavors of the meats and vegetables and therefore make them more palatable.

Here follows a listing of, and commentary on, various foods in general—with particular regard to the problems posed by the necessity of holding sodium intake down to as low a level as possible.

Breads: Salt-free bread, 6 slices per day.

Cereals: Cooked cereals (do not use "quick-cook" brands) prepared without salt. Shredded Wheat, Puffed Wheat, or Puffed Rice may be used, but do not use any other prepared cereal.

Dairy Products: Milk—2 glasses daily, to be taken as a beverage or used in cooking; 1 serving of vanilla ice cream may be substituted for 1 glass of milk. One egg daily—cooked without salt. ¼ cup coffee cream daily. Salt-free butter as desired. Salt-free cheddar cheese as meat substitute.

Fruits: Three servings daily. Any fruit—fresh, frozen, or canned—to be used unless a preservative agent has been added; read the labels to determine whether or not a preservative has been added. Serve a citrus fruit at least once daily.

Meats: 2½ ounces twice daily. Salt-free canned chicken, salmon, or tuna. Lamb, veal, beef, chicken (white meat only), or fresh fish (do not use frozen fish).

Bake, broil, or fry in vegetable shortening. Do not use salt in preparation. Onions, garlic, herbs, paprika, and pepper may be used as seasoning.

Do not use batters, bread crumbs, or other sauces.

Potato or Potato Substitutes: ½ cup serving twice daily. White potato, sweet potato, macaroni, rice, or spaghetti; dried beans, prepared without salt, seasoned with fresh pork.

Cook without salt, and do not use cream sauce or cheese sauce. Fresh tomatoes, peppers, and onion may be added to give variety.

Other Vegetables: Two servings (½ cup) daily. Asparagus, beets (salt-free canned only), broccoli, Brussels sprouts, cabbage, cauliflower, corn, cucumbers, carrots, eggplant, green beans, lettuce, Lima beans, okra, onions, peas, peppers (red or green), parsnips, mushrooms, squash, tomatoes, and turnips.

Do not use spinach, chard, fresh beets, or celery. Vegetables should be fresh, canned without salt, or frozen; do not, however, use frozen peas or Lima beans. Cook without salt. Vegetables may be cooked or served as a salad. If served as salad, a vinegar dressing, lemon juice, or any oil-and-vinegar dressing without salt may be used. Do not use commercial dressings.

L.T.B. (LARYNGOTRACHEOBRONCHITIS) This condition usually occurs in a child less than three years of age who has had a cold and cough with hoarseness. As the infection progresses, there is more and more difficulty in breathing, and the larynx, trachea, and bronchi produce heavy, thick mucous secretions.

Treatment. This inflammation of the larynx, trachea, and bronchi responds to high humidity, antibiotics, and maintenance of fluid intake. Tracheotomy is sometimes necessary.

LUNG ABSCESS This term refers to

a localized area of inflammatory destruction and suppuration within the lung which enlarges by progressive tissue-death (necrosis) and formation of infected cavities. When the process has been present for more than six weeks, it is considered a chronic abscess. Most abscesses are localized in the right lung, more specifically in its posterior areas. In the past twenty years the incidence of lung abscess has decreased considerably, probably as a result of antibiotic drugs.

Abscess is caused by infectious agents, notably bacteria. Many types of bacteria, fungi, or parasitic infestations are capable of producing an abscess; but most commonly responsible are the bacteria which live in or invade the respiratory system. Interestingly enough, there is frequent association with the bacteria which normally live in the mouth and become virulent due to poor hygienic conditions of the teeth, gums, or throat. In the genesis of a lung abscess, there must exist certain pathological conditions which favor bacterial attack upon the lung: among the most common are the sucking of stomach contents into the lung during prolonged periods of sleep (such as may follow an alcoholic bout); or the accidental inhalation of a foreign body into the lung, thus creating a state of acute bronchial obstruction. In either case, some areas of the lung are insufficiently ventilated and the stagnation of materials favors the growth of any bacteria which may be present. (In other cases, lung abscess may be the result of uncontrolled pneumonia, lung tumor, injury, etc.)

Symptoms. Temperature peaks, cough, and expectoration are the most outstanding symptoms, and their intensity related to the severity and toxicity of the infection, the patient's natural resistance, and the freedom of the airways as a coughing-outlet for sloughed material. One can picture lung-abscess evolution by analogy with a deep abscess under the skin, before and after it has opened its way to the surface and draining has started.

Many complications can attend the presence of a lung abscess, notably its extension to the pleura (empyema), its dissemination by way of the bronchi into other lung areas, and development of hemorrhages because of erosion of blood vessels. Even after the abscess is cured, the formation of thick—and sometimes extensive—fibrous tissue may severely restrict future lung activity.

Treatment. Some years ago the prognosis in cases of lung abscess was very poor and hopes were mostly pinned on surgery. Today, however, the treatment is mostly medical and this should always be attempted first. It consists of intensive administration of antibiotics and maintenance of open airways for discharge of the necrotic, sloughed debris. The latter is accomplished by inhalations of bronchodilator drugs, repeated sucking-out of bronchial secretions, and—most important—use of postural drainage as described in the treatment of bronchiectasis. It is generally agreed that if the abscess has not been cured or definitely controlled after six weeks of such intensive medical treatment, surgery may be indicated. If feasible, the best surgical procedure is minimal removal of the destroyed area.

LUNG CYSTS These are air-containing spaces or cavities which develop abnormally within the lung and do not follow the ordinary arrangement of normal lung structure. The abnormality may be present from the time of birth (congenital) due to arrested development of certain areas of the lungs. Most lung cysts, however, are acquired during life as the result of destructive lung diseases such as emphysema, bronchiectasis, traumatic wounds, etc. Thus the nomenclature of air cysts includes such names as bleb, bullae, pneumatocele, emphysematous cysts, and cystic fibrosis.

Symptoms. The nature of symptoms

depends on the cause leading to the formation of the cyst, its size, and the condition of the rest of the lung. Congenital cysts, for instance, are usually "silent" and may be discovered only during a routine chest X-ray. Acquired cysts exhibit symptoms characteristic of the causative disease and will tend, when large enough, to decrease breathing capacity and express themselves by breathlessness; this is the result of the fact that the cyst does not itself participate in ventilation and also because its size tends to compress the surrounding normal lung areas and render them airless (compression atelectasis). Three important complications may attend the presence of a cyst: rupture into the pleural space, with formation of a pneumothorax—air in the lung-covering; hemorrhage within the cyst; and infection. If the cysts result from obstruction of the airways, they may enlarge progressively, reach enormous size, and even occupy most of the lung space (giant tension cysts).

Treatment. Surgical removal is indicated only for the very large cysts, tension cysts in which acute complications have arisen, or in chronically infected cysts. Otherwise, the cyst is treated as part of the background disease.

LUNG EMBOLISM A lodgement of a blood clot or other foreign material in a branch of the pulmonary artery, lung embolism produces interruption of the arterial blood supply to a certain area of the lung and leads to a lung "solidification," usually hemorrhagic in nature, called lung infarction.

Since venous blood from all parts of the body must return through the lung, any abnormal material discharged into the circulation may finally lodge in the pulmonary arterial circulation. The most common cause is the formation of blood clots due to inflammation of a vein in the leg or following an abdominal operation (thrombophlebitis). A failing heart which cannot adequately maintain the circulation may also be the source of blood clots. Other materials, such as large parasites, globules of fat, and even air which accidentally find their way into the venous circulation may also produce embolization of the lung arteries. Emboli may range in size from microscopic to a huge, long strip. They may be single or multiple, and may occur simultaneously, in regular series, or at irregular intervals.

Symptoms. Diagnosis is difficult or even impossible in the case of small-size embolisms, which may be single or repeated over a period of several years. In such cases, ill-defined symptoms of breathlessness, chest-pain, or heart-failure will focus attention on such a possibility only after multiple embolisms have occurred and curtailed circulation irreparably through more than half of the lung arteries.

On the other hand, a large single embolus produces a dramatic picture of acute chest-pain, cough and blood-tinged sputum, rise in temperature and pulse, and rapid breathing. Bluishness (cyanosis) is also usually present, in addition to the appearance of sudden apprehension. This combination of symptoms and signs leads the physician to search for an inflamed or painful leg-vein or for any of the other possibilities mentioned among the causes. Most episodes of lung embolism are not immediately fatal and will resolve in a period of days or weeks. The most common complications are formation of a lung infarct which may become secondarily infected; pleurisy with or without fluid-formation; and acute heart-failure. Most dangerous, however, is the repetition of small series of emboli which are not clinically recognized until later, when they ultimately lead to an established and progressive chronic heart-failure called cor pulmonale.

Treatment. Aside from the rare cases of a very large embolus which is recognized immediately and removed surgically, treatment is mainly directed to the original cause. If this is an inflamed vein, appropriate rest position for the leg, antibiotics, etc., are employed. Often, anticoagulants should be used; these are drugs (such as heparin and dicoumarol) which decrease the capacity of the blood to clot. If embolization continues despite these measures, the physician may be forced to tie off a large common vein such as the inferior vena cava. More important is consideration of prevention of embolization. Older, bedridden individuals, patients with any serious prolonged disease, or patients who are being operated upon for any reason should be encouraged to move their legs, should have them moved at frequent intervals, or wear elastic stockings. These measures are designed to prevent stagnation of the circulation, the common forerunner of the vein inflammation or thrombosis from which emboli are subsequently released to lodge in the lung.

THE LUNGS

RIGHT (3 LOBES)

LEFT (2 LOBES)

LUNG FIBROSIS This is a term applied to a number of diseases which lay down appreciable amounts of scar tissue in the lung. Such conditions include tumors, degenerative and allergic conditions of the lung, chronic inflammatory diseases, and pneumoconiosis. To a large degree, lung fibrosis is a token of defense mechanisms, past or present, employed by the lung against multiple offenders. Eventually, however, the residual marks of such fight (scar tissue) are large enough to supplant the delicate elastic network of the lung and become a burden to the breathing or circulation, leading to respiratory or heart-failure.

Symptoms. The amount, distribution, and localization of fibrosis in the lung varies considerably, to the same degree as do the symptoms and complications. The fibrosis may be focal (circumscribed) or diffuse. It may encroach preferentially upon the airways, producing symptoms of obstructive lung disease; along the blood vessels, giving rise to pulmonary heart disease; or produce a scarred, rigid pleura that restricts lung expansion. The most common symptom in any given cause of lung fibrosis is breathlessness (dyspnea).

Treatment. Already-established fibrosis is irreversible. Treatment may be effective only when the original disease is promptly recognized and further spreading can be controlled, preventing formation of new scar tissue. In a few cases, when a relatively localized amount of fibrosis has distorted the structure of neighboring normal tissue, surgical removal of the worthless area of fibrosis may restore the lost function of the normal adjacent lung.

LUNG INFARCT See LUNG EMBOLISM

LUPUS ERYTHEMATOSUS, ACUTE DISSEMINATE Previously thought to be a predominantly dermatologic disease, it has in recent years become clear that the cutaneous manifestations of acute disseminate lupus erythematosus may appear many years after the disease has been present in other organs and has given rise to a multiplicity of symptoms. Long-standing fatigue, low-grade fevers, joint pains, epileptiform seizures, abdominal cramps, chest pains, recurrent attacks of pneumonia are among the symptoms that can precede involvement of the skin, and may indeed remain undiagnosed and unattended until the skin lesions afford a clue for investigation.

Occurring in all age groups and in both sexes, this condition is so much more common in young women that many investigators have fruitlessly looked into the possibility of a causal connection with some ovarian disturbance. The cause of the disease remains unknown, except for the observation that exposure to ultraviolet light almost invariably worsens the condition or precipitates an attack. Prior to the advent of cortisone, the condition was fatal after a few months, or at most two years. Treatment with one of the many available cortisone drugs has afforded years of productive life to many patients with this disease. It has also been possible, through the relief of symptoms and the prolonging of life, to better differentiate this disease from the subacute form, a vastly different disease of almost identical appearance but with no systemic involvement.

Symptoms. The lesions are usually symmetrically distributed on the "exposed" surfaces of the body (face, neck, arms, and legs), but in severe cases occur over the entire body, including the palms and soles. The reddened swollen papules appear diffusely in these areas and only seem to have a border of demarcation on the face, giving a butterfly appearance. In addition to feeling moderately or acutely ill, the patient has symptoms reflecting the presence of the disease elsewhere (joints,

lungs, kidneys). Diagnosis can be confirmed by several types of studies of the blood (lowering of the white-cell count, disturbance of clotting, changes in gamma globulin) and in the finding of the lupus erythematosus cell in the bone marrow and the blood. The lupus erythematosus cell is formed when an unusual substance in the blood (probably an enzyme) causes a disintegration of lymphocytes (a type of white blood corpuscle). The disintegrated nucleus is quickly surrounded by neutrophiles (another type of white corpuscle) which engulf the material and form an abnormal but characteristic cell, the lupus erythematosus cell. The discovery and elucidation of the lupus erythematosus cell constitute a great advance in the diagnosis, and hence the treatment, of this and other collagen diseases.

Treatment. Except under unusual circumstances, treatment consists of administration of the cortisone drugs, the selection and dosage of which can vary considerably not only with the phase of the disease, but also with the response of the particular patient. In addition to strict avoidance of exposure to ultraviolet light, avoidance of fatigue, stress, and drugs (unless considered absolutely necessary) appear to be essential both to effectiveness of treatment and to maintaining improvement

LUPUS ERYTHEMATOSUS, CHRONIC DISCOID
A disease of young and middle adult life, and more common in women, chronic discoid lupus erythematosus can nevertheless begin at any age. Of unknown causation, both the initial appearance of the eruption and subsequent flare-ups may follow excessive exposure to the sun. The relationship of this disease to ultraviolet light has not yet been established; but it is very clear that patients already affected must avoid any deliberate sunning and must seek protection from even casual sun exposure encountered in

ordinary daily activity. The condition is often difficult to differentiate from polymorphous light eruption and from acute disseminate lupus erythematosus, both of which have entirely different courses and prognosis. It is therefore essential that insofar as possible a definitive diagnosis be established.

Symptoms. The eruption is most commonly found on the face (cheeks) and anterior chest, and on the exposed surfaces of the arms. The lesions first appear as small plaques of reddened papules and scales with sharp, slightly elevated borders. As the lesions become more extensive, the central portions become depressed from atrophy (loss of tissue). When all activity has stopped, the area appears scarred and not infrequently is hyperpigmented at the borders. The course and extent of the disease are very variable, lasting from months to years, and consisting of a single bean-size lesion to extensive involvement of all the susceptible areas.

Treatment. Although this is not a disease of specific photosensitivity, the regularity of exacerbations following exposure to ultraviolet light (sun or artificial) make avoidance of such exposure urgent. The antimalarial drugs (Chloroquine®, Atabrine®, etc.) have largely replaced the previously used bismuth, gold, and arsphenamines. However, the latter group of drugs are of some benefit and can be used when the antimalarial drugs are not tolerated or are ineffective. Local treatment consists of using sun screens in an attempt to avoid the sun exposure of ordinary living. The sun screens, applied as lotion or cream, can also be used to cover the lesions and achieve some cosmetic improvement. It is possible to destroy small lesions with the application of carbon dioxide (dry ice) in the hope of forestalling progression. In rare cases, when destruction of the skin has been extensive and the disease appears to be "burned out," reconstructive surgery may afford the patient cosmetic improvement.

MALARIA   Malaria (Italian *mala aria*, meaning bad air) is an acute, often recurrent, sometimes chronic parasitic disorder marked by paroxysms of chills followed by a high fever, the presence of the parasites in the red blood cells, profuse sweats, often with enlargement of the spleen, and, at times, jaundice.

Cause. The cause of malaria is a protozoan, the plasmodium. Man is infected by the bite of the malaria-infected anopheles mosquito, or (among drug addicts) by the use of a common hypodermic syringe and needle, or by receiving blood in a transfusion from an infected donor. Malaria has become a very rare disease in the United States. However, due to the frequency with which troops and tourists visit tropical countries, this cause of hemolytic anemia continues to be important.

Symptoms. Within ten to thirty-five days after inoculation, symptoms appear as a relatively mild fever, chilliness, headache, and malaise which last for about a week and usually regarded as and treated as influenza. Suddenly the patient is seized with a violent chill followed by profuse perspiration and fever that is extremely high. The fever lasts from one to eight hours, subsides, and the patient now states that he feels well. Then, every two days (or more, depending on the type of plasmodium with which he is infected) he is stricken by an attack of chill-fever-sweats. The high fever may be accompanied by severe headache, drowsiness, delirium, confusion, and even convulsions. In the chronic form, the fever is not as high, attacks are milder and shorter, and the patient is fatigued, listless, lacks appetite, and complains of headache. If malaria persists long enough, jaundice may develop, the spleen may become enlarged, and less frequently, the liver may enlarge.

Treatment. Treatment is most successful with quinine (obtained from the cinchona bark) and several synthetic antimalarial preparations such as quinacrine, pyremethamine, Primaquine, and chlorguanide.

Persons who contemplate travel in malarial countries can prevent malarial infection if any of the above mentioned antimalarial agents are taken in prophylactic dosage before, during, and for two weeks after such a journey.

MALNUTRITION See UNDERFEEDING

MALOCCLUSION Abnormal positioning of the upper and lower teeth, so that they do not "mesh" properly when the jaws are closed, is known as malocclusion. The offending deviations from acceptable normal standards may result from malpositioned and misshapen individual teeth; improper size, shape, and relation of the jaws; congenital deformities; cleft palate; and fractures of either or both jaws.

MANDIBLE The mandible is the horseshoe-shaped lower jaw which forms the movable part of the masticatory mechanism and which supports the lower teeth.

MANIC-DEPRESSIVE PSYCHOSIS This psychosis typically involves a cycloid (cyclic) pattern of alternating periods of excitement and depression. Typically, excitement lasts for several weeks or months, followed by normality for several months, then a period of depression. These cycles tend to recur, although a few patients may have only one or two episodes during a lifetime. The disorder frequently occurs relatively early in life, between ages fifteen and thirty-five, and is more common among upper class persons, particularly women. Approximately one-third of patients have a family history of cycloid disorder. However, many attacks appear to be stimulated by environmental factors, involving personality conflict.

Symptoms. In the manic or excited phase, increased activity and heightened emotionality are principal symptoms. The patient becomes overactive and excitable, talking excessively, singing, shouting, and engaging in frenzied activities which often are quite destructive. Sexual drive tends to be heightened and the person may engage in obscene acts or proposals. Flight of ideas and easy distractibility accompany heightened activity levels. During the acute phase the patient may be too excited to eat, sleep, or take care of himself properly, requiring mental hospitalization.

During the depressive phase, the person tends to become melancholy and depressed, crying, losing interest in the environment, and expressing feelings of unworthiness and inadequacy. In extreme depression, the patient shows retardation of all mental and physical functions, sitting alone in a withdrawn manner and expressing sadness and melancholy. He may appear stuporous, giving no response to the environment, showing mutism, and requiring forced feeding.

Treatment. The discovery of psychic tranquilizers and energizers has completely revolutionized the treatment of states of excitement and depression. Formerly it was necessary to hospitalize manic patients both for their own protection and that of society; today many cases can be completely controlled at home with tranquilizers. Psychotherapy is also of great value in helping the excited person to understand and control his state of emotional overexcitability. The excited person should be encouraged to exercise several hours a day in order to reduce physical tensions; hydrotherapy in the form of long, soothing baths may also be effective in calming disturbed emotions. The excited patient should be protected against making unwise business decisions and kept from taking other actions stimulated by excessive self-confidence.

Depressive symptoms are well controlled by psychic energizers, which stimulate more positive feelings and emotional tone. The depressed patient should be encouraged to maintain his usual pattern of living, working as much as possible and avoiding unhealthy brooding. The main danger, which must be carefully guarded against, is that of suicide during periods of extreme depression. Any patient who expresses suicidal ideas should be placed under psychiatric treatment immediately, preferably in a mental hospital where twenty-four hour supervision can be maintained.

Fortunately, the outlook for manic-depressive reactions is very good, most episodes being self-terminating—even without psychiatric treatment—within a period of several weeks or months. Ordinarily no mental deterioration occurs following manic or depressive episodes, and the patient typically returns to complete normality. Modern tranquilizing and energizing drugs are valuable chiefly in cutting short manic and depressive episodes.

Recently lithium carbonate has been shown to have both therapeutic and prophylactic benefit for many sufferers, and an increasing number of patients are on daily dosage of this newer drug.

MASTITIS   Mastitis is acute infection of the breast, and may occur in breast-feeding mothers a week or more after delivery. It is characterized by swelling, redness, and tenderness of the breast, accompanied by high fever and general malaise. Treatment consists of interruption of lactation, antibiotics, breast-support, and ice bags. Very often a breast abscess will form which will require incision and drainage of the pus.

MASTURBATION   Revolutionary changes have occurred during the last fifty years in medical-psychiatric attitudes toward many types of sex behavior formerly thought to be perverted and pathological.

First, anthropological cross-cultural studies have shown the wide range of social and ethical attitudes towards various ways of expressing sexuality, demonstrating that there is no universal agreement on what a culture permits or considers pathological.

Secondly, Freudian discoveries concerning normal patterns of psycho-sexual development have greatly increased acceptance of behaviors formerly considered completely abnormal and perverted. Freud was the first to point out the facts about infantile sexuality and the various phases of interest in different sex-objects shown by normal children. He showed that erotic sensitivity usually appears early in infancy, young children first developing sexual gratification from the oral regions in feeding and sucking activity. Later, the child may be erotically stimulated by excretory functions and zones—a stage labeled by Freud as the anal-erotic phase of normal development. Still later, usually around puberty, sexual interests become fixated on genital areas as the child discovers normal heterosexuality.

Freud pointed out that every normal child usually experiments with many types of autoerotic (self) sexual stimulation, and he insisted that many older terms such as masturbation or self-abuse were illogical and inexact, expressing moralistic religious taboos which are scientifically untrue. Social repressions of sexuality reached their peak in the Victorian era, when popular authors wrote books threatening young children with mental deficiency or insanity if they indulged in any form of masturbation. Actually, there is no scientific evidence of any causative relationship between autoeroticism and any form of mental disorder. Though mentally disturbed persons characteristically show poor judgment in expressing sexuality, this may be understood as a symptom rather than a cause. Each child must, however, learn the appropriate social and legal limitations relating to expressions of sexuality.

Treatment. In the past, overly strict taboos and superstitions concerning a supposed relationship between uncontrolled sexuality and mental disorder caused masturbation to be severely punished and suppressed. It is now understood that punishment or severe repressive measures simply create neurotic conflict and further exaggerate the problem. Parents should regard children's developing sexual interest as completely normal, to be channeled into socially acceptable directions rather than to be completely repressed. The child must learn not to become socially conspicuous or a public nuisance. Ordinarily, the child's sexual development takes place most smoothly when parents show a tolerant, accepting attitude, patiently helping in the channeling of impulses in socially acceptable directions without creating conflicts in the child by becoming over-anxious or openly disturbed by its behavior. In extreme cases, where a child has developed such conflicts over problems of sex development that he expresses sexuality in socially unacceptable ways, it may be desirable for the parents and child to go to a child guidance clinic where the problems can be solved under psychiatric supervision.

MAXILLA   The maxilla is the upper jaw—the fixed part of the masticatory mechanism which supports the upper teeth in an arch-like arrangement.

MEASLES   Measles is an acute communicable disease which runs a characteristic course.

Symptoms. On the tenth day after exposure, a susceptible child will develop a fever; then each day for the next four days the patient becomes progressively sicker, with increasing fever and dry, hard cough, bleary eyes, and lethargy. Finally, on the fourteenth day, a rash begins to break out around the hair line which takes about twenty-four hours to spread from the face to the feet. The rash is intensely pink,

flat and solid on the face, and more scattered and spotted further down the body.

The patient does not feel any improvement until the day after the rash has appeared on the feet. At this point, the cough loosens up and diminishes, the fever subsides and the rash begins to fade from the face. Should the fever climb again, the cough get worse, or an earache develop, this usually means that a germ-caused complication has occurred, in which case an antibiotic may be prescribed by the physician.

Treatment. Since measles is caused by a virus, there are no specific measures against it except aspirin, fluids, rest, and comfortable baths. There is no truth to the old wives' tale that light will injure the eyes of a measles patient. The disease itself might cause a nerve injury in a susceptible person, but not the light itself: light may irritate the eyes, but cannot damage them.

If parents are aware that their child has been exposed to the "hard" measles (as distinct from roseola), they should have their doctor administer a modifying dose of gamma globulin. If given at the proper time and in the right amount, this substance will reduce the infected child's measles to a mild, yet immunizing, case.

Both the live and dead types of measles vaccine furnish good immunity for the uninfected child. (If a mother has had the measles, her baby is immune until the fourth to fifth month of life.)

As mentioned before, failure of the measles to improve on the day following complete appearance of the rash means that some complication has set in. If it is bronchitis or otitis media, the child should be given antibiotics. If the child develops measles encephalitis, the symptoms may be severe headache, coma, convulsions, or other signs of nervous-system irritation. Measles encephalitis is a particularly distressing complication because it may leave the child with some neurological damage. However, this possibility should no longer be a threat because modern measles vaccination is so effective in preventing the original disease. Every parent therefore owes it to the child to make certain that measles immunization is carried out.

Note: Measles should not be confused with German measles. Despite the similarity in names, the two diseases are entirely different in many important respects, particularly in the fact that German measles during the first trimester of pregnancy constitutes a specifically grave threat to the fetus.

MECONIUM This is a brownish or brownish-green material defecated by the newborn during the first three to four days of life and representing cellular debris from the baby's intestines, swallowed amniotic fluid during intrauterine life, and bile. After the third or fourth day of life this is replaced by normal, yellowish baby stools. Passage of meconium in the amniotic fluid during pregnancy or during labor makes the fluid appear brownish or green and is a possible sign of distress of the fetus. The only time that passage of meconium during labor may be considered normal is when the baby is coming breech-first.

MEDIAL TIBIAL TORSION This is a common cause of "in-toeing" in childhood. When this condition exists, the ankle joint and the foot face further inward than the rest of the leg. Tibial torsion is frequently self-correcting with growth, but severe cases may require brace or cast correction. Its cause is unknown, but in some cases at least there is good evidence that it is due to immobilization of the developing fetus in the uterus.

MEDIAN NERVE The median nerve supplies important muscles relating to flexion of the fingers. It also carries sensory impulses from the skin over the thumb, index, and middle fingers.

MEDICAL QUACKERY Although everyone is presumably against quackery,

it is by no means a dying business; its cost to the American people is estimated to be one billion dollars a year. This figure includes the purchase of some surprising items as well as some old "stand-bys." The American Medical Association believes, for instance, that most Americans buy vitamin pills not because they actually believe their diet requires this supplementation, but only in response to advertising which convinces them that the daily cost is so low that it is economical to be "on the safe side." The A.M.A. also considers the millions spent on laxatives and patent medicines almost entirely unnecessary.

Of course, the "cures" for arthritis and rheumatism—for which no true cures exist as yet—fall in a class of worthless medications second to none; nevertheless, they alone cost two hundred and fifty million dollars a year.

Surprisingly, the money spent on other false "cure-alls" is a comparatively small amount. In this category fall the more brazen quacks who appeal to those people who, for one reason or another, must surely have missed the point of all their high school biology and chemistry classes: such "cure-all quacks" peddle brass bracelets, magnets, boxes with colored lights, packages with bits of radioactive ores, and—most recently—concentrated sea-water.

In addition to this group there are, of course, the cancer-cure peddlers. Here the yearly "take" is fifty million dollars. The only cheery word in this otherwise dismal and dirty business is the A.M.A.'s opinion that most of the fifty million is spent by people who do not really have cancer, but only imagine they do. Thus the source of testimonials—the quack's so-called "proof" of effectiveness—are claims of recovery from a non-existent ailment brought about by nonsense medicine. In reality the effects produced are no different from those obtained by the witch doctors. A moment's reflection should convince any adult that a true cancer cure would not need to be peddled—there is infinitely too much demand for it. The scramble for a cancer cure is now so universal that almost anything with even the faintest possibility of effectiveness is snapped up by industrial or government laboratories for evaluation.

But should the individual be so temporarily foolish as to seek the advice of a quack, let him immediately regain his senses if the quack offers testimonials as proof of effectiveness—especially if the quack laments the fact that "big-shot" doctors refuse to recognize him or his cancer cure. The quack really hasn't a leg to stand on; he depends upon his victims' ignorance of facts available to any reader of the daily newspaper.

The quack is dangerous because he may deprive his customers of proper medical care, especially in cases where time is of importance. Since he works on a personal basis, the quack's services are usually expensive. His operations are never advertised nationally, and as a result, he is actually difficult to track down, and even more difficult to convict. Unfortunately, conviction carries no heavy penalties and is not a real deterrent. More than any other single factor, it is probably the justified harassment by Federal agencies that has served to keep the quackery business down to its present level.

The American Medical Association has suggested that laws with stricter penalties for unlicensed practice of medicine be passed and enforced as a means of dealing with authentic quacks; the Food and Drug Administration (FDA) has added to this a law requiring proof of the effectiveness of a drug before it can be released for public use and marketed. So it is that the burden of proof of effectiveness now rests with the individual who administers or sells a drug. In the absence of such proof, its sale becomes illegal, thus permitting the FDA to prosecute on this basis—a much easier and potentially more successful course of action, according to the FDA itself.

MEGACOLON In the congenital condition megacolon (literally, huge intestine), there is a narrowing of the rectum due to a nerve deficiency in one section of the bowel-wall; stool, of course, packs up behind this stricture in the large intestine (colon) and leads to severe, chronic constipation.

Symptoms. Sometimes the infant exhibits a very distended abdomen and there is usually a history of never having been able to have a bowel movement without the help of an enema, a suppository, or a finger. Psychosomatic (psychogenic) constipation can be distinguished from megacolon in that the former does not start so early in life, and no rectal stricture can be demonstrated.

Treatment. A barium-enema X-ray is usually used to detect the characteristic rectal stricture, and a clever operation has been devised in which the abnormal segment of intestine is removed and the normal portions of bowel at each end of the nerveless section joined together.

MELANIN Produced in the basal cell layer of the epidermis of the skin by the pigment-producing cells, the melanocytes, this pigment is largely responsible for the color of human skin. It is a relatively inert protein substance produced by the amino-acid tyrosine through the intervention of the enzyme tyrosinase, both of which substances are themselves colorless. The intensity of skin color is governed by the amount of melanin distributed in the cells of the basal layer, since the number of pigment-forming cells (melanocytes) is relatively constant in all people.

The activity of the melanocytes is governed by the anterior pituitary gland through the action of its hormone (melanocyte-stimulating hormone).

Disturbances of melanin production can be either that of increase or of decrease, and can be of local or systemic causation. Although the primary function of this pigment is protection against the damaging effects of solar radiation, changes in pigmentation can be symptomatic of specific (systemic) diseases, such as vitiligo, chloasma, and Addison's disease.

MEMBRANES While the baby is carried in the mother's womb it is surrounded by the amniotic fluid, which is contained within a thin sac (the membranes, or bag of waters). The membranes may rupture before or during labor; it is very important that the patient notifies her doctor as soon as the bag of waters breaks and fluid runs out through the birth canal. Once the membranes have ruptured, sexual relations, douches, or other vaginal manipulations are contraindicated.

MENARCHE This is the onset of menstrual periods. (See MENSTRUATION.)

MÉNIÈRE'S DISEASE Labyrinthine hydrops, or Ménière's disease, is thought to be due to excess fluid in the inner fluid system of the labyrinth.* The cause of the excess fluid is not definitely known and may be due to a number of factors.

Symptoms. Tinnitus (noise in the ear), hearing loss, episodes of dizziness, distortion of sound, and sensitivity to loud noises are all symptoms. The dizziness is true vertigo and manifests itself by the patient's sensation of his environment whirling around him or the patient whirling around the environment. Incapacitating episodes of vertigo can occur, associated with nausea and vomiting.

Treatment. The usual medical measures are low-salt diet, cessation of smoking, drugs to dilate the blood vessels, and anti-vertigo and antinausea drugs. In addition, a special vitamin is now also available, but this must be taken over a period of at least six weeks before it is possible to tell whether it is being helpful or not. Very dilute histamine injections are also used by a few physicians. Medical measures are said to control the symptoms satisfactorily in more than 85 per cent of cases, but no one medication is 100 per cent effective.

The physician must continue to try different medications until satisfactory control has been achieved. In those cases where the disease is incapacitating and will not respond to medication (the hearing in these cases being usually below serviceable level), surgery is considered. The surgical procedures are divided into two classifications: destructive and nondestructive. Destructive:

1. Labyrinthectomy. This procedure involves removal of the membranous labyrinth through the oval window or through a window drilled into the horizontal semicircular canal. Today the former operation is performed more frequently. Both methods destroy the patient's balance mechanism and hearing.

2. Ultrasound. Very high frequency sound is applied to the horizontal semicircular canal via a mastoidectomy approach. This attempts to destroy the balance mechanism while preserving the hearing. Recent analysis of a number of cases has shown a relatively high recurrence rate of vertigo. This procedure offers a good potential but must be further developed.

3. Drugs. Drugs, taken both systemically and by direct injection into the middle ear have been used to destroy the balance mechanism. Streptomycin has been used with some success.

---

* The labyrinth is the term applied to the cochlea and semicircular canals, and their connections and dilatations.

Nondestructive:

Doctors Howard P. and William F. House of Los Angeles, California, world famous ear surgeons, have developed a shunt operation which continuously drains the excess fluid from the inner ear into the fluid system of the brain (the two fluids are very similar). This operation is a promising one, although the evidence is not yet conclusive, since the procedure has thus far been performed on less than one hundred people.

Destructive surgical procedures (and the drug method which sometimes adversely affects the hearing) can clearly be used only if the hearing is already quite poor, and then only in one ear. For patients with intractable Ménière's disease who have useful hearing, the most promising procedure, and the newest, may prove to be the shunt operation.

MENINGES   The meninges are three membranes which cover the brain and spinal cord: an outer fibrous membrane, a filmy middle membrane, and a delicate inner membrane. (The space between the middle and the inner membrane is called the subarachnoid space and contains cerebrospinal fluid.) Infections of these membranes result in meningitis.

MENINGITIS   Meningitis is an acute infection of the meninges (the covering membranes of the brain). It is caused by a wide variety of infecting organisms, including bacteria and viruses. Meningococcic meningitis occurs in epidemic form; other types of meningitis usually occur as isolated cases.

Symptoms.   The acute onset of headache, fever, and stiff neck are characteristic findings in meningitis. The patient may become drowsy or stuporous and may have nausea and vomiting. With progression of the infection, the cranial nerves may be involved and result in double vision, facial

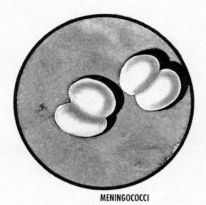

MENINGOCOCCI

weakness, deafness, or other findings. Some types of infection are associated with skin rash. Convulsions and coma may develop.

Treatment.   Bacterial infections producing meningitis are treated with antibiotics and chemical agents, such as penicillin, sulfadiazine, chloromycetin, and tetracyclines. If the causative organism can be isolated from the cerebrospinal fluid, the drug or drugs which are most effective in treating this bacterial infection are administered; if the causative organism cannot be immediately identified and if a purulent infection is present, drug therapy is immediately instituted. Early treatment of bacterial infections is of the greatest importance in lowering the mortality rate and the incidence of complications. Prior to the discovery of the drugs which are currently available for treatment of meningitis, most forms of bacterial meningitis were almost uniformly fatal. With modern therapy, the mortality rate has been decreased to 20 per cent.

No specific drugs are available for the treatment of virus infections producing meningitis. In all patients with meningitis, hospitalization and expert nursing care are mandatory. Intravenous fluids are usually required.

MENOPAUSE   Termination of the reproductive period in the life of a woman —the "change of life"—is called the menopause or female climacteric. The average

age for the menopause is fifty, although it may occur a few years earlier or later. The menopause is caused by cessation of the normal function of the ovaries, resulting in gradual or sudden disappearance of menstrual periods. Surgical removal or sterilizing irradiation of the ovaries will result in an artificial menopause.

Symptoms. The symptoms of menopause vary. In some cases cessation of menstrual periods may be the only change. On the other hand, the change of life may be accompanied by excessive physical, functional, and emotional disturbances that require prompt recognition and therapy. The commonest symptoms are: (1) sudden or (more often) gradual cessation of menstrual periods; (2) hot flushes—or flashes as they are sometimes called—with the patient feeling a wave of heat passing over her body, sometimes accompanied by actual flushing of the face and neck followed by sweating; (3) weight-gain; (4) generalized weakness of the muscles with frequent disturbances of normal vision; (5) atrophic changes of the genital organs, the change sometimes being experienced in the form of itching in the genital area and dyspareunia (pain during intercourse); and (6) psychological symptoms, headaches, dizziness, depression, and insomnia. The symptoms become worse because of inherent fears that the patient is getting old, is losing her sex appeal, and is no longer able to bear children. Most of these fears are unfounded. A menopausal woman with a healthy attitude towards this physiological stage of her life may be as happy and active in all her activities as before. *Warning:* Any amount of vaginal bleeding or spotting occurring after the definite cessation of the menstrual periods should be considered abnormal and potentially dangerous; the woman should seek medical advice immediately, to check for the possible presence of cancer of the female organs (usually womb or ovaries).

Treatment. The fact that the menopause is a normal biological phenomenon should not be taken for granted, and all means available for the well-being of the patient should be utilized. All the symptoms of menopause can be relieved with a daily intake of one of the ovarian hormones available commercially at very low cost. Used properly, they offer a sense of well-being to the postmenopausal woman for many more years. Many patients, of course, can do quite well without hormone therapy or without sedative and antidepressant drugs.

MENORRHAGIA See UTERINE BLEEDING, ABNORMAL

MENSTRUATION   Menstruation begins with puberty, usually between the ages of twelve to fourteen, continues throughout the woman's childbearing years and terminates with the onset of menopause (usually between the ages of forty-five and fifty). Several factors affect the onset of menstruation: race, nutrition, genetic inheritance, etc. Beginning of menstrual function under the age of eight or its delay beyond the age of eighteen should be considered abnormal and should be investigated.

The menstrual flow usually occurs every twenty-eight days and lasts for three to five days; the amount of flow is relatively heavy for the first two days and then gradually decreases. It is not abnormal for a woman to have menstrual periods closer together or further apart (ranging from twenty to thirty-five days or more), so long as they come at regular intervals. During the first year or two after the onset of menstruation there may be considerable irregularity in the interval, duration, and amounts of menstrual periods; this is due to the lack of ovulation, and corrects itself within time.

The monthly menstrual periods (menses) are the result of a very complex interaction of hormones from several

352

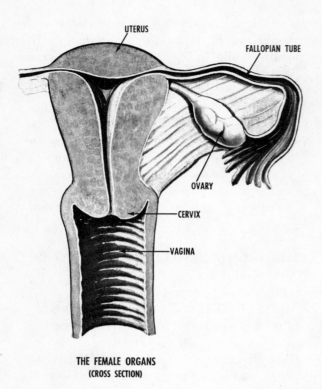

UTERUS

FALLOPIAN TUBE

OVARY

CERVIX

VAGINA

THE FEMALE ORGANS
(CROSS SECTION)

glands, mainly the ovaries and the pituitary. With the approach of puberty, the pituitary produces special hormones which make the ovaries and the uterus mature and become ready for subsequent cyclic changes that will enable the female to start her reproductive career. The rhythmic changes of the pituitary, ovaries, and uterus that result in the monthly menstrual flow may be outlined as follows: The pituitary secretes follicle-stimulating hormone (FSH) and stimulates the ovary to produce estrogens, which in turn stimulate the lining of the uterus (endometrium) to proliferate (grow thicker). The high levels of estrogens then act as a block for the further production of FSH by the pituitary, which now produces another hormone, the luteinizing hormone (LH), which promotes maturation of one out of thousands of eggs (ova) in the ovary. Ovulation then occurs, usually on the fourteenth day after the last menstrual period. If conception takes place, the

menstrual periods stop for the next nine months.

In the absence of pregnancy, the pituitary secretes still another hormone, the luteotrophic hormone (LTH), which results in the formation of the corpus luteum in the ovary; this new glandular structure starts producing another hormone, progesterone, which again stimulates the endometrium to further growth. At this point estrogen levels have dropped to their lowest levels, and the pituitary once more secretes more FSH and less LTH; progesterone levels drop; and the endometrium (which is now at the peak of its growth), losing its hormonal support, breaks down and is expelled from the womb together with blood in the form of menstrual bleeding. By this time the pituitary again produces large amounts of FSH, the estrogen levels rise once more, and the endometrium starts a new cycle. (See also PREMENSTRUAL SYNDROME [PMS].

MENTAL HYGIENE This is a branch of preventative psychiatry dedicated to the prevention of mental disorders and to the development of mental health. The founder of the modern mental hygiene movement was Clifford Beers who, early in the 1920s, wrote of his experiences as a mental hospital patient and led a movement for the establishment of child guidance clinics, adult psychiatric clinics, and improved mental hospital facilities. (The mental hygiene movement in the United States has achieved great advances, particularly since World War II, when government agencies made available large sums of money for psychiatric research and mental health projects.)

It is now widely accepted that a person may be free of mental defects or disorders and still be relatively inefficient, unhappy, and spiritually bankrupt unless he can live positively and fulfill his potential.

Mental health research has proved that a large number of social, economic,

REPRODUCTION AND FETAL DEVELOPMENT

THE FEMALE REPRODUCTIVE ORGANS

ON THE LEFT, THE ORGANS ARE SHOWN FROM BEHIND IN NATURAL
POSITION; ON THE RIGHT THE ORGANS ARE IN CROSS SECTION.

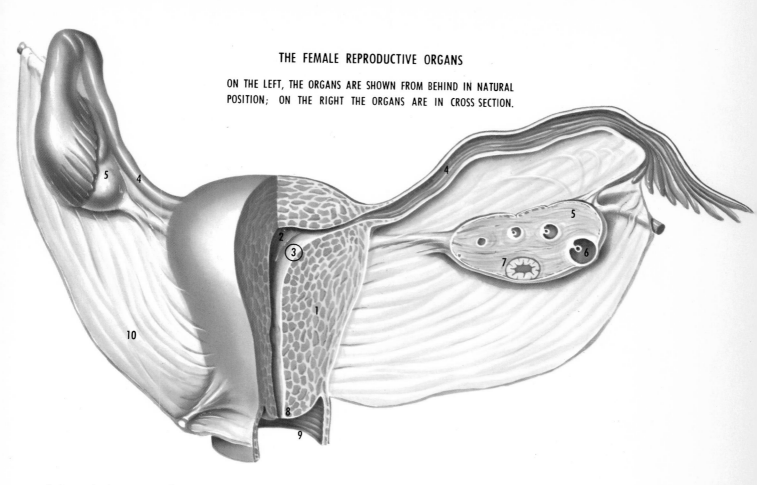

Each month the ovary produces an ovum
(egg) which develops within a hollow follicle.
When ripe, the ovum bursts out of (ovulates)
the follicle, enters the mouth of the tube, and
is fertilized by male sperm. The follicle remnants form the corpus luteum. The fertilized
ovum, developing as it travels, takes 10
days to traverse the tube and implant in
uterine lining.

1   UTERINE MUSCLE
2   UTERINE CAVITY
3   IMPLANTATION SITE
4   FALLOPIAN TUBE
5   OVARY
6   OVUM WITHIN FOLLICLE
7   CORPUS LUTEUM
8   CERVIX
9   VAGINA
10 BROAD LIGAMENT
11 BLADDER

SIDE VIEW IN CROSS SECTION

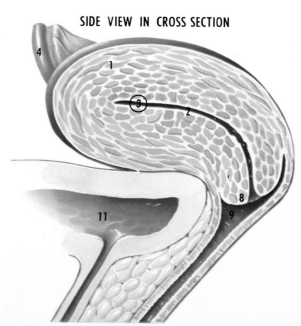

ILLUSTRATED BY

LEONARD D. DANK

ST. LUKE'S HOSPITAL
NEW YORK CITY

THE MENSTRUAL CYCLE

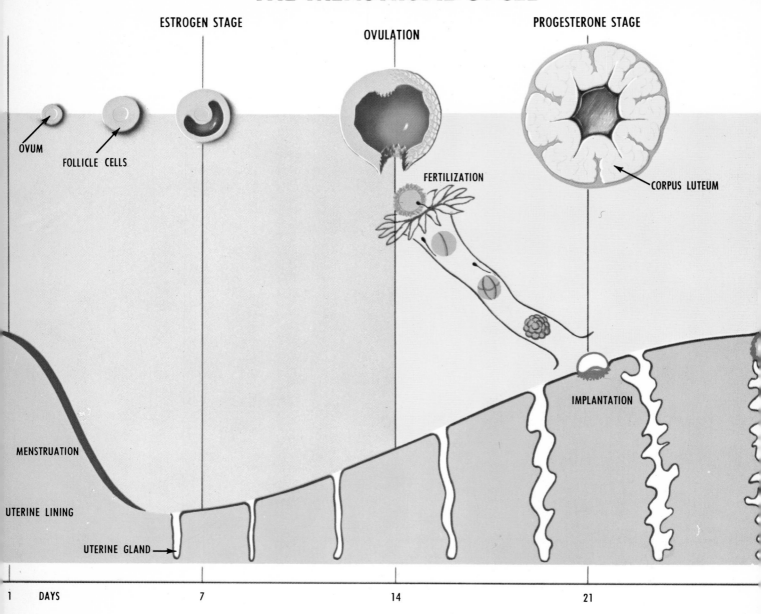

ESTROGEN STAGE

OVULATION

PROGESTERONE STAGE

OVUM

FOLLICLE CELLS

FERTILIZATION

CORPUS LUTEUM

MENSTRUATION

IMPLANTATION

UTERINE LINING

UTERINE GLAND →

1 DAYS   7   14   21

The 28-day cycle involves the simultaneous growth of an ovum within the ovary, and the thickening of the uterine lining in preparation for receiving the ovum. The cycle can be divided into 2 equal stages.

ESTROGEN STAGE, DAYS 1 TO 14
As the ovum develops, the follicle cells secrete the hormone, estrogen, which travels via the blood stream to the uterine lining. After the cessation of menstrual flow, estrogen causes the lining to thicken. The glands are straight tubes during this stage.

PROGESTERONE STAGE, DAYS 14 TO 28
When the ripe ovum is shed, it enters the fallopian tube, is fertilized, and travels down the tube to become implanted in the uterine lining. After ovulation, the follicle cells form a new structure, the corpus luteum, whose yellowish cells secrete the hormone, progesterone. Progesterone continues the uterine lining build-up in preparation for implantion, and persists until late in pregnancy.

PREGNANCY

(FIRST WEEK)

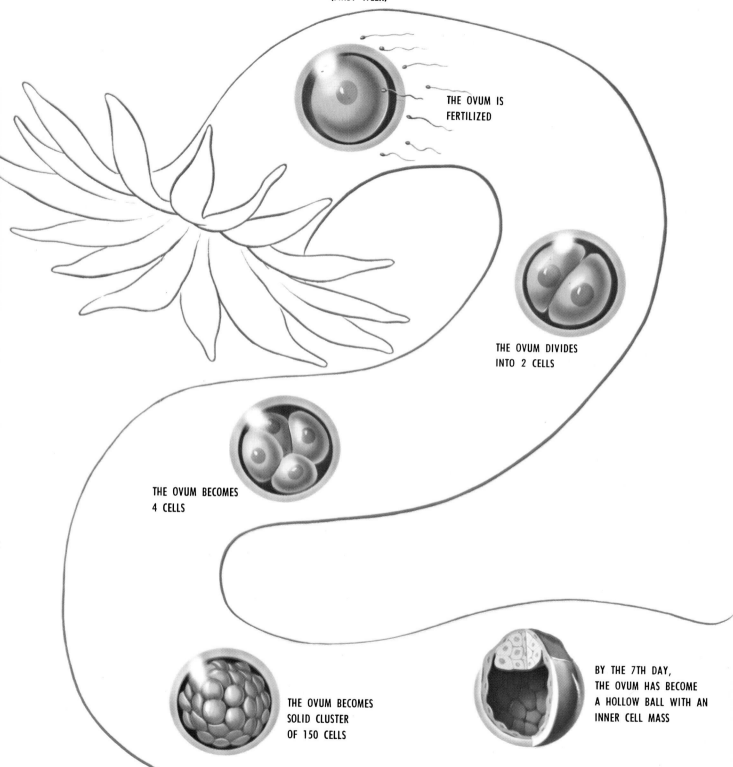

THE OVUM IS
FERTILIZED

THE OVUM DIVIDES
INTO 2 CELLS

THE OVUM BECOMES
4 CELLS

THE OVUM BECOMES
SOLID CLUSTER
OF 150 CELLS

BY THE 7TH DAY,
THE OVUM HAS BECOME
A HOLLOW BALL WITH AN
INNER CELL MASS

IMPLANTATION

PREGNANCY
(SECOND WEEK)

Pink — Maternal uterine lining
Red — Permanent placenta
Yellow — Embryonic temporary placenta
Blue — Embryo
Grey — Endoderm
Orange — Mesoderm

8TH DAY
The hollow ball of embryonic tissues pierces the uterine lining. A new cell layer, the endoderm, is formed by the embryo. Magnified 300 times.

9TH DAY
The embryonic tissues are completely implanted. The temporary placenta has established a blood supply for all the embryonic tissues. Magnified 230 times.

11TH DAY
The permanent placenta grows and forms a new tissue, the mesoderm. The embryo enlarges, and is now roofed over by the amnion. The endoderm develops a cavity, the yolk sac. Magnified 150 times.

14TH DAY
The permanent placenta lined by mesoderm is forming the villi. The amnionic and yolk sac cavities are well developed. Magnified 50 times.

PREGNANCY

(THIRD AND FOURTH WEEKS)

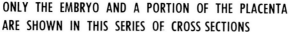

ONLY THE EMBRYO AND A PORTION OF THE PLACENTA
ARE SHOWN IN THIS SERIES OF CROSS SECTIONS

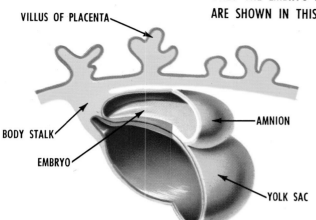

VILLUS OF PLACENTA

BODY STALK

EMBRYO

AMNION

YOLK SAC

16TH DAY

The flat embryo is roofed over by the amnion, and attached to the endoderm which forms the yolk sac. The mesodermic body stalk connects these tissues with the developing placenta. The embryo is 1/20 of an inch long.

19TH DAY

The embryo is beginning to curve. The mesoderm is pushing between the embryo and the endoderm.

22ND DAY

The mesoderm has pushed between the curved embryo and the endoderm. Head, tail, heart, and gut regions are defined. The yolk sac opening to the gut is narrowing.

28TH DAY

By the end of the first month, the embyo is 1/5 inch long. The head, heart, and gut are more advanced.

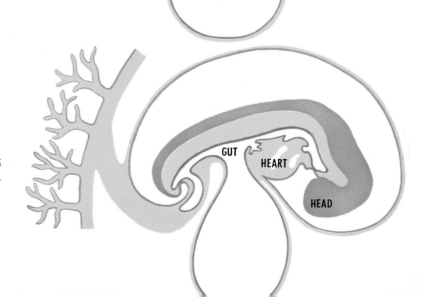

GUT

HEART

HEAD

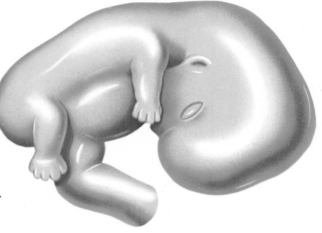

THE SECOND MONTH

EXTERNAL APPEARANCE
OF 35–DAY–OLD EMBRYO.
SIZE IS 1/3 INCH.

1   BRAIN
2   HEART
3   LIVER
4   SPINE
5   YOLK SAC
6   BODY STALK

EXTERNAL APPEARANCE
OF 45–DAY–OLD EMBRYO.
SIZE 4/5 INCH.

COMPARATIVE SIZES
IN 3-12 WEEK EMBRYOS

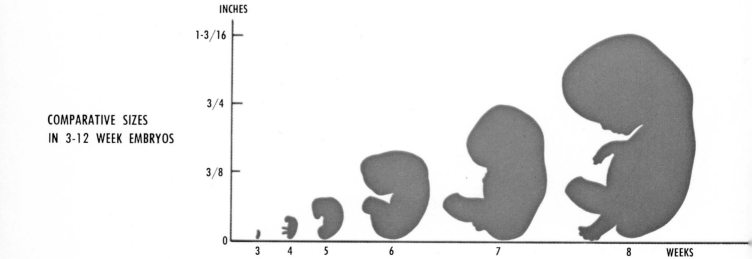

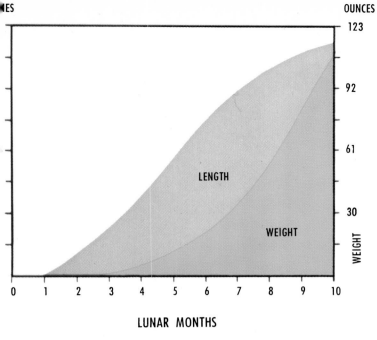

LUNAR MONTHS

Comparison of length and weight of embryo and fetus. For example: In 5th month fetus is 7-7/8 inches long and 61 ounces in weight.

PERIOD OF THE FETUS

After the end of 8th week, the embryo, complete in external form, with all organs in place is called a fetus.

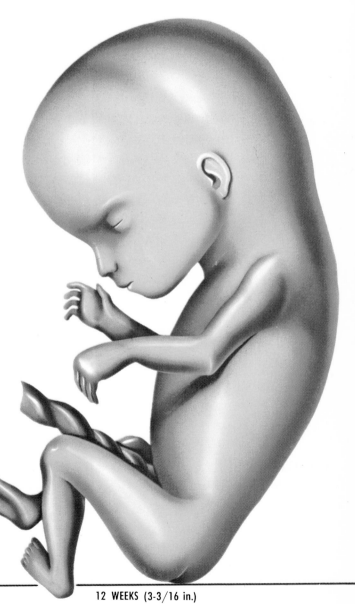

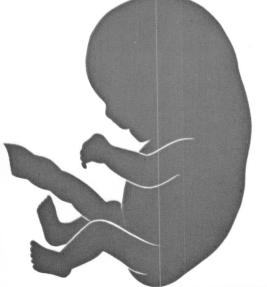

9 WEEKS (1-3/4 in.)

12 WEEKS (3-3/16 in.)

THE TENTH MONTH

FETUS WITHIN AMNION
IN 38TH WEEK

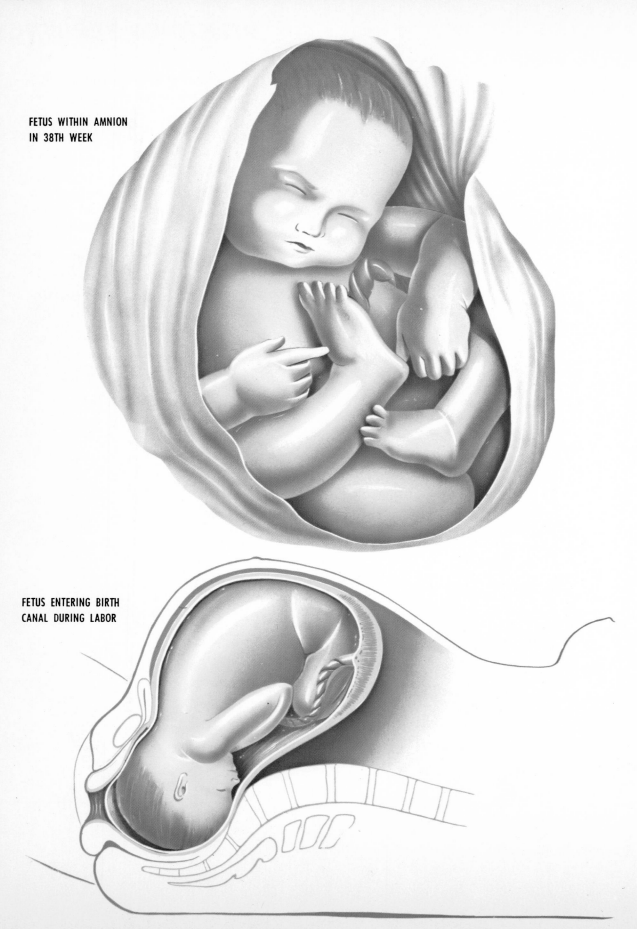

FETUS ENTERING BIRTH
CANAL DURING LABOR

and political factors determine mental health, and that such public welfare advances as higher wages, better living standards, more educational facilities, and more opportunity for rehabilitation and recreation are very important factors in mental health. Preventative social psychiatry has also made great progress in discovering interpersonal social factors causing epidemic ill health.

MENTAL ILLNESS   As recently as the nineteenth century, mental illness was not well understood and was treated by superstitious, unscientific methods which in many cases only made the mental patient worse because of mishandling. The major breakthrough occurred with public recognition that mental disorder was a medical, not a criminal, problem. Formerly, mental patients were handled like criminals, often housed in prison-like institutions and punished, rather than treated. (Even the legal procedure for committing a mental patient usually required the assistance of a sheriff.)

Particularly since World War II, there has been more general acceptance of the idea that mental patients should be given the same type of sympathetic care customarily given patients with physical disease. With the advent of tranquilizing drugs and the understanding that a mental patient is ill rather than evil, there has been a progressive liberalization and improvement in community methods for dealing with psychiatric problems. Padded cells, straitjackets, locked wards, and lifetime custodial institutionalization have largely been abandoned in most enlightened mental hospitals.

In most states a mental patient can now be voluntarily admitted to a psychiatric ward without having to go through an embarrassing court procedure. In the best mental hospitals patients are handled with such understanding and tact that violent episodes are becoming less frequent and are controlled by tranquilizing drugs

rather than by force. Patients are now kept largely in unlocked, open wards in pleasant, homelike surroundings and with a full daily program involving intensive psychotherapy, occupational therapy, recreation, and opportunities for gainful employment.

As a result of psychiatric advances, it is now no longer necessary for the milder cases even to be sent to a mental hospital, while a large percentage of first admissions to psychiatric hospitals are being routinely discharged as cured after a few months of intensive treatment. It can truthfully be said that now there is great hope, not only for cure, but also for prevention of many psychiatric conditions.

METATARSUS VARUS   This is a congenital deformity of the foot in which the inner part of the fore region of the foot is elevated, the heel remaining in a normal or slightly turned-in position. Treatment consists of corrective plaster casts which, as they are changed, gradually return the foot to normalcy. The sooner this therapy is instituted the better the prognosis.

MINERALS   Most of the minerals (see also VITAMINS) are found in such profusion in all foods that, save for a few substances, it is impossible to have a deficiency. Sodium and chloride are of course present in common table salt. Calcium, important for the formation of teeth and bone, is found chiefly in dairy products. Since vitamin D is required for the absorption and utilization of calcium, it is today ordinarily added to commercially-distributed milk. Phosphorus, magnesium, manganese, potassium, zinc, sulfur are all essential to the diet but are readily available in the child's average diet of meat, fruit, vegetables, grains, and dairy products.

Certain minerals, though normally present in sufficient quantities, may be brought to the doctor's attention by a condition caused by their very deficiency.

354

Thus, an insufficiency of iron will result in anemia. Furthermore, trace elements of copper and cobalt are apparently necessary for optimum utilization of the iron itself. A deficiency of iodine will lead to a goiter condition; but today this is almost unheard of, because of the universal use of iodized salt. Lack of fluoride in the diet will result in increased incidence of dental cavities (caries); many wise communities have voted to add this substance to their water-supply, with universal improvement in the soundness of teeth.

Many parents have been deluded by food faddists into believing that giving their children this or that element will increase pep, provide strength, and even forestall arthritis, hypertension, and the like; there are those who will go so far as to drink sea water or diluted mud if bottled attractively! The salesmen for these elixirs-of-life reap huge profits and the victims only lose money—as most of these remedies are at best no more effective than the soup one may have had for lunch.

MOLARS   The large posterior teeth having four or more cusps are the molars. There are eight in the deciduous dentition (replaced by the eight permanent bicuspids) and twelve in the permanent dentition which have no primary predecessors. The first adult tooth to erupt is the first permanent molar (six-year molar). The second permanent molar erupts at about age twelve and is referred to as the twelve-year molar. The permanent third molars are the wisdom teeth, usually the last teeth of all to erupt.

MOLDS   Molds and fungi belong to the plant world but do not contain chlorophyll. Many fungi live on decaying material, some are plant parasites, and a very few cause disease in man. They reproduce by spores and although they grow in the soil, their spores are air-borne like pollen.

The important molds causing allergic reactions are: *Alternaria, Hormodendrum, Helminthosporium, Pullaria, Aspergillus, Penicillium, Chaetomium, Phoma, Fusarium, Rhizopus, Mucor,* dry rot fungus, smuts, and rusts. Allergy to molds is more common in adults than in children.

The mold-spore content of the air is lowest during a snowfall. It is highest during the dry weather that follows the first heavy frost. April through November is the "mold season."

Symptoms. Mold sensitivity will cause such allergic disorders as conjunctivitis, perennial and seasonal rhinitis, asthma, atopic dermatitis, and croup. Diagnosis is made by skin-testing.

Treatment. Avoiding such sites as damp basements and swampy areas is important. There should be frequent vacuum-cleaning of upholstery, rugs, draperies, bedding, etc., and moldy items should be exposed to sunlight. Air conditioning is also helpful. Hyposensitization is frequently beneficial.

MOLES, PIGMENTED   Often referred to as birthmarks, but rarely present at birth, pigmented moles, or nevi, are tumors made up of pigment-producing cells (melanocytes). The lesions begin to appear in childhood and continue to grow in size and number through adult life. They range from flat to warty, dome-shaped, and pedunculated brown tumors of various shades, some of which also contain hair.

The problem of classifying the large variety of tumors in this group, many of which have overlapping characteristics, is complicated by the fact that nonpigmented moles are of the same basic structures as the pigmented ones, but without evident pigment to help in the differential diagnosis. It is obviously neither practical nor useful to remove the literally countless moles as a prophylactic measure against the rare occurrence of malignant change which occurs almost exclusively in the "junction type." Differentiation between the three main classes (intraepidermal, junction, and compound) can be made with a high degree of accuracy, and changes in the pigmentation with fuzziness at the borders, irregular coloring with speckling, or change to black or very dark brown, are indications for considering surgical removal. Hairy pigmented nevi almost always remain benign. Moles situated in areas of trauma (feet) should be removed unless removal will itself cause disability. So large a percentage of the population has moles of the toes and feet, and so low is the incidence of malignancy, as to afford a statistical reassurance and warning against unnecessary (and possibly disabling) surgery.

The intraepidermal type of nevi are more likely to be dome-shaped, globular, and pedunculated, as contrasted with the flat or slightly elevated junction type (with the exception of warty lesions which are usually junction type also). It must be emphasized that classification of nevi is possible only after it has been determined that the lesion concerned belongs to this group of growths. The skin abounds in different kinds of growths of various size, shapes, and degrees of pigmentation having no relationship in structure or significance to moles. Since it is well within the ken of the layman to recognize the common mole, expert advice should be sought either when a long-standing lesion becomes altered in appearance, or when either a new or an old lesion does not readily lend itself to a "usual" diagnosis. Warty lesions which are obviously not really warts; bleeding lesions which are not really the result of immediate injury; and inflamed lesions with no apparent explanation for the inflammation present the type of situation requiring considered diagnosis.

Treatment. Moles known to be benign and known not to undergo malignant degeneration can be removed for reasons of convenience and for improved appearance by surgery or electrocautery. Moles of known potential danger or of undetermined

classification should be excised surgically and sent to the pathologist for review. Prophylactic removal of warts is neither practical nor desirable except in instances of known potential danger.

MOLLUSCUM CONTAGIOSUM
This condition occurs most often in children. When its incidence is high in a community, the "epidemic" is usually attributed to contacts in swimming pools, gyms, and dormitories. It also occurs both in children and in adults as an isolated happenstance, without the source of infection being detected.

Symptoms. The lesions are characteristically button-shaped papules with hard rims and relatively large depressed centers. The smaller lesions are more dome-shaped. They are skin colored and appear on almost every part of the body, including the eyelids. Other than the continued growth of the individual lesions and the spread of the eruption, only occasional secondary pustular infection is a bothersome feature.

Treatment. The molluscum body, that self-contained mass under the upper-most layer of the skin which gives the lesion its form, disintegrates on even slight injury. Pricking the lesion with a sterile needle or with a smooth round toothpick is usually sufficient to cause its disappearance. More destructive measures such as electrocautery are rarely needed for cure.

MONGOLISM
Mongolism, also called "Down's syndrome" and "trisomy 21," is a congenital condition caused by faulty chromosome behavior in the fertilized human egg. The usual chromosome inventory for humans is 23 pairs. The Down's syndrome individual, however, has an extra chromosome, creating a total of 47, instead of the normal 46. This abnormality produces an individual characterized by a broad face, stubby fingers, and upward-slanting eyes, plus various degrees of mental retardation and vulnerability to infection. Dwarfism,

poor neuromuscular coordination, and congenital heart damage are also possible. Because of the genetic nature of the condition, there is no cure. Close to half of all Down's syndrome children die before adulthood, often because of their susceptibility to lung and intestinal infections.

The incidence of Down's syndrome is about one in every 600 births. However, as the age of the mother increases the chances of a Down's syndrome child also increase. For women over the age of forty-five the incidence rises to about one in every forty births.

Down's syndrome children are usually pleasant and affectionate, as well as easily managed; but although they are docile, they can be a source of strain in the family because of their retardation. Even in adulthood, the average mental age is about eight years. However, cases have been documented showing that Down's syndrome children are capable of developing vastly improved intellects when given increased parental attention, patience, and encouragement. In cases where retardation or other congenital defects are severe, or when financial requirements for medical care can not be met, parents may decide to institutionalize their Down's syndrome child.

For some parents, who must deal with the birth of a Down's syndrome child, guilt feelings and self-recrimination must be overcome. Consultation with one's physician and with other parents of mentally impaired children will help. If the decision is made to rear the child, then measures can be taken by all family members to encourage the child to develop as much as he or she possibly can. Families should be aware that there is no treatment, contrary to the claims of unscrupulous hucksters, that transforms an afflicted child into a completely normal one. Parental patience, love, and encouragement are possibly the most appropriate therapy.

Because the risk of having an afflicted child greatly increases if the mother is over thirty-five, or if a family history of the condition exists, physicians may advise couples to obtain genetic counseling or, if the woman is pregnant, to undergo amniocentesis to determine the likelihood of producing a Down's syndrome child.

MONONUCLEOSIS   See GLANDULAR FEVER (INFECTIOUS MONONUCLEOSIS)

MORBIDITY RATE   The ratio of the number of cases of a disease to the number of well people in a given population during a specified period of time, such as a year.

MORNING SICKNESS   This is a very common symptom of early pregnancy, and occurs more frequently in patients who are pregnant for the first time. It usually disappears after the first three months, although in some cases it may last throughout the entire duration of pregnancy. Morning sickness may vary from mild nausea to very severe and persistent vomiting in which the patient can not retain any food, and a dangerous degree of dehydration may develop because of the loss of body fluids and minerals. This last condition is called hyperemesis gravidarum.

The cause of morning sickness in pregnancy is not definitely known. There is little doubt that in the majority of cases purely psychosomatic factors are the only cause. Whether the physiological changes of pregnancy, and the adjustment of the body to a new balance of hormones and electrolytes, are manifested in the form of nausea and vomiting is not known.

Treatment. Most patients will respond well to reassurance and mild sedation; others will require special drugs for nausea; while the more severe cases with prolonged vomiting and dehydration will require hospitalization and treatment with intravenous fluids until tolerance to food intake is gradually reestablished. It is generally advisable to avoid any nonessential drugs during early pregnancy, and the too liberal rule-of-thumb administration of anti-vomiting agents for morning sickness is to be condemned.

MOSQUITO BITES The large zoologic division of Diptera includes several types of mosquitoes, night-flying moths, and gnats.

Symptoms. Almost all the members of this group of insects produce hive-like lesions with central puncture and occasional small local hemorrhage, the result of reaction to the contents of the insect's saliva deposited into the skin. The contents of the saliva vary according to the species. It is quite likely that almost all species produce saliva containing both an irritating substance and a material which is capable of producing an allergic response in susceptible persons. Both types of substances can be the cause of the usual insect bite. However, it is probably only the allergenic material which is capable of producing the large hives with disfiguring swelling of ears, eyelids, and other affected areas, along with general symptoms of varying degrees of shock (chills, sweating, faintness).

Treatment. Soothing lotion (calamine), antihistaminic drugs, and application of ice-cold water will control the usual mosquito bites. Symptoms of shock should be treated as in any other condition. For prevention, it is advisable to apply insect repellants to skin and clothes. Patients who are very susceptible to insect bites may find it necessary to take antihistaminic drugs by mouth prior to expected exposure to insects to render the bites innocuous.

MOUTH The oral cavity is the main point of contact with the outside world in the newborn infant. While its importance diminishes as times goes by, the mouth continues to be the source of many pleasurable sensations. Because of the rich nerve-supply, taste and the perception of texture are highly developed. The lips, tongue, teeth, palate, and salivary glands all help in the preliminary preparation of the food before swallowing. The extensive blood supply to the structures of the mouth aids in preventing most infections that might be expected from the constant minor burns and scratches to which the area is ordinarily subjected. Interestingly, a bite inflicted by another individual usually becomes severely infected, but one's own germs seldom cause trouble. Various difficulties peculiar to the mouth and its structures are discussed under their appropriate headings. (See HOME NURSING CARE.)

MOUTHWASH In general usage, this term implies a liquid with a pleasant taste or odor for rinsing the mouth. However, the council on Dental Therapeutics of the American Dental Association "does not accept mouthwashes for unsupervised use by the lay public." Routine rinsing of the mouth is not a substitute for proper toothbrushing, although at times a dentist may prescribe the practice in relation to individual needs.

MULTIPLE SCLEROSIS Multiple sclerosis is one of the common chronic disabling disorders of the central nervous system. It is characterized by recurring symptoms with progression of disability. The white matter of the brain and spinal cord is damaged through spotty destruction of myelin, which coats the nerve fiber. The cause of this malady is unknown.

Symptoms. The initial symptoms depend upon the portion of the central nervous system involved. A frequent early symptom is the rapid onset of blurred vision and decreased visual acuity due to disordered function of the optic nerves. Involvement in the brainstem may produce double vision, facial numbness or weakness, vertigo, or slurred speech. Sudden weakness, numbness, or bladder disorder may be due to spinal-cord damage. Symptoms and findings characteristically progress for a period of days or weeks and then recede, with partial or nearly complete recovery in subsequent months. With recurrence, more residual disability persists. The diagnosis is based primarily on the clinical findings. Many other neurologic conditions present a similar medical picture, however.

Treatment. Although there is no specific treatment for multiple sclerosis, supportive care is most important. It is explained to the patient that a single episode of disability may be followed by complete, or nearly complete, return of function. Then too, the interval between recurrence may vary from less than a year to many years. Thus, the patient may frequently enjoy many productive years before severe disability occurs. With an acute attack, bed rest (followed by limited activity) is important. A nutritious diet and supplementary vitamin therapy are indicated. Steroid drugs are of value in selected cases. Physical therapy enables the patient to improve his gait and strength, and occupational therapy is of value in improving hand coordination.

MUMPS   An acute, communicable virus disease, mumps is manifested by swelling and tenderness of the salivary glands, the parotid (cheek) glands being the most commonly affected.

Symptoms. The child will complain of a headache and/or an earache and run a fever of 100° to 101°, but will not be too sick. He is usually given an aspirin and sent off to school, for the characteristic swelling of the face does not develop for several hours. This is the reason that such diseases as mumps keep circulating throughout the community; no one realizes the child has a communicable illness at the very time he is highly contagious.

Usually the swelling of the parotid glands is immediately below the earlobes. It feels like hard gelatin, is tender, and fills in the "pocket" at the earlobe, going back over the tip of the mastoid bone and then straight forward to swell the cheek, like that of a chipmunk. The only condition mumps is sometimes mistaken for is swollen lymph glands of the neck caused by infected tonsils.

Mumps virus may invade the submaxillary glands and the sublingual glands producing a double-chin effect. These swellings may occur simultaneously or one after the other, so that the disease may last for two to three weeks. In four to five days the swelling reaches maximum size and in about the same length of time disappears. Once subsided the swelling cannot be seen but is still felt and the patient is no longer contagious.

Two rare but distressing complications are possible in children's mumps. These are pancreatitis, which causes severe stomachache and often vomiting, and encephalitis with extreme headache, stiff neck and back, and lethargy. In the adult male and in older boys the sex glands (testes) may also be involved and fertility may be jeopardized. Because of these complications, it is of some importance that children be immunized with mumps vaccine before maturity. Mumps vaccine should not be administered during pregnancy and pregnant women should avoid a child who has mumps if they have never had the disease themselves.

Treatment. There is no specific medication for mumps. Aspirin alone is often recommended and may prove helpful. If the patient feels poorly, he or she should stay in bed. However, if the child feels well enough to move about the house, this can be permitted, for it will not affect the likelihood of complications. Consultation with a physician concerning a vaccination schedule for childhood disease is advised.

MURMUR   An extra heart sound, sounding like fluid passing an obstruction, heard between the normal heart sounds.

MUSCULAR DYSTROPHY This is a genetic disease with a hereditary characteristic. The disease is marked by a progressive atrophy of the muscles. As the weakening and wasting progresses the patient becomes confined to a wheelchair and ultimately to bed. As yet no cure is known.

MUSHROOM POISONING Mushroom, or toadstool, poisoning is commonly due to consumption of the species of mushroom (toadstool) known as *Amanita muscaria.*

Symptoms. Symptoms begin within a few minutes to two hours after eating. There is formation of tears, salivation, sweating, vomiting, abdominal cramps, diarrhea, thirst, dizziness, confusion, collapse, and sometimes coma and convulsions.

In the form of mushroom poisoning produced by *Amanita phalloides* and related species, symptoms occur after six to fifteen hours and are announced by the sudden onset of abdominal pain, nausea, vomiting, and diarrhea. There is often blood in the stools and dehydration may be extreme. Jaundice due to liver damage follows in a few days. The liver itself is enlarged, the pulse is rapid, the blood pressure falls, and the temperature is below normal.

Treatment. In cases of poisoning from *A. muscaria,* atropine is a specific antagonist of nervous-system overstimulation. Where *A. phalloides* is the cause, a high carbohydrate intake—some via intravenous injection—is indicated to prevent severe liver damage.

MYASTHENIA GRAVIS Myasthenia gravis is a disorder associated with weakness and easy fatigability of muscles. It is related to a defect in the transmission of impulses from the nerve fiber to the muscle fiber, and occurs both in children and in adults. The cause of myasthenia is not known.

Symptoms. The initial symptoms of myasthenia gravis frequently relate to a disturbance in function of muscles supplied by the cranial nerves. Drooping of the eyelids may occur. With weakness of the muscles which move the eyeball, double vision may be a prominent symptom. The facial muscles may be weak. Swallowing may become difficult due to weakness of the throat muscles. The voice may be hoarse. Weakness may also be noted in the muscles of the neck, shoulders, arms, and legs. Characteristically, the muscles become weaker with prolonged use; for example, the patient may initially have little difficulty in chewing, then note progressive weakness as he eats a meal. Such muscular weakness diminishes with rest and there is no wasting of muscles.

In some patients weakness is confined to only a few muscle-groups, whereas in others generalized weakness is present. During the course of myasthenia severe attacks of generalized weakness or paralysis may occur, producing weakness of the muscles of respiration. The reflexes remain normal and sensation remains intact.

Treatment. Several drugs are available to improve conduction from the nerve endings to the muscles, such as Neostigmine®, Mestinon®, and Mytelase®. These drugs are taken daily, several times a day, in order to prevent muscle weakness and easy fatigability. Given the proper dosage of medication, the majority of patients with mild or moderate myasthenia are able to carry out their normal activities. Patients with severe myasthenia will show significant improvement but may continue to have partial disability in spite of large amounts of one or more of these medications. Removal of the thymus gland has been the recommended treatment in selected cases.

Patients with myasthenia have spontaneous flare-ups and remissions of their disorders; in severe flare-ups, present methods of therapy may be unsuccessful. The mortality rate in myasthenia gravis is still high.

MYCOSIS FUNGOIDES This disease belongs to the lymphoma group whose characteristic disturbance is that of the reticulo-endothelial cells which are present in the skin, lymph nodes, bone marrow, and spleen. Unlike other lymphomas, mycosis fungoides is always seen in the skin first, and remains predominantly though not exclusively in the skin throughout the course of the disease. Much more common in males, this disease rarely begins before the age of forty.

Symptoms. The lesions first appear as oval-shaped, pink, slightly scaly plaques of the face, torso, and extremities. The number of lesions can be very variable. Gradually there is a thickening of the areas, and the color becomes more intense and tends to have a violet hue. Finally, the lesions enlarge and take on the appearance of tumors, reddish-brown in color, and often ulcerated.

Treatment. Localized irradiation of small individual tumors with X-ray and generalized beta ray irradiation for patients with more general involvement constitute the current treatment for this disease.

MYOCARDIAL INFARCTION See CORONARY OCCLUSION

MYXEDEMA When thyroid activity is very low or absent, the skin becomes thickened and the tissues under the skin become filled with a mucinous thick substance. This condition is spoken of as myxedema. The same term is also often used to refer to the entire symptom complex of hypothyroidism.

NAIL-BITING This is an early symptom of emotional conflict and anxiety in young children and has significance only

as a symptom of the underlying neurotic condition. Nail-biting frequently develops during periods of increased tension and conflict when the child is under emotional pressure from the environment. Usually it is only one of a group of nervous symptoms including eating and sleeping disturbances, nose-picking, thumb-sucking, skin-picking, and tics.

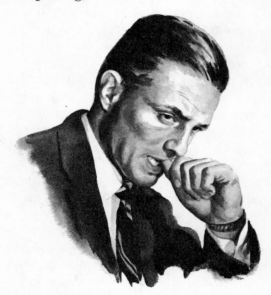

Treatment. There is no specific treatment for nail-biting, which usually disappears spontaneously as the child becomes older and more mature. If this and other neurotic symptoms interfere too seriously with adjustment, the child should be referred to a child guidance clinic for psychiatric treatment for deeper underlying causes.

NARCOANALYSIS Narcoanalysis is a method of analyzing unconscious conflicts, in which the patient is studied while under the influence of hypnotic drugs. In World War II it was discovered that psychiatric patients who had had severely disturbing war experiences (about which they were not able to talk while in a normal waking state) could be made more accessible under heavy sedation by hypnotic drugs which inhibited conscious defenses and brought repressed experiences to the surface. By this method, patients suspected of harboring repressed traumatic experiences in the unconscious are given heavy sedation and then asked about their deepest problems as they are about to fall asleep. This method is frequently very economical and time-saving, making possible examination of repressed experiences which would ordinarily take months of orthodox psychoanalysis to uncover.

NARCOLEPSY   A sudden overwhelming desire to sleep, regardless of where the person is or what he is doing. It is not caused by physical fatigue or sleep deprivation. Unlike syncope (fainting), the sleeping state is natural, lasting from seconds to a few minutes. If the slumberer is wakened, he promptly falls asleep again; upon awakening spontaneously, he feels refreshed. This bizarre affliction usually affects obese young men, who often also complain of sexual impotence. The drug amphetamine controls the condition quite effectively.

NASAL POLYPS   Polyps are pale pink (sometimes gray), soft growths in the nose. They are the most common growth of the nasal interior. Removal can give great relief from the symptoms of nasal blockage. Many, if not most, nasal polyps are the result of nasal allergy and they will quickly recur if the allergy factor is not controlled.

NASOPHARYNX   The nasopharynx can be described as a funnel-shaped cavity with five openings. The posterior nares of the nose are two of the openings; the two Eustachian tubes are two more; and the oropharynx is the fifth opening. The adenoids, when present, sit on the back wall near the roof.

The position of the openings of the Eustachian tubes in children and adults is worth noting. In infants the openings

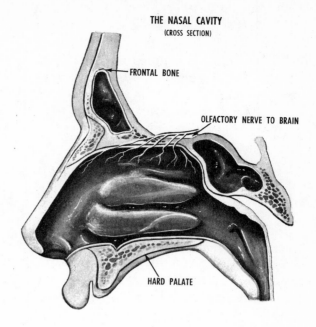

THE NASAL CAVITY
(CROSS SECTION)

FRONTAL BONE

OLFACTORY NERVE TO BRAIN

HARD PALATE

OLFACTORY SENSE
Specialized sensory neurons, capable of being stimulated by airborne odor particles, are located in the roof of the nasal cavity. The neurons collect into numerous small nerves which form the olfactory nerve. The odors most recognized are floral, fruity, herbal or spicy, resinal, and smoky.

are on a level with the floor of the nose. As the child grows older the relative position rises until in adulthood, the openings of the Eustachian tubes are as high as the lower (inferior) turbinate. The infant and younger child are therefore more prone to middle-ear infections because the wide, horizontal tube, with its opening at the floor of the nose, allows infected nasal secretions to enter the ear easily. The elevated angle of the Eustachian tube of the adult makes the middle ear less susceptible to contamination from nasal secretions.

NAUSEA AND VOMITING   Nausea and vomiting may occur independently of each other, but are usually closely associated symptoms. Nausea commonly precedes vomiting; however, this is by no means the rule. Many types of stimulation, such as severe pain or disagreeable sights or odors, may provoke nausea and subsequent vomiting. Stimulation from the organs of balance in the middle ear may cause nausea, as in seasickness. The actual act of vomiting requires a center of the brain for coordination and is therefore rather complex.

A type of vomiting not preceded by nausea, in which the stomach contents are ejected forcibly, sometimes occurs after severe head injuries, and is thus a valuable diagnostic sign. Acute infectious diseases, too—particularly in children—very often have vomiting as one of the preliminary symptoms. Practically all diseases and conditions affecting the upper digestive tract may also cause nausea and vomiting. The vomiting of early pregnancy is little understood but widely experienced. Certain types of heart or endocrine disease can be associated with nausea and vomiting. In sensitive individuals, mere stimulation of the rear portion of the throat may cause gagging and vomiting. In some persons nausea and vomiting seem to be psychogenic or emotional in origin; these patients rarely suffer malnutrition because of it, since the actual amount of food lost is negligible.

The material actually vomited up is called vomitus, and its characteristics can be of importance in diagnosing possible underlying conditions. Thus, vomitus with the odor of feces may indicate the presence of an obstruction in the small intestine. Although streaks of blood usually have no significance (mere irritation due to the vigorous muscular action may cause a small amount of bleeding), larger quantities of blood—either bright red or dark brown—usually indicate significant bleeding into the stomach or the esophagus. If vomiting is prolonged, bile is commonly present. Nausea and vomiting are usually nonspecific symptoms and the underlying cause must always be determined. Most cases are due to a transient viral gastritis or gastroenteritis, and are self-limiting. Occasionally, nausea and vomiting may provide a clue to the presence of underlying metabolic disturbance such as diabetes.

NAVEL (UMBILICUS) The navel, often called the belly button, is the mid-abdominal depression which is actually a scar indicating that point where blood vessels from and to the mother entered and left the unborn child's body. For ruptured navel see HERNIA.

NEARSIGHTEDNESS (MYOPIA) In this condition light rays from a distant object come to focus in front of the retina. It occurs because the ratio between the bending of light rays and length of the eye is not proportionate, either because of too much bending or too long an eyeball. An object which is located close to a nearsighted eye is focused on the retina so that one can see objects clearly from this point.

Symptoms. Nearsightedness causes an inability to see clearly at a distance. Objects may be brought close enough to the eye to be in focus, but may be so close that eyestrain occurs.

Treatment. The condition is neutralized by concave lenses. Most individuals are farsighted at birth and become nearsighted between the tenth and twentieth year. Thereafter, there may be minor changes, but the condition is stabilized.

Temporary nearsightedness may occur in diabetes or be associated with excessive use of the eyes which remain focused for near vision (spasm of accommodation). The condition disappears when the underlying cause is removed. In some types of cataract in the aged, nearsightedness occurs so that vision is clear for close work without lenses. However, there is a parallel reduction of vision for distance, and if the cataract progresses, near vision is also disturbed.

NEPHRITIS Inflammation or destruction of the interior of the kidney by disease is known as nephritis. If the disorder is chiefly in the glomerulus, the term employed is glomerulonephritis; if in the collecting portion of the kidney and caused by infection, the term employed is pyelonephritis.

Nephritis produces a complex of symptoms composed of high blood pressure, weakness, easy fatigability, swelling of the tissues of the body (edema), and hemorrhages—especially in the interior of the eye. Glomerulonephritis is often caused by an allergic-type reaction to the streptococcus; it is best treated by rest, careful regulation of diet, and general health measures. Pyelonephritis is treated by identification of the infectious agent and its elimination by means of antibiotics. With pyelonephritis there is also usually an obstruction somewhere in the urinary tract which must be removed before there can be permanent healing.

NEPHROLITHIASIS   This is the medical term for the presence of kidney stones.

NEPHRON   The microscopic functional unit of the kidney is the glomerulus, a filtering device. This consists of a small bundle of blood vessels and a cup-like structure which accepts blood plasma and passes into a tubular structure (nephron). This nephron has straight and looped portions and ends in the collecting duct which empties into the pelvis of the kidney.

The function of the nephron is to clear the blood of poisonous substances and products of normal metabolism which the body excretes as waste. It also functions as a regulator of the level of blood alkalinity.

NEPHROSIS AND NEPHROTIC SYNDROME   Damage to the kidneys from disease or toxins results in an inability of the kidney to prevent loss of protein from the blood; examination of the urine will reveal large quantities of albumin. This condition is known as nephrosis. The nephrotic syndrome includes all the systemic effects of this disorder. Because of loss of protein from the bloodstream, fluid collects in the tissues of the body, giving rise to a condition called dropsy (edema). This is particularly apt to occur in the face and about the eyes, helping to distinguish it from heart conditions, in which edema of the lower extremities is more common.

NERVE CELL (NEURON)   A neuron, or nerve cell, includes a cell body and long receiving (afferent) and transmitting (efferent) extensions from that body. It is the cellular unit of the nervous system. Nerve cells are designed for the reception and transmission of sensory and motor impulses throughout the entire body. Within the central nervous system, neurons are arranged in networks which transmit impulses from one transmitting extension (axon) across a gap (synapse) to a receiving extension (dendrite), and so on through an entire series of cells.

The primary motor neurons in the spinal cord have their cell bodies located in the anterior grey matter. These cell bodies contain nuclei and cytoplasm. Their dendrites form a network of receptors, which extend locally within the cord. Their axons, or motor fibers, leave the cell-body and pass through the anterior root, the spinal nerve, and the peripheral nerve to the muscle fibers, which they innervate. These axons are covered with a fatty material called myelin.

The primary sensory neurons together with their sensory fibers are the receptors in the skin, the muscles, the viscera, and elsewhere. Secondary and other sensory neurons relay these impulses to the cord and brain.

NERVE FIBERS   Nerve fibers are the long processes which extend from the cell-bodies of neurons. Nerve fibers transmit sensory and motor impulses throughout the nervous system. These fibers are of microscopic diameter, but may be as much as several feet in length.

Columns (tracts) of fibers form the white matter in the brain and spinal cord.

The cranial and peripheral nerves consist primarily of bundles of nerve fibers. Each motor fiber in a peripheral nerve connects by way of a microscopic endplate with a muscle fiber, whereas sensory nerve fibers extend from sensory nerve endings through peripheral nerves.

Damage to bundles of peripheral sensory and motor nerve-fibers results in decreased sensation and weakness of muscles in the area supplied by the nerve.

"NERVOUS BREAKDOWN" This is a nonmedical term referring to all types of neurotic disorders in which emotional instability and conflict seriously incapacitate the person in normal life. The term has many unscientific implications which do not describe the situation accurately. Breakdown implies that the person has "gone to pieces" or otherwise "lost his mind," though this is actually not the case. (No one ever loses his mind in any true sense.) What is actually involved—as in all forms of nervous and mental disorder— is some loss or absence of normal self-control.

It is more exact to refer to "a period of emotional instability" or "a period of neurotic incapacitation." Modern psychiatry is now able to diagnose all kinds of personality disorders in more exact terms which are more hopeful because they imply that causes are known and can be treated with appropriate methods.

"NERVOUSNESS" Nervousness is a nonmedical term applied to many nervous and emotional symptoms occurring in neurotic conditions and personality disorders. More specifically, the symptoms of nervousness are standard symptoms of neurotic anxiety tension states.

Symptoms. The underlying cause of emotional instability is usually fear, which produces psychosomatic symptoms of restlessness, irritability, disturbing sensations from all parts of the body, nervous tremors or twitchings, feelings of generalized muscular tension, physical weakness, and vague fears of impending illness or doom. Most laymen are aware of the psychological origin of such symptoms and fear impending mental "breakdown" or insanity. Frequently a vicious circle of increasing emotionalism and psychosomatic symptoms makes the person aware of an impending psychological crisis, as when the patient complains, "I feel I'm going to blow my top," or, "I feel something terrible is going to happen to me mentally." This rising crescendo of emotional instability associated with disturbing psychosomatic symptoms may lead to acute anxiety states associated with panicky feelings.

Treatment. Psychiatrists try to teach neurotic patients that nervous symptoms are an inevitable accompaniment to modern living and should be regarded as annoying but not dangerous. Psychiatric studies of modern, high-pressure civilization indicate that emotional instability and tension symptoms are inevitable products of stressful living conditions. One should learn to regard nervous symptoms almost like one's shadow: constantly present, but not necessarily dangerous. Modern educational methods attempt to teach children to function under increasing levels of stress and to tolerate nervous and emotional symptoms without becoming anxiously demoralized.

NERVOUS SYSTEM The nervous system is a highly integrated mechanism for the central control of the activity of all of the responsive (excitable) tissue of the body. Microscopically, it is composed of millions of nerve cells with their long processes. These cells constitute a conducting system for receiving and sending impulses throughout the body.

Although it functions as a unified system and is an integral part of the body as a whole, the nervous system may be arbitrarily divided into anatomic parts. The two major anatomic portions are the central nervous system and the peripheral nervous system; the central nervous system consists of the brain and the spinal cord, and the peripheral of outlying nerve fibers.

Certain portions of the nervous system are more susceptible to specific diseases than others. For example, certain substances, such as diphtheria toxin and arsenic, primarily damage peripheral nerves. In contrast, poliomyelitis virus involves the central nervous system.

NEURALGIA   Neuralgia is pain which lies along the path of a cranial or peripheral nerve, or posterior root. It is not associated with any change in the function of the nerve.

Symptoms. Trigeminal neuralgia is a recurring, sharp, knife-like pain along the paths of the trigeminal (fifth cranial) nerve. Frequent severe bouts of pain may be temporarily disabling. Periods of recurring pain may last for several weeks or months and may then be followed by periods of remission. (See TRIGEMINAL NEURALGIA.) A similar neuralgia, involving the ninth cranial nerve, occasionally occurs and produces severe sharp pain in the throat with spread to the ear on the same side. Intercostal neuralgia produces pain extending from the back (at the level of the affected segment) to the chest or abdomen.

Treatment. Medicines which relieve pain are needed for relief of recurrent neuralgia. It is important, however, to avoid the repeated use of narcotic drugs. Sedatives to induce sleep are required in patients with prolonged severe attacks of neuralgia. In selected patients, injections of alcohol into the involved nerve are followed by prolonged relief of symptoms. (However, alcohol-injection results in loss of sensation in the distribution of the injected nerve.) In other severe cases, direct surgical treatment is indicated. Dilantin®

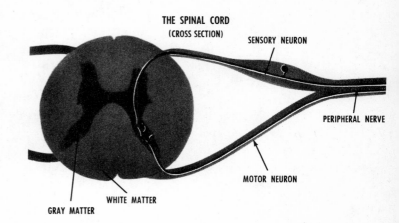

THE SPINAL CORD (CROSS SECTION)   SENSORY NEURON   PERIPHERAL NERVE   MOTOR NEURON   WHITE MATTER   GRAY MATTER

Sodium, which slows the rate of peripheral nerve conduction, has been recommended in the treatment of trigeminal neuralgia; vitamin B_{12}, given in large doses by injection has also been reported to be associated with remission of trigeminal neuralgia.

NEURITIS   Neuritis is an inflammation of one or more cranial or peripheral nerves and is associated with disturbance of sensation and strength in the muscles supplied by the involved nerve or nerves. Damage to a single nerve (mononeuritis) is frequently the result of local nerve injury. Involvement of multiple nerves (polyneuritis) occurs with severe nutritional deficiencies often associated with chronic alcoholism, or with poisoning by such substances as lead, arsenic, and chemical compounds.

Symptoms. The symptoms of mononeuritis are related to the sensory and muscular (motor) control activities of the particular nerve involved. This neuritis involving the radial nerve in the arm results in weakness of extension of the wrists and fingers; while neuritis of the peroneal nerve at the side of the knee results in foot drop and numbness over the lateral aspect of the lower leg and foot.

Polyneuritis produces decreased sensation and weakness in the distribution of multiple nerves. Usually numbness and weakness occur in both legs, or in the arms and legs. With severe weakness, the patient is unable to walk or stand. With severe involvement in the hands and arms, he may be unable to write or to feed himself.

Treatment. If an external poison is responsible for polyneuritis, this is removed. In arsenic-caused polyneuritis, BAL is used to increase urinary excretion of arsenic; to treat lead poisoning, Versene® is used. The administration of pyridoxine will prevent the appearance of polyneuritis in patients who are being treated with large dosages of isoniazid. Nutritional polyneuritis is treated by use of a high-protein, high-caloric, high-vitamin diet, with supplemental oral or peripheral vitamins. Diabetes mellitus associated with neuritis is controlled by diet and insulin. Symptomatic therapy includes physical therapy, occupational therapy, the application of supports and braces, and rehabilitation.

NEUROLOGIST The neurologist is a specialist who deals with organic diseases of the nervous system and is specially trained in the appropriate anatomy, physiology, and pathology. (A neurological surgeon or neurosurgeon is a specialist who combines training both in neurology and in brain and spinal cord surgery.) Competence in the field is recognized by certification by the American Board of Neurology and Psychiatry.

NEUROSIS (See also PSYCHONEUROSIS) Neurosis and psychoneurosis are almost synonymous psychiatric terms, describing a large number of functional disorders in which physical and mental symptoms are caused by emotional upsets. (The term functional refers to the fact that there is no permanent organic damage, but rather that the organism is simply functioning improperly.) The term neurosis is generally used to refer to minor functional disorders of emotional origin, the term psychoneurosis being reserved for more serious functional disorders which may incapacitate the person to a greater or lesser degree. (Still more serious disorders, the psychoses, are described elsewhere.)

Everyone may be called neurotic to some degree, since every person has some emotional conflicts or instability which interfere with normal adjustment. Usually neurotic disorders do not involve the whole personality but are limited to some functions. In general they may be regarded as reactions to life-stresses, in which one or another psychological function breaks down under excessive pressure; for example, psychiatric studies in World War II showed that every soldier had his own characteristic threshold of neurotic breakdown when life-pressures become too great.

Symptoms. Each person tends to show his own characteristic pattern of neurotic reactions, depending partly on inherited weaknesses and partly on injurious emotional experiences in early childhood. The situation is comparable to a chain which gives way at its weakest link when excessive strain is placed upon it. The most disagreeable symptom in many neurotic states consists of emotional anguish, involving terrifying sensations and feelings that the person is about to go insane. (The neurotic rarely, if ever, becomes insane; symptoms should be looked upon as annoying rather than dangerous.)

One of the most common patterns of neurotic disorder consists of psychosomatic symptoms developing in various organs in the body when a person becomes too emotionally conflictual. (The term psychosomatic refers to the fact that emotional upsets tend to disrupt the functioning of various organ-systems of the body, producing physical symptoms.) The most common psychosomatic symptoms occur in the gastrointestinal tract, where emotional conflicts produce a wide variety of symptoms including nausea, vomiting, gas, excess acidity, constipation, or diarrhea. The second most common type of psychosomatic disorder involves circulatory symptoms such as fast pulse, irregular heartbeat, high blood pressure, vascular flushing or paling in various parts of the body, fainting spells, and headaches.

Other types of (psycho)neurotic disorder include anxiety states, hysteria, obsession-compulsion neurosis, psychasthenia, neurasthenia, and psychoneurotic character disorders. In anxiety states, the basic pattern consists of symptoms of conscious and unconscious fear and anxiety. In obsession-compulsion neurosis, the characteristic symptoms involve obsessive ideas which the individual cannot get out of his head and irrational compulsions to commit acts which the person would not ordinarily perform. Hysteria is characterized by the conversion of emotional conflicts into a wide variety of physical symptoms such as hysterical blindness, deafness, and so forth. Psychasthenia is characterized by symptoms of extreme worry and guilt, reflecting an over-strict superego. Neurasthenia is a psychosomatic syndrome involving feelings of excessive fatigue, weakness, and lack of energy, usually accompanied by circulatory symptoms of low blood pressure and irregular heart action. Formerly, it was believed that these various kinds of psychoneurotic disorders represented essentially different conditions, but more recent psychoanalytic evidence indicates that they are only different manifestations of one basic process involving unconscious conflict.

Treatment. Most vital in getting the neurotic to accept treatment is to help him to accept the fact that his condition is completely psychological and that physical treatment can have no effect. This is often a problem, since neurotics are very sensitive and embarrassed about their symptoms and reluctant to admit that they do need psychological treatment.

Many neurotics would be greatly helped simply by accepting the fact that every person has some neurotic symptoms which he must learn to accept and live with. In certain instances treatment may teach the patient to be neurotic and like it; that is, to learn not to be panicked by neurotic symptoms. The patient should be reassured that he is not going to "lose his mind" and that the worst that can happen is that he will "feel bad" for a while.

Treatment of (psycho)neurotic conditions is a very complicated process which should be undertaken only by certified psychiatrists or clinical psychologists. It may require long and intensive specialized techniques to uncover the unconscious conflicts producing neurotic symptoms. Ultimately successful treatment usually involves some type of psychoanalysis in which the deep unconscious conflicts underlying neurotic symptoms are brought to light and dispelled after being consciously recognized.

NEUROTIC EXCORIATIONS   These lesions are usually present on the face, shoulders, arms and legs, and consist of small ulcers usually covered with a bloody crust. They are produced by the patient's picking, digging or scraping the skin in an attempt to remove a real or imagined substance from the skin. Whatever the initial cause of the need to excoriate the skin, a habit of doing this becomes established. As in nail-biting, the habit is difficult to break. The psychologic mechanisms capable of inducing neurotic excoriations are numerous but this condition is made even more difficult to resolve because both the patient and the accessibility of the skin are conducive to a habit mechanism. Whereas at first the patient picks on a pimple while washing the face in the bathroom, soon the turning on of the bathroom light results in an almost reflex picking of the skin.

Treatment. Seldom can the patient be convinced of the damaging effect of excoriating the skin, nor is the patient often convinced of the need for psychiatric care. Occasionally the patient can be persuaded to try devices for avoiding picking while the skin is being treated. The use of gloves securely fastened with adhesive tape, low-watt bulbs in the bathroom, and handiwork while looking at television can be suggested to the willing patient.

NIGHT BLINDNESS (NYCTALOPIA)

Night blindness is a condition in which sight is deficient in reduced illumination or in the dark of night, although it is normal in good illumination. It sometimes occurs in atrophy of the optic nerve, abnormality of the retina (in anemia, scurvy, etc.), and in vitamin A deficiency.

NIGHTMARES AND NIGHT-TERRORS

Insomnia, disturbed sleep, bad dreams, night-terrors, and nightmares all occur in neurotic anxiety states. They are symptomatic of deep unconscious fears and insecurities. States of emotional upset involving fear or anger tend to persist over long periods, causing anxiety symptoms during the day and sleep disturbances at night.

Symptoms. Nightmares and bad dreams usually involve horrible or tragic experiences, or fear of impending doom. They have the same psychiatric significance as daytime anxiety symptoms. The child with nightmares usually can be shown to be deeply conflictual emotionally.

Treatment. Since all anxiety symptoms are due to fear and insecurity, anything which contributes to feelings of security tends to counteract them. Specific treatment of nightmares and other anxiety symptoms involves psychotherapy directed

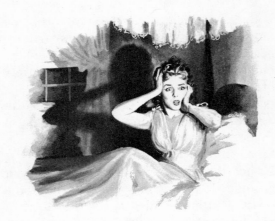

at discovering and removing sources of deep emotional conflict. It may, however, require months or years for an insecure person to develop sufficient self-confidence to feel secure.

NOCTURNAL EMISSIONS   When sexual activities or masturbation have not been engaged in for a period of time, an automatic discharge of semen may occur during sleep. This is often accompanied by dreams of an erotic nature and is sometimes referred to as a wet dream.

NONCONDUCTIVE (NEUROSENSORY, PERCEPTIVE) HEARING LOSS   Neurosensory hearing loss does *not* respond to surgery; and only Ménière's disease sometimes responds to medication. (Psychological hearing loss, of course, is a separate category and requires the services of a psychiatrist. It responds to psychotherapy and drugs, although the drugs tend only to facilitate psychotherapy rather than act directly on the nerves or blood vessels of the hearing mechanism.) (See MÉNIÈRE'S DISEASE; PRESBYCUSIS; DRUG TOXICITY; VIRAL DISEASES; ACOUSTIC TRAUMA; ACOUSTIC NEUROMA; HEAD INJURY TRAUMA; VASCULAR ACCIDENTS.)

NOSE AND PARANASAL SINUSES

The nose is composed of skin-covered cartilage, bone, and an inner lining of delicate tissue—mucous membrane (mucosa).

A bony-cartilagenous partition (septum) divides the nose into two nearly equal parts. The nostrils are the front openings of the nose, while the posterior nares are the back openings leading into the highest part of the pharynx (the so-called "back of the throat") called the nasopharynx. (The middle part of the pharynx can be seen if one looks into a mirror and says "aahh.")

The nasopharynx is just above and behind the soft palate, which may be seen in back and at the top of the mouth by looking at the open mouth in a mirror. The nasal lining (mucosa) covers all the surfaces of the sinuses, mouth, pharynx, larynx, Eustachian tubes, and middle ear, then extends throughout the lower respiratory tract. Although the mucosa varies in structure and thickness in different locations, due to the various roles it plays, essentially it is all the same membrane.

Within the nose, projecting out into the nasal space on either side toward, but not touching, the septum, are three—sometimes four—bony shelves covered by relatively thick mucosa. These shelves are called the turbinates.

The special features of the respiratory-tract mucosa are its cilia and mucus "blanket." The cilia, not visible except under a microscope, are tiny hair-like structures which beat constantly toward the mouth. This ciliary movement carries a blanket of mucus up from deep inside the lungs, as well as from the nose and sinuses downward, into the mouth, where it is swallowed. The function of the mucus blanket and the cilia is to catch foreign material, bacteria, and viruses and to carry them to a place where they will do no harm. This is a remarkable cleansing mechanism and an efficient body defense, since the swallowing allows the body effectively to eliminate unwanted material from the respiratory tract.

When the quantity of mucus becomes excessive, we may cough and spit out

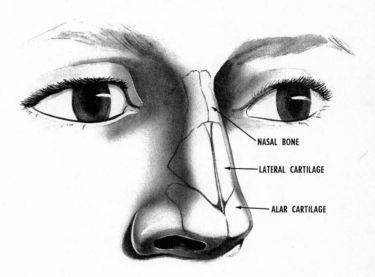

THE EXTERNAL NOSE

NASAL BONE

LATERAL CARTILAGE

ALAR CARTILAGE

some material, but this only occurs in conditions of illness. Some people suddenly become conscious of the great quantity of fluid put out by the mucosa of the respiratory tract and may begin to complain, hack, and spit. If, after examination, the physician explains there is nothing wrong and the spitting has merely become a habit, the patient is usually able to break it.

The nose also warms the air we breathe to the proper temperature for the bronchi and lungs. Inhaled air, no matter what its temperature on entering the front of the nose, is about 96.8° F. at the back of the nose. Furthermore, almost all the foreign material—bacteria, dust—in the air is gone and the relative humidity of the air is 75 per cent. All this is accomplished in about one quarter of a second by the nasal mucosa and turbinates within the four inches of space between the front and back of the nose! Every twenty-four hours about 1,000 milliliters (one quart) of fluid is mixed into the inspired air by the nose. (This figure varies with the environmental air, but is a fair estimated average.)

NOSEBLEEDS (EPISTAXIS) Epistaxis

is simply the medical term for nosebleed. Children seem to have more bloody noses than do adults, probably because they are continually falling on them or picking them. A nose will also bleed if a fever is high enough to dilate the capillaries within. Since children get many colds and upper-respiratory infections, the mucus secreted will often erode the lining.

Many people have a very red nose lining (nasal septum) with the capillaries very close to the surface. In these people, the slightest jar, or sneeze or just dry air will cause this area to split and pour out the blood. Sometimes a respiratory allergy may aggravate this tendency (see ALLERGIC CORYZA).

It is often thought that if a child has many nose bleeds he has either rheumatic fever or leukemia. This can be so; but there are so many nosebleeds as against so relatively few cases of these serious diseases that the diseases are last on the list of possibilities.

Treatment. The most important thing to do for nosebleed is to put pressure where the leak is—on the septum (the bony partition that divides the nose into two nearly equal parts.) Cold wet rags on the back of the neck, forehead, top of the nose, or under the lip are of little use, since the victim is not bleeding from these areas.

Wet a piece of clean absorbent tissue paper or cotton and press it to the size of the nasal passage. Push it up the canal and squeeze the nose from the outside hard for ten minutes; then leave the pack in place for ten minutes more and slowly withdraw it. This procedure will stop 90 per cent of nosebleeds and will leave a clear open passage without a hard, dry clot. If the condition is recurrent, a simple ointment should be applied twice daily for a week (the crack takes this long to heal) to keep the area soft and pliable. If episodes of nosebleed are too frequent, the doctor may need to cauterize the blood vessels of the septum with silver nitrate or a hot needle

—not really a painful procedure. (See also FIRST AID AND EMERGENCIES.)

NOSE, FOREIGN BODIES IN THE Just as children sometimes place small objects in the ear, they may also place them in the nose. Easily distracted from one activity to another, children shortly forget the button, bean, or pebble placed there. After a few days, one side of the nose becomes obstructed, and a purulent (pus) discharge which has an unpleasant odor becomes noticeable. These foreign objects should be removed as soon as possible and the child strongly cautioned against putting things up the nose. The habit is dangerous because there is always the possibility of suction of the foreign body into the lungs or of serious nasal infection.

NOSE INJURY The nose is the most prominent and unprotected part of the face and has the highest incidence of all fractures. The most frequent signs of nasal-bone fracture are swelling, black and blue discoloration, nasal bleeding, and movable nasal-bone fragments. X-rays are frequently needed when injury occurs. Ice compresses are helpful until the doctor is seen. A simple, small fracture is not difficult for the physician to set; extensive fractures, however, may require extensive surgery. It is important in either case that fractures not be neglected, either in adults or in children.

Often the septum is displaced during injury, and sometimes a hematoma, which is a localized collection of blood under the septum lining, occurs. If this happens, evacuation of the collected blood is necessary. An abscess can form if infection takes hold in an injured septum. This is treated with incision, drainage, and antibiotics. Neglect by the patient of a hematoma or abscess of the septum can result in permanent perforation of the septum.

NYSTAGMUS This is a rapid to-and-fro movement of the eye which is not performed voluntarily. It is seen in normal individuals as they gaze at telephone poles from a rapidly moving automobile. Rapid rotation of the body causes nystagmus, as does stimulation of the inner ear with warm or cool fluid. Eyes which have had extremely poor vision since birth also jerk irregularly back and forth, and diseases of the brain may also cause nystagmus. Symptoms may or may not occur. Attention should be directed to the cause.

OBESITY　Obesity, or the state of being overfat, is not the same as overweight. This subject is one of the most important, common, and controversial in all medicine. It is important because it is well recognized that excessive weight is a detriment to good health. Obesity aggravates heart disease and arthritis, and increases the possibility of high blood pressure, atherosclerosis, hernia, and gallbladder disease. It may bring out latent diabetes, it makes surgery and pregnancy more hazardous, and increases the mortality rate. In spite of this, perhaps 20 per cent of adults in the United States are significantly overweight, that is, more than 15 per cent above average weight for their height and age.

It is important to accept the fact that obesity is not entirely due to overeating. In spite of what is being written in various publications, people who are already overweight may actually be eating no more than those whose weight is normal. It was during the period when they were in the process of gaining weight that their food consumption was more than they could use, and they must now cut down in order to get rid of the surplus.

Obesity seems to run in families, but this may be so because of the establishment of familial eating patterns. It has been well established that the total number of fat cells in the body is the same despite weight fluctuations. After strenuous reduction, the fat cells are smaller but still capable of being repleted. Overfeeding in childhood may spur the body's production of fat cells and leave the adult with an increased base for his obesity. Increasingly, nutritionists believe that plumpness in children should be actively discouraged as a long-term prophylaxis against the problem of obesity.

Emotional and psychological factors are extremely important in the overall picture of obesity. There is gratification and pleasure in eating. Eating also offers relief from unsettling experiences such as home sickness, death of a dear one, and so on. Metabolically speaking, there is the fact that some patients may be converting more of their total caloric intake into fat deposits than others do. The fact remains that one cannot lose weight unless one reduces his caloric intake.

Treatment. The treatment of obesity is generally unsatisfactory. A long-range project, it will invariably be unsuccessful unless the patient is adequately motivated —that is, if he really and sincerely wants to lose weight and is willing to undergo a long period of discomfort in the process.

Although dietary manipulation is the simplest and easiest part of the therapy, it is not the most important one. A low-calorie diet, that is, a diet lower in calories than the body needs, is considered essential. (The usual recommendation is a 1,200 to 1,500-calorie diet, high in protein and moderately restricted in fats and carbohydrates.) Equally essential, however, is some form of increased physical activity, be it merely an hour's walking a day or participation in some mildly active sport. It is more important to maintain physical movement frequently and regularly during the day, every day, than to perform strenuous exercises intermittently.

As essential as the reduction in diet and the increase in exercise is some attempt, generally made with the aid of the physician, toward psychological re-training.

The use of bulk-producing substances or of drugs such as those said to be appetite suppressors has not been successful. Thyroid extract is no longer prescribed in obesity therapy. Responsibility for the ultimate solution of the problem remains with the patient.

Prevention is always the most desirable approach in the treatment of this stubborn condition. Therefore, any weight gain in children and young people should be carefully watched by parents in order to forestall obesity in the first place.

OBSESSIONS   Repetitious ideas which constantly return to consciousness in spite of a person's efforts to put them out of mind, are one of the main symptoms of obsession-compulsion neuroses. Obsessive ideas may occur in all degrees of severity and extensity. Most normal people experience mild obsessions in the form of worries which they cannot put aside or musical tunes which run constantly through their heads. In more serious states the obsessive idea may be so intense that the person can think of nothing else. It is generally believed that obsessive-compulsive states are produced by intense unconscious conflicts involving forbidden impulses, which are striving to enter consciousness in a struggle with conscience (superego), which is striving to repress the socially undesirable impulses.

Treatment. As with all other psychoneurotic conditions, basic treatment consists of psychiatric evaluation and psychoanalytic therapy. Symptoms invariably reflect deep unconscious conflicts which cannot be uncovered save by psychiatric methods. The general principle of treatment is to teach the patient to ignore the symptoms and try to discover the unconscious causes. Psychiatric experience has proven the futility of dealing primarily with symptoms, since, until the basic causes are removed, removal of one symptom is usually followed by the appearance of others.

OBSTETRICS   Obstetrics is the medical specialty concerned with the management of pregnancy, labor, and delivery—both normal and complicated. Physicians specializing in obstetrics are known as obstetricians. Today obstetrics and gynecology (medical and surgical) are combined in one specialty, known in abbreviation as OB-GYN.

OBSTRUCTIVE LUNG DISEASE   This is a general term applied to a group of respiratory diseases whose most common prevalent characteristic is the presence of chronic impairment of airflow into and out of the lungs. Most conspicuous in the obstructive-lung-disease group are bronchial asthma, emphysema, and bronchitis.

Obstruction to airflow may be due to many factors. Some of these are of a physical, anatomic nature, such as tumors, foreign bodies, fibrosis, or postinflammatory scars, which decrease or close down the bronchial passageway. By present-day agreement, however, the term obstructive lung disease is mainly reserved for airflow-obstructing conditions caused by one or more of the following factors: (1) broncho-constriction (active narrowing of the bronchi due to excessive contraction of the muscular coat present in their walls); (2) edema (excessive thickening of the inner layer [mucosa] of the bronchial tubes due to inflammatory or allergic fluid-accumulation); and (3) secretions (produced excessively by the mucosal glands and which mechanically impair the flow of air).

It is characteristic of this group of diseases that they are insidious and chronic in nature. Although the obstruction is usually reversible in the early stages, it becomes fixed as time goes on. The diseases of this group are usually prone to complication by bacterial infection and in their final stages, lead to progressive lung destruction and a parallel decrease in breathing capacity. Symptoms include wheezing, cough, expectoration, and shortness of breath (which may be of a paroxysmal, choking, and transient character at first, but later becomes permanent). In advanced states, the right side of the heart is pumping against increased pressure, and cardiac decompensation may occur.

OCCUPATIONAL THERAPY Psychiatrists long have recognized the importance of healthy work habits in mental health. Often one of the first symptoms of an incipient mental disorder is the breakdown of work habits; conversely, as mental patients begin to improve, one of the first symptoms of recovery is a return of an interest in working.

Occupational therapy consists of a comprehensive program of work projects in the arts and crafts to which mental patients are assigned as part of an overall plan to get them back into community living. Mental patients should be assigned during their waking hours to an activity program which keeps them busy and gainfully employed. Occupational therapy has been found to be one of the most important elements in the rehabilitation of patients, retraining them in work habits suitable for their return to community life.

OCULAR MUSCLES Movement of the eye is provided by six ocular muscles responsible for fine adjustment. Generally the eyes remain directed approximately straight ahead and the head rather than the eyes moves when objects are located far to one side. Four of the muscles, the rectus muscles, arise deep in the orbit from a tendon surrounding the opening through which nerves and blood vessels enter and leave the orbit. They attach to the outer covering of the eye, the sclera.

Two other muscles, the oblique muscles, arise from the roof and the floor of the orbit. Except for the two muscles which move the eye inward and outward, the others function in elevating and lowering the eyes, holding the globe steady when it is turned in or out, and rotating the eye when the head is tilted toward either shoulder.

OEDIPUS COMPLEX The Oedipus complex refers to the strong emotional attachment and love relationship developed by male infants towards their mothers. This complex received its name from the ancient Greek legend which was the basis for Sophocles' tragedy, *Oedipus Rex*.

Freud early recognized the clinical significance of mother-son relationships, particularly in reference to the potential triangle of jealousy and conflict involving mother, son, and father. The loving care and feeding provided by the mother often have strong sexual components, so that the male infant's first sexual contacts occur in relation to the mother. Frequently a young father becomes hostile and jealous toward a newborn son who takes up an inordinate amount of his mother's attention.

Normally the male child breaks away from the Oedipal situation during adolescence and is able to develop normal sex relations with other females. In some cases, however—particularly when a mother is openly seductive to her son, or otherwise encourages excessive dependency relationships—the son may never be able to break the bond and may maintain lifelong excessive dependence on his mother, with many kinds of undesirable psychological results.

Female infants are less susceptible to developing such intense pathological relationships with mothers, both because of the absence of heterosexual interest and because of a strong instinctive antipathy which can often be observed among females toward each other. (See, however, the entry for the ELECTRA COMPLEX.)

Treatment. Handling an unresolved Oedipus complex is always a difficult psychiatric problem, requiring the cooperation of all concerned, including mother, father, and son. Where the father is absent from the family, Oedipal complexes are usually more severe, since mother and son tend to develop excessive dependence on each other. As in other neurotic disorders, treatment, which is psychoanalytic in nature, is aimed at bringing the unconscious motivations to light.

OMENTUM The omentum is a double-layered membrane extending from the liver, then separating to encompass the stomach and transverse colon from which it then descends, apron-like, to hang within the abdominal cavity and cover the coils of the small intestine. The main function of the omentum is fat storage. A membranous structure, the omentum can be involved in any generalized peritonitis in the abdominal cavity.

OPEN-HEART SURGERY Through the use of a mechanical pump that imitates heart action, and an oxygenating chamber that temporarily assumes the function of lung tissue, the function of both heart and lungs may be suspended for several hours (cardiopulmonary bypass). During this interval, the nearly-bloodless heart can be opened and defects in the muscular or valve structures restored to more normal condition.

Congenital inborn defects, rheumatic valve damage, aneurisms, and even the coronary arteries lend themselves well to open-heart correction. The procedure of cardiopulmonary by-pass carries little risk when compared to the difficulties caused by the kind of heart damage remedied.

OPTIC NERVE The retina is connected to the brain by the optic nerve. This is about one-fifth of an inch in diameter and consists of numerous fine fibers from all portions of the retina. Shortly after leaving the bony orbit and entering the brain cavity, the inner half of the optic nerve from each eye crosses to the opposite side and joins optic-nerve fibers from the outer half of the eye on that side. Each eye is thus connected with each side of the brain. In side vision, objects on the nose-side of the eye's field of vision are perceived by the half of the brain on that eye's side; while objects towards the outer (temple) part are perceived by the portion of the brain on the opposite side of the head.

OPTIC NERVE, DEGENERATION (ATROPHY) OF Fibers of the optic nerve may die or never develop because of retinal disease, glaucoma, infection, inflammation, loss of blood supply, injury, poisons, or brain tumors.

Symptoms. The outstanding symptom is visual loss which may involve only side vision, central vision, or both. The optic nerve can be seen by means of an instrument, the ophthalmoscope, and appears white. A large number of serious conditions must be differentiated in making the diagnosis.

Treatment. This is directed to the cause. Frequently it is not possible to restore vision, but correction of the disease causing it will prevent further loss. Diseases which must be considered in the diagnosis of optic atrophy include syphilis, vitamin B (particularly thiamine) deficiency, multiple sclerosis, methyl (wood) alcohol poisoning, blood-vessel disease, meningitis, and encephalitis.

OPTIC NERVE, DISORDERS OF The optic nerves convey signals stimulated by light from the eye to the brain. Just after entering the skull, the inner half of each optic nerve crosses to the opposite side, and from this point on each optic nerve carries fibers from the nasal half of the retina of the eye on the opposite side and from the temple (temporal) half of the eye on the same side. Thus, diseases of the optic nerve back of this crossing cause a loss of half of the vision in each eye. Diseases in front of the crossing affect only one eye. Abnormalities in the optic nerve may arise because of brain tumors, inflammation of the central nervous system, infections, and diseases of the eyes.

OPTIC NERVE, INFLAMMATION OF THE (OPTIC NEURITIS)

The optic nerve may become inflamed anywhere in its course, from back of the eye to deep in the brain. Usually inflammation can be diagnosed only if it occurs in front of the crossing of the nerves in the brain. When the inflammation occurs on the surface of the nerve within the eye, it is called papillitis. If it occurs in the course of the optic nerve, it is called retrobulbar neuritis.

Symptoms. In each case, the chief symptom is loss of central vision with retention of side-vision. Retrobulbar neuritis may also cause pain upon movement of the eye. The disease usually occurs suddenly, with rapid loss of vision in one eye. The visual loss may range from slight dimness to complete blindness. The condition arises from a variety of diseases: multiple sclerosis, virus infection, malnutrition, syphilis, and others. Frequently a cause can not be found or can not be diagnosed until long after the attack.

Treatment. There is a marked tendency for recovery with or without treatment. ACTH or a steroid is commonly used internally. There is a tendency for recurrence, and as each attack causes some damage to the optic nerve, there may be permanent change.

OPTIC NERVE, SWELLING OF THE (PAPILLOEDEMA)

The optic nerve may become swollen in inflammations (pa-

pillitis) and secondarily to interference with drainage of blood in its veins. Papilloedema occurs in conditions in which the pressure within the brain is elevated, and in local conditions within the orbit which disturb venous drainage from the eye.

Symptoms. Vision is good until late in the disease. Frequently it is a sign of brain tumor or other serious intracranial disease. There are associated symptoms of the primary disease.

Treatment. This must be directed to the cause. If not relieved, the papilloedema causes optic atrophy. If corrected, it recedes and leaves no signs.

ORBIT

The orbit is the bony cavity which contains the eye. It is approximately pear-shaped, with a central expansion in the middle to contain the eye, the stem being the apex of the orbit where nerves and blood vessels enter and leave. The front margin of the orbit is composed of heavy bone which surrounds the eye except on the outer side, where it is deficient so as to permit side vision. The orbit is recessed deeply within the head. Above and on the outside, it is adjacent to the brain; inside and below, it is adjacent to the nasal sinuses. The lacrimal gland, which forms tears, is located in the upper and outer portion of the orbit.

ORBIT, ABNORMALITIES OF

The bony orbit which contains the eye is slightly more than a fluid ounce in capacity. In addition to the eye, it contains muscles, blood vessels, nerves, and fat. Most diseases and abnormalites of the orbit cause mainly a bulging-forward of the eye or eyes, called exophthalmos or proptosis. This appearance can be caused by retraction of the upper lid, which makes the eyes appear more prominent, or by an unusually enlarged eye. The symptoms of proptosis arise from exposure of the eye to irritation and sometimes from infection. Treatment must be directed to the cause.

A wide variety of congenital defects cause orbits which are too shallow or too far apart. Generally the cosmetic defect cannot be corrected.

Both eyes or one eye may become prominent in thyroid overactivity. Correction of the thyroid disease may sometimes be followed by bulging forward, so that surgery is required. Almost any new growth may occur in the orbit, and many inflammations also cause prominence of an eye. Hemorrhages and blood-vessel defects also cause proptosis.

ORCHITIS   Inflammation of the testicles is known as orchitis and is most commonly seen in mumps. When inflamed, the testis becomes exceedingly painful and tender. Orchitis is usually treated by rest, application of cold packs, and occasionally by the administration of hormones.

ORGANIC BRAIN SYNDROME   The human brain is subject to many types of physical injury and disease which can destroy its substance. Organic brain syndrome is a general classification of such conditions, which result in irreversible chronic impairment of mental functions; in extreme degree, such a syndrome produces complete loss of mental functions, a state formerly known as dementia.

It is now known that a large number of diseases and injuries can cause permanent organic damage to brain cells, which unfortunately are unable to reproduce themselves. Organic brain damage may occur even in pregnancy, if the mother contracts infectious diseases such as measles, German measles, scarlet fever, or whooping-cough, which attack the unborn child. Birth injuries to the central nervous system are estimated to occur in 10 per cent of all deliveries, and childhood accidents and diseases may also involve brain damage.

In later life, the most common causes of organic brain damage are cerebrovascular accidents such as "stroke" (embolism or hemorrhage).

Treatment. The main hope in treatment programs consists in teaching the patient to compensate for lost functions by overdeveloping his remaining resources.

ORTHOPEDIC CONDITIONS, CHILDHOOD   Congenital and acquired childhood musculoskeletal deformities are not uncommon. Some of these may be relatively minor, and may be self-correcting through normal growth and development. Others (for example, clubfeet) require vigorous therapy and all the ingenuity of the orthopedic surgeon to achieve good results.

ORTHOPEDICS   Orthopedics is the surgical specialty concerned with the care of the musculoskeletal system. The word orthopedics is derived from the Greek words meaning straight child, and from the time of Hippocrates to the end of the nineteenth century orthopedists were concerned with the care of children afflicted with congenital or acquired crippling deformities. More recently, orthopedists have also assumed the care of fractures and other injuries to the limbs and spine in adults as well, and presently orthopedic surgeons are making major advances in the surgical management of patients with arthritic conditions.

OSTEITIS   Osteitis is a general term describing inflammatory changes in the bones. A common form of osteitis called osteitis deformans is also known as Paget's disease, and produces characteristic bending and bowing of the extremities with irregular thickening of the skull, visible by X-rays. In osteitis fibrosa cystica the bone has areas of spongy tissue which by X-ray look like holes. This condition is still seen in patients with hyperparathyroidism, but is not as common as in former years, probably because of the greater availability of calcium in the diet.

OTITIS MEDIA This common cause of earache is an infection in the middle ear just behind the eardrum, seen most commonly in children following a cold. It is almost always caused by bacteria which seem to build up in the small space behind the eardrum because the cold has closed off the Eustachian tube. (This tube leads out from the middle ear to the back of the throat and allows for proper drainage and equalization of air-pressure on the two sides of the eardrum.)

Symptoms. Because the eardrum is very sensitive, not much inflammation is required here to cause excruciating pain, and the affected child who seemed almost recovered from a cold may suddenly scream out and clutch the ear.

If there is fever the infection has usually progressed to the point of abscess; this may cause the eardrum to bulge and burst, exuding a surprising amount of pus and blood. The fever may then fall and the earache disappear. One may then think that the ear has healed, but the situation remains serious and should be treated. Although not every earache demands treatment, any persistent one accompanied by fever is potentially dangerous, and a doctor should be put in charge of it. A simple earache without fever may for a time be treated by home methods, but if pain is recurrent or deafness supervenes, it is obviously not a simple case and requires serious medical attention.

Treatment. The common feelings of "fullness" in the ear experienced during a respiratory infection are often helped by decongestant pills (many of which are sold over the counter), nose drops, and aspirin. When pain and diminished hearing are complained of, home treatment is treading on dangerous ground. The doctor should be consulted, and it is customary to rely on the use of an appropriate antibiotic.

Otitis media and its sequel, the "running ear," have become rare with the advent of antibiotics. Only occasionally is it necessary to puncture the drum (an office procedure) to permit drainage of fluid in the middle ear.

OTOLARYNGOLOGY The term otolaryngology refers to the surgical specialty devoted to diagnosis and treatment of the ear, nose, and throat. (The name is actually a shortened version of the full name, otorhinolaryngology, oto-referring to the ear, -rhino- to the nose and sinuses, and -laryng- to the larynx.°) This field also includes the pharynx and almost all the structures of the neck. Otolaryngology is an immense field and many books have been written on only parts of the ear or parts of the nose and throat. There are, for example, several large books on the ear alone and several on only the middle ear.

OTOSCLEROSIS See DEAFNESS, CONDUCTION

OVARIES Two in number, one on each side close to the womb, the ovaries are the main female glands, responsible for the production of eggs (ova) and the two major female hormones: estrogen and progesterone. Through these hormones, the ovaries are responsible for the development of the girl into a normal woman; for the maturation of her womb (uterus); and for the further response of the uterus to changing hormone levels in the form of menstrual flow. The ovaries produce the ova and (after conception has occurred) will help maintain the pregnancy for the first few months.

As all other organs, the ovaries may

°As in many similar technical terms, -ology simply indicates "the science of" some particular specialty.

be involved in a variety of acute and chronic diseases. Infections, cysts, and other tumors—both benign and malignant—are liable to involve them. Most ovarian tumors are benign, but can become enormously large in size.

Cancer of the ovary is usually discovered in advanced stages, too late for it to be treated. This is one reason why every woman should have regular gynecological examinations. This is true both *before* and *after* the menopause. Many ovarian tumors arise postmenopause. Thus, unlike the common fibroid tumors of the uterus, which often produce changes in the menstrual cycle, ovarian tumors can grow silently and first become manifest by pressure on the adjacent bladder or bowel.

"OVERACTIVE THYROID" (HYPERTHYROIDISM)

Excess secretion of thyroid hormone is characterized by intolerance to heat, increased sweating, loss of weight with increased appetite, shakiness, muscle weakness, and—in some patients—diarrhea, staring eyes, and enlargement of the thyroid gland. The most common cause of hyperthyroidism is the release of excessive amounts of thyroid hormone into the circulation by a diffusely enlarged gland. (See GRAVES' DISEASE.) When excess hormone is secreted by a portion of the gland, usually felt as a nodule, the condition is called Plummer's disease.

Diagnosis is made by discovery of a high blood iodine level (PBI test), elevation of the amount of radioactive iodine taken up by the gland during a six or twenty-four hour period, and elevation of the basal metabolic rate. In Plummer's disease (nodular hyperthyroidism) a scintiscan of the gland after administration of radioactive iodine helps to outline the nodules.

Treatment. For treatment of diffuse hyperthyroidism see GRAVES' DISEASE. Nodular hyperthyroidism is usually best treated by surgical removal of a solitary nodule, or subtotal removal of a multinodular gland.

After treatment of hyperthyroidism, it is necessary to observe for signs of low or absent thyroid activity (see UNDERACTIVE THYROID), which is treated by administration of thyroid hormone.

OVERPROTECTION, PSYCHOLOGICAL

A common cause of neurotic dependency reactions and disabilities is overprotection of the child from the normal stresses of living by parents during early life. Many parents mistakenly believe that children can be protected or shielded from all that is evil in life and thereby avoid possible future mental illness. The overprotective parent overregulates the child's life and is excessively careful about anything considered undesirable.

The pattern of maternal overprotection has been described by psychiatrists as "momism." Studies of soldiers who broke down mentally under conditions of stress during World War II indicated that many of them had been overprotected as children by their parents and were totally unprepared to face any hardships in adult life. The overprotected child tends to break down emotionally under stress, crying and otherwise using immature methods to escape from facing difficult life-problems. The antidote for overprotection is gradual exposure of the child to increasingly stressful life situations so that he learns to cope with them.

OVERWEIGHT

Overweight is not the same as obesity (overfatness). It merely means that a person weighs more than the average range of the so-called "normal" for the same age and height. The excess weight may be due to heavy musculature.

The average body consists of about 20 per cent fat; 38 per cent muscle; 42 per cent bone, blood, organs, and other tissues.

DESIRABLE WEIGHTS

Weight in Pounds According to Frame (In Indoor Clothing)

	HEIGHT (with shoes on) 1-inch heels Feet Inches	SMALL FRAME	MEDIUM FRAME	LARGE FRAME
Men of Ages 25 and Over	5 2	112—120	118—129	126—141
	5 3	115—123	121—133	129—144
	5 4	118—126	124—136	132—148
	5 5	121—129	127—139	135—152
	5 6	124—133	130—143	138—156
	5 7	128—137	134—147	142—161
	5 8	132—141	138—152	147—166
	5 9	136—145	142—156	151—170
	5 10	140—150	146—160	155—174
	5 11	144—154	150—165	159—179
	6 0	148—158	154—170	164—184
	6 1	152—162	158—175	168—189
	6 2	156—167	162—180	173—194
	6 3	160—171	167—185	178—199
	6 4	164—175	172—190	182—204

	HEIGHT (with shoes on) 2-inch heels Feet Inches	SMALL FRAME	MEDIUM FRAME	LARGE FRAME
Women of Ages 25 and Over	4 10	92— 98	96—107	104—119
	4 11	94—101	98—110	106—122
	5 0	96—104	101—113	109—125
	5 1	99—107	104—116	112—128
	5 2	102—110	107—119	115—131
	5 3	105—113	110—122	118—134
	5 4	108—116	113—126	121—138
	5 5	111—119	116—130	125—142
	5 6	114—123	120—135	129—146
	5 7	118—127	124—139	133—150
	5 8	122—131	128—143	137—154
	5 9	126—135	132—147	141—158
	5 10	130—140	136—151	145—163
	5 11	134—144	140—155	149—168
	6 0	138—148	144—159	153—173

For girls between 18 and 25, subtract 1 pound for each year under 25.

Reprinted from *Four Steps to Weight Control* by permission of the Metropolitan Life Insurance Company.

If the body-fat content is normal, but the bony frame heavy with much muscle development, a person may be overweight as determined by the usual height-weight-age tables. In contrast, another individual may be "overfat" (obese) with poor muscle development and more fat, yet his total weight may be "normal" according to the standard tables. By and large, however, the person who is overweight is also overfat.

The problem of normal or ideal weight is very complex. The young man of today is somewhat taller and heavier than a man of the same age one or two generations ago. Is this good? We do not know, since we do not know what weight is most conducive to good health. Many people gain weight as they grow older. This may be the average situation, but probably represents an accumulation of fat and a decrease in muscle-mass.

The table on page 379 gives average (not necessarily ideal) weights in "ordinary clothing." It merely represents what a large number of Americans weigh. A deviation of 10 per cent above this may be overweight. A deviation of 25 per cent represents obesity.

What a person should weigh at age twenty-five to thirty is probably the ideal weight no matter what the age. It should be noted, however, that these averages are collected from a mixed population. In some racial groups the average weight for a certain age and height may be considerably different than for other groups.

OVULATION   This term means the production of eggs (ova) by the ovary. During the reproductive span of the woman's life (from onset to cessation of menstrual periods), one egg is released monthly by the ovary. In the majority of women, ovulation occurs approximately fourteen days before the onset of a menstrual period. This is the most fertile period for a woman—in fact it is believed to be the only fertile period—and if pregnancy is desired, sexual relations should be regularly undertaken during the period of six to seven days in the middle of the menstrual cycle.

Many women can actually pinpoint the day of ovulation by a sudden acute pain felt in the lower abdomen, sometimes on the left and sometimes on the right side. There are several methods of discovering whether ovulation has occurred or not; the most convenient and popular of these methods is the basal body-temperature record, which will show a sustained elevation of temperature of about one degree from the time of ovulation until the beginning of next menstrual period. Other methods consist of special tests carried out by the physician, such as vaginal smears, analysis of mucus from the mouth of the womb, and examination of uterine (endometrial) tissues by biopsies.

OXYTOCICS   These are drugs used to produce contractions of the pregnant uterus. Since they can be very dangerous to both the mother and the baby if improperly used, their use is limited to the medical profession.

PANCREAS   The pancreas, a long slender organ, lies on the rear wall of the abdominal cavity behind the stomach, and has two major functions. The first is secretion of pancreatic juice, which aids in the digestion of the intestinal contents; this is carried to the first part of the intestine (the duodenum) by way of the pancreatic duct. The second pancreatic secretion is insulin, which is concerned with the metabolism of sugar. When insulin is insufficient or is altogether lacking, the result is diabetes.

Because of the inaccessibility of this organ, a tumor of the pancreas is very difficult to diagnose until it has progressed to dangerous proportions. Infection of the pancreas (pancreatitis) can be

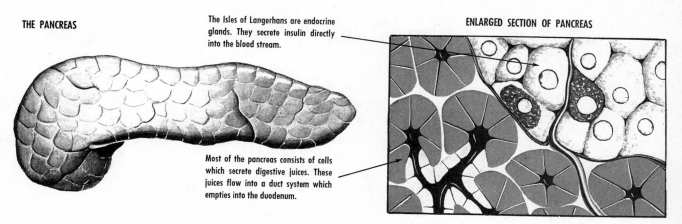

THE PANCREAS

The Isles of Langerhans are endocrine glands. They secrete insulin directly into the blood stream.

Most of the pancreas consists of cells which secrete digestive juices. These juices flow into a duct system which empties into the duodenum.

ENLARGED SECTION OF PANCREAS

quite severe and is often caused by blockage of the pancreatic duct. Occasionally, pancreatitis becomes chronic, and because of the diminished amounts of pancreatic juice formed, the patient is likely to have severe digestive difficulties and intermittent bouts of abdominal pain. Pancreatitis may also be caused by acute or chronic alcoholism.

The pancreas is also involved in cystic fibrosis, a childhood condition due to abnormal function of various glands throughout the body. Malnutrition, retarded growth, thick mucus, and lung infections are common and are particularly difficult to care for.

Occasionally, fluid-filled cysts are formed in the pancreas, and these may reach rather large proportions.

Symptoms of cysts are pain in the abdomen, nausea, weight-loss, vomiting, and jaundice. Treatment is surgical removal.

PARANOID STATES   Paranoid thinking involves the psychological mechanism of projection, in which a person "projects" his own feelings and attitudes, mistakenly imputing motives to others which are actually his own. Paranoid thinking is always delusional in the sense that real events are misinterpreted by having the individual's own feelings and motivations projected onto them.

Symptoms. The most common type of paranoid thinking involves the persecution complex, in which a person develops ideas that other people are "after him," saying untrue things about him, or otherwise persecuting him and causing him trouble. The paranoid may think that others are following him, watching him, trying to influence him over television, trying to poison him, or otherwise causing damage.

Paranoid thinking may be organized into complexes of all levels of severity and extensity, ranging from single paranoid ideas (such as that one's teacher is hostile) to the full-fledged psychosis known as paranoia, involving complex and systematized delusions. Paranoid thinking may be understood as involving defensive attempts to rationalize one's own personal inadequacies by blaming all failures on others. In extreme cases, paranoid states may be regarded as extensive reconstruction efforts, in which the patient tries to reorganize the world in line with his own motives.

A common symptom of paranoid states is auditory hallucinations, in which a person hears voices directing him to commit some act, such as killing another person, or setting fire to a building. The paranoid patient is always potentially dangerous because of his known tendency to take matters of law and order into his own hands in an attempt to correct fancied injustices or to punish or otherwise eliminate those he mistakenly perceives as enemies.

Treatment. Paranoid thinking is always unhealthy, and paranoid ideas should be corrected when first noted. One should always carefully examine any temptation to believe that others are the cause of failure or of systematic hostility, though in very occasional cases this may actually be true. Psychiatric experience indicates that paranoid states become increasingly difficult to treat and correct once paranoid ideas become incorporated into systematic and organized delusions that "the world is against me."

Paranoid conditions are among the most difficult to treat psychiatrically, and chronic paranoid states frequently never respond to treatment. Patients with well-established paranoid delusions of persecution are potentially socially dangerous and should be committed to mental hospitals for observation and treatment for as long as they remain delusional.

PARATHYROID GLANDS These glands are usually four in number and lie just behind the thyroid gland in the lower neck. Their function is quite well understood: they secrete a substance known as parathormone which regulates the level of calcium in the blood. This activity is accomplished by the hormone's effects on the kidneys and on bone. The parathyroid glands may become completely inactive or may be removed surgically, producing a state of hypoparathyroidism, characterized by painful muscle spasms and convulsions.

PARESIS, GENERAL General paresis is due to infection of the central nervous system, particularly the cerebral cortex, by syphilis. It is a chronic, infectious process which results in organic mental deterioration. General paresis was much more common in the nineteenth century, before its cause became known; today it is only rarely observed in untreated or inadequately treated syphilitic patients.

Symptoms. The onset is usually gradual and insidious, involving slow changes in personality and character which include deterioration of personal habits and cleanliness. A common symptom is delusions of grandeur, in which the patient, suddenly boastful and grandiose, believes that he has suddenly become very wealthy or powerful. The mood is usually one of euphoria and satisfaction with life. Subtle impairment of memory and judgment may result in irrational behavior and loss of normal self-control and inhibition of impulses.

Relatively late in the disorder neurological signs begin to appear, including abnormalities in eye-response and generalized skeletal muscle weakness or rigidity. If the syphilitic process also involves the spinal cord, tendon reflexes are disturbed and knee-jerks absent.

Treatment. Successful treatment always depends on definite early diagnosis, easily made by tests performed on the blood and/or spinal fluid for the presence of syphilis. (This is the reason why premarital and prenatal blood tests should be legally compulsory in order to detect the presence of syphilis before marriage and before birth.)

Once a positive Wasserman reaction has been obtained, the patient should be put on intensive anti-syphilitic treatment; this must be continued until repeated spinal-fluid tests are negative. Fortunately, modern treatment is very effective and most cases can be completely controlled if early diagnosis has been made.

PARKINSON'S DISEASE Parkinson's disease (shaking palsy) is a common chronic disorder associated with rhythmical tremors of the hands and rigidity of muscles. Post-encephalitic Parkinsonism occurs in young adults after encephalitis. Parkinsonism in individuals from forty to eighty years of age is usually due to arteriosclerosis. Damage to large masses of cells in the central portion of the brain also produces this disorder.

Symptoms. With the arm at rest, a rhythmical pill-rolling type of tremor of the fingers is present. When the patient walks, he has difficulty in initiating movements, he takes small steps, and his trunk is flexed. The face shows little expression and the eyelids blink infrequently. If the arm is moved at the wrist or elbow, cogwheel rigidity is present with increased resistance to passive movement. Although speech and writing are slowed, normal intelligence is preserved.

Treatment. An important advance, with fundamental implications for Parkinsonism, was the introduction of the drug l-dopa. L-dopa passes from the brain circulation into the cells involved in the disease. When given in slowly increasing amounts (thus lessening the troublesome side-effects of nausea and blood-pressure drops), l-dopa is capable in many instances of reversing Parkinsonian symptoms in a manner unrivaled by any other available agent. Some other useful drugs, however, are Artane®, Cogentin®, and Benadryl®.

PARONYCHIA This infection of the skin surrounding the nails is much more common on the fingers than the toes, and is usually the result of invasion by two types of organisms: pus-forming staphylococci or streptococci and a yeast (*Monilia albicans*).

Symptoms. It is likely that there is injury to the nail fold, which is followed by redness, swelling, and the formation of pus. Simultaneous involvement of several fingers is common. Recurrence of the condition is also common in susceptible persons.

Treatment. Soaking in hot water and frequent applications of antibiotic ointment in the intervals between the soakings usually effectively relieve the infection. Occasionally it becomes necessary to release the pus by means of surgical incision.

Recurrences of paronychia may require investigation to attempt to determine the cause(s) for susceptibility to this infection. But often care of the hands with special attention to avoiding injury to the cuticle will suffice in removing the provocative factor of infection.

PAROTID GLANDS Located in the cheek at the angle of the jaw, the parotids are the largest of the salivary glands. The saliva which they secrete is transported by a duct which opens into the mouth opposite the second upper molar on each side. The parotid glands are primarily affected in mumps, and the swelling is characteristic. In elderly people, acute infections of the parotid glands may result from inadequate fluid intake. Because of the heavy concentration of various salts in the saliva, it is not uncommon for stones to form in the duct, giving rise to rather severe pain and inflammation.

PARROT FEVER (PSITTICOSIS) Parrot fever (psitticosis or ornithosis) is caused by a virus contracted from certain birds, notably of the parrot family, and manifested as a form of pneumonia. Parrots and parakeets sold by reputable dealers in the United States are uninfected due to stringent health laws. When the disease appears in this country it is most often due to contact with birds that have been brought into the United States by unscrupulous dealers who smuggle the birds, chiefly across the Mexican border.

Symptoms. After one to two weeks exposure to an infected bird, the individual suffers, with gradually increasing intensity, headache, malaise, chilliness, backache, and fever. Within a short time a cough develops. X-ray examination may reveal pneumonia, but the diagnosis of what type of pneumonia is often a challenge. Early in the disease, it is easily confused with typhoid fever and influenza. The clinical picture and the history of

384

contact with a bird of the parrot family are highly suggestive of parrot fever. Specimens of blood, in succession, are required by law to be sent to the Communicable Disease Center through the Laboratory Director of the state in which the patient resides or may be.

Treatment. The outlook for psitticosis has materially brightened since the advent of antibiotics, particularly tetracycline, the treatment of choice.

PATCH TESTS   This type of skin test is used extensively to determine the cause(s) of contact dermatitis, an eruption caused by the application of a substance to which the patient has become allergic. If the suspected substance is a liquid, a drop of the original solution or of a known nonirritating dilution of the solution is placed on the skin (back or arms). Over this is placed a bandage whose gauze surface has been previously covered with an impervious material (cellophane, wax paper). If the suspected substance is a solid (cloth, plastic, etc.), the material is moistened with a small amount of water and covered with a bandage as outlined above. If several substances are applied at the same time, each bandage should be numbered to make identification possible. The most useful and practical sites for application of patch tests are the inner sides of the upper arms, the upper chests, and the upper back.

The band-aid patches are removed in forty-eight hours, unless itching or burning at the site indicates an early reaction and makes prompt removal of the bandage necessary. The reactions range from faint pinkness to blistering, and are some indication of the degree of sensitivity that the patient has developed. False positive reactions are usually the result of application of an irritating (not sensitizing) substance, and may require dilution of the material if further study is indicated. False negative responses are the result of a variety of factors and may mislead the patient in discarding

the tested material as a possible cause of the dermatitis.

Only contact dermatitis can be studied with the patch test procedure. Drug eruptions (other than those producing contact dermatitis), hives, infantile eczema, and atopic dermatitis are, for varying reasons, not clarified by patch test studies. Patch tests are useless if the allergy is to something inhaled or eaten. It is essential that the substance be applied in a dilution not irritating to the skin and in a diluent not itself irritating or capable of altering the test substance. Interpretation of the result is often complicated by redness resulting from pressure of the bandage, or from slight heat rash due to the tight fit of the patch, or from irritation caused by the adhesive material.

Patch tests can be used with considerable skill by the layman. They are of inestimable value to the dermatologist and the allergist. Although a negative result can usually be interpreted as an absence of allergy to the test substance, a negative result does not constitute evidence of the inability to develop an allergy to that substance at a later time.

PEDIATRICS   Pediatrics is the branch of medicine that deals specifically with the health care of children from birth through adolescence. The pediatrician is especially concerned with aspects of proper growth, the prevention of common childhood diseases, and advising parents concerning a wide range of physiological and psychological factors in child development.

PEDICULOSIS (LICE-INFESTATION) There are several different forms of pediculosis, including pediculosis capitis, or louse-infestation of the head. This is more common in children than in adults. Both the adult louse and the nits can be found without much difficulty. Itching can be intense, secondary infection common, and enlargement of the lymph glands of the neck a serious complication.

If the hair is long and thick, there is considerable advantage in cutting it prior to the application of remedies (mercury solution, 25 per cent benzyl benzoate, benzene in liquid petrolatum). Application of vinegar will help to loosen the nits which can then be removed with a fine tooth comb. Reapplication of the remedy six days later will insure the destruction of newly hatched young (if a nit was not removed or otherwise destroyed).

Another form, pediculosis corporis, is that in which the body louse lives in the seams of clothing and attacks the skin only to feed. Pinpoint marks are produced, followed occasionally by small hive-like lesions. The intense itching and consequent scratching result in deep excoriations and in irritation of the skin.

Removal of the infested clothing results in effective cure. The clothing should be boiled, or cleaned, or ironed with a hot iron. For the occasional remaining nits of the hair of the armpits, soap and water washing and the application of a mercury solution are effective. Soothing lotions are useful for the remaining irritation and itching.

Pediculosis pubis, except for the difference in location (genital area, abdomen, and occasionally the eyebrows and lashes), has the same symptoms as those produced by the body louse.

Soap-and-water washing and application of the above-mentioned remedies are effective.

PELLAGRA Pellagra is a serious disease characterized by mental, nervous-system, and skin symptoms produced by the deficiency of niacin (nicotinic acid) or its related substances, niacinamide and nicotinamide. Such deficiencies are usually associated with a diet overly rich in corn, and pellagra may be endemic in areas where this food plays a large part in daily nutrition. Secondary deficiency may result from prolonged diarrhea and certain forms of liver disease. (Protein containing the amino-acid tryptophan protects against low niacinamide intake because tryptophan is a raw material from which niacinamide is formed.)

Symptoms. In advanced pellagra the tongue is red, swollen, and tender, and the whole mouth appears inflamed. There is a characteristic skin lesion which forms at similar sites on both sides of the body at exposed areas such as the hands and face. The bright scarlet color of the tongue and mucous membranes of the mouth, together with soreness of the mouth and increased salivation, are characteristic findings. Diarrhea is also a serious sign.

Among the nervous-system disorders that may be found in pellagra are non-specific weakness or apathy, and later, psychoses characterized by impairment of memory, disorientation, and confusion (sometimes with excitement, mania, and delirium). The extremities may be rigid, and there may be uncontrollable sucking and grasping reflexes in more advanced cases. In pellagra, the "three d's" are diarrhea, dementia, and dermatitis—although many cases do not show these features.

Treatment. Specific therapy includes niacinamide in large doses, both by mouth and by injection. However, the total nutritional state must be corrected because the patient who develops pellagra has generally been on an inadequate diet for a long time. Pellagra-preventive foods include liver, lean meat, peanuts, potatoes, legumes, milk, and eggs. The last two furnish little niacin but are excellent sources of tryptophan, an amino acid which is the precursor of niacin. The minimum niacin requirement of the adult is about 9 to 13 milligrams a day. The requirement of an infant is about 5 milligrams a day.

Fortunately pellagra is no longer common in this country, a fact which points out the advantages of widespread preventive measures and dietary supplementation.

PELVIMETRY

Pelvimetry is the measurement of the dimensions of the female pelvis after X-ray films are taken. It is a very important examination for the discovery of disproportion between the size of the baby and that of the mother's pelvis. Decisions concerning caesarean sections are often made after study of pelvimetry films.

PELVIS (FEMALE)

This represents the lowest part of the abdominal cavity and is formed by a rigid bony girdle which is firmly attached to the spine at the back, being hinged on the sides to the bones of the thighs (femoral bones). The floor of the female pelvis is formed by several layers of muscular and connective tissues and is penetrated, from the front backwards, by the opening of the bladder (urethra), the birth canal (vagina), and the rectum. The floor of the pelvis is known as the perineum.

In addition to the bladder and loops of intestines, the female pelvis contains the womb (uterus) and ovaries. When pregnancy occurs, the pelvis plays a particularly important role in the accommodation and protection of the pregnant uterus.

The size of the bony pelvis is an all-important factor for the normal progress of labor and delivery. Disproportion between the size of the pelvis and that of the baby's head will cause difficulties in labor and delivery, and caesarean section will often be required for the baby's delivery.

PEMPHIGUS

A disease of unknown causation, occurring almost exclusively in adult life, pemphigus primarily affects the skin and the mucous membranes. Prior to the advent of cortisone therapy no treatment was effective in altering the usually —but not invariably—fatal outcome after a course ranging from several months to two or three years.

Symptoms. Usually gradual in onset (though occasionally rapid and fulminating), blisters appear on any part of the body including the mouth and nose. The blisters enlarge rapidly and become sagging, finally breaking and becoming emptied of fluid, leaving a stretched, folded mass of skin. The blisters arise on normal-appearing skin and can be produced in unaffected areas by gentle stroking of the skin. Other than a feeling of weakness, the patient presents no complaints. Secondary infection, pneumonia, and severe anemia are encountered in the terminal phase of the disease, and death is usually

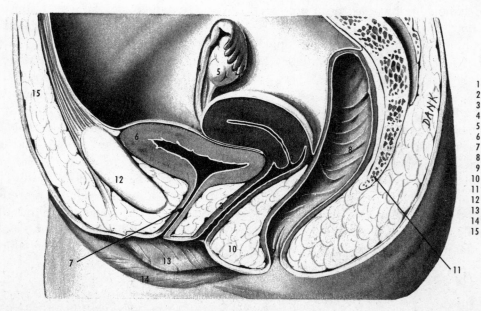

THE FEMALE PELVIS
(CROSS SECTION)

1 UTERUS
2 CERVIX
3 VAGINA
4 FALLOPIAN TUBE
5 OVARY
6 BLADDER
7 URETHRA
8 RECTUM
9 ANUS
10 PERINEUM
11 COCCYX
12 PUBIS
13 LABIA MINORA
14 LABIA MAJORA
15 ABDOMINAL WALL

attributed to these although the actual cause of what appears to be a "toxic" death is not known.

The disease is neither contagious nor inherited, and there is no sex preponderance. Variants of the disease also occur, most common among them being a scaling and crusting eruption.

Treatment. The cortisone drugs (corticosteroids) act in an almost specific manner and are life-saving. Patients have been sustained for many years and have been able to pursue a normal life. Occasional change in the particular drug may be necessary, and the precautions usual in the use of these drugs must be maintained.

PENIS The male sexual organ is known as the penis. It contains large spaces (sinuses) that are capable of filling with blood and producing a state of erection. The expanded tip of the penide shaft is known as the glans penis. Erotic sensations in the organ are due to specific nerve endings called genital corpuscles. Surprisingly, sensitivity to heat and cold is less developed in the penis than in the skin elsewhere. The fold of skin that covers the glans is known as the prepuce (foreskin) and is removed in circumcision. The adult penis varies considerably in size; an average penis is about four to six inches in length, increasing somewhat when erect.

PEPTIC ULCER Peptic ulcers are erosions of one or more layers of the stomach or duodenum (the first portion of the small intestine). Depending on their location, they are therefore classified as either gastric or duodenal. These lesions result from an inability of the mucous-membrane lining of these organs to withstand the powerful digestive action of the enzyme pepsin and an increased amount of hydrochloric acid; these overabundant secretions from the stomach are uniformly found in peptic ulcers. Occasionally, if the ulcer is found in the stomach, it becomes important in the older-age group to determine if acid is being produced at all. In its absence other diagnoses must be considered.

In times of particular emotional turmoil, acid secretion tends to become excessive—hence the common belief that the hard-driving executive type is especially prone to develop an ulcer. Recent studies have shown, however, that persons in all walks of life are susceptible. Moreover, many cases have been seen in newborns and very young infants.

Symptoms. Ulcer pain is usually very characteristic. It tends to be sharply localized in an area just below the tip of the breastbone and is often described as feeling like a red-hot poker. The pain is noteworthy for its predictable appearance at specific times of the day or night. Typically it comes on an hour or so before lunch and dinner and often around 2:00 A.M. Strangely, pain is rare before breakfast. In uncomplicated cases the burning discomfort is usually relieved promptly by food or antacids such as bicarbonate of soda. This "pain-food-relief-pain" cycle is so characteristic that a diagnosis can be strongly suspected from this history alone. Confirmatory X-rays are desirable to make sure that other conditions requiring different treatment are not present.

Rarely, an ulcer can attain a large size without pain. The first indication that there is anything wrong in these instances may be a sudden vomiting of blood or other indications of internal bleeding, such as severe weakness or fainting and the passage of black, tarry stools. Bleeding as a complication of an ulcer results from the actual destruction of a blood-vessel wall in the ulcer crater. This should be considered an emergency, and prompt medical attention is mandatory. If the crater becomes too deep, the wall of the stomach or duodenum may actually perforate. The spillage of gastrointestinal contents into the abdomen can cause severe peritonitis. If a perforation occurs in the rear wall of the duodenum, the pancreas—which is adjacent at this point—may become involved. The ensuing pancreatitis, while uncommon, can be a very serious complication. In long-standing chronic cases of duodenal ulcer, the passageway may become so scarred and/or swollen with inflammation as to be completely obstructed. The resulting constant vomiting, pain, and dehydration point to another grave complication of peptic ulcer.

Treatment. The vast majority of peptic ulcers can be treated by diet and medication. The nature itself of the disease-process suggests the proper treatment, namely: neutralization of stomach-acid; a bland diet to prevent irritation of the injured tissue; and attainment of a measure of tranquillity and freedom from emotional stress. The usual program consists of hourly feedings of milk or cream, alternating with one of the many available antacid preparations. Medications designed to reduce the secretion of acid and to relieve spasm of the affected tissues are often helpful (as are mild sedatives). This regime is rapidly successful in relieving the pain, and in a few days the diet can be gradually made more liberal. Soft-boiled eggs, puddings, bland soups, and similarly prepared foods can be included. The essence of a successful course of treatment is having something bland and soothing in the stomach at all times—either food or an antacid. All spicy and heavily seasoned foods must be avoided. Alcohol in any form is contraindicated, as it is known to be one of the most powerful stimulants to the acid-producing cells. The use of tobacco should likewise be greatly curtailed.

The length of time necessary to heal an ulcer may vary from a few weeks to several months. Since recurrences are notoriously common, certain dietary restric-

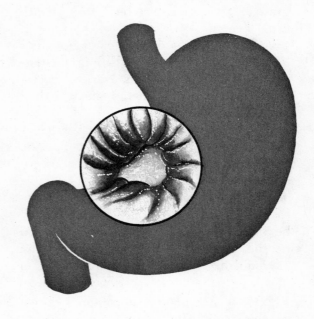

PEPTIC ULCER

A peptic ulcer is a benign crater in the mucous membrane of the stomach or duodenum, caused by the action of the acid gastric juice.

tions may be required indefinitely. Sometimes it becomes necessary to recommend a change of employment or some other alteration of a hostile environment so as to aid the healing process. In selected cases a recently perfected technique of gastric freezing has been of some use in relieving pain. The management of the previously discussed complications often requires surgical intervention. Prompt diagnosis and judicious surgery may be lifesaving. In middle-aged or older patients, an ulcer in certain locations in the stomach may require surgery if at the end of two weeks of medical treatment little progress is seen, because of the possibility of cancer. In a small percentage of chronic and recurrent ulcers surgery for the ulcer itself may be required; but most authorities agree that medical management must be given a fair and adequate trial before resorting to these more drastic procedures.

Two procedures currently have their advocates, and both are designed to cut down on the secretion of acid. The more direct approach consists of the removal of a portion of the stomach—a partial gastric resection. There are certain complications which occasionally result from this procedure (see Dumping Syndrome). Vagotomy and pyloroplasty, the other commonly performed operation, consists of interrupting the fibers of the vagus nerve (which controls the secretion of acid in the stomach) and widening the pyloric canal, the narrow band of tissue that separates the stomach from the duodenum. Ulcers have gained a certain amount of respectability in our society as the mark of the successful man. Most patients would agree that the price is exorbitant.

PERICARDITIS An acute or long-standing inflammation of the external coverings of the heart and the sac in which it lies is called pericarditis. The inflammation and disease may involve only these membranes, or may be a part of disease elsewhere in the heart, particularly the heart muscle or valves. Fluid may accumulate in the sac that encloses the heart; it may be watery fluid (perhaps blood tinged), or it may be rather thick and even purulent.

Accumulation of fluid in the pericardial sac will, of course, make difficult the normal filling of the heart, for the pericardial sac is tough and inelastic, and every ounce of fluid in it can potentially deny space to an ounce of blood entering and passing through the heart with each beat of the cycle.

Acute pericarditis may be a complication of rheumatic heart disease, tuberculosis, or blood poisoning (septicemia); or it may occur in persons with a healthy heart, as in a sudden illness with mild symptoms of vague distress or (at the other extreme) profound prostration.

After the acute phase of the disease is over, a chronic stage may begin. The membranes covering the heart can become thickened and adhere.

In healing, a fibrous process develops that will tend to shrink and contract the size of the pericardial sac. When this occurs, a constrictive pericarditis is said to be present. The heart is held in a rather rigid envelope of relatively small size. Blood cannot enter the heart chambers in quantities set by tissue demands, but is instead determined by the abnormal anatomic limitations of the constricted sac. Output of the heart, of course, diminishes and blood pressure falls below reasonable levels. Blood that should be readily drawn into the right auricle for passage to the lungs is denied adequate entrance by the constricting pericardium, and the blood dams up in the veins that supply the heart. The liver and spleen become swollen and engorged with blood; neck veins stand out like thick cords, and arm veins are very prominent and fail to empty completely until raised abnormally high.

Treatment. Permanent relief from the very inadequate and disabling circulatory state of chronic pericarditis can only be satisfactorily accomplished by surgical removal of much of the pericardium. This releases the heart, giving it relative freedom to fill properly. Sometimes the surgical relief is so dramatic that it seems as though the patient is rescued from imminent death, and he may be restored to full employment after just a few weeks of postoperative care.

PERICORONITIS This condition is an inflammation of the soft tissue covering the crown portion of a partially erupted tooth. Most commonly it involves the permanent third molars (wisdom teeth).

Symptoms. The soft tissue may swell to the point that the jaws can not be completely closed without striking this swollen area, which further injures the inflamed tissue. If untreated, the infection may spread into adjacent tissues, producing swelling which results in difficulty in opening the jaws (trismus) and swallowing.

Treatment. Treatment usually involves the use of antibiotics, irrigation of the area, and perhaps surgical removal of the soft-tissue covering (operculum) or the tooth itself.

PERIODONTAL DISEASE (PERIODONTITIS, PYORRHEA)

This is the term given to the progressive destruction of the periodontal structures (supporting structures of the teeth) which originates in the gingiva (gum) and involves the periodontal membrane, epithelial attachment, supporting bone, and the cementum.

The root of a tooth is surrounded by bone and attached to the bony socket (alveolus) by means of the fibers of the periodontal membrane which runs from the cementum of the root to surrounding bone. The gingiva is also attached to the tooth by means of a band of tissue, the epithelial attachment. Between the tooth and the gingiva is a normal space, called the gingival sulcus.

The healthy gingiva normally fits snugly around the tooth, but if for any reason the epithelial attachment is broken and moved down the root toward the tip (apex), the depth of the sulcus increases and a pocket is formed. This pocket provides an area for the accumulation of food, other debris, and calculus which further reduces the resistance and health of the adjacent tissue. The inflammatory process is progressive, and the periodontal membrane and bone surrounding the tooth are destroyed. This wave of destruction continues moving apically (tipward), the involved tooth eventually becoming loose and possibly assuming a slightly different position. Once the bone around the root has been destroyed, it cannot rebuild to its original height. The supporting structures may become so damaged that the teeth cannot be maintained and must be removed.

It is difficult to imagine, but a tooth which shows no evidence of dental caries can be lost as a result of this insidious process. In fact, periodontal disease is the major factor contributing to the loss of teeth in people past thirty years of age.

The major causative factors in periodontal disease may be classified as irritational, (dys)functional, and systemic. Some examples of local irritation are: deposits on the teeth (calculus), packing of food between the teeth, malformed or malpositioned teeth, and mechanical irritation (cavity margins, damaged fillings, and improper tooth-brushing). Overfunction (excessive stress on the teeth, excessive muscular pressures), underfunction (lack of contact between opposing teeth), and abnormal habits (clenching or grinding of the teeth) are examples of dysfunctional factors. Among the systemic causes of periodontal disease are faulty nutrition, allergies, psychosomatic factors, and hormonal imbalance related to the menstrual cycle.

Treatment. The treatment of this disease, as of all others, involves removal of the cause, restoration of normal function, increase of tissue-resistance, and stabilization of the health and integrity of the tissue. This may be accomplished by procedures performed primarily by the dentist or primarily by the patient.

Those accomplished by the dentist are scaling, which is the mechanical removal of calculus, diseased cementum, and soft tissue, and surgery, which is conservative surgery, permitting the scaling to be done more thoroughly. (In more serious cases the affected bone and the soft tissue overlying it may be removed or reshaped.)

Those accomplished by the patient upon instruction from the dentist are mechanical in nature: stimulation of the soft tissue by various means, such as with toothbrush, toothpick, pipe-cleaners, rubber stimulators, and finger-massage.

PERIPHERAL NERVES

Nerve cells

in the spinal cord are in contact with muscles and sensory receptors throughout the body by way of the peripheral nerves. Each spinal nerve is formed from an anterior motor and a posterior sensory root. The spinal nerves are divided from above to below into eight cervical, twelve thoracic, five lumbar, and five sacral nerves, plus one coccygeal nerve. In the cervical and lumbar regions, groups of spinal nerves form the brachial and the lumbar plexuses, from which peripheral nerves arise. In these areas, the disturbance of function of muscles and of sensation will vary somewhat, depending upon whether the damage is to the root, plexus, or peripheral nerve. In other areas the spinal nerves continue as the peripheral nerves and the damage to an individual nerve will result in a uniform segmental loss of function.

Unlike the nerve fibers in the spinal cord, the peripheral nerves are capable of regeneration after interruption. Peripheral nerves may be injured by pressure or may be partially or completely severed. These injuries may be related to fractures of bones in the area. The function of peripheral nerves is also sometimes affected by diabetes mellitus, nutritional deficiency, diphtheria, and other disorders.

With complete damage to a peripheral nerve, the muscles supplied by the nerve are useless, and sensation is lost in the distribution of that nerve. With partial damage, weakness and decreased sensation are observed.

Transection of a nerve may require surgical treatment. Disorders of nerves related to systemic diseases, however, may respond to treatment of the primary disorder, and recovery may be partial or complete.

PERIPHERAL VASCULAR DISEASE

When any thickening occurs in the arterial wall, the size of the opening (lumen) within the vessel through which blood passes will become narrowed, even completely closed. Peripheral vascular disease includes all types of change, whatever their causes, that produce these obstructions to adequate blood flow:

1. Raynaud's disease. In this disorder, the clinical picture is produced by arterial spasm rather by organic vascular disease, the arteries narrowing as a result of the spasm.

2. Arteriosclerosis obliterans. This term is used to designate arteriosclerosis which causes complete blockage of the lumen of vessels in the extremities, either because of the arteriosclerotic hardening process itself or because of thrombosis (blood clotting) within the vessel. It is the most common type of occlusive vascular disease in the lower extremities. Sometimes both the intimal (atherosclerosis) and the medial (senile) type of sclerosis are encountered at the same time in affected vessels. The causes of the atherosclerosis have not been made completely clear, although nutritional, endocrine, biochemical, and local vascular phenomena (as well as tissue changes in the intiminal lining substance of the vessels) are known to be implicated in its organization and development.

If vessel blockage completely cuts off the blood supply to an extremity, gangrene will occur in the toes, the foot, and sometimes even at higher levels. Death of the tissue imparts a black, mummified appearance to the skin. If the gangrene is complicated by infection, the affected part appears moist and foul-smelling. There may be considerable sloughing-away of tissue.

3. Buerger's disease (thrombioangiitis obliterans). In this form of blood-vessel disease toxic agents such as nicotine have been implicated, although it is now generally agreed that this drug represents only an aggravating or accelerating influence. Buerger's disease is a condition affecting medium-sized and small arteries, and not

infrequently the veins.

In its early stages the affected vessels contract by individual segments, particularly at sites of occlusion. The veins may be similarly involved, and in rare instances may even be the earliest site of involvement. A soft but adherent red-purple clot may be seen within the passageway (lumen) of the affected arteries. Later the clot becomes yellow-gray. Proliferation of vessel-lining may be observed in portions of arteries in which blockage has not occurred. When the lesion is advanced, the lumen is blocked by a thrombus containing vessel-lining cells, clot-related materials, and some red and white blood cells. The musculature of the middle layer of the vessel is well preserved, but the inner lining is thickened by proliferation of connective tissue which in long-standing cases includes adjacent veins. Oxygen-lack changes such as gangrene, softening of the bone, and muscular atrophy may also be present in this disorder.

In addition to the above, there are a number of rare afflictions that may cause arterial obstruction; some of these are attributed to hypersensitivity (allergy) phenomena, others to tissue (collagen) disorders and diseases of the neurological system.

PERITONITIS This condition—while still extremely serious and requiring prompt and early medical attention—is fortunately much less common and dreaded than in the days before the sulfas and antibiotics. Peritonitis is a widespread inflammation of the membranous lining of the abdominal cavity (peritoneum). Because of the extensive surface-area involved, it is a very generalized infection and causes profound symptoms.

Peritonitis is caused by infectious agents or foreign material within the abdominal cavity. Practically any type of bacteria gaining entrance will multiply rapidly, since the peritoneum and its lu-bricating secretions make an ideal growth-medium. Bacteria may gain access by perforation of the intestinal tract resulting from appendicitis, peptic ulcer, diverticulitis, severe gallbladder disease, typhoid fever, bowel obstructions, or dysentery. (Occasionally bacteria may gain access through the female genital tract.) A chemical peritonitis may result if bile or pancreatic juices are spilled into the abdominal cavity. Occasionally the infection is not generalized and a local abscess will form.

Clinical features are quite variable, since they depend upon the cause of the infection. A localized peritonitis is common with appendicitis, and in this instance pain is confined to the inflamed area. If the appendix then ruptures, the peritonitis may spread rapidly.

Symptoms. The inflammatory process usually causes a rising temperature, chills, an increase in the number of white blood cells, vomiting, and severe pain. Because of the discomfort, the abdominal muscles are usually very rigid—this being a valuable sign to the physician. Peritonitis is most often a complication of an underlying condition in the abdomen, and signs of appendicitis, gallbladder disease, intestinal obstruction, or other such conditions are also present.

Treatment. A localized peritonitis may result in spontaneous recovery, but a generalized condition requires prompt and vigorous treatment. Appropriate therapy depends upon the underlying condition and may require surgical intervention. Vigorous and prompt administration of appropriate antibiotics has reduced the incidence and gravity of the disease immeasurably, but prompt recognition and treatment are essential.

PERITONSILLAR ABSCESS (QUINSY)
See ABSCESS, PERITONSILLAR

PERSONALITY CHANGES IN ALLERGY

The personality changes that can occur in an allergic person may be due to: (1) the allergy itself; (2) the symptoms present; or (3) the treatment employed.

Confusion and unpleasant behavior may be due to edema of the brain, which in turn is caused by an allergy to some food (as in certain cases of migraine). An allergic response of the nervous system can cause symptoms such as irritability, depression, and restlessness.

An atopic child, because of all the attention his illness brings him, can become self-centered and selfish. Persons with severe allergies may be so afflicted that they avoid people and stay by themselves, becoming overwhelmed with self-pity in an almost schizophrenic manner.

Emotional disturbances such as drowsiness, irrational behavior, hysteria, or confusion, can be caused by medications that are used in treating the allergic state. (See EMOTIONS, ROLE OF.)

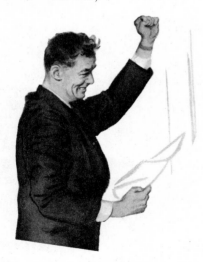

PERSONAL SOCIAL BEHAVIOR

Mental-hygiene experience indicates that getting along with others is a vital factor in mental health; studies of the development of neurotic behavior in infants and very young children indicate that such problems often originate in early disturbed human relationships. Since every child is socially trained (conditioned) by his early contacts with parents and relatives, where parents or other important adults are neurotic or emotionally unhealthy, young children tend toward the same abnormal behavior patterns.

There is considerable evidence that many neurotic patterns are transmitted from older to younger generations by imitation and conditioning; for example, the neurotic mother who is fearful of many things in life such as darkness or water tends to communicate fears and anxieties by imitation in children who develop the same pattern.

It is now generally accepted that one of the major purposes of all social institutions—the family, schools, the church, law-and-order—is the conditioning of the child in healthy personal social behavior. Getting along with others is probably the most difficult psychological problem in life, and perhaps the most common cause for neurotic conflict when a person becomes socially maladjusted. To like other people, it is first necessary to like and respect one's self; those who are difficult to get along with frequently do not like themselves and are frustrated by their own behavior.

Treatment. A basic method in child guidance clinics (and psychotherapy in general) is the conditioning of the individual who is not getting along well in new kinds of personal social relationships. Frequently the therapist is able to establish a friendly, accepting, noncritical, and helpful relationship with the patient for the first time in the latter's life. Various forms of group play and therapy provide opportunities for the socially ill-adjusted to learn to relate in healthier ways than formerly.

PERSPIRATION, EXCESSIVE

Excessive perspiration or hyperhidrosis is observed in fevers, when a high fever breaks (especially in influenza), with or following physical exertion or emotional stress, when induced by physiotherapeutic apparati such as inductothermy, steam baths, and heat lamps, in hot weather and climates, or in a humid atmosphere. Severe pain, such as colic, and shock and collapse may also cause sweating. The sweat-producing drugs (diaphoretics), ipecac, camphor and pilocarpin, cause profuse sweating. Excessive perspiration occurs in hyperthyroidism, chronic tuberculosis of the lungs (especially nocturnally, the so-called "night sweats"), psychoneurosis, acute rheumatic fever, bacterial invasion of the bloodstream, malaria, chronic myocarditis, and, less commonly, in bronchiectasis (also at night), epilepsy, gout, morphinism, and other minor conditions.

Hyperhidrosis due to emotional stimulation is often localized (perspiration under the armpits, the palms of the hands, the face, feet, etc.). In this type of sweating the stimulation to sweat glands originates in the sympathetic nervous system which responds to emotional stimuli.

Human sweat is odorless. The unfavorable scent, often referred to as body odor or "b.o.," is due to the bacteria which flourish in perspiration. A good deodorant measure (and the safest) is a bath followed by thorough toweling and dusting susceptible areas of the body with powder that tends to promote dryness of the skin regions commonly affected by perspiration odors (armpits, crotch, etc.).

PERTHES' DISEASE

This is the most common hip malady in the two-to-six-year-old group. The head of the femur bone, set in the hip, temporarily loses its blood supply and the bone softens, crumbles, and deforms. The usual symptom is the gradual onset of a painless limp. At the same time, the child may complain of inability to spread his legs as far as usual and of mild pain in the knee. (This knee-pain originates in—is "referred" from—the hip and is not a sign of knee involvement. Many children have had only knee

X-rays by mistake when the true seat of disease was in the hips.)

In mild cases, Perthes' disease is a transient problem and may even go unnoticed. In several cases, however, it requires several years to resolve. If untreated it results in destruction of the hip joint and in incapacitating degenerative arthritis in adulthood. Since the bone is softened while the deforming force itself is the weight of normal walking, treatment of the disease involves putting the child to bed for several months in order to remove the weight-stress and to allow the femoral head to re-form under the stimulus of its new blood supply. A gradual increase of weight bearing is then allowed, using crutches and an ischial weight-bearing brace, a Sam Browne sling, or an abduction device.

PHARYNGITIS

Because of its location at the back of the mouth, the pharynx (throat) is subject to "bombardment" by many bacteria and viruses from the outer air and the nose. If the host is susceptible and the bacteria are numerous enough, germs will establish a foothold and multiply to a point where symptoms of infection (pharyngitis) are noted: malaise, difficulty in swallowing, headache, and perhaps fever and swollen glands. If the tonsils are present, they will also become infected; even though other areas are also involved, the resulting condition is usually referred to as tonsillitis, because the tonsils appear most dramatically inflamed.

PHARYNGITIS, STREPTOCOCCAL

Streptococcal pharyngitis or septic sore throat is inflammation of the pharynx (throat) due to the streptococcus germ. It is a common ailment with local and generalized indications. If the disease occurs with a body rash, it is scarlet fever. While the disorder is most often caused by the streptococcus, it also occurs with pneumococcal and diphtheria infections.

Symptoms. The dominant complaint is a sore, burning, dry throat. Often a patient complains that he feels a "lump" in his throat. In addition, there are chills and fever, difficulty in swallowing, swelling of lymph nodes of the neck, and difficulty in speaking. The mucous membrane of the throat is red and swollen; there may be an obvious exudate (secretion). The pharyngitis may involve lymph nodes of the throat to the point where abscesses (singly or in a group) may form, or these may follow inflammatory implication of the tonsils and sinuses. Usually there is swelling on one side of the neck.

Treatment. Antibiotic therapy is the treatment of choice. If the pharyngeal abscess does not rupture spontaneously, surgical intervention is required. Other measures include palliation of the sore throat (chipped ice, analgesics, ice collar, chilled fluids, etc.). Sedatives are given to allay anxiety. Fluids, fortified with vitamins, are given during the period the patient is unable to swallow solids. For treatment of diphtheritic pharyngitis, see under DIPHTHERIA.

PHARYNX The pharnyx has three divisions, which may be observed if one looks into the open mouth with the help of a mirror. Following the tongue to the back of the throat, and looking a little beyond, will lead the eye to the very back of the throat, the oral pharynx. Up above the palate and in back of the nose is the nasopharynx, while the laryngopharynx lies below the base of the tongue. (Both the naso- and laryngopharynx can be seen with special instruments.)

PHARYNX, GENERAL BACTERIAL INFECTION OF THE A bacterial infection can occur which is not localized in the tonsils. A relatively common variety is streptococcus infection of the throat (strep throat). Before antibiotics and sulfa drugs were available, bacterial in-

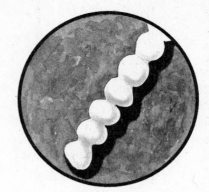

STREPTOCOCCI PYOGENES

fections of the pharynx resulted in many dangerous complications. Now in the vast majority of cases these drugs can control infections.

Symptoms. The beginning of strep throat is sudden. In addition to headache and a general feeling of ill health, a high fever (associated with chills and pain on swallowing) occurs.

Treatment. Bed rest, good nourishment, hot gargles, and antibiotics are the preferred therapy. (See TRENCH MOUTH; DIPHTHERIA; RETROPHARYNGEAL ABSCESS.)

PHOBIA Phobias are intense, unreasoned fears, usually symptomatic of deep neurotic anxiety states. Contrasted with ordinary fears, in which there is usually a recognized conscious cause for the apprehension, phobias usually reflect deep anxieties of unconscious origin, so that the sufferer may not be consciously aware of the causes or sources of his irrational behavior.

Symptoms. Phobias may appear in early childhood in the form of unreasoning fear of darkness, mice, snakes, enclosed or high places, water, or disease. Frequently, all of a child's deep anxieties and insecurities are displaced onto one phobia. The form of any particular phobia is often a matter of chance, although conditioning and imitation of similar fears in adults may be predisposing causes.

Treatment. Since phobias are always indicative of underlying unconscious conflicts, some form of psychotherapy or psychoanalysis is indicated. The child should be referred to a child guidance clinic for psychiatric evaluation.

Specific phobias, such as fear of darkness, should not be reinforced in unhealthy ways as by taking the child into bed with the parents; this may only increase the child's neurotic dependency-needs. (It sometimes helps to leave the child's room dimly lighted, but otherwise the child should be calmly and firmly induced to stay in bed by himself.)

PHONOCARDIOGRAPHY Heart murmurs can be detected by a specially constructed microphone applied to the chest wall in the same way as a stethoscope. The noise of the murmur can be permanently recorded on moving paper, together with the electrocardiograph (EKG) tracing. This procedure is somewhat greater in sensitivity than the human ear and detects sounds too faint for the ear. Also, it makes possible a permanent record, in case surgery is done or there are changes —as in the case of bacterial endocarditis. Furthermore, a very accurate relationship of murmur to the exact phase of the cardiac cycle is made possible by use of phonocardiograph tracings superimposed on the EKG tracing.

PHRENIC NERVES The phrenic nerves arise from the roots of the spinal cord in the mid-portion of the neck and descend through the central portion of the chest to supply the muscles of the diaphragm. In normal breathing, the diaphragm contracts on inspiration and allows the lower portions of the lungs to expand. With paralysis of the diaphragm, breathing is limited.

PHYSICAL ALLERGIES Some people are allergic to such natural phenomena as light, heat, cold, and pressure. This hypersensitivity is called physical allergy. Physical allergy can cause such diverse symptoms as asthma, rhinitis, urticaria, gastrointestinal upsets, tremors, weakness, headches, convulsions, and shock.

Allergy to light is an interesting phenomenon. The combination of certain drugs plus exposure to sunlight will cause a marked sunburn reaction in susceptible persons. Exposure to the same amount of sunlight—but without the drugs—causes no reaction. Antibiotics, sulfonamides, tranquilizers, antidiabetic drugs, and sedatives are a few of the groups of drugs that may be involved.

In certain cases the presence of specific chemicals or plant-life in contact with the skin will produce an eczema only if sunlight is present; in the absence of one or the other there will be no reaction. This is known as a phytosolar reaction. Limes, figs, meadow grass, wild parsnips, lady-slippers, and gas plants are some of the plants involved. Bithionol is a common chemical producing a similar effect.

Some individuals develop hives (urticaria) on exposure to sunlight, with or without drugs or chemicals; and—although not exactly an allergy—there are those in whom exposure to sunlight produces paroxysms of violent sneezing.

Heat, too, will cause small red wheals (hives) over the body in certain persons.

Cold allergy may be due to the presence of abnormal proteins in the body. The hives associated with this physical allergy are large and may be accompanied by swelling of the lips, tongue, and face. Exposure to cold may also flare up as an asthmatic attack. Cold allergy is especially dangerous in the summer, when the afflicted person goes swimming. The sudden change in temperature can cause the cold allergy to manifest itself, and the sufferer may even drown while undergoing the reactions.

Pressure urticaria occurs after prolonged intense pressure. The parts involved become swollen and sometimes painful. Dermographism (literally skin-writing) is a milder form in which wheals may be induced by stroking the skin.

Treatment of the physical allergies depends on the type and severity. Antihistamines and some form of hyposensitization may be employed.

PHYSICAL THERAPY AND EXERCISE

Physical therapy is the technique by which physical means such as light, heat, electricity, and exercise are utilized to help patients overcome pain and increase the strength and mobility of the involved parts. Heat is widely used to relieve tension, relax tense muscles, and increase joint mobility. It may be applied superficially, with a hot-water bottle or heat lamp; or deeply, with shortwave diathermy or ultrasound. Massage, as applied by a trained therapist, may be very helpful in reducing muscle spasm and in freeing tightened structures. Well-performed massage should be vigorous enough to achieve its goal without being so violent as to inflict damage.

Exercises are planned muscular activities designed to increase limb strength, joint control and motion. Active exercises are those in which all muscular effort is expended by the patient, while passive exercises are those in which the joint is put through a range of motion by the therapist. Active exercises are superior because the patient, limited by his pain, is unlikely to damage the limb. Passive exercise is hard to control, and the patient is dependent on the therapist's experience.

Walking is considered an excellent exercise for persons in the older age group. In recent years, jogging has been heralded as an important exercise, especially for its tonic effects on the heart and the increment in cardiac capacity that results. A hoped for, although still unproven, effect

NORMAL AND ABNORMAL POSTURE

The normal vertebral column has three curves — a forward cervical, a forward lumbar, and a backward thoracic. Lordosis is an excessive forward curvature of the cervical or lumbar curves; kyphosis is an excessive backward thoracic curve.

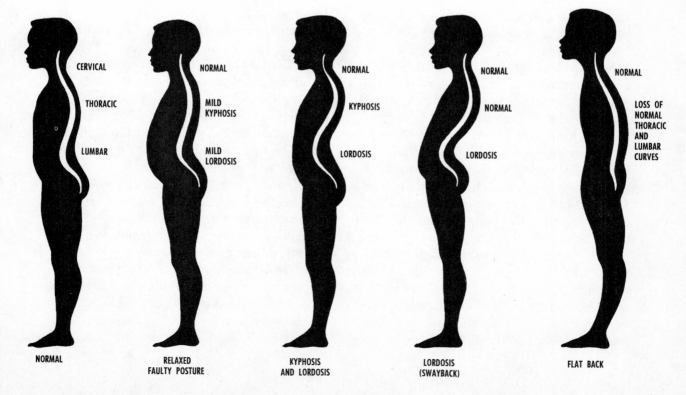

NORMAL

RELAXED FAULTY POSTURE

KYPHOSIS AND LORDOSIS

LORDOSIS (SWAYBACK)

FLAT BACK

398

might be a decrease in coronary artery disease. Progressive jogging should not be undertaken by sedentary or middle-aged persons without prior medical clearance.

Sedentary people may benefit from conditioning exercises, such as those illustrated in "Physical Fitness and Reducing Exercises" (color plates E1 through E8) and ISOMETRICS (pages 319-322).

PILONIDAL CYST A pilonidal cyst is a result of congenital folding-under of tissues which are normally at the surface. As a result, skin-like structures—including hair and epithelial cells—are enclosed within a cyst located at the base of the spine. After repeated irritation, the area may become inflamed and cause a draining abscess.

Pilonidal cysts are most commonly seen in young males, particularly those who have more than average amounts of hair on the body.

Symptoms. The symptoms of this type of cyst are pain and tenderness at the base of the spine and repeated episodes of pus drainage.

Treatment. In chronic cases of pilonidal cyst the only treatment likely to give lasting results is surgical removal.

PINEAL GLAND The pineal gland is an interesting structure about which little is known, located deep in the brain, above and behind the pituitary gland. In animals such as lizards, the pineal is known to be an organ receptive to light. It has also been determined that numerous metabolic substances are manufactured in this gland. As improved techniques become available, it will be possible to study its function more adequately. Since tumors of the pineal gland which produce active metabolic substances have not been described, the chief importance of this structure, as seen in man at the present time, is as an indicator of the skull midline in X-rays, since it calcifies after adolescence.

PITUITARY GLAND, ANTERIOR The pituitary gland at the base of the skull is divided into two portions, the posterior and the anterior. It is the anterior or forward portion which is responsible for secreting the hormones regulating the function of the thyroid gland, the adrenals, and the sex glands; in addition, it secretes growth hormone. The anterior pituitary is made of several cell-types, some of which have a secretory function. It may be the site of tumor, hemorrhage, or atrophy, all of these causing it to lose its characteristic function, thus also depressing the function of the glands which it controls.

PITUITARY GLAND, POSTERIOR The rear part of the pituitary gland is a direct extension downward of the brain and is richly supplied with nerves. It is responsible for secreting hormones with powerful effects on the uterus and the smooth muscle of blood vessels. It is also the site of secretion of the antidiuretic (anti-urination) hormone which acts to keep the body from losing too much water through the kidneys. Destruction of the posterior portion of the pituitary gland produces a tremendous increase in the output of urine (diabetes insipidus) together with thirst.

PITUITARY TUMORS Tumors of the pituitary gland are classified according to the type of cell which predominates. Most common is the chromophobe (color-fearing) tumor, so called because the cells do not take up the high color stain which is usually used in the laboratory.

Inasmuch as these cells do not secrete any of the known hormones, this tumor does not affect the other endocrine glands except by destruction of normal pituitary cells when the tumor becomes large. Treatment is by radiation or surgical removal.

Other types of pituitary tumor do have endocrine effects. Eosinophile tumors of the pituitary produce gigantism or acromegaly. Basophile tumors are thought to be responsible for the production of Cushing's syndrome, and sometimes appear after treatment of this syndrome by removal of the adrenal glands.

PITYRIASIS ROSEA   Although the causative agent has not been isolated, it is not unlikely that this disease is of viral origin.

Symptoms. The initial or "mother" plaque is red, scaly, oval or round, and about the size of a half-dollar. It has been known to occur on almost any part of the body and is followed in two or three weeks by a generalized eruption of similar but smaller lesions distributed on the trunk, upper arms and thighs—the face, neck, and legs being infrequently affected. It is a common observation that lesions are less likely to appear on portions of the body with recent tanning from the sun. The lesions continue to appear for a period of from two to four weeks, after which they begin to fade. The disease has a total course of from six to ten weeks, with occasional instances of much shorter or much longer duration. There is almost always a lifetime immunity to subsequent attacks. The disease recurs rarely, and even more rarely a patient may have an attack every few years. There are usually no symptoms other than itching. The patient is able to pursue normal activities, especially since the disease is most often confined to the covered portions of the body.

Treatment. No treatment is usually necessary in this spontaneously involuting disease. However, it may be necessary to control itching and hasten the clearing up of lesions with oral antihistaminic drugs, emollient baths, drying (plain calamine) lotion, and exposure to sun (when possible) or sunlamp (with great precaution against burn).

PLANTAR WARTS   Plantar warts can be confused with callusses of the soles and not infrequently the two conditions co-

exist. The virus which causes plantar warts is apparently "triggered" into producing the lesions by irritation (from shoes, pebbles, splinters).

Other than eliminating the most usual precipitating factor of friction from shoes (either by going barefoot or by wearing shoes molded to the exact shape of the foot, thus simulating the barefoot state), treatment must necessarily be left to the specialist.

PLEURISY   The term pleurisy refers to an inflammation of the chest structure known as the pleura. The pleura is a two-ply membrane, one layer of which neatly encloses each lung-surface, the other layer lining the inner side of the chest wall. Normally there is no free space between these two layers; a thin amount of lubricant fluid contained between them allows for free movement of the lung during breathing. So it is that pleurisy may be merely a dry inflammation of the lining, or it may progress to the formation of increased amounts of fluids, separating the layers and creating a true space in between.

Pleurisy is usually a complication or extension of diseases affecting the lung or chest wall; but once established, it may run a course independent from the original disease. Pleurisy is most commonly secondary to pneumonia, tuberculosis, lung tumor, abscess, chest wounds, or rib fracture. Primary pleurisy, in which the disease begins in the pleura itself, is rare.

Symptoms. The disease may be acute —the symptoms and course being of short duration—or chronic, lasting for months or years with exacerbations and remissions. The chief manifestation is always pain. In a typical case of pleurisy the pain develops progressively over a period of hours or days, is jagged and shooting in quality and intensified during deep breathing, cough, or sneezing. (Patients instinctively curtail the depth of breathing or lie over the affected side.) The pain is due to the continuous rubbing together of the inflamed pleural layers. As the inflammation continues, fluid begins to accumulate in the pleural space, thus separating the inflamed layers, and thereby somewhat reducing the pain. If fluid-formation is large, the breathing expansion of the lung is decreased and breathlessness may ensue. Fever may or may not be present. (Other concurrent symptoms, such as cough, expectoration, and malaise, are usually features of the primary disease in the lung or chest wall.)

Depending on the cause and nature of the inflammation, the disease may subside completely; if the fluid is clear, it may be reabsorbed without further consequences. In other cases, when the fluid is itself infected (empyema) or bloody (hemothorax) spontaneous reabsorption is difficult and slow, and the ultimate result is formation of adhesive bands which will continue to "imprison" the lung, severely limiting breathing capacity.

Treatment. Fundamentally, treatment is aimed at therapy for the primary disease whether in the lung or the chest wall. In cases of pneumonia, tuberculosis, lung abscess, a fractured rib, or penetrating chest-wall injury, which cause the pleurisy, proper autibiotic treatment will take care of the pleural inflammation as well.

Sometimes symptomatic treatment of the pleurisy itself is necessary to relieve pain or breathlessness. If fluid-formation is large, or if it is purulent or bloody, thoracentesis is indicated. This consists of removing the fluid by means of a needle puncture or by inserting a rubber tube which will drain the fluid continuously into a sealed bottle. The latter is usually left in place for several days or weeks until the fluid stops reaccumulating and the lung has re-expanded. In cases where the lung will not re-expand after fluid-removal because fibrous adhesions "imprison" the lung, a decortication should be performed; this operation strips the lung from the pleural peel.

PNEUMOCOCCUS This word refers to a bacterial microorganism, conical or lance-shaped and usually appearing in pairs, which takes on a bluish color when stained by the Gram method (Gram-positive). About seventy-five types or strains of pneumococcus have been isolated by laboratory tests, the type depending on the composition of the bacterial capsule. Also depending on the capsular material is the differing virulence of various pneumococcal strains.

The pneumococci are normal inhabitants of the upper respiratory tract of most individuals. Under stress situations, they may become virulent, multiply rapidly, invade the lower respiratory tract, and produce disease. The exact reasons for this transformation are not clear at present.

The pneumococcus is responsible for more than 95 per cent of lobar pneumonias and is also a common cause of bronchopneumonia. Most pneumococci are extremely responsive to penicillin therapy, the drug of choice in lobar pneumonia. (See PNEUMONIA; RESPIRATORY TRACT INFECTIONS.)

PNEUMOCONIOSES This word was coined in 1866 to describe all lung diseases caused by inhaled dust. Even at that time several specific "industrial diseases" were already known, including anthracosis (in coal miners), silicosis (in mine, quarry, and road workers), and siderosis (in foundry workers). Early medical studies also indicated that inhalation of any dust in excessive concentrations, if continued long enough, might lead to manifest disturbances of lung function. It was also learned that the lungs of most individuals living in largely populated areas would always show the presence of dust during post-mortem examination.

As modern industry expanded, new

materials and new means of processing old materials considerably complicated and enlarged the pneumoconioses hazard, either in the form of direct inhalation of comparatively large particles or through fine breakdown and subsequent inhalation as fumes. In the United States, silicosis is still the most prevalent pneumoconiosis, and more than 3,000 cases (chiefly in the mining industry) are reported and compensated annually. Other relatively common pneumoconioses and their causes are: asbestosis (magnesium silicate fibers), talcosis (talc), diatomaceous earth pneumoconiosis, berylliosis (beryllium oxide fumes), and byssinosis (cotton).

Different offenders may produce different types of pneumoconioses. The most important factors relating to disease are the physical form, chemical state, and particle-size of the dust, as well as duration of exposure to it. For instance, dust particles greater than 20 microns in diameter° will not cause disease because they will be trapped in the upper respiratory tract and will never reach and settle in the lung. (An exception to this is the long, thin asbestos fiber.) The chemical state is important: the more soluble the offender, the greater the chance it has to produce chronic inflammation. Obviously, the higher the concentration of the dust per unit of air volume and the longer the time of exposure, the more likelihood there is of producing disease. An important and variable factor is the biological response of the respiratory system to the ability of the offenders to induce toxic tissue-reactions: some individuals are susceptible and respond early; others, under the same conditions, are more resistant.

Symptoms. Pneumoconiosis is usually a disease of slow and insidious nature, diagnosis of which is generally made only after several years of exposure to the harmful dust. The most common symptoms are breathlessness and cough. Certain types of pneumoconioses do not produce symptoms at all, although considerable deposit of dust has taken place in the lung. (These are the benign or inert pneumoconioses, such as the siderosis of welders, steel-burners, and some grinders.) On the other hand, certain types of dusts tend to produce complications. Complicated silicosis, for instance, is frequently associated with infections, bronchitis, emphysema, and tuberculosis. In such case the manifestations of pneumoconiosis and the respiratory disability become dependent on the course of the superimposed diseases.

Fibrosis of the lung (replacement of its normal elastic structure by nodules and strands of solid, coalescent, inextensible material) is a distinctive characteristic of pneumoconiosis. This material curtails the capacity of the lung to expand and contract and contributes to breathlessness. As time goes on, crippling respiratory invalidism becomes more severe and a bluish color of the skin (cyanosis) and heart-failure appear. This latter is called pulmonary heart disease because heart function fails as a consequence of, and secondary to, lung disease.

Treatment. In the symptomatic or complicated pneumoconioses, both cessation of exposure and treatment of associated disease are mandatory. Any favorable results achieved are due to effective treatment of the infection or bronchitis and not of the dust disease itself (which is usually of a non-reversible nature and whose disability effects tend to increase with time).

Considerable controversy may, from the legal standpoint, arise regarding compensation. To validate a claim, there must be sufficient proof of the relationship between the type of employment and length of exposure to the symptoms, signs, and X-ray manifestations observed in the patient. Not every X-ray shadow, although

°1 micron = approximately 1/25,000 inch.

due to dust deposits in the lung, implies that the person is or will be affected by continuance of his present occupation.

Most important are the preventive measures which are the responsibility of industrial hygienists. It is the responsibility of these persons to collect the proper information concerning the processing and production equipment of industrial concerns and to analyze the physical, chemical, and toxicological properties or harmful materials likely to be present in the air. In addition, they also study the characteristics of exhaust-ventilation and sample and determine the concentration of dust which is representative of habitual working conditions during different shifts or times of day. Based on such studies the degree of hazard can be properly estimated and preventive measures (in terms of general exhaust-ventilation and individual filtering devices) can be instituted.

PNEUMONIA   This word comes from the Greek word meaning lungs. The disease is an inflammation of the lung during which the normal "beehive," air-containing lung structure is consolidated into a solid mass. This mass may vary in size according to the structural lung unit it occupies: lobule, segment, or lobe. Not every lung consolidation is a pneumonia. Tumors, non-infectious processes, atelectasis (airless lung due to bronchial obstruction and subsequent air reabsorption), and lung fibrosis (replacement of the normal elastic lung structure by scar tissue) can mimic, or be complicated by, pneumonia. Pneumonitis is an ill-defined term simply meaning lung inflammation.

The classical pneumonia is most commonly lobar in size, but may be bilobar (involving two lobes) or larger. The disease is more prevalent in late winter and early spring and attacks more men than women, particularly in the fifteen to forty age-range. Prior chronic respiratory or cardiac disease, poor nutrition, alcoholism, and exposure to sudden changes in temperature particularly predispose persons to the disease. Although it is not considered highly contagious, pneumonia may spread in small epidemics. There is no absolute immunity against the disease, and healthy individuals may be stricken.

More than 95 per cent of all classical primary lobar pneumonias are due to pneumococcus bacteria, of which there are numerous strains of different virulence. This characteristic, together with the previous state of health of the patient, will eventually determine the seriousness of the infection, the capacity of the organism to fight it, the severity of the possible complications, and the effectiveness of treatment. A nonbacterial type of pneumonia, caused by a virus, is called primary atypical pneumonia.

Symptoms. The clinical picture of lobar pneumonia is often dramatic and its onset sudden. Usually a mild head cold has been present for several days; the disease may also strike "out of the blue." The patient is attacked by shaking chills shortly followed by very high fever. Symptoms center in the chest in rapid succession: cough becomes troublesome (first dry and then slightly productive of mucus which may be red or rusty in color); breathing becomes labored (dyspnea); and chest pain may be intense—usually of a stabbing or constricting nature and intensified by deep breathing and by changing position in bed. Air-hunger may be intense and frequently the patient needs to sit up in bed to relieve it. The color of the nail beds and the lips becomes dusky or bluish (cyanosis), reflecting an inadequate supply of oxygen to the body tissues. Serious complications may ensue: (1) local spread of the disease to the pleura (pleurisy) and formation of fluid which may become infected (empyema); (2) invasion of the blood vessels producing a blood infection (bacteremia); (3) subsequent localization of the bacteria in other organs such as the brain-covers (meningitis), heart (endocarditis, pericarditis), etc. As a result, the patient may become unconscious (coma) or go into shock (blood pressure drop). The diagnosis is usually easy to establish on the basis of physical examination, study of the sputum, and especially the chest X-ray findings.

Treatment. The seriousness of the disease and its potential complications in most cases warrant immediate hospitalization. The basis of modern treatment rests on the antibiotics—in this case particularly penicillin, which will be effective against most strains of pneumococcus. (Occasionally, other antibiotics need to be employed because of the patient's allergy to the drug or because of complication of the infection by other bacteria. Under antibiotic treatment the results are usually dramatic: the fever disappears in twenty-four to forty-eight hours and the symptoms (chest pain, cough, malaise, dyspnea) are promptly relieved. Nevertheless, treatment should be continued for at least one week after the fever disappears. Notwithstanding the importance of antibiotics, other supportive measures are also employed, particularly to relieve the pain and cough temporarily, to decrease the fever, and insure rest. Adequate fluid intake is important and oxygen is often needed. The complications should be treated selectively as they appear.

PNEUMONIA, ATYPICAL   Similar to the classical lobar pneumonia in its physical characteristics, this condition differs in other aspects. The cause is a virus, or group of viruses, which spreads from person to person via infected discharges from nose and mouth. This disease is most common in middle age, but has no predilection for race, color, or sex. It produces extensive patch areas of lung consolidation, is hemorrhagic in nature, and tends to regress without complications.

Symptoms. These are similar to pneumonia, but the patient appears less seriously affected. Cough and expectoration is always a prominent feature in addition to fever, malaise, and chest pain. The severity of symptoms varies from a mild feverish illness of a few days' duration to a severe disease with high temperature lasting several weeks. In the average case, the temperature lasts approximately ten days and declines slowly. Convalescence is attended by prolonged weakness; there are comparatively few complications.

Treatment. There is no specific treatment for this disease and the patient should receive therapy directed to the prevailing symptoms (particularly the cough and fever), adequate fluid intake, and medicines to insure rest. Thus, aspirin, salicilates, codein, and barbiturates are commonly employed. Where bacterial infection has complicated the typical picture, antibiotics, particularly tetracyclines are indicated. Early ambulation (moving or walking about) is to be discouraged because it accentuates and prolongs the weakness which characteristically follows the period of acute illness.

PNEUMOTHORAX   Pneumothorax indicates the abnormal presence of air within the two layers of the pleura (see PLEURISY). Normally the pleura is a virtual space containing only a very small amount of lubricating fluid to favor lung movement during inspiration and expiration. If air (or fluid) occupies this space, lung expansion is impaired, leading to its collapse. Hydropneumothorax, pyopneumothorax, and hemopneumothorax indicate the combination of air with water, pus, or blood respectively in the pleural space.

Pneumothorax may occur spontaneously because of rupture of internal blisters (bullae) or cysts into the pleura of the lung. It may be traumatic, the result of a chest wound; or it may be induced by the physician for therapeutic purposes. Spontaneous pneumothorax may occur in otherwise perfectly healthy individuals, but most commonly in patients already afflicted by chronic pulmonary emphysema, lung cysts, or pulmonary fibrosis.

Symptoms. If pneumothorax occurs suddenly and in large amounts, the onset will be abrupt and marked by severe pain, breathlessness, cyanosis, and a shock-like state. These symptoms may progress rapidly and threaten the patient's life because in some cases, the air continues to enter the pleural space but is prevented from leaving it (tension pneumothorax). Chronic pneumothorax renders the collapsed lung useless, and if left untreated for long periods of time the organ may never re-expand. Any pneumothorax, although composed at the beginning of air only, has the potential for complication by the addition of clear or infected fluid.

Treatment. If the amount of air is small no active treatment is necessary. With increased amounts immediate suction (aspiration) is indicated, either through repeated needle aspirations or preferably by continuous suction. (The latter is the treatment of choice when tension pneumothorax is suspected.) Early aspiration of the air will prevent chronic lung collapse and failure to re-expand. Artificial pneumothorax is a therapeutic procedure which was very popular in the past for the treatment of pulmonary tuberculosis. The lung was collapsed selectively in the diseased area to arrest the activity of the inflammation. Although the method was effective in many instances, complications were frequent, some of them very serious. Today this procedure is seldom employed.

POISONING Any substances which may prove harmful to the body are considered poisons; they are particularly apt to affect children because the young do not understand the dangers involved. Without going into statistics, it is important for parents (and other adults handling children) to remember that the incidence of accidental poisonings is needlessly high, and also that the highest rate of poisoning accidents occurs among the two- to four-year-olds.

So many of the medicines and chemicals available today for home and household use can harm or kill human beings that just to list them would require a book of the present size. Suffice it to say that if there are small children about, they will surely find whatever poisons are available—therefore the best possible treatment is prevention. Among the most common poisons taken by children are various solvents, soaps, and of course medicines, with aspirin heading the list chiefly because candy-flavored aspirin seems to be a favorite hazard; chocolate-flavored laxatives are another danger. Therefore the intelligent mother will not allow any medicine in the form of candy in her house; when her child needs aspirin, she will make up the proper dose with sugar and water in a spoon.

Treatment. Call your doctor *immediately*. Then, if it is known what the child ate, antidotes for temporary relief are given in the FIRST AID AND EMERGENCIES section. While waiting for the doctor, temporary measures may often be obtained by calling the Poison Control centers, which exist in many large cities. A phone call to a hospital or city health department is another quick means to obtaining instant advice or help.

POISON IVY (OAK, SUMAC) See CONTACT DERMATITIS

POLIO See INFANTILE PARALYSIS

POLLEN Pollen is a dust-like, powdery material produced by seed-bearing plants. The important pollens in inhalant allergies are those that are air-borne. Hay fever, asthma, and allergic rhinitis are

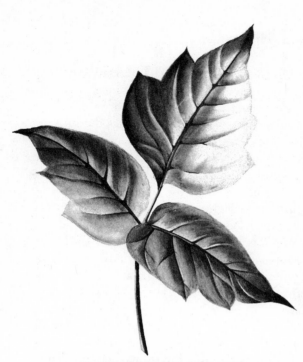

THE COMMON POISON IVY (RHUS RADICANS)
The common poison ivy grows as a small plant, vine, or bush. Its foliage consists of three glossy leaves.

diseases that can be caused by inhaling pollen. There is also one form of contact dermatitis known as ragweed dermatitis in which the eruption is caused by exposure of the skin to ragweed pollen.

Trees pollinate in the spring and early summer, grasses in the late spring and summer, and weeds in the late summer and autumn. The amount of pollen in the air at any one time depends on a number of factors. The pollen count increases with heightened wind velocity or temperature, with sunshine, and at altitudes under 5,000 feet. It decreases with increased rainfall or atmospheric humidity, with decreased temperature, and at altitudes over 5,000 feet.

Pollen counts are taken by exposing a glass slide covered with a very thin layer of some sticky substance, such as petrolatum, to the atmosphere. The air to be sampled is permitted to flow over this surface, the pollen adhering to the slide.

The number of pollen grains per square centimeter of slide, as counted under a microscope, is then defined as the pollen count.

The grasses whose pollens cause the most difficulty in the United States are bluegrass (June grass), timothy, orchard, redtop, Bermuda, Johnson, sweet vernal, rye, and corn.

There are eight groups of trees whose spring pollinations have caused symptoms: (1) the birches, alders, and hazels; (2) beeches, oaks, and chestnuts; (3) the elms and hackberries; (4) the mulberries; (5) the walnuts, hickories, and pecans; (6) the poplars, aspens, cottonwoods, and willows; (7) the maples and box elders; and (8) the ashes, olives, and privets.

Many kinds of weeds cause trouble among allergic persons. In the ragweed family are the short ragweed, giant ragweed, Western ragweed, Southern ragweed, cocklebur, rough marsh elder, and tall povertyweed. The wormwood and sage group consists of annual sage, biennial sage, sagebrush, pasture sage, sand sagebrush, prairie sage, and tall wormwood. In the pigweed family there are pigweed, spiny pigweed, and western waterhemp. The goosefoot group includes lambsquarter, sugar beet, shadscale, Russian thistle, and summer cypress. The English plaintain is the most important representative of the plantain family. Hemp and hop belong to the hemps, while sorrel and rhubarb are included under the docks.

When one is allergic to one of the grasses one is usually also allergic (in different degrees) to other members of the grass group. Timothy is often employed as the grass representative. (This type of cross-reactivity also occurs within the different groups of trees and weeds.) (See ASTHMA; HAY FEVER.)

POLYMORPHOUS LIGHT ERUPTION
This eruption occurs at all ages and in both sexes. It can make its first appearance

notwithstanding the patient's previous uneventful exposure to ultraviolet light. Not infrequently, however, the initiation of the photosensitivity may have been preceded by the taking of drugs capable of inducing or eliciting the eruption. Among the known photosensitizing drugs are the sulfonamides, antibiotics, and tranquilizers, and no doubt a host of other substances less well known and less frequently encountered (for example, diagnostic fluorescent dyes).

Symptoms. The lesions appear on the parts of the body usually exposed to the sun (upper chest, face, neck, arms, and legs). The eruption consists of red papules irregularly distributed and giving a measles-like appearance. The course is short, the eruption lasting a few days or weeks after removal from ultraviolet light exposure (and elimination of the drug in cases in which this has been an eliciting factor). There are usually no concomitant systemic findings.

Treatment. On eliminating the provocative agent(s), palliative soothing lotions suffice in treatment. Because of the possible photosensitizing potential of many drugs, some presently unknown, the usual remedies for sedation and control of itching are better avoided. In some patients it is possible to determine the particular wavelengths of ultraviolet to which the patient has become sensitized, and it is then possible to find lotions containing sunscreening substances (to screen out the offending bands of ultraviolet light) for the patient to apply before exposing himself to the sun. Difficulties attend such a procedure, and the patient must continue to be cautious in further exposing himself to ultraviolet light.

POLYPS   Polyps are nonmalignant tumors. They generally grow on the surface of various body cavities in mushroom-like shapes. They are found in the nose, intestines, the rectum, etc.

Treatment. Surgical removal of the polyps by a physician surgeon is the approved treatment.

PORTAL VEIN   The portal vein is a large vessel which collects blood from the gastrointestinal tract and transports it to the liver, where absorbed foodstuffs can be extracted and stored until needed. Harmful substances which may have been absorbed into the bloodstream are rendered harmless in the liver before entering the general circulation. Obstruction to the flow of blood in the portal vein may occur from cirrhosis or hardening of the liver, cancer of the pancreas-head, and rarely by a clot (thrombus-formation). If the flow through the portal vein is completely obstructed, the blood must find other routes to gain access to the general circulation; swollen or varicose veins of the esophagus, the rectum, and the anus (hemorrhoids) may result.

PORT-WINE STAIN (NEVUS FLAMMEUS)   This type of blood-vessel birthmark is extremely common on the nape of the neck and occurs less commonly over the bridge of the nose, on the forehead, and elsewhere. The bluish-red, flat, irregularly shaped lesion of varying size becomes exaggerated on crying,

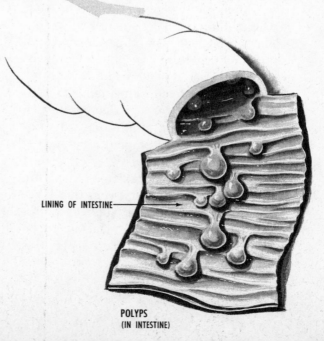

LINING OF INTESTINE—

POLYPS
(IN INTESTINE)

coughing, or blushing, and can also fade appreciably. Not infrequently the smaller and less intensely red lesions will completely disappear. Some lesions extend and grow in size in proportion to the growth of the child.

Treatment. Because this type of birthmark is of importance only as a cosmetic defect, it is essential that no treatment be undertaken which might produce further disfigurement. Hence surgical procedures which necessarily produce scarring are not useful, since scars cannot be covered with makeup as effectively as the smooth surface of the lesion. Even a very young child can accept the application of a cosmetic lotion or cream, and should be instructed in the use of one early in order to avoid disturbing comments from playmates. The possibility of treatment with thorium X should be considered in extensive cases involving exposed parts and producing much disfigurement.

POTASSIUM Potassium is an important electrolyte in the body which is intimately associated with sodium metabolism. The normal intake of potassium is about one to four grams and is related largely to the meat and fruit content of the diet. Unlike sodium, which is extracellular (in the external body fluids rather than in the cell), potassium is to a great extent intracellular.

Potassium deficiency develops through excessive loss from the kidneys or bowels. It occurs in certain types of complex kidney disease and in various types of overactivity of the adrenal gland. Patients with diarrhea or those who chronically use cathartics may lose potassium in excessive amounts in the stool.

In severe potassium deficiency, muscle weakness and paralysis may develop, leading to difficulties in breathing and changes in the heart.

In certain diseases, both potassium and sodium concentration need to be ad-

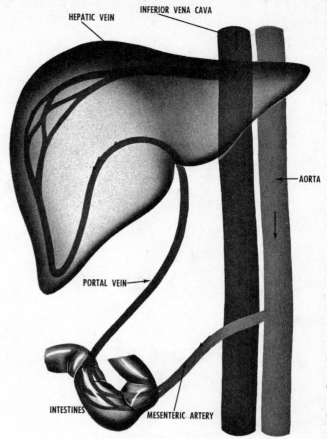

THE PORTAL VEIN CIRCULATION

justed. For this the physician uses certain drugs (diuretics) or hormones to stabilize the electrolyte pattern of the body. He often replaces deficiencies in these substances by administration of intravenous fluids in the hospital.

PREGNANCY Pregnancy is the result of conception and subsequent implantation of the fertilized egg (ovum) inside the womb cavity. The tubes, ovaries, or even the abdominal cavity are occasionally sites of implantation and development of the fertilized ovum (see TUBAL PREGNANCY). The average duration of the human pregnancy is 280 days (ten lunar months or nine calendar months).

Signs and symptoms of early pregnancy are: (1) cessation of the monthly menstrual periods; (2) morning sickness; (3) enlargement and soreness of the breasts, with milky discharge; (4) enlargement of the womb; (5) perception of fetal movements. None of these subjective symptoms is a definite sign of pregnancy,

FERTILIZATION

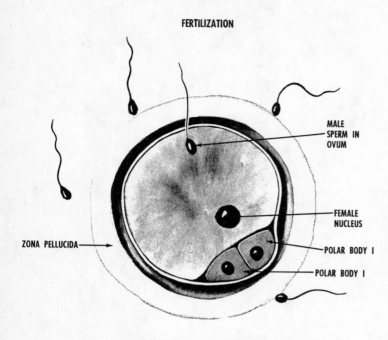

MALE
SPERM IN
OVUM

FEMALE
NUCLEUS

POLAR BODY I

POLAR BODY I

ZONA PELLUCIDA

THE EVENTS OF FERTILIZATION

The female ovum (egg), surrounded by a thick, transparent Zona Pellucida, divides unequally, producing Polar Body I. At this point, a single sperm penetrates the Zona. The ovum again divides, producing Polar Body II. The female nucleus migrates toward the male sperm. The union of the two completes fertilization.

and the presence of one or more of them is merely suggestive, but not diagnostic, of pregnancy. Probable diagnosis of early pregnancy can be made by uterine palpation and verified by laboratory tests available for this purpose. The most widely used are chemical tests performed on a small amount of urine placed on a slide. Unlike the older biological tests using mice or rabbits, the new tests can give diagnostic results in a few minutes.

PREMATURE BABY   Any baby whose birth-weight is less than five and a half pounds is today called premature. This arbitrary definition makes it easier to compile statistics, but fails to take into account babies which are mature but small, or those which are immature but large.

The true premature infant has a higher death rate than the full-term baby,

usually has some difficulty with respiration because of incompletely developed lungs, and is more likely to have some nervous-system damage (at birth or later) which can involve vision, hearing and speech difficulties, and/or behavior and personality problems.

The "preemy's" immediate survival depends on many factors: if prematurity is suspected during labor, it may be considered advisable to give the mother very little in the way of pain-killing drugs or sedatives in the early stages, and only the lightest possible anesthetic—rarely gas or ether—later on. (If the mother is in active labor, these drugs may affect the baby's respiratory center, with the result that it may become difficult—or sometimes even impossible—to resuscitate the baby.)

At birth, as soon as an airway has been established, the premature baby is placed in an incubator which provides mist and oxygen; this is preferably done in a special premature nursery staffed with trained personnel. Too much oxygen is now known to damage the premature retina, so the concentration of this gas in the incubator must be measured. The baby is carefully watched, but is not disturbed unless respiratory trouble is noted.

Premature babies are rarely fed until forty-eight hours after birth. Another general rule is that if the premature survives until the forty-eighth hour and color and respiration are reasonably normal, the child should continue to do well. It is at this point that feedings may be started. Usually only sugar-water in half-teaspoon amounts is given at first; if this is tolerated, some form of human or cow's milk is then begun.

The baby is fed through a thin tube which is passed down the esophagus for each feeding, usually every three hours. These babies generally take at least three to four weeks to achieve normal birth-weight. If doing well, the premature child will grow at about the rate of one ounce a day, or about one-half pound a week.

At about four pounds, an attempt is made to have the child drink from a bottle. For the first time, he may be dressed and taken out of the incubator. Premature infants are usually allowed home when they are eating and gaining well, maintaining their body-temperature, and when weighing close to five pounds.

PREMENSTRUAL SYNDROME
(PMS) The condition of mental tension, irritability, headache, depression and a feeling of "bloatedness," with some evidence of edema, that begins in the week prior to menstruation and usually resolves completely the day after a menstrual period's flow has begun.

It is a common condition which causes a good deal of distress to those affected by it—which includes women of all ethnic groups. It is *cyclical* in that it may occur before the menarche, after the menopause and even after a hysterectomy. Hormonal origins are the obvious cause, with water and salt retention as the consequence of a hormonal imbalance; but psychogenic causes play their part in initiating a behavioral response to physical changes in the body.

Treatment. In severe cases, treatment is often effective with hormonal supplements of the progesterone type, with the initiation of anovulatory cycles by use of the oral contraceptive pill and with diuretics ("water pills") taken for the immediate premenstrual period.

PRENATAL CARE
Most of the serious complications of pregnancy, which may endanger the health and even the life of the baby and the mother, could today be prevented or controlled with regular prenatal care. Facilities ranging from private obstetricians to municipal or county prenatal clinics, are available for every socioeco-

nomic group, and there is hardly any excuse for the expectant mother who neglects to register for prenatal care. The benefits for both the mother and the baby are numerous, while the potential risks of neglect can be truly dramatic. On the average, a total of ten to twelve visits during the entire nine months of pregnancy are adequate as excellent preparation of the expectant mother for a smooth pregnancy and delivery. Initially, monthly visits suffice; during the seventh and eighth months, they should be scheduled every two or three weeks, and during the last month every week.

In the course of the visits, several important blood and urine tests are done by the obstetrician and repeated if necessary; the baby's growth is carefully followed; the mother is given instructions on diet, exercise, and rest; vitamins and mineral preparations are prescribed, and any deviation from normal is thoroughly investigated and properly treated. The returns on this very intelligent investment are an expectant mother who is physically and emotionally well prepared to go through the wonderful experience of childbirth with the least possible risks for herself and her baby.

To meet the nutritional requirements of pregnancy, to insure that the newborn will have had available the best dietary constituents, and to correct any existing dietary deficiencies, it is recommended that a prenatal diet be of wide variety and well-balanced. (See DIET IN PREGNANCY.)

PRESBYCUSIS
Presbycusis refers to old-age hearing. This condition, which may begin as early as age thirty-five and as late as sixty-five, is the most common cause of hearing loss in the older age group. A neurosensory type of hearing loss, it is sometimes complicated by an inability to discriminate correctly between similar sounds. When discriminative faculty of the hearing mechanism is functioning poorly, merely increasing the loudness of

the voice is ineffective in helping the hard-of-hearing person. The problem is one of insufficient signals leading to understanding. Speaking slowly and clearly, and letting the hearing-impaired person watch the speaker's lips, will aid materially in achieving understanding of speech. This problem—of not understanding speech even if it is made loud—can occur in many types of neurosensory hearing loss and is not restricted to presbycusis. This phenomenon does not occur in purely conductive loss.

PRESBYOPIA   The power of accommodation (focusing for close work), is gradually lost, and at about the age of forty-five it is no longer possible to do close work comfortably.

Symptoms. The chief symptom of presbyopia is gradual increase in the distance from the eye at which close work can be seen clearly. There may be difficulty in seeing small print or seeing clearly in poor light.

Treatment. The condition is neutralized by convex lenses which must be made stronger as the condition progresses.

The lenses used to correct presbyopia cause blurring for distance, so that bifocals are frequently used for clear vision both near and far. If glasses must be worn at all times, bifocals are preferable to single-vision lenses. If a lens is required only for close work, a reading-glass may be preferred. Presbyopia occurs in all eyes, but the nearsighted individual may achieve clear near vision by removing his glasses. Selection of single-vision or bifocal lenses is a personal preference only; but usually, if it becomes evident that a glass is required at all times, it is best to adjust to bifocals as early as they are required.

PRIAPISM   Persistent erection of the penis, unrelieved by sexual intercourse or masturbation, is abnormal and is spoken of as priapism. It is a rare complication in patients with leukemia and blood disorders in which the blood collects in the large channels of the penis and is unable to return to the normal channels. Priapism may also occur in spinal-cord injuries.

PRICKLY HEAT (MILIARIA)   Prickly heat is a plugging of the openings of the sweat glands which results in the damming back and enlargement of the glands and the consequent formation of pus from resident bacteria. This condition has always been an important occupational disease in industries of high environmental humidity caused by geographic conditions (tropics, sub-sea level) or the nature of the industry (steam process or other heat mechanisms).

Symptoms. The lesions can appear singly or in groups evenly or irregularly distributed over the body, but chiefly on the face, neck, and upper chest. Each lesion consists of a tiny pustule surrounded by a flush of redness. In infants, the redness of adjacent lesions merges, especially in the folds of the neck, and forms a confluent mass of redness and moisture. This also happens in adults where moisture accumulates in folds of skin (under the breasts, in the groin).

Treatment. Care consists of drying each lesion by using simple agents, such as corn starch, talcum powder, or plain calamine lotion. If the pustular portion does not respond to the drying agents, local antibiotics (bacitracin, Neosporin®) will be required. Removal of the patient from the humid (for him) environment is essential. Also frequent sponging, the use of air-conditioning, dehumidifiers— and where the condition is endemic in an industry, changes in the industrial process —may be necessary for prevention.

PROCTITIS   Proctitis is an inflammatory disease of the rectum which may be due to various agents. Frequent enemas or cathartics, heavy pinworm-infestation, and chronic constipation may be causes. Irritating discharges from diseases higher up in the intestinal tract (such as ulcerative colitis and diverticulitis) can cause a secondary proctitis.

Symptoms. Symptoms vary, depending upon the cause. In general, diarrhea, occasionally blood and pus, rectal discomfort, and pain are the common manifestations. Chronic proctitis may occasionally lead to the development of inflammatory polyps which have a tendency to become malignant.

Treatment. The diagnosis depends on inspection of the area and treatment is directed towards the underlying cause.

PROGESTERONE This hormone is secreted by the corpus luteum (yellow body) of the ovary and is commonly known as the hormone of pregnancy. It is produced after ovulation—during the second half of the menstrual cycle. If conception occurs, this hormone is essential for the maintenance of pregnancy. Eventually the placenta also participates in the production of progesterone and of the other hormones necessary for the normal development of pregnancy. Progesterone deficiencies may be a cause of occasional or habitual abortions. This abnormality can be detected through special laboratory tests and the patient treated with progesterone, orally or through injections, to achieve full-term delivery. Progesterone is now available in tablet form and, combined with a small amount of astrogen, is being used, under various trade names, as a birth-control pill.

PROLAPSE Sometimes due to complications in childbirth, or because of other disorders, the uterus may become displaced and drop into the vagina. This situation is known as a prolapsed uterus.

Prolapse of the rectum is also relatively common, especially among the elderly. This condition occurs when the rectum falls through the anus. It may be brought about by the muscle strain of chronic constipation, parasitic infections, or hemorrhoids.

Women are six times more likely to suffer some form of prolapse than are men. Most cases of prolapse can be corrected either by the implantation of a supportive appliance (a pessary), or by reconstructive surgery. As soon as a prolapse is discovered, a physician should be consulted.

PROPHYLACTIC The term "prophylactic" generally refers to any device or method that is used to prevent disease. Thus, vaccines can be considered prophylactic measures. The term may also be used in a specific sense referring to a device or technique that prevents pregnancy. The condom, a sheath usually of rubber, which is worn over the penis during sexual intercourse, is an example of a prophylactic device in that it protects against the spread of venereal disease as well as being a device used to prevent pregnancy. The I. U. D. (intrauterine device), which is inserted into the womb, and the diaphragm, which is used with spermicidal gel and fitted into the vagina, are also examples of prophylactic devices in that they prevent pregnancy. (See also CONTRACEPTION.)

PROPHYLACTIC ODONOTOMY This term refers to those procedures, whether mechanical or chemical, which have as their objective the prevention of dental decay. This particularly applies in areas of the teeth which appear to be likely sites of decay and also in those teeth with developmental faults. These areas may be reshaped or restored by fillings.

PROPHYLAXIS (ORAL) Oral prophylaxis describes those measures aimed at the prevention of oral and dental diseases—especially the mechanical cleaning of the teeth by the dentist, utilizing scaling and polishing techniques.

PROTEINS Proteins are an essential constituent of all living things, from bacteria to man. Every cell contains some members of this large family of complex molecules. For growth; for maintenance and replacement of loss by "wear and tear"; for the creation of enzymes which initiate chemical reactions; and for hormones (such as insulin) which direct how, when, and where these reactions proceed, proteins are essential. About 17 per cent of an adult body is protein tissue, chiefly muscle tissue.

Chemically, proteins consist of hundreds or thousands of small units, (its "building blocks"), known as amino acids, all of which contain nitrogen as well as the usual elements, carbon, hydrogen, and oxygen.

Tissue proteins such as albumin cannot be formed unless all the essential amino acids are present in the diet and sufficient calories are supplied from fats and carbohydrates to provide the energy needs. If there is a deficiency in intake of either proteins or calories, the body tissues waste away. One ill effect of protein deficiency is that the formation of protective antibodies against infection is lessened and the malnourished patient may become more susceptible to infectious conditions.

Protein requirements vary in health and in disease; they also vary at different ages. They are proportionately highest in infancy, when the body is rapidly creating new cells and tissue (that is, during growth). Under certain circumstances such as pregnancy and breast-feeding, infections, burns, serious injuries, and hyperthyroidism, the protein requirements also rise.

The recommended daily average protein requirement is about 1 gram per kilogram (2.2 pounds) of body weight. Thus a man weighing about 150 pounds needs about 70 grams of protein a day.

The daily intake in our country varies from about 50 to 100 grams; occasionally wider variations are seen. However, these requirements apply to "good" protein—that is, protein high in essential amino acids. Animal sources, chiefly meat, fish, and poultry, supply these in well-balanced amounts. The protein of vegetables is less satisfactory.* (The precise needs for protein in terms of quality and amino-acid balance are still uncertain.)

Unlike fat, protein cannot be stored in appreciable quantities. Excess dietary amino acids are metabolized, and it is therefore not economical to feed the relatively expensive high-protein foods in very large quantities.

Because protein is so basic to the living processes, deficiency symptoms are widespread and varied. They include weight loss, stunted growth, fatigue, lack of energy, slow wound healing, and prolonged convalescence. The liver does not function normally. The serum albumin falls and edema develops. Infections are another common symptom. The resulting anemia is a reflection of inadequate formation of the critical blood protein, hemoglobin. In certain tropical areas a serious disorder of protein malnutrition, known as kwashiorkor, occurs in young children; there is wasting, liver damage, accumulation of fluids (edema), growth-failure, and changes in skin and hair. Unless vigorously treated, this may prove fatal.

A well-balanced diet will protect against protein deficiency. High-protein diets, often used in convalescence, consist of larger proportions of meats, fish, poul-

---

*Because starches, rice, roots, fruits, and vegetables form the basic diet in many Oriental and African regions, millions over the world today suffer from inadequate protein intake.

try, milk, cheese, and eggs. (Egg white is pure protein.) Products made of wheat, rice, and potatoes contain some protein, but not in large amounts. Because high-protein foods are also usually more expensive than foods rich in starches or fat, many people, even in this rich country, do not eat enough protein.

PRURITUS   See ITCHING

PSORIASIS   The cause of psoriasis is unknown. This noncontagious disease occurs in both sexes and usually first appears in adults but is occasionally present in very young children. Although the hereditary nature of the disease has not been established, there is a tendency for it to be more prevalent in certain families. Psoriasis is not associated with any other medical condition (except for the rare combination of arthritis and psoriasis known as psoriasis arthropathica). The accumulated information on the influences and mechanisms of what psoriasis is not related to is so extensive that it is often referred to as a disease of persons in good health—a view not shared by the afflicted.

Symptoms. The silvery-scaled red lesions range from pinhead to silver-dollar size and larger, and are most often present on the outer sides of the elbows and knees and on the scalp. The areas are sharply outlined and the skin is thickened and raised. When the body and other portions of the arms and legs are involved, it is usual for the lesions to begin small and very slightly raised. They then become enlarged, join with adjacent lesions, and become so thickened and leathery that the skin can "crack" and bleed on little provocation. The disease is accompanied by itching of varying degree. Aside from the tremendous inconvenience that an even limited form of the disease imposes, the patient suffers no concomitant disorders and there are usually no secondary complications unique to this disease.

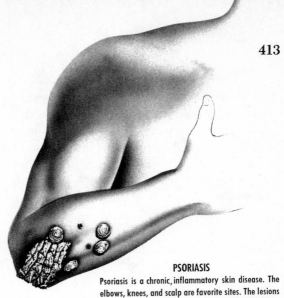

PSORIASIS
Psoriasis is a chronic, inflammatory skin disease. The elbows, knees, and scalp are favorite sites. The lesions are reddish, dry, rounded, or sharply defined patches covered with abundant scales.

One of the more distressing features of psoriasis is the presence of the disease in the nails. This can occur at any time in the course of the disease and is occasionally present in patients with no other evidence of this condition on the skin. Diagnosis is often made difficult, not only when the disease is not evident elsewhere on the skin, but also because lesions of the nails of the toes are often complicated by infection with fungi. Psoriatic nails are characterized by pinpoint depressions arranged in fairly symmetrical horizontal and longitudinal pattern throughout the nails, and greyish heaped-up scaling in small plaques under the nail at the side margins. Except for irradiation (X-ray, grenz ray), local remedies are not effective. Systemic treatment is that of the generalized disease.

The course of psoriasis is quite varied, as is the response to treatment. Its duration is from months to years to a lifetime, with periods of remission of the same order. Recurrences are more common in the winter, or in climates in which exposure to the sun is not possible. Recurrences have also been attributed to many generalized conditions including tension, changes in diet, infection, and pregnancy.

Treatment. In spite of the patient's quick discouragement—usually the result of well-intentioned lay opinion—control of the eruption is possible in most cases.

Types of management of the disease are numerous, though the response of the patient to a particular type of treatment is unpredictable. It is not unheard-of, for instance, for a previously much-treated patient suddenly, for no apparent reason, to respond to an old and simple remedy like mercury ointment. Conversely, even the most sophisticated and well-designed course of treatment may fail. Among the effective remedies are ultraviolet light, tars, combinations of ultraviolet light and tar application, vitamins given singly and in combination (A, B, D), local and systemically administered cortisone drugs, arsenic in the form of Fowler's Solution, irradiation (X-rays, grenz ray), nonspecific immunization (autohemotherapy, immune globulin), hospitalization or other environmental change, baths for the softening of the scales, antihistaminic drugs for control of the itching, supportive measures (sedatives, stimulants, tranquilizers), and finally the newer drugs which are toxic to cellular proteins (Methotrexate®).

What should be made eminently clear is that an energetic and diligent pursuit of relief from the symptoms can be rewarding. The fact that cure is not obtainable under current circumstances should not be a deterrent to the seeking of relief in this disease, any more than it is in such other diseases of unknown cause and long duration as stomach ulcer, with its need for continued therapeutic vigilance.

PSYCHIATRIST   The psychiatrist is a physician specializing in the diagnosis and treatment of mental disorders. Under present qualifications, the psychiatrist must have had four years of medical education leading to a medical degree; an internship in general medicine of at least a year; one year of training in neurology; and at least three years of specialized psychiatric internship and residency involving mental-hospital and out-patient experience with children and adults. Certification in psy-

chiatry by the American Board of Neurology and Psychiatry is achieved by passing examinations in all branches of the study of neurology and psychiatry.

PSYCHOANALYSIS; PSYCHOANALYST
Psychoanalysis involves specialized theory and methods of treatment developed for the study of the unconscious and conditions caused by unconscious conflict. The specific term, psychoanalysis, usually refers to orthodox Freudian methods as further developed by students adhering to Freudian theories. However, the situation is complicated by the fact that many former pupils of Freud split away from his theories to form their own schools, so that today there are many types of psychoanalysis, labeled with confusingly similar titles.

All psychoanalytic methods involve "depth-analysis" of unconscious levels of personality integration. Psychoanalysts seek to discover the hidden (latent) unconscious meanings of overt manifest symptoms—which are regarded as only symbolic of the underlying unconscious processes.

Four of the special methods devised by Freud for psychoanalytic study of mental processes are described in the following paragraphs.

Free association: The patient lies down on a comfortable couch and is instructed by the analyst simply to say anything which comes to the mind. This process of undirected free association results in progressively deeper uncovering of forgotten memories, unpleasant experiences; personal conflicts, and a general reporting of all the contents of consciousness. The analyst usually assumes a more or less passive role, simply stimulating the patient to talk about himself on deeper and deeper levels and only occasionally interpreting the unconscious significance of the associations produced by the patient.

Dream interpretation: Freud early recognized that the obvious contents of dreams are heavily loaded with latent symbolic significance, reflecting unconscious conflicts. Through the interpretation of unconscious significance in dream symbolism the patient becomes aware of some of the underlying conflicts of his life.

Transference mechanisms: As a natural part of the psychoanalytic process, the patient tends to bring out and transfer to the analyst many of the key problems and conflicts which he has had with others. In the more healthy and healing atmosphere of personal relationship with his analyst, the patient learns more appropriate patterns of reaction.

Analysis of psychological abnormality (psychopathology) in everyday life: During the course of psychoanalysis the patient gradually develops deep understanding of the unconscious significance of such activities as symptom-formation, humor, wit, errors, slips of the tongue, and other forms of psychopathology in everyday life.

Although Freud did not require his own students to be physicians and argued that medical training might actually be a handicap in becoming a competent psychoanalyst, modern psychoanalysis has largely become a medical specialty in the field of psychiatry. The theories and methods of psychoanalysis largely remain scientifically unproven; the psychoanalytic movement has, however, achieved wide acceptance and recognition as a necessary foundation for modern psychiatry.

There are those who consider psychiatric training incomplete until the psychiatrist has become adept in psychoanalytic methods by being analyzed himself. There is increasing evidence, however, that although psychoanalysis has made invaluable contributions to modern psychopathology, it does not provide the complete answer to all psychiatric problems and must eventually take its place among a wide variety of other methods, all of which have specific application.

PSYCHOBIOLOGY; PSYCHOBIOLOGIST   Psychobiology is a school of psychiatry which was led by the late American psychiatrist Adolph Meyer. In contrast to psychoanalysis, which is concerned primarily with the study of the unconscious, psychobiology teaches that each person should be regarded as a biological organism in which physical and mental functions are integrated as a unit. The psychobiological method is based on the recognition that every person is a biologic organism which must be studied by all possible biological and psychological methods, in order to obtain a comprehensive understanding of all levels of behavior. Meyer emphasized a broad-spectrum approach, simultaneous study of all levels of behavior integration by suitable biochemical, physiological, neurological, psychological, psychiatric, and biosocial methods.

PSYCHODRAMA   Psychodrama is a form of group therapy in which mental patients are encouraged to take part in amateur plays or dramas related to their own problems. Psychiatric experience indicates that patients often derive great benefit from acting out their problems with other people who have lived through similar experiences. Often the psychiatrist supervising psychodrama assigns themes to be acted out which are close to the patients' own problems, so that each patient learns to express himself more openly and arrive at new solutions to his problem(s).

PSYCHOGENIC   Psychogenic is an adjective applied to symptoms or clusters of symptoms (syndromes) of psychological origin, as distinct from those produced by physical causes. Psychogenic disorders are usually caused by unconscious conflicts and complexes of emotional origin. Thus, psychogenic vomiting refers to vomiting caused by underlying emotional conflicts or unconscious complexes, while psychogenic headaches are psychological symptoms of anxiety tension states.

PSYCHOLOGICAL EXAMINATION AND TESTING

The use of scientific psychological tests by scientifically trained clinical psychologists for the purpose of testing higher mental functions has become increasingly common. Psychological testing usually involves the following special examination methods: (1) life history studies, relating particularly to patterns and rates of development and maturation of the different processes and abilities; (2) direct behavior observations, in which objective ratings made on all types of personal social behavior, are often later compared with ratings made by the subject himself; (3) introspective reporting, in which the individual is encouraged to report in detail all the feelings, thoughts, and experiences of his life; (4) objective tests and measurements, by means of which standardized tests are used to measure intellectual abilities and personality factors; and (5) projective tests—the use of ambiguous (unstructured) test-stimuli, such as the Rorschach ink-blot test, to draw forth purely subjective responses which reflect the deep psychic organization of the person.

Psychological tests may be employed in many special situations, such as schools, hospitals, clinics, military service, courts, prisons, industry, and so forth. They are used to measure special abilities or disabilities which may have vital bearing on a person's functioning in the appropriate context. In all testing situations, psychological examinations should be administered by qualified psychologists with specialized scientific training.

PSYCHOLOGY; PSYCHOLOGIST

Psychology is the science of behavior. It is basic to psychiatry and concerned with the innate and acquired factors which or-

ganize the normal personality. Modern psychology stresses the use of special experimental and statistical methods for the objective study of sensation, perception, learning, memory, thinking, feelings and emotions, judgment, and higher mental processes.

Training as a psychologist consists of at least four years of graduate study in normal, experimental, developmental, abnormal, clinical, applied, physical (physiological), educational, and animal psychology; the course of study leading to the A.M. and Ph.D. degrees. After completing formal academic study of basic psychology, many psychologists seek further training in special applications of their field—clinical, educational, industrial, business, advertising, personality-counseling, and so forth. Competence is attested by certification of a psychologist by the American Board of Examiners in Professional Psychology after demonstration of suitable qualifications and satisfactory completion of required examinations. In contrast to the psychiatrist, whose training is basically medical, the psychologist's training is basically academic, and oriented within the specialized field of psychology.

PSYCHONEUROSIS

The term psychoneurosis is almost synonymous with neurosis. The only distinction involves a matter of degree, with the psychoneuroses including the more severe and incapacitating functional mental disorders involving only part functions of personality, and the neuroses referring to less serious functional disorders of everyday life.

PSYCHOSES

Psychiatric classification of mental disorders involves two major groups: (psycho)neuroses and psychoses. The psychoneuroses include minor reactions, usually involving only part of the personality. They are generally considered as functional disorders, not involving organic disease or lesions, and caused by un-

CLASSIFICATION OF FRACTURES

DIRECTION OF FRACTURE

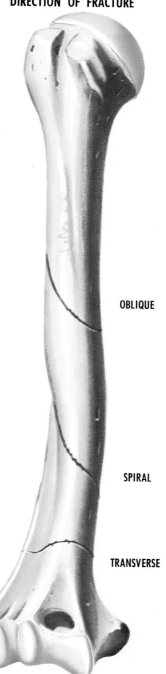

OBLIQUE

SPIRAL

TRANSVERSE

A fracture is classified according to direction, extent, and displacement, i.e., a simple, spiral complete fracture, etc.

EXTENT OF FRACTURE

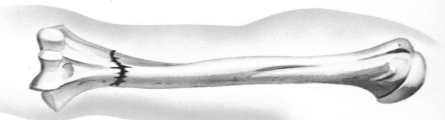

COMPLETE   Bone is broken entirely across.

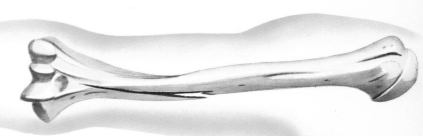

INCOMPLETE   (Linear or Greenstick)

A fracture which does not destroy the continuity of the bone.

EXTENT OF DISPLACEMENT

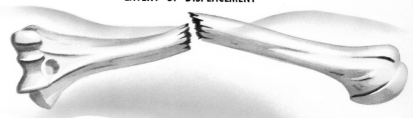

COMPOUND

Bone penetrates overlying structures, causing external wound. A simple fracture does not penetrate.

INJURIES PRODUCED BY A FALL

POSSIBLE INJURY SITES FOLLOWING A FALL

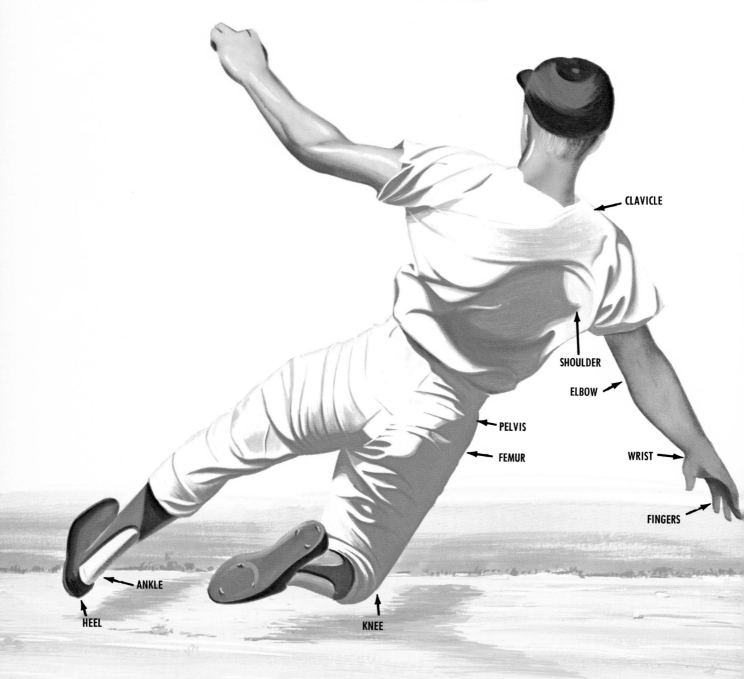

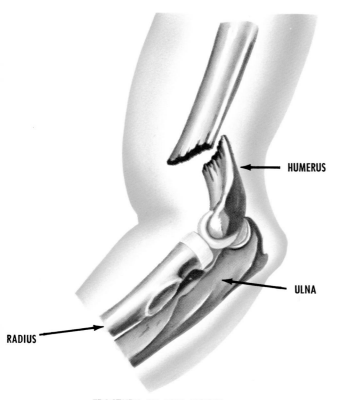

HUMERUS

ULNA

RADIUS

FRACTURE OF THE ELBOW

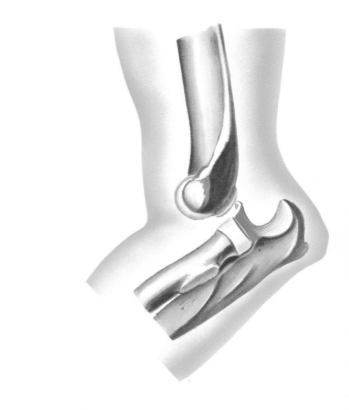

POSTERIOR DISLOCATION OF ELBOW

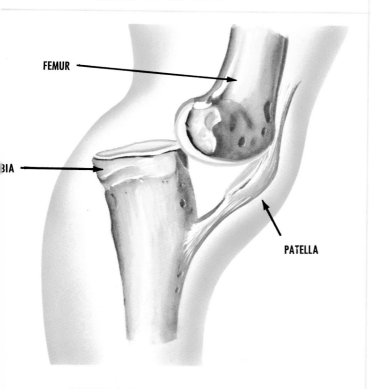

FEMUR

3IA

PATELLA

POSTERIOR DISLOCATION OF KNEE

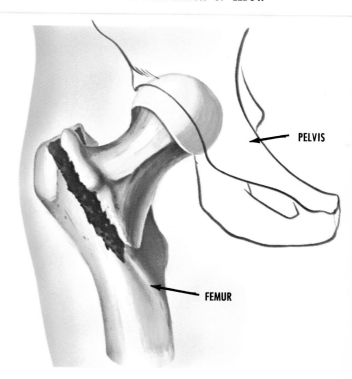

PELVIS

FEMUR

FRACTURE OF FEMUR

ACQUIRED TRAUMATIC DISEASES

Curvature of spine (scoliosis) lateral displacement of vertebrae commonly due to poliomyelitis.

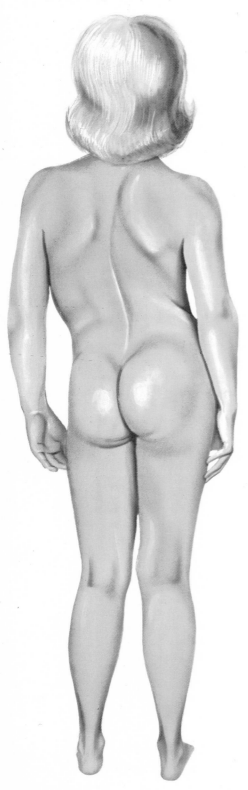

Traumatic torticollis is a scoliosis of the neck vertébrae due to an injury (blow on head). Congenital torticollis is due to an injury to the neck muscles. Both produce an outwardly similar deformity.

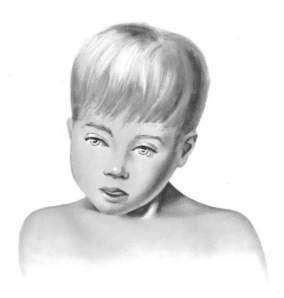

Ankylosis is the fusion of bones at a joint, due to an injury. Here the jaw and skull have fused, causing immobility.

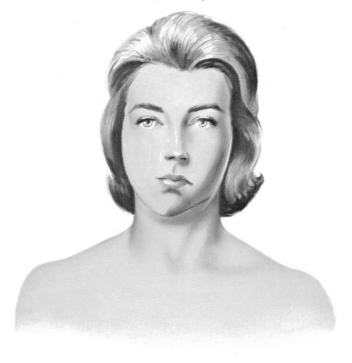

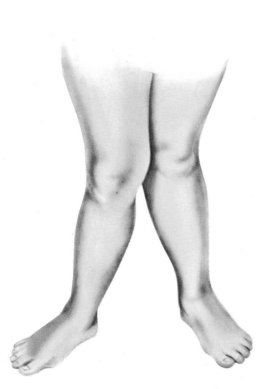

Knock-knees in which the leg bones angle outward is generally due to rickets.

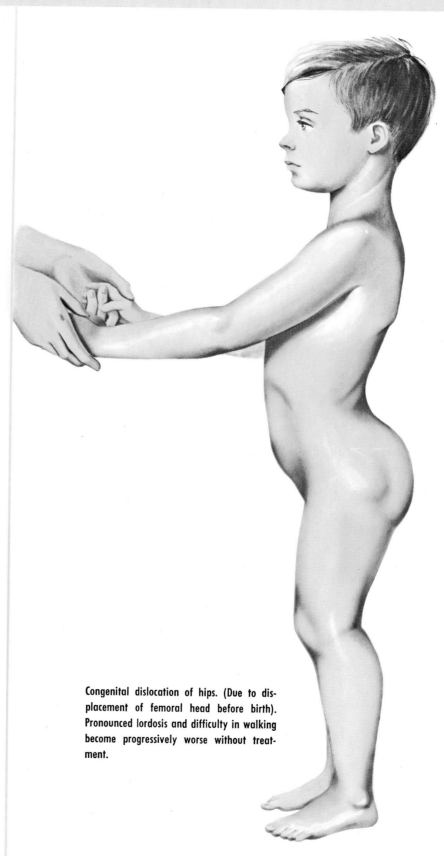

Congenital dislocation of hips. (Due to displacement of femoral head before birth). Pronounced lordosis and difficulty in walking become progressively worse without treatment.

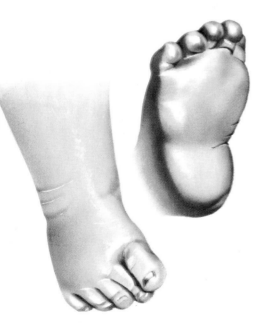

Clubfoot is any congenital turning of the bones of the foot. The foot may turn in, out, up, or down. The heel is also misplaced.

BIRTHMARKS AND WARTS

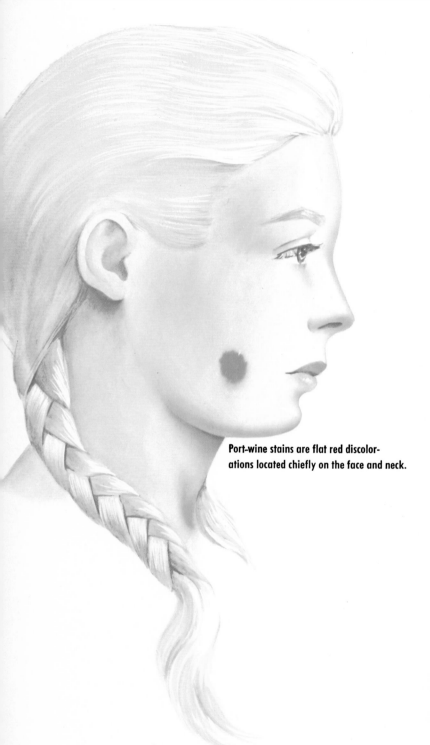

Moles can be flat, raised, rough or smooth, hairless or hairy. Their color varies from brown to black. Hairy moles are apt to be congenital.

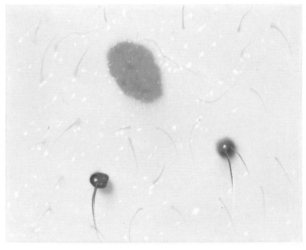

Port-wine stains are flat red discolorations located chiefly on the face and neck.

A wart is a virus-caused infection of the skin. Round, pea-sized, rough or smooth, yellow or brownish elevations occur singly or in groups, commonly on the hand.

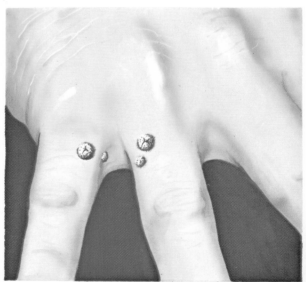

SKIN RASHES

Contact dermatitis is an inflammation due to contact with irritant material. Poison ivy is an example.

Lupus erythematosus is a chronic skin disease. Patches with raised red edges, and depressed scaly centers commonly are found on the face.

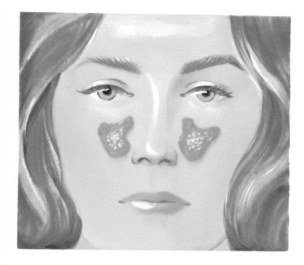

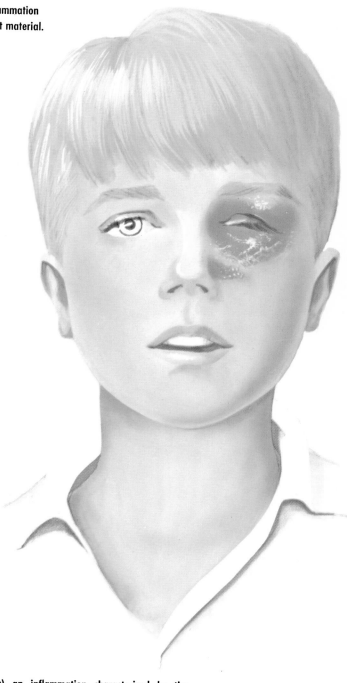

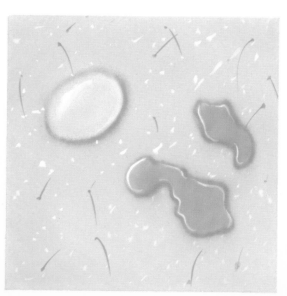

Urticaria (Hives) an inflammation characterized by the sudden appearance of pale, or reddish flat, smooth elevated patches or wheals. Severe itching and stinging is experienced. The wheals last minutes or hours, but disappear suddenly without a trace.

COMMON NASAL DEFORMITIES

Typical s-shaped nasal fracture causes a deviated septum, with resultant breathing difficulties.

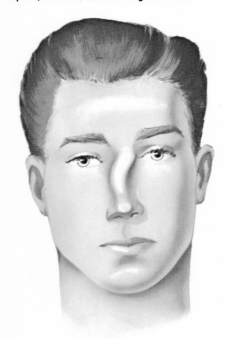

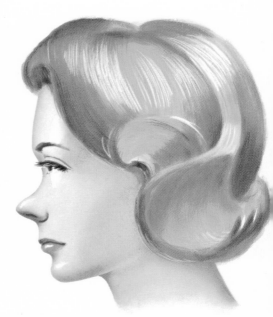

Typical saddle-nose is result of depressed fracture of nasal bones

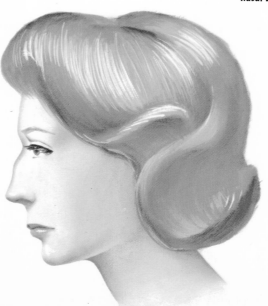

Typical nasal hump is produced by outward displaced fracture of nasal bones.

ILLUSTRATED BY LEONARD D. D.

resolved unconscious conflicts of emotional origin.

Symptoms. The psychoses, by contrast, involve deeper disintegration of the whole personality, to such an extent that mental functions are distorted in comparative entirety. The psychotic individual usually shows greater or lesser disintegration of normal personality functions and is recognized socially as not being responsible for what he does. Loss of control is a constant symptom.

Psychoses may be either organic or functional, depending on whether the causes lie in physical damage to the central nervous system or are determined by psychic conflicts. Any organic impairment of brain function due to circulatory disease, infections, brain tumor, metabolic disease, physical injury, or toxic conditions can result in more or less permanent disruption of mental functions. In the so-called "functional" psychoses—schizophrenia, paranoid states, manic-depressive psychoses, and the involutional psychoses—disruption of mental functioning by psychological conflicts is not ordinarily accompanied by demonstrable physical damage. The condition may be reversible, normal functioning usually returning once psychic conflicts have been resolved.

Treatment. The outlook in many psychotic conditions is much more hopeful than was previously believed. Although prognosis for organic psychoses is generally relatively poor, anything that can be done to prevent or control further extension of the organic process can result in some improvement. With the recent development of behavior-controlling drugs, many severely psychotic patients in this category can be kept sufficiently tranquilized to live in the community.

Functional psychoses, which are presumably caused by psychological conflict, are best treated by psychotherapy and some form of depth analysis. Even in the functional psychoses, however, tranquilizing or antidepressant drugs have proved to be of great value in calming the patient to the point where he is able to accept and benefit from psychotherapy.

PSYCHOSES IN PREGNANCY   Pregnancy involves many changes in metabolism, glandular balance, and physical status, and sometimes psychological conflicts, one or more of which may bring on psychotic reactions. These can occur at any stage of pregnancy, or during the period following it. It is generally agreed, however, that such psychotic reactions do not differ in kind from ordinary mental disorders, but rather involve standard reactions to periods of increased life stress.

To many a young woman with underlying personality weaknesses and immaturities, pregnancy comes as something unwanted, about which she may feel conflict and ambivalence. Frequently she may not really have wished to become pregnant, is not really ready for it, and develops hostility towards the husband as a consequence.

Symptoms. Psychoses of pregnancy may take the form of schizophrenic withdrawal from an intolerable situation, psychotic excitement expressing anger and hostility, or depressive reactions in which suicide is regarded as an escape. In psychosis following birth of the child (postpartum psychosis), aggressive impulses toward the baby, often of homicidal intensity, are very common; the young mother may be afraid to be with her child for fear that she will not be able to resist them. Also common are feelings of anger and resentment toward the husband, whom the young mother may not wish to see again. Neurasthenic states, in which the young mother does not feel she has the energy to return home and take care of the infant and her family, are also frequently met with.

Treatment. Treatment for psychoses of pregnancy is the same as for similar

418

disorders occurring in other periods. Experience indicates that many psychoses of pregnancy are self-limited, disappearing spontaneously within a few weeks or months. It is very important that the young mother be protected from her own hostile impulses until she feels completely able to handle herself. Psychiatric treatment should be directed towards discovery and removal of underlying emotional conflicts so that the psychosis does not recur during succeeding pregnancies.

PSYCHOSOMATIC   Psychosomatic refers to the functional unity of physical and psychological components of the human organism. It is recognized that somatic conditions may determine psychological states and, conversely, psychological states may influence somatic conditions. Psychosomatic symptoms involve physical disorders reactive to psychological states. For example, gastric ulcers may be caused by chronic psychic tension states. Hypertension may develop in reaction to chronic anger and irritability. In other words, mind and body are inseparable; what affects one also influences the other. Mental contents influence the condition of the body, and the condition of the body influences the state of the mind.

PSYCHOSURGERY   Psychosurgery involves the use of brain surgery for the treatment of various mental disorders.

Historical studies indicate that brain operations were used in ancient Egypt for the relief of symptoms caused by tumor and physical injuries to the brain. Furthermore, skulls recovered from prehistoric times indicate that early man understood the relation between disorders of the brain and mental illness, attempting to treat mental disorders by opening the skull.

Modern neurology has developed much of its knowledge of the location of brain functions by the study of localized injuries to the brain, and by experiment-

ing with surgical operations on various parts of the brain. Within modern times, study of rare injuries and damage to the brain has resulted in the discovery that normal functioning can apparently be recovered after extensive injury; and that even mental disorders can in some cases be symptomatically "cured" by operations which destroy an entire lobe of the brain. Thus, certain types of chronic schizophrenics show mental improvement after lobotomy, a surgical severing of the nerve fibers serving an entire lobe of the brain—a procedure largely equivalent to lobe-destruction.

A large number of experimental operations have been performed severing connections to the frontal lobes, and beneficial results have been obtained in some cases. Psychosurgery is still, however, in an experimental stage of development. It is recommended only in chronic cases where all other methods of psychotherapy have failed, since all forms of psychosurgery are highly dangerous and associated with the risk of worsening symptoms and producing permanent loss of mental function.

PSYCHOTHERAPY   Special psychological methods for treating mental conditions by purely psychological techniques as contrasted with physical or chemical treatment. It is now generally accepted that functional psychological disorders respond only to distinctive psychological methods of treatment. Since most personality problems and psychoneurotic disorders are caused by disorders of learning or conditioning, and involve habits, ideational complexes, and emotional conflicts which exist on purely psychological levels, they can be treated only by psychotherapy.

All forms of psychotherapy ultimately depend on retraining methods whereby the patient learns how to solve life's problems in healthier ways. All psychotherapy involves: (1) some type of diagnostic process to discover the psychological causes of disorder; (2) suitable conditions of rapport and understanding so that relearning can take place; and (3) the use of suitable retraining methods by means of which the patient learns to cope more efficiently with his problems.

Among the more important established methods of psychotherapy are: psychoanalysis, involving the "depth" study of unconscious complexes; personality counseling, involving specialized psychological tutoring in problem areas to help the client actualize himself in all areas of life; marriage counseling utilizing special methods for dealing with situational problems in marriage; vocational guidance, helping the client to discover what kinds of work he is suited for, and adjusting to work situations; group therapy where groups of patients with similar conditions meet with a psychiatrist to discuss mutual problems; psychodrama involves the use of plays and dramatic productions where mental patients can act out their problems; play therapy, usually with children, provides an opportunity to act out deep emotional problems; and behavioral and emotional retraining are used to recondition behavior patterns in persons with conduct or personality disorders.

PUBERTY   Puberty is that stage of growth and development when the generative organs achieve the capability of functioning reproductively. In the boy, this is accompanied by the discharge of semen (physiologically observed usually by nocturnal emission—the so-called "wet dream"), deepening of the voice, and development of pubic and facial hair.

In the girl, it is marked by the menarche (onset of menstruation), development of the breasts, and an interest in feminine attractiveness (dress, hair-care, cosmetics, etc.).

In psychiatry, puberty is the physiological milestone on the road of psycho-sexual development heralding the advent of heterosexuality.

PUERPERIUM (POSTPARTUM PERIOD)   This is the interval between delivery and the reversal of all the changes caused by pregnancy to normal levels. The process takes approximately six weeks, and the interval has been traditionally set for the reevaluation of the mother and the detection of any persisting changes or abnormalities connected with her recent pregnancy and delivery. Resumption of normal menstrual periods usually takes place seven to eight weeks after birth, unless the mother is breast-feeding the baby, in which case several months may elapse before menstruation begins again.

PULMONARY ARTERY   The pulmonary artery conducts the blood from the right ventricle to the lungs. It is separated from the right ventricle by a valve that prevents ejected blood from returning to the ventricular pumping-chamber. A short distance from the heart, the pulmonary artery divides into a right branch that supplies the artery branches in the right lung and a left branch that serves the arteries in the left lung.

Blood pressure in the pulmonary artery is much lower than in the arterial system of the rest of the body. Unless pulmonary-artery disease is present, there is great adaptability to large changes in blood-flow during exercise, with little increase needed in pulmonary artery pressure to insure prompt passage of blood through the capillaries of the lung.

PULMONARY EMBOLISM   If a blood clot (thrombus) is present in the veins of the legs or pelvis, it can break away and migrate in the blood to the right auricle, pass through the right ventricle and pulmonary artery, and then come to rest in a major vessel of the lung, where the diminishing diameter of the vessel finally traps it and prevents further travel.

If a medium-sized vessel is blocked, there is usually sudden pain in the chest over the area of lung involvement, some spitting of blood, and variable signs and symptoms that accompany tissue destruction—for inevitably there will be some death of tissue in the lung that is being denied proper circulation by the thrombus. An X-ray of the chest usually shows the involved area as a wedge of airless lung rather clearly demarcated from unaffected pulmonary tissue.

If very small fragments of clot pass into the lungs at repeated intervals, a somewhat different disease of pulmonary vessels can occur. In this case a progressive pulmonary hypertension appears. When a number of arteries become blocked in the lungs, high pulmonary-artery pressure will be needed to move along the same quantity of blood per beat; because fewer blood channels are available, extra force is needed to push blood through the remaining few pathways.

Occasionally, a very large clot breaks away from a pelvic or leg vein, passes into one of the main pulmonary arteries, and blocks it. When at least two-thirds of all pulmonary blood-flow is blocked, death can occur in a few minutes.

PULMONARY INFARCTION See PULMONARY EMBOLISM

PULMONARY HEART DISEASE
Strictly speaking, pulmonary heart disease (often termed chronic cor pulmonale) is that form of enlargement of the right side of the heart that develops as a result of diseases of the lung, rib-cage, pulmonary blood vessels, or from primary pulmonary hypertension. Cor pulmonale may also follow mitral stenosis and some types of congenital heart disease.

Development of heart disease following lung involvement depends mainly upon the degree and duration of the resistance to the usual free flow of blood through the lungs at relatively low pressures. Increased resistance to flow through the lung (pulmonary circulation) is usually referred to as pulmonary vascular disease, or pulmonary hypertension.

Cor pulmonale caused by pulmonary vascular disease is seen in such lung diseases as obstructive emphysema and any other structural derangement in lung anatomy that mechanically obstructs the pulmonary blood vessels in such ways that pressure must necessarily rise to force blood through those narrowed vessels. Obstructive emphysema is now recognized as a most common and important cause of cor pulmonale.

Sometimes industrial dusts and chronic infection can affect the lungs and cause cor pulmonale, especially when the disease involves both lungs and produces structural narrowings in the vessel system. Occasionally, multiple blood clots that come into the lungs over a period of weeks and months from a diseased heart or even from distant veins can gradually block the free flow of blood through the lungs. Pulmonary heart disease will then follow.

PUPIL, ABNORMALITIES OF The central black opening in the colored iris is the pupil. It controls the amount of light entering the eye by becoming small in bright illumination and large in dim. Usually the pupils are large in youth and become smaller with the passing years. They are small in sleep, following medicines used in glaucoma treatment, following the use of morphine, and when bound to the iris after iritis. The pupils markedly enlarge in death, in dim light, when the eye is blind, and following medicines used in the treatment of certain eye inflammations. Most medical attention is directed to whether the pupils constrict with light directed into the eye and dilate when it is discontinued. Failure of the pupils to react may occur with many serious diseases of the eye and the nervous system, and is a signal for careful study.

PUS The formation of pus is known as suppuration. Pus is the waste product of inflammation which includes fluid, dead white blood cells, fibrin, which is the threadlike, insoluble protein formed by the interaction of thrombin (a clotting element of the blood), and fibrinogen, which is a protein derivative found in the watery part of the blood (the plasma or serum).

PYELITIS The term pyelitis applies to the presence of an infection (pus) in the kidneys. The disease is almost exclusively seen in females (see CYSTITIS).

Symptoms. Pyelitis often begins suddenly with a chill followed in an hour or so by a high fever. It may or may not be accompanied by backache (just below the floating rib), or frequent and/or burning urination. Usually the child is prostrated and has a headache. A urinalysis will reveal pus.

Treatment. Because these patients are nauseated and often vomit, they often need antibiotic injections for the first day or so of treatment (which treatment is much the same as that given for cystitis). Patients with pyelitis should have thorough urological examination when the condition has subsided.

PYLORIC STENOSIS Between the stomach and the duodenum (the first part of the small intestine) there is a slightly narrowed segment called the pylorus. In its wall are a large number of muscle fibers which run in circular (sphincter) fashion around this area. (It is assumed that the chief function of the pylorus is to keep food in the stomach until its digestive activity is complete.) A few newborn babies develop an enlargement of these muscle fibers, so that the passage-

way from the stomach is narrowed (becomes stenotic) to such an extent that little or no milk or food will move into the duodenum.

Symptoms. The condition occurs almost exclusively in first-born males in the first six weeks of life. Sometime in the first two or three weeks the infant begins spitting up; this is assumed to be a feeding problem and the child may go through several milk-changes, always with the same result. The spitting becomes vomiting and the vomiting material may be shot out two to four feet. Stools become hard and infrequent and the urine scanty. The child loses weight and may become severely dehydrated. If proper care is not given early he may die. The diagnosis is made on the basis of these symptoms and confirmed by the doctor, who can feel the swollen muscle and also observes the abdominal waves moving across the upper abdomen. Spasm of the pylorus (pylorospasm) due to irritation or emotional stresses can similarly cause symptoms of bloating, belching, and mild pain. Simple medications are usually effective for relief.

Treatment. After fluids have been restored by injections and the baby is in better general physical condition, the surgeon treats pyloric stenosis by making an amazingly small incision to find the tumor; he then partially cuts the fibers. Within just a few hours the baby is eating normally. There seem to be no residual effects. Recurrences of pyloric stenosis are practically unknown.

"QUICKENING" In pregnant women quickening means the perception of fetal movements. This "feeling of life" appears in the form of intermittent, fluttering movements in the lower abdomen near the fourth month of pregnancy—occasionally as early as two and one-half to three months. Many patients describe it as "butterflies in the stomach." This is by no means a definite sign of pregnancy, since it has been known to be experienced by women who were never pregnant (false pregnancy).

RABIES (HYDROPHOBIA)   This virus-caused condition may be one of the most widespread sources of potential infection known, although public attention is focused on it only during sporadic outbreaks of alarm when one or more cases are reported in a community. Although the so-called "mad" dog is popularly believed to be the carrier, plentiful evidence would seem to show that many wild animals, such as foxes, wolves, skunks, and bears, also harbor the virus. Indeed, one of the most important carriers (vectors) has been shown to be the bat; infection from bat excrement and/or urine ejected during the creature's flight may be a possibility, and occasional instances of attack by a "mad" bat have also been reported.

Rabies is produced by a virus with a specific affinity for tissue of the nervous system. The virus migrates from the entry-point (scratch or bite-mark) along the peripheral (outlying) nerves until it reaches the spinal cord and the brain. Within the brain it multiplies, and some of the "descendant particles" migrate to the salivary glands. It is this migration which makes the bite of an infected animal so potentially dangerous.

Symptoms.   In human beings, rabies has a flexible incubation period ranging from about ten days to as much as two years; the average is perhaps a trifle less than two months. Since the appearance of symptoms depends on the length of time it takes the virus to move from the site of entry to the brain, the closer the wound is to the head, the shorter the incubation period.

In man, rabies is generally marked by symptoms of moodiness, restlessness, a feeling of unease, and fever; this phase, however, lasts only a short while. As time goes on, the restlessness changes to frenzy and excitement which cannot be controlled. There is increased output of saliva, together with muscular spasms of the throat. These spasms are unbelievably painful, and since they are the result of the virus's infection of brain centers controlling breathing and swallowing, they can easily be triggered by such simple actions as attempting to swallow water. This phenomenon is what has given the disease its name, hydrophobia (Greek for water-fear) although a term meaning water-hatred might be more descriptive.

Since the patient discovers that drinking can be painful, dehydration is a factor often encountered: he simply refuses to drink liquids. There is, in addition, a progressive weakening which stems from increased difficulty in breathing, paralysis, and general exhaustion. Once overt symptoms appear, death usually occurs within a week.

Treatment.   Aside from making the patient as comfortable as possible, there is no effective curative treatment of rabies once symptoms have made their appearance. Therefore, if there is any evidence that the attacking animal may be rabid, thoroughgoing treatment must be started immediately—that is, before symptoms have a chance to develop. If at all possible, the animal should be caught and kept a week for observation, in order to learn whether or not it is rabid; if there is the slightest doubt, and/or if the animal is not available, a program of injection of rabies vaccine should be instituted immediately. (An initial dose of "antiserum" may be given before the vaccine, to "buy time" while the animal is being observed.)

The schedule of vaccine injections lasts for fourteen days, followed by a "booster" shot three weeks following the last regular injection of the vaccine itself. Although the treatment can be a trying one, it is effective—and if not used, death is inevitable.

Since, as was already mentioned, little can be done for the patient who has developed frank rabies, complete with symptoms, except to make him comfortable, the care indicated is that which would be given to any sufferer from convulsive disorders.

RADIAL NERVE   The radial nerve supplies muscles in the arm and hand. Extension of the elbow, wrist, and fingers is carried out by muscles supplied by this nerve.

RAGWEED POLLEN   Members of the ragweed family (short ragweed, giant ragweed, Western ragweed, Southern ragweed, cocklebur, rough marsh elder, and tall povertyweed) pollinate from summer until frost.

Persons allergic to ragweed pollen develop what is commonly called hay fever by inhaling the pollen.

The symptoms of hay fever or pollinosis (the more correct term) consist of itchy, red, tearful eyes with an itchy, burning nose. There occur multiple attacks of severe sneezing.

RATIONALIZATION   Rationalization is a form of mental defense mechanism (originally described by Freud) in which a person seeks to excuse or defend his conduct by providing plausible, seemingly rational explanations. One may blame errors on others, depict one's self as the victim of circumstance, and attempt to invent reasons for explaining bad conduct.

Psychologists believe that the best defense is no defense at all, but rather a frank admission of error and the taking of steps to prevent its repetition in the future. The person who rationalizes is unconsciously seeking to avoid blame or responsibility for his own conduct; however, the only result is continuance or intensification of the original difficulty.

RECOMMENDED DAILY ALLOWANCES   In 1941 the Food and Nutrition Board of the National Research Council established a guide for nutritional recommendations. These have been called Recommended Dietary Allowances, and have been revised periodically since that time. It is important to note that the specific recommendations are designed for the maintenance of good nutrition of practically all healthy persons in the United States; but because of individual variations and requirements, these figures do not cover every person. Furthermore, it is not true, as is sometimes stated, that amounts below the RDA are inadequate.

The recommended allowances can be attained with a variety of common foods. Other nutrients, vitamins, and minerals for which human requirements are uncertain at this time are not included. When used as suggested (see table, page [621], the recommended dietary allowances offer the best available estimate of dietary recommendations for the average healthy American. His needs in illness or under unusual circumstances may be different.

RECTUM   The rectum is the final portion of the large intestine, which leads to the anus. Its function is primarily the storage of feces until evacuation is convenient. As the rectum becomes distended with feces, the urge to move the bowels is created. Disregarding this urge repeatedly may lead to chronic constipation. Bleeding from the rectum may be the first sign of rectal cancer and demands investigation. It can be a dangerous mistake to ignore such a sign by assuming the source of the blood to be piles or hemorrhoids. Fissures and abscesses in the rectal area can be the source of much discomfort, as can internal and external hemorrhoids. Irritability and irritation of the rectal area in children should raise the possibility of pinworm infestation. The diagnosis is sim-

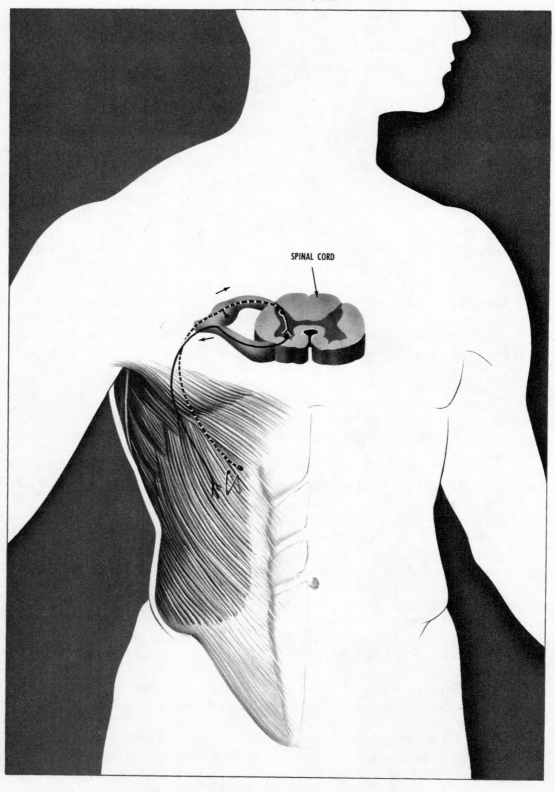

SPINAL CORD

ple and the treatment, while occasionally tedious, is effective and well worth the trouble.

RECTUS MUSCLE　　This is a long, flat muscle which arises from the pubic bone and is inserted into the cartilage of the lower ribs. It affords protection and aids in bending the trunk. The rectus muscle is divided in its mid-portion by fibrous tissue. After repeated pregnancies, this tissue occasionally separates allowing the abdominal contents to protrude, and thus causing a ventral (belly) hernia. A binder may help keep the abdominal contents in place, but surgical repair is often required.

REFLEX ARC　　A reflex arc consists of the transmission of impulses across two or more neurons. The simplest type of reflex arc occurs in the spinal cord and involves only one synapse. A sensory impulse is transmitted along a sensory fiber to the cord; this impulse then crosses a synapse to a motor neuron, whose axon stimulates a muscle fiber. By such simple reflex arcs, the spinal cord carries out certain functions, such as some aspects of the maintenance of posture.

Most reflex arcs involve three or more neurons. Some involve many chains of neurons within the cord and brain.

A reflex arc can be demonstrated by the response to a sharp scratch of the skin on one side of the abdomen. Impulses are thereby sent to the cord, where they pass through several intermediate neurons to the motor cells controlling the muscles of the same side of the abdomen. The axons of these cells stimulate the abdominal muscle, and a visible brief contraction occurs. This skin reflex is called the abdominal reflex.

If the tendon below the kneecap is tapped with a rubber hammer, the reflex response is that of transient extension at the knee. This tendon reflex is called the knee-jerk.

REGRESSION　　A mental mechanism by which people retreat (regress) to more primitive stages of development on encountering frustration or failure in their attempts to adjust at higher levels of development. Thus a child experiencing severe emotional conflicts may show regression to infantile behavior such as bed-wetting, baby talk, increased demand for protective care from the mother, and thumb-sucking. Masturbation or homosexual interests, after one has supposedly reached adult heterosexual levels of adjustment, may be regarded as regressive behavior in reaction to failures to adjust normally to the opposite sex. Since it is a constant struggle to maintain adult levels of adjustment, many types of regressive behavior are commonly seen in everyday life.

REHABILITATION　　One of the most important public health and educational problems is rehabilitation of those suffering from physical or mental disorders so that they may resume working and supporting themselves. It is now recognized that most handicapped people have both physical and psychological problems and require psychiatric as well as physical rehabilitation.

Among the more important methods of rehabilitation are retraining of the blind; provision of hearing aids and of artificial limbs; muscular retraining for the physically crippled; special job situations for those with physical handicaps; and psychotherapy for those among them who are too emotionally disturbed to be able to work. Perhaps most important in rehabilitation is improvement of self-confidence and morale to such an extent that one wishes to become self-supporting and independent again.

REPRESSION　　A mental mechanism described by Freud to explain the dynamics of unconscious mental conflict. According to Freudian theory, every child develops a conscience (superego) by internalizing moral codes imposed by society. The superego then operates by excluding (repressing) socially forbidden impulses from consciousness. To Freudians, the unconscious consists of unacceptable impulses, strivings, and painful memories which have been repressed from conscious expression and which can gain outlet only in disguised form, such as symptom formation, dreams, errors, or other types of everyday psychopathology. Repression mechanisms play an important role in the causation of functional mental disorders, where unconscious conflicts and complexes can be discovered and treated only by psychoanalytic or related methods.

RESPIRATION (BREATHING) Although the function of breathing is performed by the integrated mechanisms of the whole respiratory system, respiration itself is accomplished only at the level of the lung, by exchanging oxygen and carbon dioxide between the inhaled air and the blood circulating through the lung. To obtain a total picture of the respiratory process, however, it is pertinent to review briefly the characteristics of the participating organs that accomplish the entire function of breathing.

The respiratory system can be pictured in simple terms as a series of tubes of progressively decreasing width (the airways): the nose, mouth, throat, voice box (larynx), windpipe (trachea), and the bronchi. The bronchi themselves subdivide into smaller and smaller tubes running throughout the lung until they reach the basic respiratory units, the alveoli.

Alveoli can be pictured as small, lobed sacs, microscopic in size, of which there are billions in each lung. Amazingly, if one could continuously "stretch out" all the alveoli in the human lungs, they would cover a surface roughly the size of a tennis court. Paralleling this branching structure, there exists a similar network of subdivisions for the blood vessels, which run throughout the lungs in proximity to the air tubes. Ultimately, tiny blood vessels called capillaries reach the air in the alveoli and it is here that gases are exchanged. Thus, joining together, alveoli and blood capillaries become the actual cross-point of respiration. Here the freshly inhaled air gives off oxygen to the blood and receives in exchange carbon dioxide, which is then expelled while breathing out (expiration). (Incidentally, this expired air passes back through the larynx and makes it vibrate, generating sounds or voice.)

Attention should next be turned to the motor forces involved in the process of breathing. Respiratory centers located in the central nervous system (brain) send orders through the nerves to both the respiratory muscles located in the chest wall between the ribs (intercostal muscles) and the muscular "tent" separating the inside of the chest from the abdomen (diaphragm). The contraction of these muscles forces the lung to "open up" in all directions. This in turn creates a suction force within the lung which produces an inrush of outside air (inspiration). Being elastic in nature, the lung when it fills up behaves like a rubber balloon under tension and will deflate by itself (expiration) as soon as the filling has ceased. Inspiration is therefore normally an active process which requires energy, while expiration is passive. The pump for the circulation of blood through the lung is of course the heart. Venous ("used," dark) blood, which returns to the heart from all over the body, is pumped by the heart to the lung through the pulmonary artery. This blood is "revitalized" (oxygenated) in the capillaries of the alveoli by inspired fresh air, and is returned to the heart by the pulmonary veins as "fresh," bright-red blood, and is thence pumped out to the entire body. There the process is reversed: the body tissues extract the oxygen from the blood and load it with carbon dioxide.

Although the true process of respiration (gas exchange) takes place only within the lung in the lower respiratory tract (at the alveoli-level), the upper airways do perform some specific work in addition to letting air pass through. The upper respiratory tract has a rich network of blood vessels which readily give off heat and bring the temperature and humidity of inspired air instantaneously to optimal levels. In addition, the airways possess numerous glands which constantly produce mucus that acts as a lubricant fluid. On the inner surface of the airways there are also numerous hair-like formations called cilia. These beat constantly, thus keeping the mucus in motion and eventually expelling it. (Another function of the cilia is to act as a trap for some of the dust particles contaminating the air.)

One can see that breathing involves many structures which strike a beautifully designed balance to satisfy changing body needs. Still, breathing is largely an involuntary function performed without our awareness, although we may change it at will. Normally an adult will breathe at a rate of about twelve to eighteen times per minute, each inhalation consisting of about 500 cubic milliliters (30 cubic inches) of air. However, like the pulse rate, this often varies.

Excessive breathing (hyperventilation) can be as deleterious as insufficient breathing (hypoventilation). When breathing becomes noticeable and creates discomfort, under otherwise normal conditions of body activity, one speaks of dyspnea or "shortness of breath." Numerous tests have been devised to measure the adequacy of the lung performance, and standards of normality have also been established.

RESPIRATORY TRACT INFECTION
Because of its easy accessibility to external

offenders, the respiratory system is the most common site of infection in the body. Thus, all sorts of viruses, bacteria, and parasites present in the environment or carried by other individuals can easily gain access to any level of the respiratory system in the inhaled air. Many of these agents are normal inhabitants of the upper respiratory tract, where they live in harmony with the body until some disturbing condition creates a favorable climate for their multiplication and attack upon the host.

The lung can also be infected from within; infections in any part of the body may gain access to the circulation and thence be carried to, and eventually lodged in, the lung.

The potential harm of any infectious agent varies with the condition of each individual and the characteristics of the body-system under stress. The respiratory tract has certain anatomical characteristics designed to provide natural mechanical defenses against the entrance and deposit of foreign materials: a temperature-control system provided by a rich network of blood vessels which almost instantaneously equalizes the temperature and humidity of the inhaled air with that of the body; hair-like structures, called cilia, which beat constantly to keep the constantly-produced lubricant fluid (mucus) in movement. This system works as a conveyor belt and prevents the deposit of larger particles at the upper levels of the respiratory tract. In addition, the cilia act as a trap for these particles; and a mechanical "wash-out" provided by the rhythmic exhalation of air.

It therefore becomes obvious that most of the infections attacking the respiratory system will be dealt with primarily by the "first lines of defense" in the upper respiratory tract; namely the nose, throat, larynx, and trachea. This also explains why the development of symptoms usually follows a descending anatomical course.

Much less frequent, but of far greater seriousness, are the infections which localize in the lower respiratory tract: the bronchi and lung tissues. To the extent that the respiratory system suffers anatomical or functional damage to its natural defenses, it becomes exceedingly vulnerable to infectious agents—and particularly to the serious consequences of bronchitis and pneumonia.

Any infectious agent can produce respiratory disease; in practice, however, viruses and bacteria are by far the most common offenders. Although either can attack any part of the respiratory system, some broad distinctions can be made: The viruses are responsible for the largest number of upper respiratory tract infections, which are usually self-limiting in nature, free of complications, and for which no specific treatment is either generally available or mandatory. Studies in the United States Army classified the upper-respiratory viral diseases in two main clinical groups: Acute Undifferentiated Respiratory Disease; and Non-Streptococcal Exudative Pharyngitis. A particular group of viruses, (adenovirus) seems to be the prevalent agent in these conditions. In addition, one should also consider the group of viruses responsible for the disease called influenza.

Bacteria which produce respiratory infections originate more distinctive types of disease, and the agent can easily be identified in the nose and throat, or by examination of the sputum. Bacteria are responsible for such potentially serious diseases of the upper and lower respiratory tract as diphtheria, streptococcal sore throat, pneumonia, and bronchopneumonia. The bacterial diseases are more prone to serious complications, nor are they self-limited; they can, however, be effectively treated by presently available specific means. The most common bacteria responsible for respiratory infections are the pneumococcus, hemophilus influenzae, and streptococcus. A respiratory disease of viral origin may be complicated secondarily by a bacterial invader, but the reverse is rare. Furthermore, any initial bacterial agent may be eventually superceded in the course of the same disease by a different bacterium. Viral respiratory diseases are usually diagnosed on clinical grounds alone, because their precise recognition and identification require highly specialized laboratory techniques. Fortunately, despite the large number of viruses hitherto identified as capable of producing respiratory infection (more than one hundred different types and strains), they all tend to exhibit similar clinical characteristics. They are world wide in distribution and appear in epidemic outbreaks involving in a short period of time many individuals in the family, at school, or at work, without regard for age or sex.

Symptoms. The most common viral symptoms are itchy and watery secretions from the nose, throat, or eyes, accompanied by pains or discomfort in the neck glands, headaches, and malaise. Fever, if present, may be high but usually lasts no more than forty-eight hours. Often these symptoms are followed by hoarseness and cough—at first dry, and later productive of sputum.

Treatment. In most cases the only treatment required for virus infections is abundant fluid ingestion, mild analgesics (such as aspirin), and simple nasal decongestants. If the symptoms are severe or the patient is debilitated, bed rest is advisable. Widely advertised "miracle drugs" have not been proved to be superior to the regimen mentioned here. Prevention of these diseases is primarily a matter of avoidance of the human source of infection. Vaccines are at present of very limited use because of the large number of viruses involved, each requiring a specific different vaccine.

The bacterial respiratory diseases primarily affect the lower respiratory tract—

with the important exceptions of the streptococcal sore throat and diphtheria. In the bronchi and lung the bacteria may produce bronchitis, bronchopneumonia, pneumonia, tuberculosis, lung abscess, and pleurisy (see the respective entries). These are serious conditions which may last from several days to weeks and longer, and are prone to complications. Most of them are characterized by fever, prostration, and productive cough. Frequently they produce respiratory difficulty leading to shortness of breath (dyspnea) and dusky lips and nails (cyanosis). The bacteria are usually easily recognized by microscopic examination of the secretions, and specific antibiotic treatment is highly effective.

RESTORATION   This is a general term in dentistry which usually refers to a filling or a bridge.

RETINA   The inner layer of the eye, the retina, is a complicated and highly organized nerve network which converts light impulses to nerve impulses by means of a chemical reaction not yet entirely understood. There are two main layers in the retina: an outer pigment layer which supports nutrition of the cells receiving light impulses; and an inner nerve layer. The nerve layer contains cells—the rods and cones—which undergo changes in chemistry in response to light impulses, giving rise to a nerve impulse. Each such impulse is magnified in the retina and conducted to the brain through nerve fibers which combine to form the optic nerve. In addition to these cells, the retina contains a supporting skeleton and a number of nerve cells the function of which is not yet known.

RETINA, BLOOD VESSEL CHANGES IN   The blood vessels which nourish the retina may be seen by means of an ophthalmoscope. Changes occurring in hardening of the arteries, diabetes, kidney

disease, blood cancers, and many other conditions can be detected by changes in the retina. Frequently, however, these diseases are not reflected in the eyes, and the presence of normal eyes is no assurance that systemic disease is not present.

RETINA, CLOSURE OF CENTRAL ARTERY OF   In high blood pressure, in hardening of the arteries, in heart disease with scarring of the valves, in certain obscure inflammation of arteries, in migraine, and in some other conditions the blood supply to the retina through its main artery may be stopped.

Symptoms.   There is a sudden loss of all vision in the eye, unless only a branch is involved—in which instance only the area of the vessel is injured. Examination indicates a spasm of the artery, with the retina milky white.

Treatment.   This must be carried out immediately. If pills have been used for heart pain (angina), they should be used. Breathing into a small paper bag may dilate the involved vessel. Rubbing the closed eye with the fist through the lids for fifteen seconds, followed by ten seconds' rest, over a total of five minutes may be helpful. Early medical care is important if vision is to improve.

RETINA, CLOSURE OF CENTRAL VEIN OF   This is most likely to occur in hardening of the arteries, glaucoma, conditions in which blood flow is slowed, and conditions favoring clotting of the blood.

Symptoms.   Vision is lost over a period of several minutes. Inspection with an ophthalmoscope shows the vein to be dilated and sausage-like, with intermittent narrowing and a large number of hemorrhages.

Treatment.   Massage as described for retinal arterial closure is of questionable value. Treatment is directed towards lowering pressure in the eye and reducing the coagulability of blood. There may be gradual improvement over many months, but the condition may be complicated by the development of glaucoma.

RETINA, DETACHMENT OF

The retina may become separated from its underlying layer of pigment in primary detachment, or become elevated because of hemorrhage or new growth in the underlying choroid. Primary retinal detachment (serous) occurs because of the formation of a hole in the nerve layer. The hole occurs because of degeneration or injury.

Symptoms. The first symptom is commonly a localized area of bright lights flashing in the eye, followed by a sudden appearance of minute "floaters"; the detachment causes a progressive loss of side vision. The condition is diagnosed by examination with an instrument which illuminates the interior of the eye (ophthalmoscope) and must be differentiated particularly from a tumor of the choroid, which causes a secondary detachment.

Treatment. The treatment is nearly always surgical. The hole in the retina is closed by creating scar tissue in the choroid adjacent to it. Sometimes the outer wall of the eye is indented by means of a plastic rod to push the wall in slightly and bring the choroid toward the retina.

RETINA, DISORDERS OF

The retina is a complex nervous structure for converting light to nerve impulses which are then carried to the brain. Because of the delicacy of structure of the retina, even minor disturbances reflect themselves in changes in vision. The change involved may be in recognition of letters or objects (form), in color, in side vision (peripheral), or in dark-adaptation. Retinal disorders themselves never cause pain or redness of the eye, although these may accompany complications or involvement of other structures.

RETINA, HEMORRHAGE OF

Bleeding into the retina may occur because of injury, congenital abnormalities of blood vessels, diseases involving a bleeding tendency, inflammations within the eye, or from rupture of newly formed blood vessels. Symptoms depend upon the area of retina involved. Treatment is directed to the cause of the disease.

RETINA, MACULAR DISEASE OF

The area of the retina at the very back of the eye contains cones responsible for clear central vision and color vision. Disturbances in this area (macula) cause dimness of vision, with an island of blindness surrounded by an area of vision. The macular area may be affected in a large variety of diseases, including congenital disorders which may occur with mental retardation and muscle paralysis.

In aging, the blood supply in the choroid which supplies the macular area may gradually fail, causing gradual loss of clear central vision. There is never complete loss of vision. Treatment is seldom effective. Some macular degenerations occur because of an inherited tendency and become evident only late in life.

RETINA, OXYGEN DAMAGE TO, (RETROLENTAL FIBROPLASIA)

Premature infants with a birth-weight of less than three pounds may, in order to survive, require oxygen in addition to that in the surrounding atmosphere. In some infants the oxygen interferes with the orderly growth of blood vessels in the retina, and the retina is converted to scar tissue. There are varying degrees of severity, and in the worst forms all vision is lost. The possibility of the disease developing is minimized by using oxygen as rarely as possible, and never in a concentration exceeding 50 per cent. However, some cases do occur in infants who have not received any oxygen, and other unknown factors are involved.

RETINA, PIGMENTED DEGENERATION OF, (RETINITIS PIGMENTOSA)
This is a hereditary disorder beginning in adolescence in which there is gradual loss of side vision and decreased night vision. In severe instances vision is entirely lost by about age fifty. The condition is diagnosed by measurement of side vision, recognition of characteristic changes in the back of the eye, and a number of special tests. There is no effective treatment.

RHEUMATIC FEVER Generally thought of as heart disease, rheumatic fever is really a general disease of the connective tissue of the body (the more serious manifestations, however, center in the heart valves). The disease is due to an overreaction or supersensitivity to the effects of toxins produced by the same variety of streptococcus bacteria which usually causes strep throat or scarlet fever. It is known that rheumatic fever will develop in 3 to 5 per cent of patients who receive no treatment for strep throat; however, if treatment is early and adequate, the incidence of subsequent rheumatic fever is only a fraction of 1 per cent. A single attack of rheumatic fever does not seem to cause heart damage, but each subsequent attack may scar the valves of the heart.

Symptoms. The diagnosis may be difficult, or it may be all too obvious. It must be made by the doctor, but important suggestive signs include: painful joints, purposeless movements (St. Vitus' dance), and recurrent fever. A number of laboratory tests, including electrocardiograms, are usually used to confirm the diagnosis.

Treatment. Once the diagnosis has been firmly established, treatment is designed to eliminate (by antibiotics) any residual streptococcus in the system and to give the heart as much rest as possible, so that it may heal with a minimum of damage. Aspirin is of great help in alleviating the pain and fever of this disease, and some believe that large doses shorten its course. Some patients require oxygen and special heart stimulants because of the severe damage. Certain authorities claim to have speeded the healing process by the use of cortisone-like drugs. Sedatives may be necessary against restlessness. Activity must be kept down to a minimum through complete rest until the heart has recuperated and laboratory tests indicate that the disease is less active.

The most important part of treatment is prevention of subsequent attacks. Rheumatic patients are susceptible to recurrence of the disease once they have had it, and since each attack creates further heart damage, the solution is prevention of the strep throat which triggers the disease. Daily oral penicillin tablets or once-a-month injections of long-acting penicillin are the methods of choice. The "sulfas" or "mycins" given daily by mouth are a poor second to penicillin and are used only if the patient has become allergic to it. Fortunately, this disease is not as common nor as devastating as it was twenty to thirty years ago.

RHEUMATIC HEART DISEASE In young adults and children heart disease is usually of rheumatic origin. The antibiotics have so reduced the occurrence of diphtheria and syphilis that rheumatic heart disease is now the only important form of heart disease primarily caused by a specific infection, but it too is becoming much less frequent as time passes.

Acute rheumatic fever is a disease affecting all tissues in some degree. The joints are usually affected and can be swollen and painful for days or weeks. The acute phase of the disease, however, may be so mild that only fatigue is noted, and the young persons so afflicted may even be accused of laziness.

Rheumatic fever is in some way caused by a specific streptococcus (the so-called "Group A beta-hemolytic type"). A sore throat caused by this organism often precedes the rheumatic fever by several weeks. While this group of bacteria does not cause changes in the heart directly, the tissue-reaction and damage related to the organisms are rather characteristic.

Although patients over the age of thirty-five have been known to suffer a first attack of rheumatic fever, it usually comes before the age of twenty. Boys and girls are equally affected. The disease seems much more prevalent in the cold, damp areas of the world where upper-respiratory infections and sore throats are common and contagious.

Symptoms. Characteristic tissue changes are seen in joint membranes, often accompanied by an outpouring of fluid into the cavity of the joint—knees, ankles, elbows, and even fingers.

All structures of the heart can be involved. The muscle fibers can show rheumatic changes, as can the valve leaflets and the membrane that covers the heart (the pericardium). With healing after an acute attack, scar tissue is deposited in the muscle, reducing its efficient contraction. Along the valves, scar tissue can cause a distortion in shape, and proper closure of the valve can be rendered impossible because the now-diseased valve is so malformed that it will not close tightly. Leakage of blood through the valve opening causes inefficient pumping of blood through the heart into the arterial system. Blood can even dam back into the lungs and cause an overfilling of the pulmonary vessels, with congestive changes and severely diminished space for the accommodation of breathed air.

Symptoms of rheumatic fever range from mild growing-pains in the muscles of the legs to a profoundly incapacitating general illness with high fever, sweating, and swollen and painful joints (especially in the ankles, knees, wrists, and fingers).

On examination there may be a heart murmur, and even enlargement of the heart. Characteristic findings may be seen in laboratory analysis of the blood (sedimentation rate and white-cell count). Although the electrocardiogram sometimes shows very little at first, before the disease has run its course many changes are usually apparent.

Treatment. Rheumatic heart patients need to have their condition followed for life by their physician. Medical treatment includes general care as well as specific and constant antibiotic attack on the bacteria that can cause and complicate further heart trouble.

Surgical relief may be needed to correct damaged heart valves. A tightly scarred mitral valve (mitral stenosis) may require opening to a nearly normal size; while a leaking mitral valve (mitral regurgitation) may require open-heart surgical repair, or insertion of an artificial valve. Aortic valves deformed by rheumatic fever may also be repaired during open-heart surgery, or an artificial valve replacement provided.

RHEUMATISM AND ARTHRITIS

The terms arthritis and rheumatism are used synonymously for afflictions of joints or supporting structures.

Arthritis is inflammation of a joint. However, because arthritis seldom occurs without pain, arthralgia (joint pain) must be linked with it.

Physicians, singly and in organized groups (such as the American Rheumatism Association), have been trying to establish a classification for arthritic and rheumatic disorders. To date there has been no success. The following classification, based chiefly on causes or alleged causes, is the one generally used.

Due to Specific Agents
(the more common ones)
    Gonorrhea

Tuberculosis
Staphylococcus (osteomyelitis)
Brucellosis
Syphilitic arthritis
Undulant fever
Rheumatoid arthritis
Paget's disease
Osteoarthritis
Rheumatoid spondylitis
Backache (lumbago and sciatica)
   Sprains, strains, and poor posture
   Spondylitis and spondylolisthesis
   Osteoporosis
   Slipped disk
Gout
Lupus erythematosus
Polyarteritis nodosa
Scleroderma
Schönlein-Henoch purpura
Hemophilia
Bursitis

RH FACTOR AND RH SENSITIZATION

In addition to the major blood groups (A, B, O), each person's red cells are characterized by the presence or absence of a specific substance, or antigen, the Rh antigen (referred to also as the Rh factor). This antigen is present in approximately 85 per cent of white people, who are then designated as Rh-positive (Rh+), and it is absent in about 15 per cent, who are designated as Rh-negative (Rh—). Among Negroes Rh-negative blood is found in only 7 to 8 per cent, while among the Japanese in only 1 to 2 per cent.

This substance becomes of particular significance mainly under two sets of circumstances: (1) in blood transfusions, where transfusion of Rh-positive blood to Rh-negative persons may cause complications, ranging from a mild sensitivity reaction to severe hemolysis (destruction of red cells); and (2) in pregnancy, where through an identical mechanism the baby may be exposed to serious damage or even fetal death. The danger arises when an Rh-negative wife gets pregnant by an Rh-

positive husband and the baby's blood happens to be Rh-positive. It should be noted that an Rh-positive husband does not always produce Rh-positive children. This will depend on whether he is Rh-positive homozygous (in this case all his children will be Rh-positive), or Rh-positive heterozygous (here the possibilities are fifty-fifty). Through special blood tests one can tell whether an Rh-positive person is homozygous or heterozygous.

The Rh disease of the fetus or the newborn is known as erythroblastosis fetalis or hemolytic disease of the newborn. An Rh-negative mother does not have to worry about erythroblastosis if she is carrying her first baby. The first baby is almost never affected unless the mother has had blood transfusions or a miscarriage in the past, so that she has been sensitized. Very often, however, she does become sensitized during her first pregnancy if the baby she is carrying happens to be Rh-positive, and this means trouble with the second and subsequent pregnancies.

Briefly, what is taking place is this: Rh-positive cells from the baby get into the mother's circulation and create antibodies. This occurs mostly during labor and delivery, but there is not enough time for harm to come to this first baby. With a subsequent pregnancy and another Rh-positive baby, more Rh-positive blood cells get into the mother's blood, and more antibodies are produced. These antibodies now go back to the baby, passing through the afterbirth, and they destroy the baby's red cells, resulting in hemolysis. Depending on the amounts of antibodies, and therefore on the degree of hemolysis, the baby becomes icteric (yellow) and suffers from severe anemia, which to a considerable extent affects his brain. If the disease is too severe, the baby dies inside the mother's womb. These antibodies may, however, be measured in the mother's blood through special tests, and when large amounts are detected and the baby is big enough to be born, then the obstetrician will usually advise interruption of pregnancy and will induce labor before term in order to prevent irrepairable damage to the baby. All such babies need to have special blood tests right after birth and, if the degree of anemia and hemolysis is considerable, their blood is replaced through exchange transfusion, that is, through gradual removal of their blood and replacement with normal, fresh, non-hemolyzed blood. This is usually effective in arresting the disease process.

The Rh problem is not really a serious one for the Rh-negative woman who is married to a heterozygous Rh-positive husband. But it often becomes desperate when the Rh-negative wife of a homozygous Rh-positive husband gives birth to a baby with severe erythroblastosis fetalis or fetal death inside the womb. In these cases, subsequent pregnancies are affected more severely and earlier, as compared with previous ones. The couple may be advised to avoid further pregnancies. Several experimental studies are carried out now and, hopefully, within a few years we may have some means of preventing erythroblastosis fetalis.

Neither Rh-positive women married to Rh-negative men nor Rh-negative wives of Rh-negative husbands have any problem with Rh disease in their children. The problem arises only when an Rh-negative woman marries an Rh-positive man, especially a homozygous one.

RHINITIS   See Atrophic Rhinitis; Vasomotor Rhinitis; Hyperplastic Rhinitis; Nasal Polyps; and Rhinitis Sicca

RHINITIS SICCA   Chronic rhinitis sicca (literally dry rhinitis) is not common in young healthy adults or children. It occurs more frequently in women at the time of the menopause, or in persons with chronic debilitating diseases such as diabetes or chronic kidney problems. The

symptoms: dryness of the nose and annoying crusting with a heavy odor. With rhinitis sicca there is no atrophy of the nasal lining or bone, thus distinguishing it from the more severe atrophic rhinitis. Treatment consists of local medication which promotes secretion of the nasal mucosa and restoration of general health as much as possible.

RHINOPLASTY   Reconstruction of the nose may be indicated either because of injury or for reasons of developmental deformity. Sometimes it is intended to aid breathing and other times is done for purely cosmetic purposes. This operation, called a rhinoplasty, is performed by the ear-nose-and-throat surgeon, who may, if necessary, straighten the nasal septum at the same time.

Rhinoplastic surgery may make the nose look more attractive, and it may make breathing easier; but it will not change life situations, open the door to romance and adventure, or solve personal problems. Given the proper motivation, this is a useful operation even when done solely for cosmetic purposes; with poor and erroneous motivation, even a beautiful surgical result may prove unsatisfying to the patient.

RICKETS   Rickets is a disease of childhood and is due to vitamin D deficiency. It is usually found in areas where the intake of vitamin D is low and where there is insufficient exposure to ultraviolet rays (see Vitamin D). At times it may be caused by failure to absorb the vitamin, as in patients with chronic intestinal disorders.

The basic disturbance is inadequate calcification of growing bones; that is, the basic bone structure is formed normally but does not become calcified or hard. There is also enlargement of the structures at the ends of the bones.

Infants with early rickets are restless

and sleep poorly. They continually move their heads on the pillow, which denudes the head of hair. Such infants do not sit, crawl, or walk at an early date. Later there may be enlargement of the frontal bones (the bones in the forehead), enlargement of the cartilage at the ribs (known as the rachitic rosary), and disturbances in the leg and hand bones. Bowlegs, knock-knees, and pigeon breast may develop. X-ray examination shows these signs early.

If vitamin D deficiency is severe but develops later in adult life, a condition known as osteomalacia occurs. This is a demineralization of the spine, pelvis, and legs, producing bowing of the legs and abnormalities in the spine and pelvis.

In rickets, the serum calcium level may fall abnormally low, and the patient may develop tetany, or muscle spasm.

This once common disease can easily be prevented by giving infants vitamin D, beginning in the third or fourth week of life. The child who already has rickets responds slowly to doses of vitamin D, and these doses have to be larger.

It is important to remember that there is danger in giving excessive amounts of vitamin D. Therefore, no parent should feel that if a little vitamin D is good protection against rickets, much more can be safely given. One should always follow the recommendations of the physician or the manufacturer of the product used.

RINGWORM OF THE SCALP

This still-common condition is due to a fungus which gets into the hair shaft and causes brittleness; the hair then breaks off, leaving quite an obvious bald spot. (The skin at the base of these short hairs may be slightly scaly.) A special ultraviolet filter (Wood's light) at the doctor's office will show these diseased hairs, and a culture can be made to confirm the diagnosis. This type of ringworm is called the human type because it comes from other infected children.

Treatment. Treatment of scalp ringworm is more satisfactory than it once was, thanks to the new drugs which destroy the fungus though taken internally. Many doctors still advocate plucking the hairs out and applying ointment in addition to giving internal medication, continuing this treatment until no more diseased hairs are found under the Wood's light. They argue that unless this is done the diseased hairs may spread the infection to healthy ones. Others argue that the same oral medication which destroys the fungus will also take care of the overall situation, preventing spread. Before the oral fungicides were developed, curing a case of ringworm of the scalp usually required at least a month or two of treatment. Today a child is given medicine for only one day; the cure, however, is not effected for two and a half weeks.

ROLE-PLAYING

Every person must learn to play many roles in life: student, wage earner, parent, marriage partner, financial manager, and social figure in the community. Many of these roles are learned in family life, others in school. Unfortunately, few people learn to play all their roles well, succeeding in some but failing in others. Psychiatrists attempt to evaluate role-playing skills and to provide special tutoring where role-playing is inadequate.

ROOT-CANAL TREATMENT

Root-canal treatment encompasses those procedures which involve removal of the entire pulp from a tooth, so that the root canal and chamber can be cleaned, sterilized, filled, and sealed. The resulting tooth will be "non-vital," since there will be no nerves or blood supply within it; hence, it will not respond to such external stimuli as heat or cold. However, the treatment does not affect the supporting structures, and the tooth can remain in the arch and

436

continue to give additional service. The tooth so treated will be subject to dental decay just as any tooth in the mouth. When the supporting structures are healthy and the pulp canal can be treated, root-canal therapy may be resorted to instead of extraction.

RORSCHACH TEST

The Rorschach test is a method for studying unconscious complexes and deep personality structure by eliciting spontaneous responses to ambiguous ink blots. The subject is presented with the ink blots, one at a time, and first simply asked to tell what they mean to him. Later the clinical psychologist administering the test, questions the subject, to discover which specific features of the ink blots elicited which responses. Clinical experience with the ink-blot responses of normal individuals and of clinical patients indicates that very important information is provided concerning deep personality-structure and unconscious conflicts, since these are projected into, and determine, the responses.

ROSACEA

This chronic reddening of the center portion of the face (forehead, nose, chin) is often accompanied by the papules and pustules of acne. More common in women of middle age, it can nevertheless occur in both sexes and almost any age. The reddening worsens on exposure to extremes of temperature, and gradually the intensity of color becomes persistent with no periods of lightening. Tiny superficial vessels become visible in the skin. When the nose is the area most dominantly affected, as is often the case in men, an overgrowth of all the components of the skin takes place, giving the lower portion of the nose a grotesque appearance.

Rosacea is often associated with lesions of the eyes (conjunctivitis, keratitis) at the same time that the skin becomes involved with blackhead formation, dilated pores and much greasiness.

Probably of multiple causation, the condition flares up on eating hot foods (both from condiment and temperature), iodides (shellfish), bromides (sedatives), chocolate, and nuts, and is thought to be associated with a lowering of the stomach hydrochloric acid.

Treatment. Avoidance of extremes of temperature, alcohol, spicy foods, and foods interdicted in acne is essential in treatment. Drying lotions, antibiotics for pustules, suitable hydrochloric acid therapy, and, finally, electrolysis or electrocautery of the enlarged vessels and surgical removal of excess tissue (nose), can prove effective. (See also ACNE.)

ROSEOLA

Roseola is an acute virus disease usually seen between the ages of six months and two years. It does not seem to be contagious even though it bears a superficial resemblance to the measles.

Symptoms. There often seems to be a triggering mechanism, in the development of roseola, such as cutting a tooth. The baby suddenly develops a high fever (and may even have a convulsion) without any other sign of symptoms. The eyes may be a little red-rimmed and there may be a trace of nasal stuffiness. Aspirin almost always brings the fever down and is an important diagnostic sign; for if the aspirin works well, and if the baby cools down and acts normally, the disease is most probably roseola. The fever lasts seventy-two hours, disappears just as suddenly as it started, and is then replaced by a rash over the trunk, neck, and face, but almost never on the arms and legs. (If however, the fever recurs once the rash has made its appearance, the illness is not roseola.)

Roseola rash is pink, often slightly raised, and each spot is one-eighth to one-fourth of an inch in diameter. There are one-fourth to one-half-inch swollen lymph nodes on the back of the head on either side, directly above the neck, where the neck cords are attached to the skull.

Treatment. Roseola is a virus disease and treatment is only for relief of the fever. In contrast to the regular "hard" measles, there are virtually no complications. Because the fever is so high and because the throat may be a little pink, some have mistaken roseola for strep throat and given the baby penicillin for the disease. When the rash broke out, it was assumed the baby was allergic to penicillin. Since roseola is the only disease in which a rash follows the fever, there should really be no confusion.

RUBELLA (GERMAN MEASLES)

German measles is a communicable virus disease characterized by the appearance of a generalized fine-pink rash, swollen glands behind the ears, slight fever (no more than 101°F.), and red-rimmed eyes. The incubation period is fourteen days.

Symptoms. The symptoms of rubella usually last three days and the majority of patients are only slightly ill. The disease may be confused with a drug rash or scarlatina, but the swollen glands behind the ears indicate that it is rubella. Complications are almost unheard of, but if a woman in the first three months of a pregnancy contracts this disease, there is a marked possiblity of producing a deformed or deaf baby; it is therefore important to expose female children to this disease early in life. Families and doctors should keep conspicuous and available records so that girl children who have had rubella and are immune will have this knowledge later if they are pregnant and become exposed. The disease leaves permanent immunity, so the diagnosis should be confirmed.

Treatment. Once the rubella is contracted there is no effective treatment, and none is needed. In the first trimester of pregnancy, however, rubella poses a serious threat to the fetus; the virus is capable of passing through the placenta to infect and damage the developing fetus. An effective rubella vaccine has been developed and is particularly desirable as part of the immunogenic program of all young girls.

SABIN VACCINE   See INFANTILE PARALYSIS

ST. VITUS' DANCE (SYDENHAM'S CHOREA)

Sydenham's chorea, or St. Vitus' dance, is characterized by the sudden onset of spontaneous movements of the face, arms, and legs associated with poor coordination and muscular weakness. One-half of patients with chorea show evidence of rheumatic infection before, during, or after an attack of chorea. The disorder affects the basal ganglia in the center of the brain as well as other structures, and is probably related to hypersensitivity to streptococcus infection.

Symptoms. Most patients develop Sydenham's chorea between five and fifteen years of age. The child may be irritable and fatigue easily. While writing, eating, or playing games, he may notice difficulty in using one or both arms. He may complain of weakness; frequent involuntary grimaces of the face are noted; there may be difficulty in speaking and in swallowing; involuntary movements occur in the arms and legs.

Treatment. There is no specific treatment available for Sydenham's chorea although sedative drugs are effective in decreasing the involuntary movements. Complete recovery from the condition is the rule. However, if chorea is associated with rheumatic involvement of the heart, complications may result then from the cardiac disorder.

SALIVA

Saliva is a mixture of clear fluids secreted into the mouth by certain glands (salivary glands). These fluids lubricate the mucosa and aid in preventing dehydration of all soft tissues of the mouth. During chewing (mastication), the saliva is mixed with food, aiding in swallowing and initiating digestion. Saliva is usually alkaline, and possesses a great capacity for neutralizing acids; in addition, it contains materials which delay or halt bacterial growth; both of these characteristics reducing the possibility of dental caries. Saliva also helps certain fillings to remain moist and thus to maintain their color, stability, and durability.

The quantity and quality of saliva varies with each individual. Its flow is stimulated by mastication or other stimuli capable of affecting the nervous system (such as the sight and smell of food). Breathing through the mouth for long periods of time may result in excessive evaporation, producing a reduction in the lubricating qualities of saliva.

SALIVARY GLANDS   These are specialized organs, associated with the oral cavity, whose function is the production and secretion of the watery fluid called saliva. The principal salivary glands are the parotid, the submaxillary, and the sublingual. These occur in pairs, and empty their saliva into the mouth through the salivary ducts.

The parotids are the largest of the principal glands. They lie embedded on either side of the face, just below and in front of each ear; the ducts carrying the saliva of these glands into the mouth course through the cheeks and empty into the oral cavity opposite the maxillary second molars. The secretion is usually quite thin and watery. Epidemic parotitis is a viral infection of this pair of glands, its more common name being the mumps.

The submaxillary glands are located, one on either side, just in front of and below the angles of the lower jaw. The saliva from these glands is emptied into the mouth through the ducts which are located beneath the tongue, one on each side of the frenulum of the tongue.

The smallest pair of salivary glands are those located beneath the tongue, the sublingual glands. These, too, empty into the mouth beneath the tongue.

In addition to the three pairs of major salivary glands, there are a number of smaller accessory glands which also produce some saliva. These are located primarily in the roof of the mouth and on the inside of the lips.

Partial or complete blockage of the ducts of the major glands may result from swelling or the presence of salivary stones (sialolith). In these conditions the glands continue to secrete saliva, but since it cannot pass out of the glands and into the oral cavity, it backs up into the gland, causing it to swell. This swelling may be especially noticeable and painful when a hungry person with this obstruction sees or smells food, inasmuch as the glands are stimulated to produce still more saliva in preparation for the anticipated food. If this obstruction prevails for long periods, the glands may be damaged and begin to shrink (atrophy).

Treatment.   The treatment of sialolithiasis involves locating the position, size, and nature of the stone or stones and removing this obstruction. Though this may occur spontaneously, frequently a dental consultation is necessary to determine if the salivary stones (calculi) should be removed surgically or expressed manually.

SALK VACCINE See Infantile Paralysis

SALPINGITIS   Salpingitis is an acute or chronic infection of the fallopian tubes. It is common during the reproductive span of the woman and is usually due to gonorrhea. If not treated early and thoroughly, this type of infection advances to the chronic stage and then causes obstruction of the tubes and secondary sterility. Chronic salpingitis is also a frequent cause of irregular vaginal bleeding because of the spread of infection to the ovaries. The infection may also end in multiple adhesions in the pelvis, with a variety of painful symptoms. Occasionally, large abscesses may form in the pelvis which rupture and cause severe peritonitis; an emergency operation and removal of the womb, tubes, and ovaries is then necessary for the survival of the patient.

This disease is also known as Pelvic Inflammatory Disease (PID).

SCABIES An intensely itchy, highly communicable disease occurring in all age groups and both sexes, scabies is caused by a mite, *Sarcoptes scabiei*, and is transmitted by direct contact from person to person. Other varieties of mite, parasitic to fowl and to domestic and wild mammals, occasionally attack human beings, but produce eruptions of less intensity and shorter duration. It is interesting to note that prior to about 1950, scabies was a common disease, both endemic and epidemic in the urban communities of the United States.

Symptoms. The mite produces small papules in which a darkened horizontal shadow (a burrow) is noted. The lesion may give the appearance of a small blister, and in young children the condition may indeed be a blistering one. The lesions occur most commonly in the bend of the wrist, the webs of the fingers and over the entire torso, but not on the neck, face, and head. In children, the palms and soles are frequently affected. Secondary pustular infection is usual. The itching is always intense, but characteristically is much worse at night (perhaps because of the warmth of bed covers).

Treatment. Sulfur ointments, solution of benzyl benzoate, or Qwell® ointment applied before bedtime and left on the next day are among the effective remedies. Reapplication of the remedy for five to seven days, and boiling or cleaning the clothes and bed linens, are necessary for cure.

SCARLET FEVER Scarlet fever, scarlatina, and streptococcus sore throat with rash are all variants of the same disease-process: a streptococcal sore throat—pharyngitis and/or tonsillitis—due to a bacterium with the ability to produce a toxin which makes the capillaries expand and cause a rash.

Symptoms. It is only two to four days from exposure to the onset of symptoms, which may be sudden and severe: chill, vomiting and fever to 105° or 106°F. A headache and prostration are usual, and there is almost always the complaint of a severe sore throat. Recently, the streptococcus infection has not been as debilitating as it once was; some patients today complain only mildly about their symptoms, and the temperature may climb no higher than 101°.

The throat is usually deep red and the tonsils blood-red often with white spots of exudate on them. The soft palate (the back part of the roof of the mouth) is usually red, and if there seems to be bleeding areas on it, the diagnosis of strep throat is most likely. The neck glands usually swell up and can be felt on the second day of sickness just under the corner of the jaw bone. A culture is sometimes taken to confirm the diagnosis.

Treatment. Standard treatment is ten days of adequate doses of penicillen, which acts specifically against the streptococcus. As yet this bacterium has not become resistant to penicillin, as has the staphylococcus. If a patient has become allergic to penicillin, one of the "mycins" is substituted with equally good results. It is important to treat the condition during the whole ten days, since complications (rheumatic fever, nephritis, abscess-formation) are virtually unheard of if this is done.

SCARS Of considerable variety and of many causes, scars are evidence of a disruption of the connective tissue of the dermis (subcutis) of the skin, with a loss of the elastic elements, hair follicle, sebaceous and sweat glands, a scarcity of blood vessels, much fibrous tissue, and a thin epidermal covering. The fibrous tissue can be so excessive as to give the lesion the appearance of a keloid, and then become flattened spontaneously (hypertrophic scar). The smooth, glossy appearance of scars and the absence of contours or surface "relief" is the result of the absence of certain tissues (gland and hair structures) in the normal skin.

Many scars can be identified as resulting from a specific preceding condition (acne, chickenpox, striae of pregnancy, neurotic excoriations, burns, lupus erythematosus, syphilis, surgery).

Treatment. Except when scarring is extensive and interferes with function, or when a scar is further devitalized and "breaks down," treatment is unnecessary. For esthetic betterment, scars can be excised, abraded, or treated with acids, depending on the configuration of the scarring and the area involved.

SCHIZOPHRENIA
Formerly known as dementia praecox (mental disorder of the young), schizophrenia is one of the more serious and common psychoses, resulting in disabling mental symptoms. The term schizophrenia means splitting of the mind and is manifested by a splitting or dissociation of emotional and rational mental processes. Schizophrenia is regarded by many as a functional reaction, caused by personality inadequacies which result in inability to meet the demands of adult adjustment. The basic mechanism appears to be progressive withdrawal from contact with the real world, with regression to infantile or childish feelings and reactions.

Symptoms. No physical or organic cause has been demonstrated in schizophrenia. (Hereditary factors have, however, been suspected, since mental disorders and schizoid personality types are frequently observed among other members of the family.) Age of onset is most frequently adolescence or early adult life, but

may occur as late as the middle years. Most psychiatrists now agree that schizophrenia is related to defects or weaknesses of basic personality structure caused by damaging childhood experiences, unconscious conflicts, and inability to express instinctive—particularly sexual—drives. Several clinical types of schizophrenia have been classically described:

Simple schizophrenia is associated with gradual personality changes manifested by increasing withdrawal from contact with external reality and a lessened response to social demands in the form of a falling-off of emotional reactivity, interests, and ability to adjust to the community. In extreme form, the person may become completely apathetic, preoccupied with an inner mental life, and indifferent to group activity.

Hebephrenic schizophrenia is characterized by silly, foolish, or inappropriate behavior; bizarre ideas reflecting an abnormal fantasy life; and frequent hallucinations, usually auditory. The patient shows a progressive disintegration of personality, becomes inaccessible to social contacts, and shows increasing immaturity and shallowness in emotional reactions, with regressive features such as failure to attend to matters of personal grooming and bowel or bladder control.

Catatonic schizophrenia is characterized by phases of truculence, silence, stupor, and excitement, frequently alternating suddenly. So-called "catatonic" symptoms include negativism, peculiar grimaces and gestures, and muscular immobility associated with inattention to bodily needs, refusal to eat, and neglect of toilet habits. In excited phases the patient is driven by purposeless overactivity motivated from within, which results in sleeplessness and rapid physical exhaustion. Catatonic patients have relatively hopeful prospects for cure, and the condition frequently clears up spontaneously.

Paranoid schizophrenia is characterized by bizarre delusional thinking combined with an otherwise relatively intact personality. The delusions, usually of persecution, apparently represent a defensive effort to "rebuild" the world in terms of the individual's own motivations, the symptoms representing a projection of inner conflict. Systematic paranoid delusions are highly resistant to treatment, and the long-term outcome is usually very poor. Paranoid schizophrenics are usually regarded as potentially dangerous because of their known tendency to take law and order into their own hands and to attempt to punish anyone they believe is persecuting them.

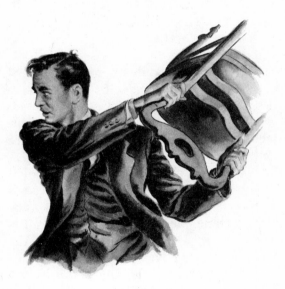

Treatment. Because of the difficulty in determining the exact cause of schizophrenia, treatment of the condition cannot guarantee absolute cure. A large percentage of schizophrenics have shown spontaneous improvement and may also have long periods of normality, although regression may take place. Drug therapies using tranquilizers such as chlorpromazine and trifluoperazine, and other substances, are an attempt to limit schizophrenic attacks, which can be aggressive, paranoic, or self-destructive in nature. Such drug treat-ment can increase the schizophrenic's contact with reality and help bring compulsive behavior under control. In combination with psychiatric therapy, which attempts to uncover the original causes of the disorder, treatment with drugs is phasing out other forms of treatment, such as electroshock therapy.

With proper treatment, usually involving both drugs and psychotherapy, and with the support of patient and understanding family and friends, many schizophrenics can improve their condition and function successfully in their community.

SCIATICA See Slipped Disk

SCIATIC NERVE The sciatic nerve supplies many of the muscles in the upper and lower leg. It also carries sensory impulses from a large portion of the skin of the lower leg to the spinal cord.

SCLERITIS Inflammation of the sclera of the eye may be superficial (episcleritis) or deep (scleritis). Causes include irritation, inflammatory infections, injury, rheumatism, gout, syphilis, tuberculosis.

Episcleritis is usually harmless and is marked by slight discomfort, tearing, and pain. Occasionally there are more severe manifestations. There may be a slightly raised patch, red or purple in color, which causes congestion of the conjunctiva and the sclera. After a few weeks this lesion disappears, but recurrences, one after the other, are not uncommon. The condition may resemble certain types of conjunctivitis; it may become a frank scleritis.

Therapy is chiefly sedative, such as warm compresses using boric acid solution. If the cornea or iris is involved, atropine is administered. Anesthetic drops relieve discomfort and pain. Antibiotics (by mouth or in drops) are also employed.

Treatment is also of the underlying condition, as mentioned above.

The symptoms of scleritis are acute, the course of the affliction is protracted, and consequences may be serious. Involvement of both eyes is not rare and relapses are usual.

Severe pain, tenderness to the examing finger, tearing, and marked sensitivity to light are the major indications. The doctor finds that the tension of the eyeball is often increased; there may be secondary glaucoma. Other elements of the eye may be involved leading to markedly impaired vision, even blindness.

Therapy is that as given above, except that it is vigorously pursued and energetic treatment of the underlying cause, if it can be determined, is followed as soon as possible. Sulfa medication and antibiotics have recently been of great help in bacterial infections.

SCLERODERMA, DIFFUSE SYSTEMIC

The cutaneous manifestation of this disease represents the visible evidence of a connective tissue disturbance of the entire body, and is usually the first symptom the patient is aware of. It is a disease of adult life, occurring earliest in adolescence and rarely in the elderly.

Symptoms. The replacement of normal pliable connective tissue by thick and brittle fibers causes a hardening of the skin which is usually noted by a restriction of muscular activity in the affected area. Thus the patient finds it increasingly difficult to smile, grin, or frown if the face is affected. Objectively, there may be an erasing of the lines and wrinkles of the face. Fine movements of the fingers are made impossible if those areas are involved. Swallowing or breathing can be labored from involvement of the skin of these areas or from lesions in the throat or the lungs.

The disease is irregular in its course; remission of many months and years are not uncommon. Although the hardness of the affected areas usually persists, extensive periods of remission of the disease may afford the patient continued "normal" activity.

Treatment. Relief of symptoms with massage, whirlpool baths, avoidance of cold (when the hands and feet are involved), and the application of drugs and physical appliances which promote increased blood circulation of the skin may be helpful. The cortisone drugs are occasionally effective and are worthy of trial in spite of the seeming contraindications.

SCLERODERMA, LOCALIZED (MORPHEA)

This benign disease affects both children and adults, but is rare in the elderly.

Symptoms. Confined to the skin, it consists of a disturbance of the connective tissue and is first noted as bluish discoloration occurring on any part of the skin surface, though most commonly on the face and neck. The area becomes enlarged, feels hard to the touch, loses its violet-blue color, becoming yellow or alabaster-like. As the lesions become firmer they also become elevated. Succeeding flare-ups produce a purplish halo around the existing lesions. The eruption can consist of a single lesion stationary in size, or the lesion can extend—usually in linear fashion—over the entire extremity. Remission can result in a moderate depression in the center of the lesion, but the hard, firm texture almost always persists, even when the lesion is "burned out" and presents a brownish hyperpigmented, and occasionally scaling area. Itching is not common.

Localized scleroderma is not associated with any known condition. While the prognosis is good, disfigurement and incapacitation can be severe and constitute a significant handicap.

Treatment. The many suggested remedies including massage, local administration of mecholyl, cortisone, and PABA (para-aminobenzoic acid) afford only questionable relief.

SCLEROMA   Scleroma is a diagnostic term indicating unusual or abnormal hardness of a part or an area of the body.

SCOLIOSIS   Scoliosis is lateral curvature of the spine which may be congenital in origin, or due to faulty posture, to organic causes such as rickets or spinal paralytic disease, or to a series of vertebrae which are constantly deviated from the normal spinal axis. Depending on cause and severity, treatment is special exercises, orthopedic braces, surgery, or a combination of all three.

SCRATCH TEST See ALLERGIES, DIAGNOSIS OF

SCROTUM   The sac suspended below the penis in the male is known as the scrotum. It contains the testicles, epididymis, and seminal vessels, as well as nerves and blood vessels. In the adult it has a somewhat corrugated surface which is capable of contraction and expansion. In a cold environment the scrotum will be markedly contracted, and in a warm environment it will expand permitting the testes to hang further away from the warm body surface. Both of these reactions are designed to provide a stable temperature for the heat-sensitive testes and the sperm.

SCURVY   Scurvy indicates vitamin C deficiency. A typical case is suggested when a baby between six and twelve months old (who has not been getting enough vitamin C as fruit juice or as vitamin supplement) fails to gain weight, becomes irritable, cries when it is moved, and seems to have pain and tenderness in its legs. There may be swelling around the knees or other joints.

Deformities at the junction of ribs and cartilage are seen. The gums are swollen and bleed easily; there is fever, increased pulse and respiration. Severe, untreated scurvy is fatal.

X-ray examination of the limb bones shows a distinctive pattern. Anemia is common, and tests for fragility of the capillaries are positive. In adults, weakness, irritability, weight loss, anemia, and muscle and joint pains come on gradually. Bleeding gums and loosening of teeth follow. The patient bruises easily. The level of ascorbic acid in the blood (white cell layer) is very low.

Treatment. Both young and old with scurvy usually respond rapidly to large doses of vitamin C. Because this serious illness is so easily prevented, it is the obligation of all parents, physicians, dietitians, and others involved with dietary planning to insure an adequate intake of this nontoxic substance for all.

SEASONAL ALLERGIES   Seasonal allergies are those allergic disorders which occur only during certain seasons: ragweed hay fever in the fall, grass hay fever in the spring, and so on.

SEBORRHEIC DERMATITIS   This is a disturbance of the hair follicle-connected sebaceous (oil) gland in which the eruption consists of round and oval-shaped plaques located chiefly over the mid-portion of the chest, the middle of the back, the shoulders, the eyebrows and eyelids, the sides of the nose, behind the ears, and the margin of the scalp where it joins the skin of the face and neck. This term also applies to a similar condition of the scalp, which in a mild form, and present in a very high percentage of persons in certain populations, is the well-known dandruff.

Symptoms. Ranging from the earliest "cradle-cap" of the newborn, and the simplest mild scaling of the scalp noted by almost everyone from time to time, to a recurrent and often persistent widespread eruption, the disease is associated with considerable itching. Remissions are common especially in the summer (during vacations, and under conditions of an improved state of health). No specific cause has been assigned to this malfunctioning of the sebaceous glands.

Treatment. For the uncomplicated dandruff confined to the scalp, there is an abundance of effective and harmless remedies available over-the-counter in the pharmacy. These remedies contain (either singly or in combination) such remedies as sulfur, mercury, tars, salicylic acid. Dandruff which does not respond to the commercially available remedies may be relieved by prescription drugs. Seborrheic dermatitis which does not respond to simple drying agents like calamine lotion requires a physician's care.

SELF-CONCEPT The newer Self psychologies teach that the central core of personality is the person's concept of himself. Every child early begins to compare himself with others and builds up positive and negative self-regarding attitudes concerning what he is (Actual Self-Concept) and what he should be (Ideal Self-Concept).

An individual with basically positive self-concepts likes himself and develops self-confidence. Conversely, the person with basically negative self-concepts tends to dislike himself and to lack self-confidence. When the discrepancy between the Actual Self-Concept and the Ideal Self-Concept is too great, the person tends to become frustrated and demoralized because he cannot be what he would like to be. Self-hate is recognized to be an important factor underlying many guilt reactions and depressive states and may lead to suicidal impulses.

SELF-CONSCIOUSNESS Heightened awareness of the self is a common symptom in neurotic anxiety states. Normally, most bodily functions are "silent" in that they operate automatically on physical levels and the person is not aware of them. Most neurotic disorders, however, are associated with emotional disturbances producing symptoms on all physical and mental levels, of which the patient quickly becomes aware.

Symptoms. Classically related to self-consciousness are emotional conflict and insecurity manifested by lack of self-confidence, stage-fright, inability to perform well in public, and specific symptoms such as stuttering and stammering, inability to remember, and concentration difficulties in thinking.

Treatment. Symptoms tend to disappear spontaneously if the individual can gain some measure of success which will give him more self-confidence and emotional security. In general, success is Nature's antidote for anxiety, and can exercise a therapeutic influence under appropriate circumstances.

SENESCENCE AND SENILITY Studies of biologic development indicate that a peak of physical health, strength, endurance, resistance to disease, and virility is reached in the late teens and early twenties, following which a slow process of aging begins to exert progressive limitations on both physical and mental functioning. Evidence from studies of the growth of intelligence in childhood indicates that maximum development of innate abilities is complete by age fourteen or fifteen, after which any improvements in performance are achieved by training rather than by further increases in native ability. However, any person can compensate for the gradual decline of physical and mental powers through increasing experience and perfection of learned controls over behavior.

Symptoms. The aging process is

manifested physically by loss and graying of hair, loss of accommodating power of the lenses of the eye resulting in progressive farsightedness, opacity of the optic lenses resulting in cataracts, progressive loss of hearing, deteriorative changes in the skin, arthritic joint changes, and a variety of circulatory changes involving hardening of the arteries, high blood pressure, and kidney impairment.

A primary cause of psychological changes in old age is circulatory change in the brain, involving hardening of brain arteries, blood clots or hemorrhage. Studies of older brains indicate a progressive loss of cells due to such damage as arterial damage, brain tumors, or post-encephalitic scarring. The speed of mental functioning tends to decrease over the years, and there is progressive loss of retentive ability manifested by inability to learn new things or remember recent events.

Treatment. Although little can be done to delay the process of aging, a great deal can be done in preserving and rehabilitating such functions as are left. There is considerable evidence that mental as well as muscular function can be retained only by means of constant daily exercise and use. The older person should make every effort to retain the habitual activities of his working life in order to remain useful and in full contact with reality. Too many older people make no plans for retirement and then feel lost when forced to give up their habitual routine, only to be left without anything interesting to do. The modern geriatric movement has made great progress in organizing activity programs and stimulating conditions of living for older people.

SENSORY NERVE CELL (NEURON) Primary sensory neurons are located in the skin, muscles, eyes, ears, nose, viscera, and elsewhere throughout the body. They receive stimuli and transmit impulses along sensory pathways to the central nervous system. Thus, the rods and cones in the retina of the eye are special cells for the reception of visual stimuli from the external environment. Taste buds in the tongue receive and transmit chemical stimuli, which the central nervous system integrates and interprets as sweet or sour. Sensory neurons in the skin receive stimuli such as a pin prick or a light touch. Sensory neurons contained within muscle bundles transmit stimuli relating to movement. Special neurons in the intestines, in the bladder and elsewhere, provide other types of sensory information.

Secondary and other sensory neurons transmit impulses to the cord and brain through relays.

SEX INSTRUCTION AND SEX-ORGAN CONCERN Concern on the part of children with sex matters and sex organs is today much more openly expressed and, by and large, given more serious thought by adults than was once the case. This holds true even with younger children. The age level of overt sex-consciousness has dropped within recent times by at least two years; children now hear much more and think much more about matters of sex —and do so at earlier ages—hence the attention of parents must be attuned to these changes.

In almost all modern school curricula, even at grammar-school level, children are taught adequate anatomy and general physiology in relation to sex. At the same time, on the outside, they are exposed to a rather alarming amount of frank discussion among their companions—revelations which most parents completely fail to realize are going on.

There are, of course, countless books dealing with sex instruction, available to parents, unfortunately not all of them well written. The present author believes that detailed teaching regarding sex physiology, love, and related topics must be skillfully—

446

and individually—handled, and should never be forced upon young children whose own curiosity has not yet been awakened. The child's wish to know should be the key to effective teaching. Given a little general reading, it should not be difficult for parents to determine the optimum method to use.

SEXUAL ACT   Sexual intercourse consists basically of contact between the male and female genitalia, the male organ (penis) being inserted into the vagina through a series of rhythmic motions. Sperm (semen) is ejaculated through the male urethra and deposited in the female vagina at the neck of the uterus (cervix). The climax of the sexual act is accompanied by an all-consuming sensation of ecstasy known as orgasm. Orgasm is felt by both the man and the woman, but may not coincide in the partners. Normally the woman is slower to reach climax and requires a longer period of preparation (foreplay). Unless measures are taken to prevent conception, the sperm passes into the uterus, and meets the ovum either somewhere in the uterus or the fallopian tube. This process is known as conception, and if it is successful the fertilized ovum is implanted in the wall of the uterus, where it then grows. (For conception to occur, however, intercourse must take place during the woman's fertile period, at a time close to ovulation. This period is generally about mid-way between successive menstrual periods.)

Many fears and taboos surround the sexual act, and it is quite common—especially on the wedding night—for either partner to be unable to complete the act successfully. Usually, however, with patience and understanding the husband and wife are able to achieve a mutually satisfactory relationship. Persistently incomplete sexual intercourse may result in tensions and nervousness in the woman and may cause her to be irritable and rejecting of her husband's attentions.

SHAKING PALSY   See Parkinson's Disease

SHINGLES (HERPES ZOSTER)   This condition, often attributed to "nerves," is actually an affliction of a particular nerve. The site of the pathology is at the point of emergence of the nerve from the spinal column or the skull, as the case may be. The inflammation of the nerve is caused by a virus closely related to the virus of chickenpox; and, indeed, the disease occurs either in people who have never had chickenpox and have therefore not had an opportunity to become immunized to the virus (and to related viruses); or in people who have lost their immunity either partially or completely. Therefore this disease occurs not uncommonly in grandparents who are exposed to the chickenpox of their grandchildren and no longer have sufficient immunity to withstand the related virus of shingles. Also, in the elderly and in the extremely and often terminally ill, activation of the virus is evidence of a general loss of immunity, hence of a poor prognosis.

Symptoms.   The eruption consists of groups of blisters surounded by some redness. The blisters are deep-seated and therefore not easily broken. The groups are found in the general distribution of a nerve. For instance, groups of blisters will form around the chest in the approximate location of one rib, or in an irregular line down a thigh or leg. There can be a scattering of smaller groups beyond the ordinary position of a particular nerve, because very small nerve-ends extend into areas seemingly beyond that of the involved nerve. And so one occasionally sees shingles appear to be present on "both sides." The legendary fatal outcome for this situation is not based on fact. Pain may precede the eruption by several days. The pain is of a dull toothache kind, but with occasional sharp, knife-like sensations. The skin condition lasts from two to three weeks, somewhat longer when the face is involved. The pain may last a much longer time. Often patients having known somebody with prolonged post-shingles pain are apprehensive about this aspect of the disease. It should therefore be noted that prolonged pain is the exception, and that patients usually recover in three or four weeks from both the skin eruption and the pain.

Treatment. Even though there is no specific treatment available, the patient is

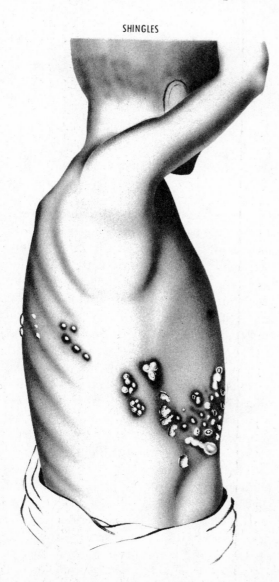

SHINGLES

well advised to seek current medical measures in the hope of ameliorating the symptoms. Steroid drugs diminish pain and shorten the course of the disease.

SHOCK TREATMENT Various methods have been used to produce convulsions artificially as a method of treating mental disorders. This is based on the clinical observation that epileptic patients rarely seem to develop schizophrenia.

Insulin shock therapy uses carefully controlled doses of insulin to produce shock and convulsions; this method is, however, potentially dangerous and requires experienced nursing personnel to administer it properly. It was later discovered that convulsions could be produced more safely and easily by administering convulsive dosages of electricity through electrodes strapped to the head. When administered properly and with suitable precautions to prevent bone fractures during the convulsive seizures, electroshock therapy is relatively safe and economical and can be used even on an outpatient basis.

During early experimentation with various methods of shock treatment, some beneficial effects were reported in treating all the functional psychoses, but overall experience indicates that they are chiefly valuable in depressive conditions. More recently, shock methods have been replaced by tranquilizing and antidepressant drugs, which in most cases, produce the same effects more safely without causing convulsions.

All forms of shock therapy have been criticized as being refined methods of punishment and, in fact, many patients come to fear electroshock treatments because of the progressive memory loss accompanying long series of treatments. In selected cases, however, electroshock still remains the method of choice in treating depressive states resistant to psychotherapy.

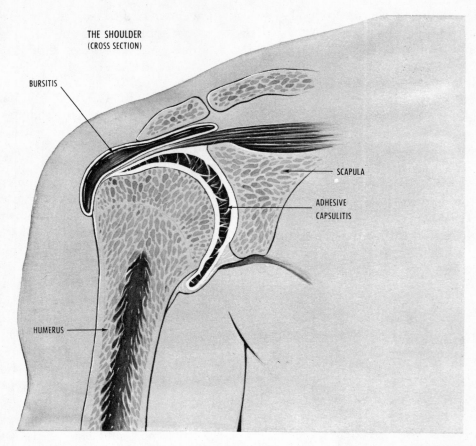

THE SHOULDER
(CROSS SECTION)

BURSITIS

SCAPULA

ADHESIVE
CAPSULITIS

HUMERUS

SHOULDER, PAINFUL   Pain in the shoulder may be due to a multitude of causes: it may be a manifestation of generalized arthritic disease, and in some cases represents pain "referred" from internal organs; heart disease, pleurisy, gallbladder disease may all present symptoms of shoulder pain.   Adults with pain in the shoulder not accompanied by tenderness on palpation of the shoulder and not accompanied by limitation of motion should suspect the possibility of internal disease and undergo careful medical evaluation. Bursitis and adhesive capsulitis are the most common local shoulder conditions.

SIBLING RIVALRY   Sibling rivalry refers to competitive reactions, jealousies, and hostility developing between children in the same family.   The first child in the family typically feels rejected and deprived when the birth of the second child diverts some of the attention he formerly received. Older children frequently become jealous of the youngest child who is treated as the baby in the family and gets the most attention.   Middle children tend to get "lost in the shuffle" and to receive less recognition than either the oldest or the youngest child.

Sibling rivalry should be recognized as a normal phenomenon and can be minimized if the parents will attempt to prepare older children for the birth of younger ones and later attempt to divide attention equally among all children.

Selfishness is a typical symptom of emotional insecurity in children who feel deprived or rejected.   It may be regarded as normal so long as the child feels insecure and usually disappears spontaneously in young adults when they become mature enough to begin sharing with others.

SICKLE CELL ANEMIA

Sickle cell anemia is an inherited disorder of the hemoglobin, the substance in blood that carries oxygen. Because of the defective hemoglobin, the red blood cells suffer a deformation and take on a collapsed, sickle-like shape. This structural abnormality, and the loss of oxygen-carrying capacity, may cause or increase the likelihood of extreme fatigue, blood clots, pneumonia, heart failure, and stroke. Many victims die before the age of twenty.

The sickle cell genetic trait occurs predominately among people of African descent. Just over 10 percent of the American Black population have this trait, usually with few or no ill effects. However, when a couple, both possessing the sickle cell trait, produce a child, the child will suffer the full effects of sickle cell anemia.

A possible reason for the high incidence of sickle cell trait among African populations is that the trait brings with it an increased resistance to malaria. This beneficial aspect is negated when two trait-possessing individuals produce offspring debilitated, perhaps fatally, by sickle cell anemia.

There is no cure for sickle cell anemia. However, treatment that may include drug therapy and blood transfusions has enabled some sufferers to lead long and relatively independent lives.

SIDEROSIS See PNEUMOCONIOSES

SILICATE

A semi-permanent filling material, silicate is used primarily in the anterior teeth because of its color-matching qualities.

SILICOSIS See PNEUMOCONIOSES

SIMMONDS' DISEASE

This term is used to describe the condition resulting from the destruction of the anterior pituitary gland either by disease or injury. It is accompanied by wasting of the body musculature, emaciation, generalized weakness, loss of body hair, thinning of the skin, with accompanying yellow coloration, low sex drive, and manifestations of deficiency in the other endocrine organs. It is treated by administration of hormones to replace the deficiencies found in all endocrine organs except the pituitary.

SINUSITIS

The air-containing sinuses of the head, situated around and emptying into the nose, are called the paranasal sinuses. They are lined by mucosa similar to that of the nose itself, but modified and much thinner.

Whenever there is an infection of the nose (such as a cold) the sinus membranes, being continuous with that of the nose, are also affected. This does not mean that every time one has a cold one has sinusitis, for sinusitis refers to retained secretions in the sinuses.

Symptoms. The most common symptom of sinus disease is discharge; head pain is much overrated as a symptom. An acute sinus infection will often give a feeling of weakness and fever.

Treatment. Treatment should be by the physician, who may use antibiotics, nosedrops, and/or drainage of the sinuses.

SKIN, FUNCTION AND STRUCTURE

The skin is not only the largest organ in the body, but also probably has the largest number of different functions, in addition to the pre-eminent one of enveloping and containing all the other organs. Its soft and elastic structure permits voluntary and involuntary motion and at the same time withstands physical trauma. Its highly impermeable outer layer seals off the body from noxious agents in the environment, and yet permits the excretion of sweat and oil for the maintenance of even body temperature by the former and lubrication of the surface by the latter. Its pigment, melanin, protects against actinic radiation, and yet permits sufficient absorption of ultraviolet light to insure the skin's production of vitamin D. The skin protects against excesses of heat and of cold, and gives notice of many forms of danger by its sense of pain. The sense of touch affords communication with the environment and fills a variety of needs, organic and emotional. The immunologic role of the skin (manifest in its reactions to substances conveyed to it directly by application or indirectly by the blood vessels after injection, ingestion, or inhalation) is another facet of its protective function. And probably most impressive of all is the skin's "memory" and "record-keeping," as revealed in the individuality of finger-prints, life-time specific allergic responses, genetic precision of distribution of pigment, hair, and texture, and the reliability of the cells to reproduce seemingly identical cells during the whole span of life.

The skin is made up of three readily identifiable parts: (1) the epidermis which is comprised of the vital stratum germinativum and stratum spinulosum, and the non-vital stratum granulosum, stratum lucidum, and stratum corneum; (2) the cutis which consists of a network of collagenous supporting tissue through which the blood vessels and nerves reach the epidermis; and (3) the subcutaneous layer composed of fat, connective tissue, and interspersed blood vessels and nerves.

The thickness of the epidermis varies considerably in different body sites, depending partially on the thickness of its four component parts. However, the stratum germinativum or basal layer always consists of a single layer of cells, except in disease. The cells of this layer constantly reproduce themselves, and in this layer are found the pigment-forming cells which produce melanin and give the unique and varying color to the skin. The epidermis also contains a varying number of nerve fibrils. This outermost portion of the skin is nourished by fluids derived from the blood vessels of the underlying cutis since there are no blood vessels in the epidermis.

The cutis is also of varying thickness and density. The blood vessel supply is of a dual nature, superficial and deep, and is augmented by a lymphatic system made up largely of "spaces" and few identifiable vessels. The two major types of nerves are seen in the cutis: the autonomic (vegetative) nerves which service the tissues themselves, blood vessels, glands, hairs, and the cerebrospinal nerves (perceptive organ) which convey sensation.

The subcutis, or subcutaneous layer, like the epidermis and the cutis is of varying thickness in different regions of the body. In addition to the blood vessels and nerves which traverse it, the connective tissue network enmeshes clusters of fat which provide padding for absorption of mechanical shock, insulation against heat and cold, and storage for food and water. The apparent difference of distribution of fat in the sexes is probably based on biologic usefulness, a factor of which is undoubtedly its esthetic satisfaction.

Of the same tissue of origin (the ectoderm) as the epidermis, and indeed an extension of epidermal development, are the skin appendages: hair, nails, sweat glands, oil glands.

Hair arises from an invagination—or dipping down—of the epidermis which extends into the cutis, and occasionally into the subcutis, at an oblique angle and is apparent at its emergence at the surface of the skin as the shaft. At its deepest portion, the epidermal lining of the shaft is enlarged to form the bulb in the convexity of which is the nourishing blood vessel network, the hair papilla. The hair-bulb is made up largely of germinating or reproductive cells which undergo cyclic periods of activity and of rest, depending on the type of hair and the area in which the hair is situated. For example, the long hair of the scalp grows for about three years, is loosened and lost when a new active cycle of hair-growth replaces the loosened hair. The rate of growth, the texture of the hair, the color, and the contour are considerably dependent on inherited characteristics.

The portion of the hair contained in the cutis is comprised of an inner root sheath attached to the hair cuticle and an outer root sheath coated by a vitreous (glossy) layer. The entire structure is encased in a dense mass of connective tissue to which are attached strands of "involuntary" muscle (arrectores pilorum), one of the functions of which is to aid in the secretion of the sebaceous glands.

The three types of hair (long, bristle, and lanugo) begin to replace the fetal hair at birth, and the replacement is complete at puberty. But even within the groups, there are apparent and functional differences. The long hair of the scalp differs from that of the beard, the armpits and the pubis; and they each differ from each other. The same is true of the eyelashes, the eyebrows, the hair of external openings of the nose and of the ears. Only the lanugo or downy hair varies little from area to area. Lanugo-like hair is also seen as the first hair growth preceding the appearance of the normal hair in alopecia areata, a disease of complete loss of hair in circumscribed areas.

The color of the hair is largely derived from the pigment melanin present in the shaft and synthesized in the upper portion of the hair bulb.

The sebaceous glands are situated in the upper part of the cutis and secrete sebum (oil) into the hair follicles to which they are attached just beneath the epidermis. Only the sebaceous glands of the border of the lips, the foreskin, and the vaginal labia (mucous membrane surface) are "free" of hair follicle association. The glands, which are grape-like in structure, vary in size inversely with the size of the follicles to which they are attached—a small gland being connected with a large follicle and a large gland being connected with a small one. Over-activity of the se-

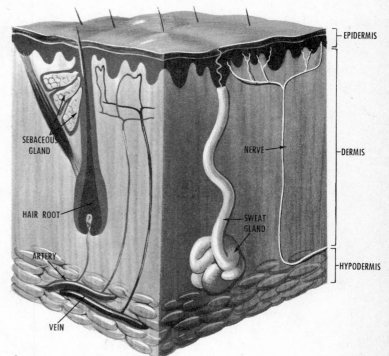

THE SKIN
(CROSS SECTION)

EPIDERMIS

DERMIS

HYPODERMIS

SEBACEOUS GLAND

NERVE

HAIR ROOT

SWEAT GLAND

ARTERY

VEIN

baceous gland, with thickening of the orifice, results in the horny plug (blackhead) of acne; overactivity and occlusion of the orifice results in cyst formation; uncomplicated over-activity of the gland results in excessive oiliness of the skin.

The sweat glands are tubular coiled structures situated chiefly in the lower part of the cutis and occasionally in the subcutis. They extend in a vertical fashion and penetrate the cells of the epidermis to empty at the surface of the skin in very small openings, the pores. Except for the apocrine sweat glands which are found in the armpits and in the pubic area, and which empty into hair follicles, sweat glands are of eccrine nature, that is, the cells secrete sweat without shedding themselves in the secretion. Disturbances of activity of these glands result in local irritation and infection and in systemic reactions resulting from interference with the sweating mechanism.

The nail consists of a nail-plate which is firmly attached to the nail bed except for its outermost portion which has a free, unattached edge. Composed entirely of closely packed keratin and growing continuously, nail is almost colorless except for the shades of color resulting from light reflection on the three different-appearing portions of the nail-plate. The moon-shaped portion closest to the cuticle is the matrix, that portion of the nail which produces the keratin nail substance. Beyond this is the pink-appearing nail bed whose color is attributable to the many blood vessels present in this area. The free edge is white or gray, the color of keratin.

The nail-plate is attached to lateral grooves at the sides and a posterior groove at the base. These are covered by nail-folds, the anterior portion of which is visible and is known as the cuticle.

Changes in the nail often reflect specific alterations in the functioning of the matrix, although distortion or infection can disturb nail growth without matrix involvement.

The blood vessels of the skin, whose primary function is the conveying of necessary materials and removing noxious agents, consist of minute capillaries and only slightly larger venules. Much of the exchange of materials is accomplished by "shunts" or "joinings" of arterioles (slightly larger than capillaries) and venules (A-V shunts).

In addition to the autonomic nerves (motor nerves) which control sweat, the skin is supplied with sensory nerves which afford the skin perception of touch, temperature, and pain. Itching is not a "primary" sensation, but is probably a low order of pain produced by tissue injury of small magnitude.

SKIN HYGIENE Were it not for man-made environmental changes, discussion of skin hygiene would be superfluous. All species of animals have cutaneous covering suited to their needs and evolved, even if somewhat imperfectly, as the result of an unmatchable evolutionary experience. Relatively little can be suggested, for ex-

ample, to care more properly for the fur of animals, or the feathers of birds, or the scales of fish. And relatively little can be suggested for the care of the skin of man that has not already been anticipated by nature, were it not for the problems created by man himself.

In health, the skin is in an exquisite state of balance: with myriads of micro-organisms living saprophytically on its surface; with the gaseous and water content of the enveloping air; with its own lubricating mechanisms giving varying textures to its different areas, depending on the local needs (compare palms and soles with eyelids, armpits, knees, ears); with radiation effects of light (tanning to protect); and environmental temperature, noxious agents, allergens, etc.

The problems arise largely from excesses: excesses of bathing, excesses of sunning, excesses of control of environmental temperature (overheating in winter and overcooling in summer); and excesses of cleansing, lubricating, de-sweating, de-odorizing; and others.

We bathe for many reasons unrelated to the requirements of skin health. We bathe because we are told as children that "cleanliness is next to godliness" (cleanliness of the skin?). We bathe to rid ourselves of normal "animal" odor, having trained our sense of smell to respond to man-made, perfume odors, or at worst, to no odor at all. We bathe to maintain a status symbol of affluence (being able to afford the plumbing, the time, and cosmetic accoutrement of the bath). We bathe to remove the stigma of the soil of labor.

But bathing does have merit. A bath supplies privacy and relaxation which are not only pleasant but also often therapeutic. Bathing cleanses the skin of air-borne industrial contaminants, the grime of urban and commercial areas, the dust of arid areas. Modern soaps are designed for frequent bathing and are not usually irritating to the normal skin. Sometimes soap-substitutes or super-fatted soaps may be necessary even for skin not obviously disturbed. Excessive drying of the skin from bathing can be modified by the use of water-softeners or bath oils, especially in areas of hard-water supply. The use of after-bath oils is unnecessary except in areas prone to dryness (shins, arms, ankles), and in cases of generalized dryness unrelieved by specific therapy. Excessive oiliness is usually confined to the face and can be controlled with frequent washing and with the use of astringents.

The frequency of hair-washing is a matter of individual taste. In most climates, weekly shampoos serve to cleanse the hair of accumulated oil and dust; but more frequent washing is not harmful. Hair pomades, waving solutions, dyes, sprays, and the like do not affect hair growth. They can cause damage to the hair, the scalp, and the surrounding skin under circumstances of excessive use (breaking of hair) or allergic sensitization (eruption of the skin and scalp and occasionally burn-like irritation from prolonged application). Mechanical devices (curlers, clips, rubber bands, brushes) can cause breaking of hair; but the damage is only to the portion of the hair that was injured and does not affect the basic growth of the hair. The wearing of wigs does not seem to alter the growth or texture of the natural hair. (See also HOME NURSING CARE.)

Sun-bathing is undeservedly popular. Notwithstanding the attractiveness of a "tan" and the luxurious circumstances under which it is acquired, no certain benefits accrue from the deliberate exposure of adults to the sun, other than the enforced rest necessary to the achieving of the desired result. Actinic radiation (sun or sunlamp) causes an aging of the skin in excess of that of the chronologic age and hastens deterioration of the skin, with re-

sultant keratoses and skin cancer in susceptible individuals. Limited sun-bathing can be enjoyed and a sense of well-being can be achieved without serious ill effects even in the fair-complexioned if the exposures are not too long or repeated too often.

Sweating is variously managed by the wearing of porous and absorptive clothing, the use of local antiperspirants, and the oral administration of sweat-inhibitors (Banthine®) in aggravated cases. Associated "strong" body odor is relieved by frequent bathing, avoidance of strong perfumes to which the body odor can cling, restriction of odor-producing foods (and consequent restriction of their excretion in sweat), removal of the hair of the armpits (and a consequent removal of resident odor-producing bacteria), the use of deodorants, and the use of pleasant perfume odors to alter or displace remnant unpleasant body odor.

Hand lotions are widely used and are often necessary for prevention of hand irritations resulting from occupational (both gainful and non-gainful) exposures to abrasives, cleansers, oils, etc. A high percentage of hand eczemas are the result of repeated washing and inadequate drying of the hands. The busy housewife, the pediatric nurse, the dentist, the bartender, are all likely to have constantly moist hands as they go from chore to chore meticulously washing but not taking the time to dry their hands. The skin tolerates wetness (total immersion) or dryness, but reacts to remnant moisture which interferes with the mechanism of sweating and evaporation. Especially in cold, wet climates, careful drying of hands, the use of mild soaps, hand lotions for excessive dryness, and gloves on exposure to the outdoors will be helpful in preventing eczema of the hands.

The large array of wrinkle creams, youth-giving lotions, mud packs, fresh-

454

eners, and restorers are of no known merit in retarding aging changes in skin.

SKIN TAGS   These small outpouchings of skin occur chiefly on the neck, upper chest, armpits, and occasionally the face of middleaged women, but not infrequently also in men. The bases of these lesions are thread-like and often do not bleed when cut off. While the usual tag is skin-colored, some are variously brown-colored. Other than being irritated or torn from the skin (with some bleeding), no serious consequences result from leaving them untreated. Simple excision or cautery is useful in this unimportant, but occasionally very disagreeable, condition.

SKIN TESTS   The skin and related organs of a person with suspected allergies may be used for testing various substances. If the allergen is a food or an inhalant (dust, dander, pollen) the scratch, intra-dermal, conjunctival, inhalation, or electrode tests may be used. If the allergen is of a contact nature (chemicals, cosmetics, toilet articles, jewelry) then patch testing is done (see ALLERGIES, DIAGNOSIS OF).

SLEEP - DISTURBANCES   Disturbances in sleeping are usually more tiring and upsetting to a child's parents than to the child itself. The newborn baby is usually wakeful—frequently at night—because of hunger; but from the age of two to three months on he is a good sleeper unless he is allergic to milk, has been fed some gas-forming food, or has pain such as an earache. There will be another period of wakefulness at about ten to fifteen months, one which may well be due to the cutting of teeth. The child will often suffer from ammoniacal diaper rash and awaken because of the pain when salty urine touches the open sores. Again, a child will often waken at about two years of age and cry out for no discernible cause.

The older child will sometimes sleep restlessly or waken if he is suffering from worms. Pinworms produce nocturnal anal or vaginal itching.

A very rare situation can cause a child to cry at night because he is having "a spell" or peculiar type of fit; a brain-wave test will be needed to determine this. Occasionally a baby or child needs merely to be put in a different bed in another room away from parents or siblings—and the problem is solved.

Parents may make the mistake of rushing into the baby's room at the first cry, picking him up, and trying to soothe him. The child that is not sick soon gets to expect and even demand this treatment every time he awakens.

SLEEPING AND DREAMING.   Studies over the past 20 years reveal that dreaming is a constant feature of normal sleep. It can be identified in the sleeping subject by picking up potentials generated by rapid eye-muscle movements (REM). REM sleep recurs approximately every 90 minutes throughout the night. Subjects awakened during the REM phase are generally able to give details of the dream. Further, if they are repeatedly awakened at the onset of REM, daytime irritability and concentration difficulties occur, and succeeding sleep is marked by greater than usual amounts of dreaming. These observations establish a role for dreaming as part of normal central nervous system functioning.

SLEEPING SICKNESS   See ENCEPHALITIS

SLEEPWALKING (SOMNAMBULISM)
Sleepwalking and other actions performed by a person while apparently asleep are evidence that certain brain areas become inhibited in sleep while others continue to function. Talking while asleep and somnambulism frequently represent automatic acting-out of dream contents. Such symp-

toms are more commonly observed in conflict-filled persons, the behavior being understood as symbolic of underlying unconscious distress.

SLIPPED CAPITAL FEMORAL EPIPHYSIS
This disease is an adolescent hip malady showing much the same symptoms as Perthes' disease. What happens is that the growth-center (or epiphysis) of the bone becomes loosened from its attachment to the shaft of the femur and slowly slips into an abnormal position. Since this malady develops in children during puberty, it is thought to be related in some manner to the sex hormones, but no definitive cause has been established. Slipping of the femoral head occurs very gradually, and the child can rarely recall an injury to the hip. If untreated, this condition also leads to degenerative arthritis of the hip. Hip-nailing is usually required to hold the femoral head and neck aligned so that no further slipping occurs.

SLIPPED DISK
This is one of the most common causes of "low back pain." The vertebrae most often involved are the fourth and fifth lumbar, which have undergone strain and degeneration with resultant displacement of their intervertebral disk. Onset may be acute and sudden (for example, while bending over to lift a weight); it may be gradual, particularly in degenerative vertebral changes when the disk protrudes more and more. Disk protrusion is known as herniated disk.

Symptoms. Pain is the dominant sign, and is one-sided, indicating the direction in which the disk protrudes. In its common location, a disk impinges on the rootlets of the body's largest nerve, the sciatic —a condition formerly called sciatica. There is compensatory muscle spasm in all cases, and the sufferer "favors" the painful side. There is tenderness all along the sciatic nerve down to the lower leg.

If the patient is asked to stand on tiptoe the pain is immediately aggravated. There are several tests that clinch the diagnosis.

Treatment. During the acute phase, complete bed rest is indicated. Heat (electric pads, hot water bottles, etc.), analgesics (aspirin, codeine, etc.), and gentle massage are prescribed. The acute attack usually subsides in a couple of weeks at which time attention is paid to correction of postural defects, and a supporting brace or corset may be needed. Sometimes traction is used in recalcitrant or repetitive cases. Surgery is resorted to when the acute attack does not yield to the usual treatment or when attacks tend to be repetitive. Operative intervention is not always successful the first time, and the procedure may have to be repeated two, even three, times. The operation consists of the removal of the protruding disk, and the vertebrae may be fused.

SMALL INTESTINE
The small intestine is a thin-walled muscular tube about one inch in diameter and approximately twenty feet in length. It is divided into three parts, the duodenum, the jejunum, and ileum.

SMALLPOX
Smallpox is rarely seen in this country today because of widespread smallpox vaccination but may be serious when it does occur.

Symptoms. The incubation period of smallpox is seven days. The disease appears suddenly with a high fever, backache, and prostration. After two or three days the fever abates and numerous pustules appear over the whole body, especially the face. The disease drags on for days, the patients are usually very sick, and the death-rate is high, though not as high as it once was. There is usually scarring of the face.

Treatment. The best treatment of smallpox is prevention, and the wise parent will insist that his child have the benefit of smallpox vaccination in the first year of life. If someone contracts the disease, skilled nursing care is necessary because it is highly contagious and complications are so common.

SMEAR (VAGINAL, CANCER, PAPANI-COLAOU, OR "PAP" SMEAR) This is the collection of cells from the vagina and the neck of the womb (cervix) of a woman, and the examination of these cells for the diagnosis of cancer. It is a very simple, inexpensive, and accurate means of detecting early cancer of the cervix or the womb. It is also useful for the study of female hormones. Similiar studies can be done on the sputum, urine, gastric juice, and other secretions for the detection of cancer of the lungs, kidneys, stomach, etc.

SMEGMA This term refers to the cheesy substance which collects between the foreskin (prepuce) and the glans penis in the male, and between the labia minora about the clitoris in the female. It is composed of the secretions of the glands in the area, together with shed-off cells.

SMOKING The use of tobacco is a widespread habit to which the human race has been exposed for many centuries. It was first introduced to the Western world in the 16th century by the Spanish explorers of America, then rerouted to England and Europe. It was first used mainly in the form of pipe-smoking, quickly spreading thoughout the Western world. For the past seventy years, cigarettes have steadily replaced other forms of tobacco and have simultaneously produced an ever-rising increase of tobacco consumption. It also seems that cigarettes made the smoking habit socially more acceptable, thereby opening the way to women and minors.

Until the early 1950's, smoking was considered and discussed mainly in terms of its social and psychological implications. Since that time, increased emphasis has been placed on its potential harm to physical health, particularly as a contributing cause of lung cancer, chronic bronchitis, and coronary heart disease. The case against cigarette smoking has been overwhelmingly established in the statistical sense, but demonstration of a direct cause-and-effect relationship is still lacking. The best assembled summaries of presently available information on this subject can be found in the reports by the English Royal College of Physicians (Smoking and Health, 1962) and the U.S. Surgeon General's Report on Smoking and Health, (January, 1963).

About 300 different compounds have been identified in the tobacco leaf and about 260 in the tobacco smoke. Due to changes produced by combustion (cigarettes burn at about 1120° F.), only 98 compounds have been found in both leaves and smoke. This shows at a glance the enormous complexity of trying to extricate the one or more agents responsible for smoking damage. Of the isolated compounds, 16 substances have the potential capacity of producing cancer in some animals. Tobacco smoke contains gases, volatile compounds, and solid matter. No filter can completely remove all particulate matter. About 50 per cent of inhaled smoke is retained in the respiratory system, mostly in the lung.

The physiological effects of smoking can be divided into local—upon the respiratory system—and general—upon the body, as a whole, after being absorbed. Local effects are mostly characterized by increase in the resistance to airflow in and out of the lung; stimulation of mucus-secretion; and delay of mucus-removal. The latter is the result of a slowing down in the beating of hair-like structures (cilia) located in the inner lining of the bronchial tubes, whose function is to remove normal mucus and to trap and expel foreign material entering with inspiration. The net result of these effects is to create a state of chronic irritation which perpetuates itself, particularly in heavy smokers. This irritation in turn is believed to initiate, by hitherto unknown mechanisms, the structural changes which may lead to chronic bronchitis or cancer.

The general effects of smoking are mainly due to the absorption of nicotine. The amount of nicotine which can be recovered from the mainstream smoke of an average cigarette is about 2 mg.; of this, the amount absorbed into the lung varies from 10 to 90 per cent, depending on the smoker's habits (depth of inhaling, breath-holding time, etc.). The main effects of the absorbed nicotine are transient increases in blood pressure and heart-rate, and decreases in skin temperature and urinary volume. The appetite is usually reduced.

There is very little exact information on the psychological effects of smoking. Smoking often relieves tension and anxiety and in some individuals provides pleasure. The pattern of smoking at different ages in the two sexes does not throw light on motivation. Studies of schoolchildren and young adults show a significant correlation between their smoking rates and the smoking habits of parents and siblings. The different ways of enjoying tobacco (cigars, cigarettes, water-pipe) bear a distinct relationship to prevalent cultural habits. Very little is known about the factors that lead people to discontinue smoking, but it seems evident that awareness and intelligent appraisal of the hazards involved are the most potent motivations for discontinuance of the habit. This decision is more frequently taken by professional and skilled workers than by unskilled manual laborers.

There is no evidence that smoking promotes physical health. On the contrary, as stated previously, the statistically overwhelming evidence indicates that smoking is a causative factor in, or the most likely cause of, the worldwide increase in deaths from lung cancer; that it is an important predisposing factor in chronic bronchitis; that it increases the risk of dying from coronary heart disease, and accentuates the symptoms of vascular disease of the limbs; and that it has an adverse effect on healing of gastric or duodenal ulcers. Cigar and pipe smoking carry less risk than cigarette smoking, probably because the smoke is not inhaled; however, local lesions of the mouth and lips are more frequent. It is also important to point out that the mentioned risks of smoking are proportional to the amount of smoking. For all practical purposes, anything above twenty cigarettes daily is considered heavy smoking.

Although many smokers may never experience any serious ill effect or shortening of life-span as the result of smoking, there is no sure way to identify the minority who will be affected. Full protection for all requires preventive measures of general application. Since at present we cannot yet identify the substance or substances in tobacco smoke which are deleterious to health, no claim of safety can be made on the basis of modified cigarette-tobacco or filters.

SOCIOPATHIC REACTIONS These are personality states formerly referred to as moral imbecility or as psychopathic personality and characterized by a wide range of anti-social behavior combined with an otherwise relatively intact personality.

Symptoms. The sociopath tries to "take" what people normally have to earn. Sociopaths show a lifetime history of lying, stealing, fraud, deceit, sexual promiscuity, alcoholism, and general personal irresponsibility—usually not corrected by punishment or experience.

Sociopathic reactions are not hereditary, since it is rare for more than one case to appear in a family. There is no evidence of underlying organic disease, except that a small percentage of cases shows abnormal brain waves, possibly indicating an underlying diffuse brain disease. Most sociopathic reactions appear to be learned, as various types of personal and social conditioning factors reinforce sociopathic tendencies. Thus, some particularly attractive children tend to be spoiled by parents, teachers, and other adults, all of whom allow the child to get his own way and escape normal punishment and corrective measures. Sociopaths in any community tend to flock together, teaching each other new methods of "getting away with murder" and encouraging each other in subtle ways to prey on the rest of the population.

Treatment. To date, only a few states have developed special resources for the treatment of sociopaths, who properly belong neither in prison, since their trouble is psychological, nor in mental hospitals, since they are not mentally ill in the ordinary sense of the term. Only a few psychiatrists have claimed much success in treating sociopathic reactions. Contrary to former opinion, which maintained that such cases did not show any normal anxiety or ability to learn from experience, the sociopath is highly adept at learning methods of swindling the public and of avoiding punishment.

Most sociopaths show improvement only when they can be led to recognize that their activities are too self-defeating and that the cost in mental anguish is not worth the gains obtained.

Many young people who are regarded as "black sheep" in early life tend to become more law-abiding as increasing age and experience result in a better understanding of themselves and of the costs of their anti-social behavior. One of the great psychiatric problems of the future is to develop special methods and resources in the community for diagnosing and treating young sociopaths before such patterns become too deeply ingrained.

SODIUM Sodium is an essential mineral that plays a critical role in normal electrolyte metabolism. The average intake of sodium in the diet varies widely: from two to perhaps 15 grams of sodium chloride (common salt) per day. Intake depends to a large extent upon the amount of table salt added to the food and is a matter of taste. Some salt is present in foods. Salt is excreted mainly in the urine, and although its content in the body depends largely on the intake by mouth and output in the urine, its concentration in the blood is regulated in part by hormones. The adrenal glands, for example, produce a salt-retaining hormone.

Because the kidneys normally are efficient sodium conservers, sodium deficiency practically never develops due to low sodium intake. If the kidneys are diseased or if there is excessive loss from the bowels in diarrhea or through the skin in sweating, there may be excessive loss of salt and sodium deficiency may develop. Adrenal disease (with accompanying loss of salt-regulating hormone) allows wastage of sodium. Such a deficit is accompanied by dehydration or acidosis. Excessive fatigue, muscle cramps, and mental confusion are characteristic of sodium deficiency. Sodium excess is accompanied by overhydration and edema.

SOMATIC SYMPTOMS Somatic symptoms refer to physical symptoms of bodily dysfunctions.

SORE THROAT Sore throat has many causes, the most common of which is acute pharyngitis (without membrane-formation). This may be caused by viral diseases such as the common cold or influenza, or by noninfectious inflammations resulting from inhalation of irritant substances, excessive dryness or ingestion of very hot foods or liquids. All of these are self-limited conditions, disappearing when the offending mechanism no longer causes pharyngeal infection or irritation. Infections of any part of Waldeyer's ring can also cause sore throat. (It should be noted that sore throat can also cause ear pain because of a common nerve supply.)

Treatment. The organisms causing syphilis and tuberculosis, as well as certain fungi, can also produce throat infections. These are not common and require special diagnostic procedures. Pharyngitis and tonsillitis can also become chronic and manifest themselves by persistent sore throat—as can certain blood diseases. Cancer frequently first shows itself as a chronic sore throat and/or a lump in the neck. A sore throat should not be neglected. If lasting more than two weeks, it should be seen by a physician. Bed rest and fluids are helpful for a sore throat. Hot salt water gargles are soothing. Further details for treatment are given under the specific ailment.

SPASTICITY Literally a drawing in, spasticity is increased tension or tonus of a muscle or group of muscles. It is marked by increase in deep reflex response, often with clonus (movements characterized by alternating contraction and relaxation, commonly referred to as clonic spasm), and a partial or incomplete loss of voluntary control. The examining physician determines the presence of clonus by suddenly putting a muscle on the stretch which, if there is spasticity, results in rapid, involuntary reflex and irregular contractions.

SPEECH DISORDERS There are three categories of speech disorder. The most common is the "functional" type; here the child appears to be quite normal in mentality and in structure, but his speech is abnormal. The stutterer, the stammerer, the lisper are examples. The second type of speech problem is seen in the child whose speech defect is due to some anatomical defect: a cleft or short palate, enlarged tonsils and adenoids, etc. In the third type there is some abnormality of the nervous system, such as mental retardation, or some forms of epilepsy; the speech may be slurred, garbled, or otherwise distorted. Then too, the deaf child may be unable to speak, since he has been unable to hear spoken words and imitate them. "Tongue-tie" may also be a cause—if, however, a child can touch the tip of the tongue to the lips the tongue is not tied and the frenulum (the membrane attached under the tongue to the floor of the mouth) need not be clipped.

If the child does not have a vocabulary of at least five understandable words by the age of two years, an effort should be made to determine in which category his speech problem lies. Much progress had been made in recent years in diagnosing and treating these handicapped children. One very common speech anomaly will disappear if parents recognize it for what it is; stammering in the three-to-four-year-old, as "I—I—I—I—go—go—go—go—out." If wise parents realize this is a normal part of maturing, they will pay no attention, and the trouble will disappear within a few months. If they draw the child's attention to it by making him repeat his remarks correctly, the child may become so upset that an otherwise insignificant deviation may become a permanent speech problem.

SPERM(ATOZOA) The normal spermatozoon is a microscopic structure consisting of an oval-shaped head and long tail, somewhat resembling a tadpole. The spermatozoa are able to propel themselves about in a liquid medium, and after ejaculation are able to travel into the body of the uterus. It is important for fertility that there be a normal number of spermatozoa present in the ejaculate; adult males should have at least fifty million sperm per cubic centimeter. (The normal average count is one hundred twenty million per cubic centimeter.) A few of the sperm may be abnormal in shape or size, or may lack the head or part of the tail.

SPHINCTER MUSCLE The anal sphincter is a well-developed circular muscle in the anal canal that closes the passage until such time as defecation is to take place; conscious effort causes the muscle to relax and allows the stool to pass. Inflammatory conditions of the mucous-membrane lining of the canal may cause a spasm of the sphincter and make passage difficult. Conditions such as hemorrhoids, fissures, and rectal abscesses are also common causes. Chronic rectal conditions may give rise to excessive scar tissue in the area and cause permanent narrowing of the anal canal. The ensuing straining necessary to force the stool past the region may then cause additional irritation, worsening the condition and causing further constipation. Surgery is sometimes necessary under these circumstances.

SPIDER BITES (BLACK WIDOW) The black widow spider (*Latrodectus mactans*), resident in all the Americas, is encountered most frequently in dark, dry places (under rocks, in trash piles, basements, tree roots), is jet black with orange-red markings, and has an hourglass pattern on the abdomen.

Symptoms. The site of the bite becomes painful, swollen, and occasionally blue-black from hemorrhage. Generalized symptoms develop rapidly and are those of shock and toxic poisoning (vomiting, sweating, aching of muscles, abdominal cramps, faint generalized rash). Not all of these symptoms may be present in each case. Suspicion that the bite is by a spider, and appearance of any of the symptoms of shock or toxicity, make treatment imperative.

Treatment. Treatment for shock and administration of the specific antiserum are highly effective. Though the symptoms are formidable, reports of fatalities are rare.

SPIDER NEVUS Occurring at any age, but not infrequently also in early childhood—most commonly on the face—the lesion of spider nevus consists of a pinhead-size enlargement of a blood vessel, surrounded by very small tentacle-like vessels. Sometimes the central raised vessel can be seen to pulsate.

The occurrence of lesions on the chest and neck is often noted during pregnancy and after sunburn in susceptible patients. Although spontaneous disappearance of the lesions is possible, it is more likely that they will persist and that new ones will appear during subsequent pregnancies and on subsequent episodes of sunburn. The condition is also not uncommonly noted in patients with diseases of the liver.

Treatment. The lesions can be obliterated with electrocautery or with electrolysis. It may be necessary to repeat either procedure several times for final removal of the vessel.

SPINAL ACCESSORY NERVES The two spinal accessory (or eleventh cranial) nerves control the trapezius and the sternomastoid (neck and high-back) muscles. Injury to these nerves results in weakness or paralysis of these muscles. The sternomastoid muscles rotate the head and the trapezius muscles elevate the shoulders.

SPINAL CORD The spinal cord is enclosed within the bony spine and is protected by meningeal coverings and the cerebrospinal fluid. It is arbitrarily divided from top to bottom into cervical, thoracic, lumbar, and sacral portions. At each segmental level, the posterior roots bring sensory impulses from the sensory

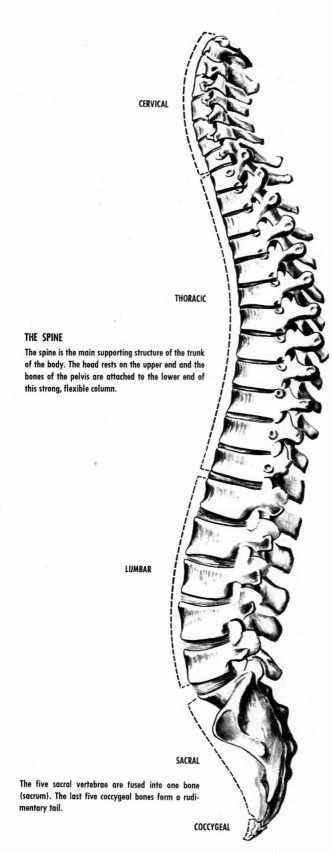

CERVICAL

THORACIC

THE SPINE

The spine is the main supporting structure of the trunk of the body. The head rests on the upper end and the bones of the pelvis are attached to the lower end of this strong, flexible column.

LUMBAR

SACRAL

The five sacral vertebrae are fused into one bone (sacrum). The last five coccygeal bones form a rudimentary tail.

COCCYGEAL

nerve endings into the cord, and the anterior roots carry motor stimuli to skeletal muscles.

At the "core" of the spinal cord is the grey matter consisting of nerve cells. This is surrounded by white matter which contains columns of nerve fibers. Some of the closely packed fibers carry impulses from the brain to the spinal cord, while others carry impulses from the spinal cord to the brain.

If the spinal cord is severely injured, the isolated portion of the cord below the level of the injury is capable of a variety of limited reflex activities. However, voluntary motor control from the brain is completely lost, and transmission of sensory impulses to the brain is blocked. If injury to the spine occurs at the level of the chest or abdomen, the patient is paralyzed in the legs, and bladder and bowel control is lost. If the injury occurs in the neck, the arms as well as the legs are paralyzed. Compression of the cord by tumor results in similar loss of function below that level. Some disorders involve only selected portions of the cord. For example, multiple sclerosis involves only white matter; whereas the virus of poliomyelitis damages the cells in the anterior grey matter.

SPLENIC DISORDERS   The spleen is an organ weighing, on the average, from three to five pounds, situated in the left upper abdomen, behind and below the stomach. It is made up of vascular components, reticuloendothelial and lymphoid elements, and connective (supportive) tissue. The reticuloendothelial system is that part of the blood's cellular elements concerned with "policing" and "cleaning" up the bloodstream and sites of invasion by foreign bodies such as germs; but it does not include the white blood cells.

The spleen destroys blood cells, an activity that is accelerated with splenic enlargement. It also stores up red blood cells. It has the capacity to "pick" de-

462

formed red blood cells out of the circulation. The spleen, it seems, plays some role in bodily defense against infection and has a function, as yet not determined, in protecting the whole blood-manufacturing process. The extent to which the spleen influences bone marrow function is not yet known.

The spleen is often involved in blood diseases, such as leukemia, anemia, and Hodgkin's disease. There are also splenic disorders due to pathology of the organ itself or localized pathology, such as cancer of the pancreas and high blood pressure in the liver's circulatory system (the portal system).

Two blood disorders in which the spleen is enlarged are Felty's syndrome and Banti's disease.

Banti's disease is a disease characterized by enlargement of the spleen, lowering of the white blood cell and platelet count, and cirrhosis of the liver. It is caused by increased congestion in the circulatory system in and about the liver, by clotting formation within the liver's circulatory system, or by cirrhosis of the liver.

Felty's syndrome is a disorder characterized by rheumatoid arthritis, enlarged spleen, and a lowered white blood cell count. Its cause is unknown.

Lowered white and/or red cell counts with enlargement of the spleen are observed in several other conditions for which surgical removal of the spleen is performed if the disease itself and the patient's condition do not make the operation unwise. On the other hand, splenectomy is rarely done in lymphomatous diseases such as Hodgkin's disease and leukemia.

"SPLIT PERSONALITY"

Cases of multiple personality are typically described as occurring in hysteria. Multiple personalities are explained psychologically as dissociation reactions, in which strong conflicting incompatible impulses or complexes in the unconscious struggle for expression and alternately gain outlet in the form of apparently incompatible personality reactions.

Symptoms. In states of multiple personality the same person may alternately act out two or even three different personalities, calling himself by different names and behaving like several different people.

Treatment. As in all psychoneurotic disorders, the preferred treatment is psychoanalytic study of the repressed unconscious impulses or conflicts underlying the dissociation reactions.

SPOROTRICHOSIS

Caused by the fungus *Sportichum schenckii,* this deep mycosis is usually produced by infection at the site of skin injury which has been in contact with infested soil or wood. The fungal spores are found all over the world but enjoy their most active growth on timber.

Symptoms. The infection is most commonly present on the hands because of their availability for the trauma necessary for the organism's entry into the skin. The lesions are usually multiple, hard, nodular, and ulcerated. The regional lymph nodes can become enlarged, and in rare instances the disease can become disseminated. When the site of the infection is the face, the disease can be mistaken for an ordinary pustular infection except for its persistence and progression.

Treatment. Iodides taken by mouth in appropriate dosage are specifically effective. If laboratory facilities are not readily available for examination of the fungus, a trial course of iodide medication can be given. If the treatment results in a cure, the diagnosis can be presumed to have been correct even without laboratory confirmation.

STAPHYLOCOCCUS

The staphylococcus is a bacterium which in the last decades has become resistant to the usual antibiotics, making it difficult to control—especially in hospitals, where it is known as "hospital staph." In some families where this germ has been introduced by one method or another, it will pass from one member to another, producing a variety of infections over the course of months or even years. Thus, one individual may have boils, another a furuncle, and a third a paronychia (infection about the nail). Still another will have a sty, then impetigo; while a staphylococcus pneumonia, with abscess-formation, may put yet a fifth member into the hospital. The germ may also cause tonsilitis and middle-ear infection.

It is now thought that one particular member of the family harbors the "staph" in his nose (where it is warm and wet) and every time he exhales, blows out germs to infect someone else. In hospitals it has been known to float about in the air, invade even clean surgical wounds and, despite careful technique, cause wound-infection and abscess-formation.

Treatment. More than routine home cleanliness is necessary to eradicate "staph" infection. The family must bathe with special surgical soaps (showers are better than bathing in the tub); and an antibiotic ointment must be used on every cut, scratch, and sore, as well as put into every member's nose daily to kill whatever germs are harbored there. These rigid measures are taken for a month, then relaxed. If the infections return as before, usually the next step is to give the victims a series of staphylococcus-vaccine shots. The theory is that these shots will immunize the patients to the bacterium and make them more resistant. Treatment of the individual infections listed above is determined by the physician, on the basis of their nature and severity.

STERILITY AND INFERTILITY   The term sterility implies the inability to conceive because of abnormalities in the male, the female, or both; while the term infertility means the inability to produce a viable fetus—either because of sterility, or because of factors operating after a pregnancy has taken place. In order to use the terms correctly, then, we should speak of a sterile person or an infertile couple.

A popular misconception has existed over the years that the wife is usually the one responsible for the infertility. This is certainly not true, since in almost 50 percent of the cases the husbands are at fault; therefore, the investigation of an infertile couple should concentrate on both husband and wife. Strangely enough, the male is often resistant to this approach, yet investigation of the husband is much easier and may save many long and unnecessary tests on the wife.

In the woman, there may be either primary difficulties in ovulation (discharge of the egg from the surface of the ovary), or blockage in the passage through the fallopian tubes due to adhesions or infections; there may also be abnormalities in the womb (uterus). Often an imbalance of hormone-regulation prevents proper implantation of the egg (ovum) in the cavity of the uterus. In some instances, lack of adequate supplies of thyroid hormone is responsible.

In the male, sterility may be the result of three general classes of misfunction: (1) inability of the testes to produce live or efficient sperm—which in turn may be due to such factors as injury, age, thyroid or pituitary hormone deficiency, mumps, nutritional deficiencies, or exposure to radiation; (2) blockage of the tract through which the sperm move, resulting from infection or after surgery performed relating to the vas deferens, the seminal vesicles, the urethra, the prostate gland, or the epididymis; and (3) defective depositing of sperm within the female genital tract—which may be caused either by impotence or by anatomical abnormalities of the male organ.

In general, before a viable baby is born to a couple the following prerequisites must be fulfilled: A woman must have ovaries that are able to produce eggs (ova); and a husband must have sperm sufficient in quality and quantity, and must be able to ejaculate without difficulty at relatively frequent intervals—depositing the ejaculate through normal sexual intercourse in the vagina. From here, the sperm should be able to travel through the womb, meet the egg, and fertilize it. Severe abnormalities in the structure and the number of spermatozoa (this latter usually runs as high as the billions in each ejaculated specimen) will result in infertility. As far as the female is concerned, in addition to being able to ovulate regularly she should have a normal vagina and possess normal secretions from the glands of the cervix (neck of the womb) which will allow the sperm to penetrate and ascend to the womb itself. The uterus must be normal and the fallopian tubes open, so that the sperm can meet the egg for conception.

After conception, the female should manufacture adequate hormones (ovarian and other) to support the pregnancy. The fetus and the afterbirth (placenta) should develop without any major congenital abnormalities, and the pregnancy should be closely traced by an experienced specialist, every deviation from normal being corrected. Finally, the mother should be well-attended throughout the labor and delivery. If all these requisites are met, the couple will be rewarded with the happy arrival of the newborn.

In short, the miracle of reproduction is far from being a simple process. The best witnesses of this are those unfortunate couples who go through months and years of medical tests and financial sacrifices for a dream that often never materializes.

Treatment. Since the causes of infertility are so numerous, the methods of treatment are proportionately varied. Existing medical complications should be treated accordingly; deficiencies in hormones of one or more glands should be rectified; infections should be treated with antibiotics; and anatomical anomalies in either the male or female should be corrected surgically. The

investigation, diagnosis, and treatment of an infertile couple usually requires the cooperation of several specialists: the gynecologist, urologist, internist, surgeon, radiologist, the laboratory technicians specializing in endocrinological tests, and so forth.

STERILIZATION, SURGICAL   An operation for the sterilization of a couple may be done either on the male or on the female. Although the operation is much simpler when performed on the male (a vasectomy—the severing of the spermatic cord), the vanity of the "strong sex" is so well established that even to suggest such a measure is not well tolerated in our present society. On the other hand, there are some definite advantages to the operation being performed on the female, since it is usually combined with plastic repair of the vagina, which undergoes relaxation after repeated childbirth. Sterilization of the female is done either by tying (ligation) of the fallopian tubes, or by hysterectomy (removal of the womb). Either of these procedures can be done vaginally or abdominally, and the choice will depend on the individual case. It is the belief of this author that when the patient has no special objections to the procedure, hysterectomy is the operation of choice for sterilization. Actually, when the real facts are explained to patients of average intelligence, hysterectomy is chosen by most of them. Since the only proven function of the womb is childbearing, once the decision in favor of sterilization is made, the only role a sterile uterus can play is to be the seat of cancer, bleeding (normal and abnormal), prolapse, dysmenorrhea, and many other undesirable complications.

STEROID HORMONES   These chemical substances consist of four rings of carbon atoms with attachments of hydrogen and oxygen. Carbon-containing side chains are present in some compounds. Metabolic reactions in the adrenal glands and the sex glands are responsible for the manufacture of steroid hormones; their configurations are characteristic of the particular gland, and each substance is able to perform a distinctive function within the body.

The chief steroid hormone groupings are the androgens (male hormones), and estrogens (female hormones); the progestins, which are responsible for maintaining pregnancy; and the products of the adrenal cortex (including cortisone). Steroid hormones are available for use in therapy by injection and by mouth. Combinations of progestins and estrogens are used as "birth control pills," and some of the adrenal-cortex hormones are used in inflammations and disease of connective tissue.

STILLBORN   Under a variety of pathological circumstances, some of them known and some unknown, a baby of considerable size may die inside the mother's womb. It is then called stillborn. If the baby remains dead inside the uterus for more than five or six weeks, it is liable to cause certain defects in the clotting mechanism of the mother's blood (hypofibrinogenemia). Special blood tests should be frequently performed for the early detection of such abnormality; in such cases the womb should be evacuated before severe bleeding complications appear.

STONES (CALCULI)   Stone formation in body fluids is hastened by stagnation of heavily saturated solutions such as are found in the gallbladder, urinary system, pancreas, and salivary glands. Chronic infection may also hasten their formation. Because of their mechanical interference with normal flow of fluids they can cause severe symptoms; the pain associated with gallstones and kidney stones in particular can be very severe. If the stones become impacted they must be removed, but often they will pass spontaneously. (See also GALLSTONES, PAROTID GLAND; PANCREAS).

STRESS   In the course of athletic activity or work, the body may be subjected to physical forces that strain muscles, internal organs, bones, and joints. The body may also have its normal metabolic functioning and internal physiology disrupted by sickness, weather changes, injury, and emotional tension. All such influences can be considered forms of stress.

When stress is experienced for prolonged periods, or when the stress is sudden and overwhelming, disorders such as ulcer, asthma, migraine, colitis, constipation, cardiac dysfunction, and hypertension may result. Mental instability leading to schizophrenia may also be induced by physical or emotional stress.

The body possesses mechanisms that attempt to deal with stress. In preparation for stressful situations the adrenal glands produce the hormones epinephrine and norepinephrine, which act to increase cardiac activity, as well as to send an increased blood supply to muscle tissue and to promote the use of stored glucose. When stress occurs over an extended period of time, the body's energy reserves may be extended and the stress-triggered mechanisms may become less responsive. An individual's physical and mental health is then in jeopardy. Stress from various causes may also affect the fertility of both men and women.

Studies concerning "life events" that cause the most stress indicate that loss of a spouse or other family member, imprisonment, childbirth, personal injury, divorce, and unemployment are among the most stressful situations individuals can encounter. Urban life is also often associated with a lifestyle that is stressful—including physical stresses connected with air and noise pollution and the psychological stresses of career competition, traffic congestion, and anxiety about one's personal safety.

Maintaining regular exercise and sleep habits and taking vacations are known to alleviate the fatigue of some forms of stress. Important, too, is the discovery of the true cause of physical and emotional stress, with treatment of the cause, rather than merely focusing on the symptoms. Psychiatric counseling and a complete physical examination may uncover the true origin of undue stress.

STRESS TEST   A diagnostic method used to determine the body's response to physical exertion (stress). Usually involves taking an ECG and other physiological measurements (such as breathing rate and blood pressure) while the patient is exercising—usually jogging on a treadmill, walking up and down a short set of stairs, or pedaling on a stationary bicycle.

"STRETCHMARKS" (STRIAE OF PREGNANCY)   These are pinkish or silvery lines over the skin of the abdomen and the upper thighs, and are probably due to overstretching of the skin because of the enlarged womb.

STROKE   Also called cerebral vascular accident. An impeded blood supply to some part of the brain, generally caused by:

1. A blood clot forming in the vessel (cerebral thrombosis).
2. A rupture of the blood vessel wall (cerebral hemorrhage).
3. A blood clot or other material from another part of the vascular system which flows to the brain and obstructs a cerebral vessel (cerebral embolism).
4. Pressure on a blood vessel, as by a tumor.

STUTTERING AND STAMMERING   Stammering is hesitant, spasmodic speech with interruptions in which no sound is produced. It is regarded as neurotic in origin, with strong emotional and environmental influences. Stuttering is a speech disorder whose chief feature is the repetition of certain consonant sounds in rapid succession. It is also known as "logoclonia." Stuttering is also used synonymously with stammering.

Treatment. The use of amphetamine in the treatment of stammering and stuttering is still undergoing investigation. It seems to be quite effective with mentally retarded children who stammer, but sufficient data are not available to conclude that it is equally beneficial among adults and normal children.

Current therapy is twofold: speech correction and psychotherapy. In the former, the accent is on slowness. That is, the subject is encouraged to speak in an exaggerated and deliberate fashion at first, to the point of breaking words down to individual syllables; later, sentences are marked by prolonged spacing of words. Throughout the National Hospital for Speech Disorders in New York there are signs bearing a single word: SLOW.

STY   A boil (sty) on the lid margin arises because of an infection in one of the glands of the lashes. There is a tendency for the infection to involve successive glands so that the sites occur in "crops."

Symptoms. The eyelid is tender and red until the sty ruptures.

Treatment. Hot compresses applied for ten minutes every hour give comfort. It may be necessary to open the sty surgically when it comes to a head. Generally it is not wise to administer antibiotics either locally or systemically.

SUBDURAL HEMATOMA   A subdural hematoma is a collection of blood in the subdural space of the meninges located between the skull and the surface of the cerebral hemisphere. One-third of subdural hematomas are bilateral. Bleeding is usually related to an external head injury, although the patient and his family may not be able to recall the injury. Rarely, subdural hematomas occur as a complication of an abnormal bleeding tendency. Usually, however, the bleeding occurs as a result of laceration of veins which bridge the meningeal coverings.

Symptoms. Subdural hematomas may

occur acutely within forty-eight hours after a head injury; subacutely from forty-eight hours to two weeks after injury; or chronically from two weeks to many months after injury. The pressure of the subdural hematoma on the brain results in mental confusion, memory defects, weakness, speech disorder, stupor, or other findings of brain dysfunction.

Treatment. The patient is admitted to the hospital for X-ray studies to locate the suspected blood clot. The treatment is surgical, the clot being removed through an opening made in the skull. This procedure frequently results in dramatic improvement in the clinical condition of the patient; but, with some patients in whom the brain is also "bruised" (contused), there may be little clinical improvement noted after removal of the blood clot.

SUDDEN INFANT DEATH SYNDROME (SIDS)

Each year as many as 10,000 infants in the United States die of a mysterious disorder known as "sudden infant death syndrome," more commonly called "crib death." In such cases an infant, rarely older than ten months, is placed in a crib or bed to sleep, perhaps with no noticeable signs of ill health, and then is found dead sometime later. Examination after death reveals, if anything, only a slight degree of respiratory inflammation. Currently, there are no methods available either to predict or prevent SIDS.

Research into case histories reveals that sudden infant death is not due to suffocation or choking and that males are more susceptible than females. Although a viral infection is a possible cause, the condition is not thought to be contagious. Investigation is underway to determine if hereditary factors, sleep disorders, respiratory immaturity, and impaired immune response are somehow involved.

Parents who suffer the loss of a child because of SIDS often have to overcome extreme depression, grief, and self-recrimination. Feelings of guilt about such a death are not justified because no preventive or predictive measures are known to be effective. More information about SIDS can be obtained from the National Foundation for Sudden Infant Death, Inc., 310 S. Michigan Ave., Chicago, IL 60604.

SUFFOCATION

Suffocation, asphyxiation, strangulation, choking, and hanging cause coma due to insufficient oxygenation in the body.

Blockage of the air passages (windpipe, bronchi, etc.) may result from water in the lungs from submersion or a foreign body in the throat. Carbon monoxide blocks air passages by keeping air from the lungs and replacing oxygen by itself. Cessation of breathing may result from paralysis of the respiratory center in the brain by tumor, injury, drugs (opium), electric shock, etc.; it may result from pressure on the chest and/or abdomen as when a person is caught beneath rubble from a collapsed building.

Choking, particularly due to a foreign body lodged in the throat (such as insufficiently chewed meat), or strangulation due to hanging requires prompt dislodgement of the foreign body in the former and cutting of rope in the latter. In either case, an emergency tracheotomy (cutting directly into the windpipe and installing a rubber tube to allow air to enter) may have to be done. Artificial respiration is then used as in suffocation. (See "Choking" and "The Heimlich Maneuver" [Plates F8B–F8C] under First Aid and Emergencies.)

SUNBURN

Caused by excessive exposure to ultraviolet light (sun or artificial), sunburn is an increasingly common disability resulting from greater opportunity for exposure to sun (ease of travel to distant places), increased open-air activity (skiing, fishing, mountain climbing), and the current social acceptance of reducing the amounts of covering clothing to what may now have become an irreducible minimum.

No portion of the body with the possible exception of the palms and soles is immune to the burning properties of sunlight. The eyelids, armpits, and the like are more readily affected because of the sparseness of the horny protective skin layer. Highly pigmented skin offers protection but no guarantee of freedom from possible sun damage. Seemingly similar exposures to sun may vary widely depending on elevation (sea level), time of day, wind, reflection (sand, water), and available shade.

Even mild redness of the skin may result in extensive blistering and be accompanied by dizziness, nausea, and much discomfort.

Treatment. Aside from the obvious wisdom of prevention, early application of wet dressings, either by immersion in a tepid bath or by placing cold water-soaked cloths on the affected parts for as long and as often as practical, is the single best remedy for sunburn. Addition of a water softener (salts, starch) is useful but not essential. During the intervals between wet applications, thin, mild lotions (preferably unmedicated and unperfumed) can be used. Blisters can be opened under antiseptic conditions; this should be followed by application of an antibiotic ointment (Bacitracin, Neosporin®).

SUPPORTIVE TREATMENT In the care of the sick person any treatment that is not specifically directed at the underlying cause (germs, for example) or at the actual relief of symptoms (pain, vomiting, etc.) is "supportive." Among the items in this category of therapy are: bed rest, diet, adequate fluid intake (unless the basic illness proscribes fluids), alcohol sponges for high fever, hygiene of the mouth and skin, routine bed bath, ventilation, encouragement, and, above all, good nursing, whether by the professional nurse or someone in the home.

SWALLOWING DIFFICULTIES Most cases of swallowing difficulty are due to obstructions in the esophagus (the tube from the throat to the stomach). Hiatus hernia may cause similar symptoms. In patients over fifty years of age a gradually progressive difficulty in swallowing should be given prompt attention, as cancer of the esophagus is a common cause. Pain is usually absent, and the diagnosis is easily confirmed or rejected. Another common cause of this distressing symptom is spasm at the entrance to the stomach. The cause is not known, but the symptoms are usually transitory. Pain and vomiting are commonly associated with the swallowing difficulty. Treatment with medications is usually satisfactory. Narrowings or strictures as a result of lye or other corrosive substances on the lining of the esophagus are a common cause of swallowing difficulty in children. Swallowing a foreign body (such as bridgework or too large a bite of meat) may cause difficulty but the cause is usually readily apparent. Occasionally, the complex nerve-control of the act of swallowing will become impaired by such diseases as poliomyelitis, diphtheria, or strokes. Rare causes can be myasthemia gravis—a poorly understood disorder of nerve-impulse transmission—or an opening (fistula) between the esophagus and windpipe. A common complaint in nervous individuals of a lump or sense of constriction in the throat is usually easily diagnosed because there is no actual demonstrable difficulty in swallowing.

SWEATING, EXCESSIVE Excessive sweating is a source of great inconvenience to many people. It constitutes an occupational hazard in a variety of types of work, especially those in which the hands or feet are in primary use, for instance, the work of musicians, mechanics, typists, dentists, artists, construction workers, dancers, and models. The condition also can cause great embarrassment when it occurs in other areas, such as the face, the armpits, and the chest. Sweating is worsened by physical exertion, fatigue, and a variety of emotions including fear, anxiety, and states of stress.

Treatment. Mild sedation, rest, and the use of sweat-inhibiting drugs (Banthine®, Prantal®) will afford some relief. However, the patient must also be made to understand the underlying emotional factors for effective management of the problem. Astringents and anti-perspirants are available commercially and have a limited usefulness.

SWIMMER'S ITCH This is caused by the larvae (cercariae) of several species of the worm Schistosoma (known also as Bilharzia) which are hatched from snails found in water which has been polluted by the parasite-laden feces of the mammalian and avian hosts.

Symptoms. The eruption appears on portions of the body which were submerged in the water. A few minutes after the patient leaves the water, there is a burning sensation, followed by the appearance of small, flat, reddened areas, in turn followed by several crops of similar lesions. These enlarge and are covered by crusts. The burning and smarting is followed by itching. Secondary infection is not uncommon. The lesions last about two weeks, leaving reddish-brown stains.

Treatment. Immediate washing with soap and water followed by thorough drying of the skin serves to remove the larvae, or to prevent their penetrating the skin. Penetration of the larvae is facilitated in the process of evaporation of the water, and quick drying effectively prevents this. Subjective symptoms are controlled with soothing lotion (calamine), oral antihistaminic drugs for the itching, and antibiotic drugs for the secondary infection. Control of further infestation from the polluted water depends on removal of the parasite's vector, the snails.

SWIMMING POOL GRANULOMA This relatively new disease entity, which apparently results from injury incurred in swimming pools, has been noted with increasing frequency. The causative organism, *Mycobacterium balnei*, either survives or thrives in swimming pool water, and closely resembles the organism causing tuberculosis of the skin.

Symptoms. The lesion appears three or four weeks after even minor injury. The most common sites for the appearance of the lesions are the bridge of the nose, elbows, knees, and feet. One or more small brownish-red nodules appear, grow slowly, extend somewhat, and usually disappear in several months. It is possible, though not usual, for other sites to become infected from the original lesion.

Treatment. Small lesions can be destroyed with electrocautery if spontaneous disappearance seems unlikely. Prevention can be achieved by lining roughened pool surfaces with smooth tile and by adequate chlorination of the water.

SYNAPSE A synapse is the microscopic space at which the end of an axon of a nerve cell comes in contact with the dendrite or the cell body of another neuron. The axon carries an impulse away from its cell body. This impulse is transmitted across the space, or synapse, to the receiving portion, the dendrite, of a second nerve cell. Transmission, (which is probably accomplished by chemical mediators) occurs at the synapse in only

470

one direction. The system of nerve fibers and synapses provides a conduction and insulation system which regulates and controls the spread of impulses throughout the nervous system.

SYNDROME A syndrome is a pattern of symptoms which together are indicative of a disease. Many diseases present characteristic syndromes (patterns) of signs and symptoms which are diagnostic.

SYPHILIS Known as the great imitator, syphilis can affect every organ of the body and has produced almost every observed medical symptom. The range of the intensity and duration of this disease varies from "early" syphilis, with its primary ulcerated tumor mass (chancre) and secondary lesions of several types of appearance, distribution, and duration, to "late" syphilis, with its destructive lesions of the skin (gumma), heart and blood vessels, bones and joints, nerves and brain (paresis). So protean are the manifestations of syphilis that it is even known to produce no significant damage in a relatively small percentage of patients who have remained untreated because of lack of medical facilities.

In addition to the types of syphilis with overt lesions of the skin and mucous membranes, the disease can exist for many years without signs or symptoms except for changes in the blood serology in congenital and in latent syphilis. Some forms of congenital syphilis, acquired from the mother during the course of pregnancy, and latent syphilis in which there are no signs of the disease other than a persistently positive blood test, constitute situations in which the diagnosis is established on the basis of the patient's history, repeated and varied blood tests, and the absence of other diseases capable of producing similar blood serologic changes (lupus erythematosus, vaccination).

The causative organism, a spirochete,

Treponema pallidum, can be obtained from early lesions with great ease, and almost not at all from late (tertiary) lesions—an indication of the immune changes resulting from the infection. Infection takes place in so high a percentage of persons exposed to the organism (usually in the primary and secondary highly infectious lesions) that for practical and preventive purposes it can be assumed that sexual contact with a known "active" syphilitic will result in infection in the non-syphilitic partner. Because of this high contagiosity, it is well to treat all known "contacts" of a diagnosed syphilitic with immediate and effective doses of antibiotic (usually penicillin), both to avoid spread of the disease in the community and to attempt to provide adequate treatment of the individual.

The advent of antibiotics has vastly altered the incidence of syphilitic infection wherever treatment is available. Antibiotic therapy has also altered the course of the disease because of the rapidity of the cure. With previous treatment (arsphenamines, bismuth, mercury), demonstrable cure was rare, and was known to have occurred only when every vestige of the disease had disappeared sufficiently so that the patient could acquire the disease again on exposure to the spirochete. Since antibiotic therapy, evidence of cure (ability to be re-infected) is usual enough to have resulted in the invention of the term "ping-pong syphilis" to designate the back and forth transfer of the disease by the presently affected sexual partner to the presently cured partner, with a reversal of the situation on treatment of the affected one.

Antibiotic therapy has had another profound effect on the management of this disease, that of the urgency of adequate treatment. It has long been known that in order to effect a cure, or at least improvement, in a disease of so many changes to so many organs, treatment must be sufficiently complete to insure at least immunologic (serologic) evidence of change to normal, that is a negative test of the blood and of the spinal fluid. If remedies are given in insufficient amounts or for too short a time, and the treatment is inadequate for cure, the immune responses of the body are interfered with. Under these circumstances, a spontaneous cure effected by the body's own protective mechanisms is rendered impossible of completion, and a treatment cure is impossible to achieve. Since antibiotic therapy is so effective in curing syphilis, it is essential that medication be given early and adequately. The taking of antibiotics in lesser doses for shorter periods of time for concurrent "minor" ailments, such as boils, infected teeth, respiratory infections, is so commonplace that if the existence of a syphilitic infection is suspected, the patient should be investigated quickly and thoroughly; and if a diagnosis of syphilis is made, adequate treatment be administered to prevent the serious consequences attending the usually lesser dosage of antibiotics given for other conditions.

Treatment. Although antibiotics are of singular merit in the treatment of syphilis, the method of administration, the dosage and the duration of treatment depend on the stage of the disease and the age, sex, and general medical condition of the patient, and include considerations of prevention (as in pregnancy).

TACHYCARDIA

Tachycardia is unduly rapid heart action. It may be caused by anxiety, excitement, fever, anemia, pericarditis, exercise, and the many varieties of stress that may occur in the human organism. The heart can speed up yet will ordinarily function quite well until it reaches a rate of 160 to 180 beats per minute; any rate beyond this is undesirable, because the heart is unable to fill itself satisfactorily and the beats will become most inefficient.

The heart rate in a resting adult varies, but on the average beats about 80 times per minute. Its pace is set in the sino-atrial node, which is under the influence of both sympathetic nerve fibers which accelerate the rate and vagal impulses from an entirely different set of nerves which tend to slow it. In addition, hormones from the adrenal glands, and even circulating thyroid hormone can alter and even determine the heart rate. In times of emotional stress, the adrenal glands may assist the sympathetic nerves in raising the heart rate. On exercise or exertion, there is an increased return of blood through the veins; this is a factor in increasing the heartbeat to prevent overfilling of the central circulation.

A rather serious type of tachycardia is due to disordered function of the heart muscle, the abnormal heart rate being set by a focus in the auricular (or even the ventricular) tissue taking over the normal function of pacemaker. Thus, rapid arrhythmias are classed as supraventricular if the rate of discharge comes from an irritable focus in the auricles. In auricular fibrillation, the auricle may beat as often as 500 times per minute, while the ventricular rate can remain anywhere between 100 and 200 beats per minute. In a flutter of the auricle the rate of both auricle and ventricle is somewhat slower. Auricular or nodal tachycardia is the usual variety of simple tachycardia. Rapid rhythms produced in an abnormal ventricular area are very rare in patients without heart disease. Very often ventricular tachycardia is related to an overdosage of digitalis but it can easily be aggravated by overexertion or coexisting serious illness. In nodal tachycardia the ventricles beat at the same rate as the abnormal focus—100 to 200 per minute.

The electrocardiogram can make the exact diagnosis and definitively distinguish whether the increased heart rate has its origin at the ventricular level or above it.

Symptoms. The tachycardias are functional disorders and symptoms are not those of organic disease, unless organic heart changes are present in association with the disorder. Tachycardia is perceived by the patient as extremely rapid heart action, referred to as "fast palpitation." The fluttering behind the breastbone or in the neck is unpleasant and as a rule begins to be felt rather abruptly. Usually the tachycardia stops as quickly as it begins. The general rhythm is regular; if it is not, fibrillation is probable rather than a simple tachycardia.

As a rule, attacks of tachycardia rarely last longer than a few hours. They often occur at infrequent intervals over many years, and the patient may learn how to terminate or tolerate them in various ways.

Paroxysmal tachycardia may be considered a rather special type of tachycardia. It rarely causes any disability except for an awareness of its presence. The awareness of rapid heart action appears without warning, and after a brief period of annoyance, suddenly disappears. Characteristically, it repeats itself throughout the lifetime of the patient which is rarely shortened by the disturbing attacks.

Treatment. If no associated organic heart disease is present, the patient may require no special medication for mild attacks of paroxysmal tachycardia. If severe however, careful clinical or laboratory study will be required to indicate the appropriate measures required for accurate treatment.

TAPEWORM Tapeworms are a common cause of human parasitic disease. These long, flat, thin worms (which *do* look like "tape") live in the human intestine. The species that most commonly infest man are the beef (*Taenia saginata*), pork (*Taenia solium*), fish (*Diphyllobothrium latum*), and dwarf tapeworm (*Hymenolepsis nana*).

Man becomes the host by consuming raw or improperly cooked flesh-food, or food or water contaminated with droppings from infected dogs, rats, etc. Thorough cooking will destroy the larvae stages.

The adult tapeworm has a head (scolex) with little hooks or sucking disks attaching it to the bowel lining. This head is followed by a long ribbon-like string of segments (proglottids), each capable of reproducing additional segments or producing eggs. The number of segments range from three to several thousand. Segments and eggs are passed in the stool, and the diagnosis is made by finding them on microscopic examination.

Symptoms. Symptoms of tapeworm are quite variable and depend on both the type and number of worms present and the general health and nutrition of the host. In fully developed cases, there is diarrhea, weakness, anemia, and weight loss despite a surprisingly good appetite.

Treatment. A number of drugs, called vermifuges, are used in an attempt to dislodge the tapeworm. Unless the head is removed, however, new segments and eggs will continue to be produced.

TATTOO A tattoo is commonly thought to be solely the result of deliberate decoration of the skin (with a variety of substances deposited deep into the skin). However, a tattoo may often be the result of accidental deposition of such substances as lead (from pencils), dye (from pens), gravel (from brushburns), and from medicinals like mercury and gentian violet applied to abraded skin.

Treatment. Extirpation by some form of surgery, electrocautery, application of acids, or blistering with the application of dry ice yield varying degrees of success. Because the tattoo is in the deep portion of skin, scarring is an inevitable result of removing the lesion. Depending on the area involved, reconstruction of the tattooed area by means of plastic surgery may be necessary to achieve cosmetic betterment.

TEAR DUCT, PLUGGED   Stoppage of the tear duct is a common affliction during the newborn period; there is a congenital blockage of the tiny canal that allows the tears to flow from the inner corner of the eye into the nose.

Symptoms. Since tears are formed at a constant rate, if dammed back they will cause a watery eye and will flow over the lid and down the cheek. There is nothing wrong with the eye itself, but because the fluid is a good culture medium for germs, babies with blocked tear duct are frequent sufferers from conjunctivitis.

Treatment. Nine out of ten babies with this problem will outgrow it by the age of ten months; a mucus plug is expelled and/or the canal simply opens up. If the stoppage persists, an eye specialist (ophthalmologist) should be seen for treatment. Mere passage of a probe may be all the treatment required.

TEARS   The tears are secreted by an almond-shaped gland located in the upper, outer portion of the orbit. Additional tears are secreted by glands on the inside of the lids. Relatively few tears are normally formed, but they are evenly spread over the globe and keep the eye moist, preventing growth of bacteria.

TEARS, EXCESSIVE   These are formed when crying, or when the eye is irritated by cold, a superficial injury, a foreign body or infection. Blocking of the drainage ducts for tears may cause overflow of a normal amount of tears. With aging, the lids become relaxed and tears may no longer be guided to the drainage ducts and overflow. Excess tears may be merely a nuisance or they may be a sign of serious disease. Tearing in an infant's eye should alert one to infantile glaucoma which requires immediate surgical treatment. However, an infant's eye may also water because of failure of the tear duct to open during the early weeks of life. Glaucoma may be recognized by the loss of clearness of the cornea and difficulty in seeing the iris pattern and pupil clearly.

TEETHING   The word teething refers to the problems associated with the eruption or "cutting" of the first teeth. Both the primary and secondary teeth must emerge into the mouth through the soft tissue that covers the bony crypt in which they develop. Although the exact process by which a tooth erupts and penetrates the covering mucosa is not known, it is understandable that more problems can be expected while this is occurring for the first time—in the primary dentition. Thus the gum at the site of cutting may become sensitive and inflamed.

In the past, many childhood illnesses (coughs, fevers, diarrhea) were attributed, without factual evidence, to the eruptive process. However, mild disturbances of the gums during this process can explain the child's slight fever, irritability, increased flow of saliva, and constant chewing of objects placed in the mouth.

Teething normally involves an orderly sequence of tooth eruption in which only a very few teeth are involved at any one time. An existing fever may accelerate the eruptive process, resulting in more than the usual number of cutting areas. Inflammation and pain may be increased (especially in the child who is already ill); however, once the tooth has erupted, the symptoms will diminish. Persistent problems require dental consultation.

Clean, soothing teething substances should be substituted for objects which can result in infection or create possible finger habits. The supervised use of ice placed in a clean towel has solved many personal problems related to teething, without recourse to other medications. A similar, though more complicated, series of events may follow the eruption of the permanent third molars (wisdom teeth) of the adult (see PERICORONITIS).

TEETH, INJURED   Injuries to teeth are usually the result of a traumatic blow. The result of such damage may be displacement of the tooth from its normal position in the socket, fracture of any or all of the hard tissues of the tooth, or a combination of the two.

Displacement of a tooth may be complete—in which case the tooth is removed from its socket—or partial, the tooth being moved from its normal position but remaining attached.

Fractures of a tooth may involve the enamel; the enamel and dentin; the enamel, dentin, and pulp cavity; or the root and its pulp canal. Due to their location, front teeth (especially those which protrude) are most often involved.

There are other possibilities, however. In some cases there is neither displacement nor fracture, but rather a rupture of the blood vessels of the pulp, producing a "pink tooth." The pulp may degenerate because of pressure from the hemorrhage, producing a "darkened tooth." Displacement of the first teeth may result in injury to the underlying developing permanent teeth.

In some instances, teeth which have been completely displaced from their socket may be replanted by a dentist. Partial displacement may also be treated by the dentist, the tooth being manually returned to its original position and stabilized by some mechanical means.

Fractures involving only the enamel may be treated by smoothing the rough edges, or by restoring the missing part. Those involving the enamel and dentin may have more serious consequences, since the dentin possesses the ability to transmit pain impulses to the pulp, and may eventually result in pulp damage.

If the fracture involves the protective wall of the pulp and exposure of it to the external environment, immediate treatment is essential if the pulp is to be preserved. Fractures of the root always involve the pulp, but healing may occur if the broken parts are joined and stabilized. Any damaged tooth, regardless of the severity of the injury, may be loose for some time; eventually, however, it usually resumes its normal stability.

TEMPERATURE CHARTS   In the investigation of sterility in the female, a record of body temperature, taken daily immediately upon awakening, and carefully studied, will give valuable information on whether the patient is ovulating or not (see OVULATION).

TEMPER TANTRUMS   Tantrums are infantile uncontrolled rage reactions used to terrorize the environment and get one's own way. Every child learns early to control adults by crying or screaming in rage to get what it wants. Once it learns that temper tantrums are successful in controlling the environment, the child tends to organize these into a terroristic life style in which the child constantly intimidates others to gain his own ends. Temper tantrums have become commoner with the advent of progressive methods of education, the child being permitted and encouraged to express himself in all situations. The over-permissive parent tends to allow the young child early to escape from discipline, using temper tantrums and other undesirable behavior in unhealthy ways.

Treatment. Temper tantrums are more easily prevented than controlled once the pattern has been established. When the child first develops a tantrum, he should not be given his own way or allowed to acquire any secondary gains. Many parents make their first mistake in attempting to argue or reason with the child, who is out of emotional control; such methods are rarely effective. The child should be handled quietly but firmly, being isolated until he quiets down and is willing to listen to reason again. Above all, the parent should keep control of his own emotions and not allow himself to shout at the child.

TENSION SYMPTOMS
States of emotional excitability tend to be expressed in muscular contractions in all systems of the body, and are experienced as unpleasant tension symptoms. In abnormal metabolic states such as hyperthyroidism, heightened metabolism in all body systems causes feelings of generalized tension.

Symptoms. Very similar symptoms occur in psychoneurotic anxiety states or anger reactions, in which an over-secretion of adrenalin causes generalized body tension. In situations of acute emotional reaction such as combat fatigue or war neurosis, the person may complain of a generalized unpleasant tension state in such words as, "I feel as if I'm going to explode, as if I'm going to blow my stack."

Localized tension states may reflect muscular contractions in any of the specific body systems. Tension headaches may be caused by spasm of the temporal or occipital muscles at the sides or back of the head. Tension in the facial musculature causes frowning or grimacing. Spasm of the throat and swallowing muscles causes the symptom of a lump in the throat (globus hystericus), with difficulties in swallowing. Spasm of the coronary arteries of the heart causes anginal chest pains and feelings of pressure in the chest; spasms of the diaphragm cause interference with breathing and sighing respirations; and spasms of the stomach or intestinal musculature cause quivering sensations ("butterflies in the stomach") or abdominal cramps. Tension in the arms, legs, and bodily musculature also frequently occurs in anxiety states as a symptom of nervousness.

Treatment. Since most tension symptoms are only symptomatic of underlying states of emotional excitement or conflict, basic treatment is to remove such causes of deep underlying conflict. However, much symptomatic relief can be achieved by learning methods of progressive muscular relaxation. This involves identifying specific muscular contractions and then inhibiting them voluntarily. The tense person may discover that he is frowning, grinding his teeth, clenching his hands, and holding himself stiffly. By recognizing

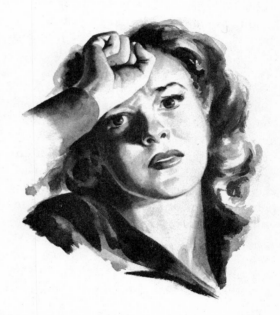

these tensions individually, it is possible for him to relax them one by one until a state of complete relaxation is attained.

Much tension can be prevented by learning to take a calm, tolerant attitude toward life, accepting what cannot be changed and attempting only what is possible. It is important to take life's problems and frustrations in stride, rather than over-reacting emotionally in ways which progressively build up tension.

In severe anxiety, tension states in which upset emotions and bodily tensions have gotten completely out of control, it may be necessary to use tranquilizing drugs or sedatives to quiet the patient

476

sufficiently so that psychotherapeutic methods can be used. In extreme cases it may be necessary to remove the person from a disturbing environment for a short period of hospitalization in order to re-achieve control.

TESTICLES (TESTES) These rounded, elongated organs reside in the male scrotum in adulthood. They are firm and covered by a tough capsule. Internally, they are composed of thousands of tiny pockets in which sperm is manufactured. At body temperature, the process of sperm-manufacture is incomplete, but at the somewhat lower temperature of the scrotum (outside the body) conditions are favorable to it.

A testicle may become twisted on the spermatic cord producing enlargement, congestion, and tension. Not uncommonly, mumps affects the testes—especially in males past the age of puberty. It is therefore important that rest and a close medical regime be carefully followed to prevent permanent damage after recovery from mumps.

Tumors of the testicles are relatively uncommon but are almost always malignant; they are usually painless, and the only clue to their presence may be a hard lump in the testicle. At an early stage, testicular tumors may be removed with a high likelihood of cure. The most malignant of these tumors, however, spread rapidly, more than half the patients so afflicted dying within five years.

TESTICLE, UNDESCENDED Before birth the testicles are developed in the lower abdomen. Prior to birth they normally descend to the scrotum. One or both testes however, may remain within the body. In such cases descent usually occurs in the first few years of childhood or may be delayed until puberty. If the testicle has not migrated to the scrotum by the age of nine or ten, it is usually considered advisable to institute treatment.

Treatment. Surgery is considered by the majority to be the recommended treatment, although some physicians consider the use of gonadotropic hormone injections. Frequently, surgery is necessary before the testis can be placed in its proper location in the scrotum. It is important to treat undescended testes to assure fertility, because development of the sperm is incomplete at the higher temperature within the body. There is also an increased incidence of tumors in undescended testes.

TESTOSTERONE This is a hormone secreted by the testicles directly into the bloodstream. It is responsible for production of a masculine body configuration and other male characteristics. Output of testosterone greatly increases at the time of puberty, and it is this substance which induces growth of the penis and scrotum, as well as distribution of hair in the pubic, under-arm, and facial areas. Testosterone is also a potent stimulator of muscle growth and power, as well as growth and length of the long bones since it influences closure of the cartilage plates (epiphyses) which are responsible for growth of the long bones.

THEMATIC APPERCEPTION TEST (TAT) The TAT is a series of pictures presenting simple scenes involving human beings, about which the subject is asked to write a brief story. The test was invented by the psychologist Dr. Henry A. Murray to reveal deep underlying needs and conflicts; in writing a story about the comparatively unstructured scene in the picture, the subject tends to project his own deep underlying personality structure, needs, conflicts, and problems ascribing his own experiences and motives to the subjects in the pictures.

THERMOMETER There are many instruments for the measurement of heat. In medicine, the clinical thermometer is a glass tube with graduated markings ranging from 94° to 108°F. (most foreign countries use the centigrade scale). The encased fluid—capable of expanding and contracting with temperature changes—is usually mercury, although other substances, such as alcohol, are used. In clinical practice and in the home mouth thermometers are used; the terminal, which contains the mercury, is thin and about three-fourths of an inch long to facilitate placement under the tongue. The rectal thermometer also has a short, spherical end for ease of rectal insertion.

Thermometers should be shaken before using until the fluid is at least as low as 96°F. The tips of rectal thermometers should be greased with vaseline before insertion. A thermometer is left in the mouth or rectum for three minutes before removing it for reading. A thermometer by mouth is not used in very young or very old persons, who may bite or swallow it.

THIRST   The sensation of thirst is regulated by a highly specialized group of nerve endings that respond to changes in the volume and composition of the various body-fluids. This is part of an intricate system that regulates urine excretion, sweating, blood volume, and the amount of fluid in tissue cells. While an individual is aware of being thirsty when his mouth and throat are dry, the degree of thirst is not dependent on these sensations, since dryness is relieved after the first swallow. Nevertheless, the total intake of fluid is generally regulated precisely so as to provide the amount necessary for maintenance of proper fluid composition. Excessive thirst may be due to a hot environment, increased perspiration, intake of alcohol or spicy or salty foods, or may herald such conditions as diabetes. Internal bleeding can sometimes be suspected in a patient

with sudden excessive thirst, because of the reduction in circulating blood. Shock due to extensive burns or bleeding from any source is usually accompanied by thirst in the conscious patient.

THORACOTOMY   The surgical opening of the chest wall and exposure of the inside structures, thoracotomy may be done as a diagnostic (exploratory) procedure to view the area directly and/or to obtain a specimen for microscopic examination (biopsy), or it may be followed by an actual removal of rib, pleura, lung, or tissue between the two lungs (mediastinum.) These procedures have different names: thoracoplasty and pleurectomy refer to removal of tissue in rib and pleural areas respectively. Segmentectomy, lobectomy, and pneumonectomy refer to the cutting-out (excision) of progressively larger divisions of the lung.

THROAT   The throat is a general term applied to the pharynx, the larynx, and the associated muscles, blood vessels, and other tissues of the neck. Infections and diseases of the entire neck are part of otolaryngology.

(THROMBO)PHLEBITIS   Phlebitis is an inflammatory disease of the vein-wall and surrounding tissues. Usually there is a thrombosis or clot of blood (thrombophlebitis) that completely blocks the flow of blood through the area of vein holding the clot. Phlebitis can occur in any of the veins of the body, but almost always appears in the veins of the legs, thighs, or pelvis.

Symptoms. An acute phlebitis will produce swelling of the extremity involved, together with fever and an elevated pulse rate. Pain may be acute in some patients, especially when motion of the affected part is attempted. Chronic phlebitis is characterized by persistent swelling and that physical disability which is caused both by the swelling and the deficient circulation in the extremity.

Treatment. In the acute stage, phlebitis will require rest in bed and careful observation of the changes produced by the blood clot obstructing the large vein. If either the life of the limb or the patient is threatened by these changes, surgical extraction of the clot (thrombectomy) may be necessary, even as an emergency procedure. Furthermore, when some of the clot threatens to break away and drift to the lungs (pulmonary embolus) one of the surgical procedures designed to narrow the diameter of the abdomenal vena cava and therefore block the passage of a large clot, may be indicated.

If the acute phlebitis subsides and a low-grade inflammation persists for many years, chronic phlebitis will need careful treatment. Although no cure can be offered, the swelling and deficient circulation can be held in control by means of elastic stockings, selective exercise, and physiotherapy.

THRUSH This is a fairly common fungus infection of the mouth, occurring in babies during the first few weeks of life. It almost always stems from the same fungus infection (*Monilia*) as that found in the mother's birth canal (vagina); hence the mother and the baby should be treated simultaneously.

Symptoms. Thrush appears as white, slightly raised areas inside the cheeks, along the gums, and the edges of the tongue. These look like small milk-curds, but if rubbed off leave a raw area. The condition is usually harmless, but can be rather persistent.

Treatment. Certain new and very effective antifungal remedies can be prescribed by the physician to clear up the condition rather rapidly.

THUMB-SUCKING This is an infantile habit which usually begins in the first three months of life. Some authorities feel that it comes from an unsatisfied sucking drive and that the milk is flowing too freely. Others feel that it comes from hunger or colic pains and that the sucking action seems to quiet the baby. Still others feel that it is an inborn trait, as it is often familial.

Most mothers encourage their babies to suck on a pacifier as it is the lesser of two evils. The baby who is not pestered about his habit will give it up when he is ready. Most avid thumb-suckers need to continue until three years or so, and many normal children will still be sucking their thumbs at age five or six when falling asleep at night.

Treatment. Children seem to sense a mother's dislike of some habit; often, they will continue it if it bothers the mother. Setting up obstacles to the sucking just seems to set a challenge for the child, and he will pursue the habit even more aggressively. Applying bandages or tapes to the thumb seems to make no difference until the child is over five years of age. If a mother could look on the habit as being as normal as wetting the diapers, she would perhaps not be so tense about it.

When babies are small, they should be allowed to be babies: suck their thumbs, wet their pants, smear things, and throw food about. Then, when they are older, they will give up these traits. The modern mother is often too eager to get her baby to grow up and assume adult characteristics. Children need discipline, but they should not be punished or reprimanded for bed-rocking, nail-biting, thumb-sucking, hair-twisting, and the holding of bits of cloth next to them. They will give up the habits more quickly if they are ignored.

THYMUS GLAND This gland is set in the anterior part of the chest known as the mediastinum, just above the heart and great blood vessels. In childhood it is quite large, but decreases markedly in size at adolescence. Until recently its function was not well understood, although it was known to be implicated in the rare disease known as myasthenia gravis in which the muscles fatigue very rapidly with use. During the past several years, however, it has been discovered that the thymus gland is important in the production of antibodies in infants and children; it is very likely that it shrinks in adulthood because antibody-producing function is well established in other tissues of the body. A number of years ago it was felt that enlargement of the thymus in infants was a dangerous condition often responsible for sudden death. In many patients this led to treatment of the gland by means of radiation therapy. It is now believed that such treatment is unnecessary and that the gland would reduce in size without it.

THYROID GLAND The thyroid gland is a structure weighing approximately one ounce and shaped roughly like an H, which is partially wrapped about the windpipe directly below the larynx (voicebox). It secretes a hormone (thyroxin) which is responsible for regulating the rate of metabolic activity in all organs and tissues. For proper functioning of this gland iodine is a necessity, and in regions poor in this element this may be easily supplied in the diet through use of iodized salt.

The thyroid gland is composed of clusters of cells arranged to form pockets filled with a gelatinous substance known as colloid, which contains stored thyroid hormone. When the gland is extremely active, the colloid disappears and the cells become tall and more numerous.

The thyroid is controlled by the pituitary gland through the secretion of thyrotropic hormone. There is also a "feedback" mechanism, whereby depletion of thyroid hormone stimulates secretion of thyro-

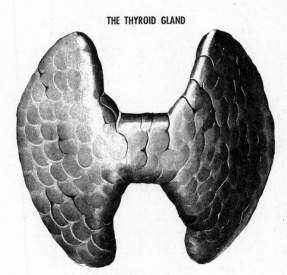

THE THYROID GLAND

The thyroid is a large reddish, endocrine (ductless) gland located in front of, and on either side of, the trachea. It consists of two lateral lobes and a connecting isthmus.

tropic hormone by the pituitary. Should the amount of thyroid circulating in the body be too high, the secretion of thyrotropic hormone by the pituitary is immediately inhibited. Thus, under normal conditions, the secretion of thyroid hormone is kept within a rather narrow range.

The blood protein-bound iodine level measures the amount of circulating thyroid hormone. The function of the thyroid gland is also assessed by measuring the uptake of radioactive iodine and by the basal metabolic rate. In "overactive thyroid," one of the standard treatments is its partial removal by surgery (thyroidectomy). Thyroid substance used as medication is prepared from dried thyroid glands of domestic animals. It is prescribed by physicians when either the thyroid or the pituitary is underactive, and also in some cases of obesity and menstrual disturbance.

THYROIDITIS In addition to the other well-known conditions which afflict the thyroid gland, it is frequently the seat of inflammation which is usually nonspecific in origin. (It may be that the gland becomes sensitive to some of its own hormone, thus setting up an inflammatory response which temporarily or permanently inhibits the secretion of thyroid hormone.) This condition is accompanied by pain in the anterior region of the neck, fever, and symptoms and signs of thyroid overactivity. If untreated, this condition slowly subsides, but the individual may be left in a hypothyroid state. Treatment is usually by means of thyroid substance, cortisone, and medication to relieve pain. It is important to distinguish this condition from hyperthyroidism or other afflictions of the gland, as inappropriate treatment may result in permanent damage. Chronic forms of thyroiditis do exist and are called Hashimoto's disease and Riedel's struma.

TICS

Tics are involuntary muscular contractions and twitchings which in anxiety tension states may occur in any part of the voluntary musculature. The most primitive form is the involuntary startle reaction, in which the person gives an involuntary jump or twitch when surprised. Other forms of tics include jerking the head, frowning or grimacing, blinking the eyes, twitchings of the facial musculature, and a wide variety of other involuntary body movements. In some cases tics may be muscular habits (conditioned reactions) duplicating patterns which originally occurred in some significant situation, as when a person reenacts his behavior during an accident.

It is generally observed that all forms of tic become exaggerated during periods of increased stress and emotional tension. The onset of a tic may thus be one of the first symptoms of states of emotional excitability.

Treatment. Since tics have only symptomatic significance, treatment should be directed primarily toward the underlying emotional causes. It usually does no good to attempt to deal with tics directly, since calling attention to them only makes the person feel more insecure and conflictual, thereby increasing levels of emotional instability. Tics tend to disappear spontaneously during rest periods and when the person achieves emotional calm.

TINNITUS

Tinnitus refers to noise in the ear. Subjective tinnitus is noise only the patient can hear, and is the most common type. Objective tinnitus is noise an examiner can hear as well. There are countless reasons for tinnitus. It is usually associated with a hearing loss. Occasionally, after the hearing loss is corrected, the tinnitus disappears.

Tinnitus is not a cause of hearing loss as many people think; it is only associated with it. Some people are sure that if they can get rid of their tinnitus, they will hear better. This is not true. If they get rid of their hearing loss, however, the tinnitus may disappear. This is particularly true of otosclerosis. The noise may be high- or low-pitched, constant or intermittent, and usually seems worse at night.

Treatment. Tinnitus is very difficult to treat. Many people simply become accustomed to it; this may be the best answer when there is a noncorrectable hearing loss. A careful examination should be made by the physician to rule out any dangerous causes of tinnitus. If the doctor's examination reveals no danger, then learning to live with tinnitus is the most effective way of handling the problem.

TOILET TRAINING

Patience, perseverance, and common sense are required to toilet train the average normal infant. This program can be initiated when the baby is able to sit up without propping or assistance; usually in the six or seventh month. The mother usually learns to predict when her child is about to move its bowels—he may grimace, grunt, or give some characteristic gesture or sound. As soon as this is noted the mother should

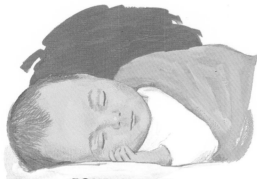

CHILD GROWTH AND BEHAVIOR

Parents should always be aware that statistics, behavior patterns, growth charts and norms for all growing children generally represent averages or medians. Parents should expect some variations from such printed data in their own children's development. Development norms are influenced by heredity, environment, nutrition, and a variety of other factors. An observable marked retardation from so-called norms should be brought to the attention of a physician.

FOUR WEEKS

Baby does not really see yet or focus the eyes but does follow a moving light. Sleep takes up on an average of twenty hours of the infant's day. Body temperature is steady and not as subject to fluctuations as it was the first weeks after birth. Baby gains about six ounces a week and has grown about one inch since birth.

EIGHT WEEKS

Baby is able to recognize familiar people and objects. Sleep has been cut to about eighteen hours a day. Weight increases at about three ounces a week. Height is still increasing at about one inch a month.

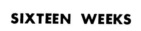

SIXTEEN WEEKS

Baby sees objects very well now and reaches for them. Length of sleep is about the same as at eight weeks. Weight is increasing at a steady rate and will be doubled at about twenty weeks. Objects now are grasped and held. Baby laughs.

SIX MONTHS

Baby still sleeps about sixteen hours a day and may sleep through the night. Weight may be increasing by two to three ounces a month. Baby probably is about six inches taller than at birth. Hearing is showing a marked development and there is a definite response to sound. Of the twenty temporary teeth baby is to get, the first two, the lower center incisors, may now appear. Baby may try to sit up without help, and may attemp to pick up and grasp small objects, and shift them from hand to hand. Baby turns over but may have started to do so even at five months.

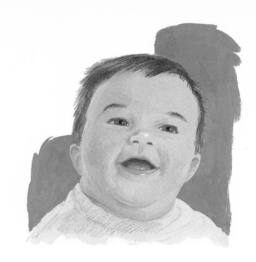

TEN MONTHS

Baby may now be sleeping only fifteen hours a day. Gets around by crawling, and can sit unsupported and also change from a sitting to a prone position. Baby generally can pull himself up to a standing position and may be able to imitate simple syllables such as "da da."

TWELVE MONTHS

The baby can now distinguish colors in this order: yellow, red, blue. Some babies now sleep about fourteen hours a day but there are some who still need sixteen full hours. The scale will show that baby's weight has tripled since birth. Height is still increasing at about three inches a year. To the two lower central incisors will have been added four upper incisors. Baby crawls and can walk by holding on to chairs and other objects nearby and some may be able to walk without support.

FIFTEEN MONTHS

In addition to the previous temporary teeth, baby has added two lower lateral incisors. Baby can walk and attempts to climb stairs. Toys and dolls are hugged and just as readily thrown away. Although baby is not talking yet, demands are made known by pointing and shouting. Some babies are now trying to feed themselves by attempting to drink from a glass or cup and by using a spoon.

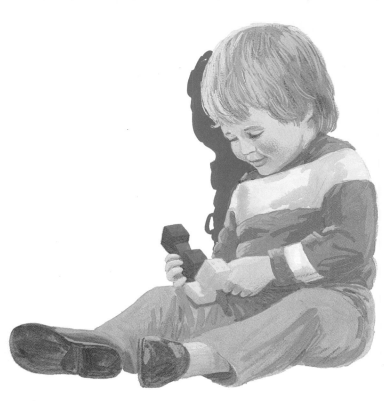

EIGHTEEN MONTHS

Baby has added the four canines to the temporary teeth already in, and is growing at the rate of about three inches a year. This is the age when being "contrary" is the normal way to be. Baby is able to climb and run and does so at every opportunity.

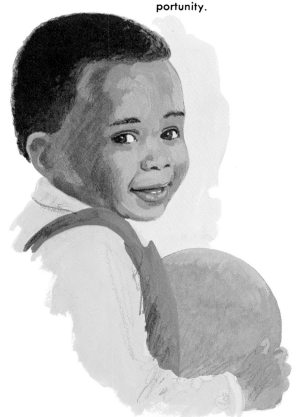

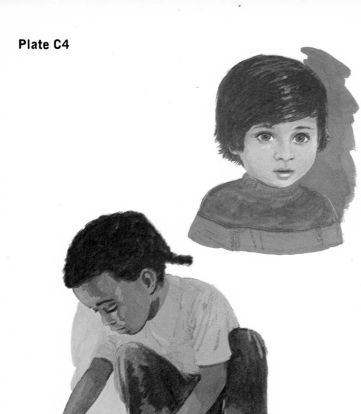

TWO YEARS

Baby is now sleeping twelve to fourteen hours and may skip the daytime nap more often than parents would like. The balance of the temporary teeth (four posterior molars) are coming in now. Motor control has improved. He points to his eyes, nose, and ears and may be toilet-trained. He understands more and makes himself understood.

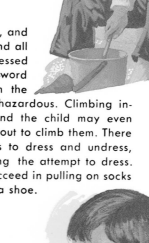

TWO AND ONE-HALF YEARS

Baby's weight has quadrupled since birth, and he probably is about thirty-five inches tall and all the temporary teeth are in. Speech has progressed to the point where the child is talking in three-word sentences. Play is very vigorous and from the parents' point of view, hazardous. Climbing instinct may show itself and the child may even grasp small trees as if about to climb them. There will be genuine attempts to dress and undress, with undressing preceding the attempt to dress. Some children actually succeed in pulling on socks and slipping a foot into a shoe.

THREE YEARS

Child feeds himself, talks in short sentences, and generally is toilet-trained by this age. Motor control is improving — he can now build and keep from tumbling a large number of blocks. He can manage physical activities that were beyond his capacity only a few months ago. Emotionally he is temporarily becoming a conformer and will follow suggestions and orders from elders. He is more cooperative and will share toys with friends.

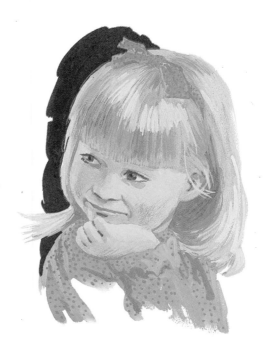

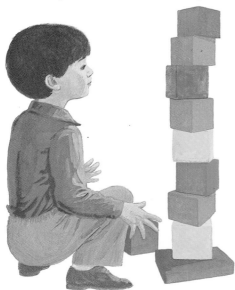

THREE AND ONE-HALF YEARS

Sudden changes occur. Child seems to temporarily slip back in motor coordination, despite the fact that for several months already he has been riding a tricycle, is now feeding himself with a minimum of spilling, and is able to put on his shoes quite well. Temporary regression shows itself in fear of heights. Stuttering may appear and temporary crossing of the eyes is also symtomatic of this strange age. The child seems to need greater expressions of affection and is constantly accusing parents of not loving him. Fortunately this "retardation" is temporary and will disappear as quickly as it came.

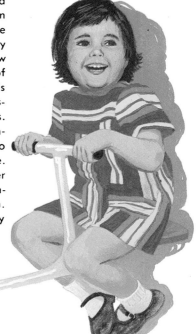

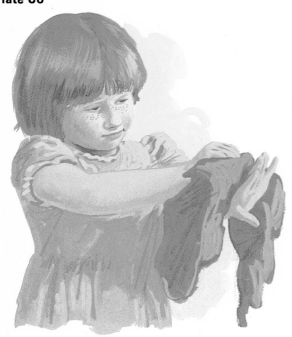

FOUR YEARS

The four-year-old can dress and undress himself and even lace his shoes. He can skip on one foot and can wash and dry himself and brush his teeth. Generally, he plays cooperatively with his friends.

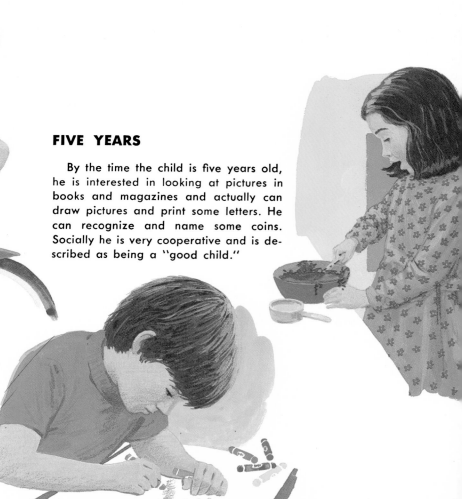

FIVE YEARS

By the time the child is five years old, he is interested in looking at pictures in books and magazines and actually can draw pictures and print some letters. He can recognize and name some coins. Socially he is very cooperative and is described as being a "good child."

SIX YEARS

The child is very active and he is occupied in running, jumping, skating, likes to wrestle and have friendly fist fights. He is using about 2,500 words and he knows his address and parents' names and how to cross streets. He is just beginning to learn to read.

SEVEN YEARS

The child seems to suddenly develop nervous habits such as nail-biting and tongue-sucking. He has begun to be keenly competitive in play and dresses like his friends. He is becoming aware of the social and economic differences between himself and his classmates. He is beginning to understand addition and subtraction concepts and is able to tell time and may know what month it is. Child may now show great curiosity about the sexes and how babies are born.

EIGHT YEARS

The eight-year-old can swim and ride a bicycle. He begins to respect the property rights of others and he is becoming more "choosy" in selecting his friends. He is beginning to read the comics and the funnies in the newspapers and attempts to spend more time watching television. This is merely an expression of a greater interest in the world about him.

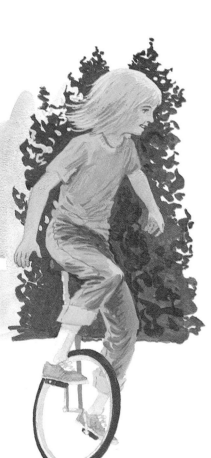

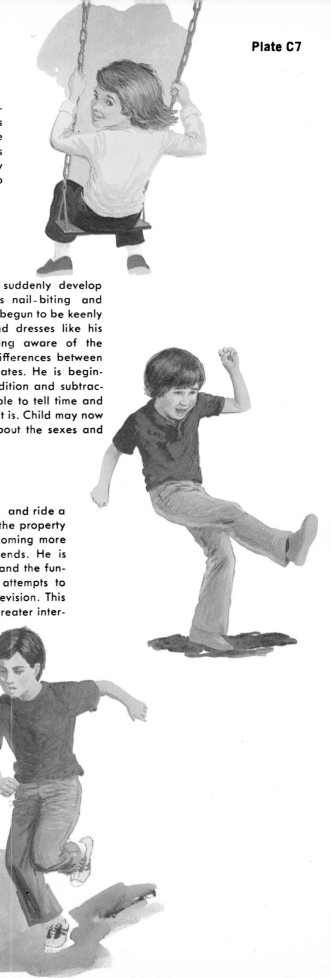

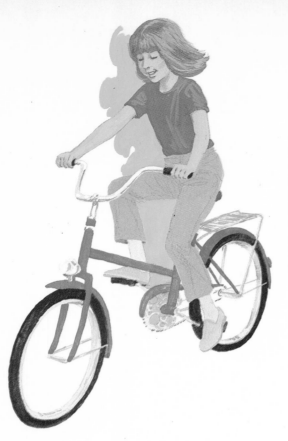

NINE YEARS

The nine-year-old can bathe, comb his hair and take care of other physical needs. He is beginning to be able to use tools very well. Boys and girls are beginning to play separately now and there is a greater variety in their play activities. There is a greater interest in visiting friends and sleeping away from home. In school work he is now able to do some multiplication and division. Generally he is interested in how things are made. There is curiosity about science, nature, and the world around him.

TEN YEARS

The ten-year-old is showing a greater involvement in hazardous games and activities. There is a greater interest in organized games and teamwork spirit is developing. In school, numbers beyond 100 are being used and examples and problems involving simple fractions are now understood. There is a growing interest in other people and their ideas.

take the infant to the bathroom immediately and place him on the toilet (usually an infant's "potty" that rests on the ordinary hopper). Then, smiling and speaking to him gently and warmly, she encourages him to evacuate. The infant cannot understand words but does interpret sounds and facial expressions; he can differentiate between love and anger. This procedure will not meet with instant success, and many repetitions will be required before the idea dawns on the child that this is what mother wants. From the very first time, even though the attempt meets with failure, the baby should be rewarded with a kiss and other expressions and words of love.

The same idea holds true for bladder control. Seldom does an infant indicate when he is wetting or has wet his diaper. The best the mother can do is learn to approximate when the child voids—the time period between urinary passages. Then, just prior to the next anticipated voiding, she should take the child to the bathroom so that by association he learns what is expected of him. In all cases of toilet training, the mother should never reveal impatience, or frustration, or disgust in angry outbursts.

TONGUE   The tongue is a muscular organ with a rich blood- and nerve-supply. Its functions include the manipulation and perception of materials placed in the mouth, the initiation of the act of swallowing, and—aided by the nose—the appreciation of taste. This latter function is important in digestion, as the sensation of taste evokes reflexes necessary for the secretion of the indispensable gastric juices. Because of its rich blood-supply, minor injuries are rapidly healed; bacterial infections are rare for the same reason. Vitamin deficiencies resulting in pellagra can cause a severe inflammation of the tongue, but this is now a relatively rare disorder in the United States. The disappearance of the

taste buds (papillae) may signal the onset of pernicious anemia, a condition caused by the individual's inability to absorb vitamin B_{12}. An interesting, but benign, condition known as geographic tongue is so named because of the peculiar map-like appearance produced.

"TONGUE-TIE"   A web of tissue is found under the front and central part of the tongue and runs to the floor of the mouth, just behind the lower teeth; called the frenulum, it serves no purpose. It is worth mentioning only because there are some who feel that the membrane has some deleterious effect on the development of speech.

If the tongue is mobile enough to reach the lips, this membrane can have no effect on a child's speech. Many doctors, however, will snip it, because of pressure from parents and grandparents. This is probably a safe procedure, although an occasional baby will bleed alarmingly when cut here.

TONSILLITIS   An acute bacterial infection of the tonsils, most often due to streptococcus, tonsillitis develops suddenly.

Symptoms. The tonsils are on either side of the throat near the back of the

TONSILLITIS

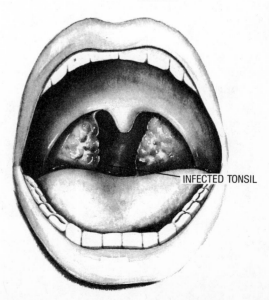

INFECTED TONSIL

tongue, and when acutely inflamed are red and swollen, and usually have white spots (follicular exudate) on the surfaces. Tonsillitis is one of the most common diseases of childhood and causes fever, vomiting, headache, malaise, sore throat, and sometimes ear pain. It is contagious, taking two to four days to transmit.

The so-called "strep throat" is usually a deep blood-red color and small red spots may be seen on the soft palate (the back of the roof of the mouth). If this is accompanied by a red skin rash, it is known as scarlet fever.

In some instances it is necessary to find out which specific organism is responsible for the infection. When this happens, a swab is used to take some bacteria from the infected tonsils. These germs are then grown in an incubator, identified, and perhaps even tested against different drugs to determine the most effective treatment for that particular case. Chronic tonsillitis implies that what started as a case of acute onset has subsided, but that some redness or dilated blood vessels remain on the tonsillar surfaces. There is usually some low-grade fever (up to 100°) and some swollen lymph glands under the corners of the jawbone.

Treatment. Baths or sponging to reduce the fever and aspirin for the relief of discomfort are the principal methods of home care. However, the doctor should decide when to treat, with what medicine, and for how long. A good general rule to follow is that if a comfortable warm bath and one grain of aspirin for every ten pounds of body-weight significantly reduce a fever within two hours, it usually means that the cause of the fever is not too serious and that a delay of twenty-four to forty-eight hours is justified before seeking medical assistance.

If the doctor decides on sustained treatment, it is important that the antibiotic drug chosen be continued for several days—usually ten—even though the patient may feel completely well by the fourth day. A significant number of complications (rheumatic fever, nephritis) may develop as a result of inadequate therapy. Some bacteria may even become resistant to the usual drugs because of early cessation of treatment.

Cases of chronic tonsillitis are often difficult to treat medically, and it is for this reason that tonsillectomy (surgical removal of tonsils) is often done. The size of the tonsils is not the sole criterion for removal; the frequency of attacks of tonsillitis and swollen glands is the best indicator for surgery. Before a decision can be made, there should be careful balancing of the risks of surgery against the risks of repeated infection.

TONSILS (See also ADENOIDS.) The lymphoid tissue at the back of the nasopharynx is really the pharyngeal tonsil; when it becomes enlarged, it is called (in the plural number) the adenoids. These can cause obstruction of the Eustachian tubes and are removed surgically when the obstruction causes hearing problems or ear infections. This lymphoid-tissue mass is part of a ring of lymphoid tissue which, unless allergy or infection is frequent, tends to grow smaller and becomes functionless as adulthood is approached. The other components of the ring (Waldeyer's ring) are the lingual tonsil, the lateral pharyngeal bands, and the palatine (faucial) tonsils. (When the term tonsils is used without qualification, it refers to the palatine tonsils, the ones we can easily see through the open mouth.)

Any of the tonsils may become infected, and any and all may have to be removed. The most common troublemakers, however, are the palatine tonsils and adenoids. It is when these tissues cause more trouble than their protective benefits are worth, that the physician recommends removal. Indications for tonsillectomy are recurrent tonsillitis and abscess in the tonsillar area. Indications for adenoidectomy are blockage of the Eustachian tube leading to hearing loss; recurrent middle-ear infection; fluid in the ear; and nasal obstruction and mouth-breathing.

These indications comprise about 90 per cent of the reasons for tonsillectomy and adenoidectomy. Frequently the tonsils and adenoids are removed at the same time, when both are enlarged and diseased, and when there are indications for surgical removal of both organs. On occasion, however, the tonsils or adenoids alone may be at fault and either one—but not both—is removed. This decision must be left to the physician.

Not all children need tonsillectomies and adenoidectomies (T-A's), and this, like any other operation, has specific indications. It is a safe procedure, but in children it is performed under general anesthesia, and any general anesthesia carries with it a small risk. The danger from T-A itself is very small, the major complication being bleeding. Bleeding can occur immediately after surgery, in the hospital, where the doctor can control it; or it can occur when the healing membrane sloughs off, about a week after surgery. The bleeding is usually controlled without great problems, but sometimes the child must be brought back to the hospital. True, bleeding of this kind does not occur often, but it will happen on occasion even to the most cooperative patient with the best doctor in the finest hospital.

TOOTHBRUSH   In spite of its name, this is a brush designed to facilitate cleansing not only of the teeth, but also of associated structures of the oral cavity. These include furrows of the tongue, the gums, and the inside of the cheeks. The brush may also serve as a means of stimulating the gums. It would therefore be better to consider a toothbrush as a "mouth-brush" or a "gum-brush."

An incorrectly used toothbrush can cause damage to the structures of the oral cavity. The dentist should therefore be consulted to assist in the proper selection of a brush, with due regard to individual differences, requirements, and needs. In general, the adult brush should consist of a long straight narrow handle (five to six inches long) and a working head of stiff bristles which are arranged in two rows, six tufts to a row. The bristles, whether synthetic or natural, should be of even height (one-half inch). Each person should preferably have three brushes, so as to allow sufficient time for them to dry thoroughly between brushings; this will insure that they are clean and maintain their stiffness. When the bristles are loose and become dislodged during use, the brush should be discarded and replaced. (A single toothbrush bristle forced into the gingiva can act as a foreign body, like a splinter, serving as a source of irritation and possible inflammation.)

A child's brush should be of a similar design, except that it is necessarily smaller and should be somewhat softer. This type of brush is usually called a junior brush.

Electric toothbrushes of various styles are available. The brushing head itself is the same as that of a manual toothbrush; the main difference lies in the mechanical action involved. The final decision as to the type of brush needed should always be decided by the dentist on the basis of the individual's needs. There are, for example, specially constructed brushes for use on dentures, bridges, for patients wearing orthodontic appliances, or for those with certain periodontal problems.

TOOTHBRUSHING   When properly manipulated, the toothbrush aids in cleaning the teeth and stimulating the gums. Improper toothbrushing implies inadequate as well as overzealous techniques. Since there are so many variations from individual to individual, the method of brushing should be determined by the dentist in order to make this procedure as effective as possible. In general, the teeth should be brushed for a period of three minutes, and this within fifteen minutes of eating. If this is done, the debris remaining after eating, as well as any by-products resulting from carbohydrate (sugar) conversion into acids, will be removed, thereby minimizing the possibility of dental caries. When brushing is done properly for three minutes, the gums will also be maintained in a healthy state, thus decreasing the possibility of periodontal disease.

Only the chewing surfaces of posterior teeth should be brushed with a scrubbing (back-and-forth) action. All other surfaces of the teeth and their adjacent gums should be brushed in the following manner: Place the bristles in line with the teeth, with the ends of the bristles pointing away from the teeth while resting on the gum; then rotate the brush in the hand, while pulling it toward the biting surface of the teeth. This enables the bristles to stimulate the gums and pass over and in between the teeth in a cleansing motion. In this manner, groups of teeth in each arch are brushed in the direction in which they "grow," by brushing down on the "uppers" and up on the "lowers."

TOOTH-SURFACES   Generally, each tooth has five surfaces, each related to the direction in which it faces. The biting surface is termed the occlusal surface; the surface which faces the midline of the face is termed the mesial surface; the surface which faces away from the midline is the distal surface; the surface which faces the tongue is the lingual surface; and the surface which faces the cheeks or lips is the facial surface. (In the posterior teeth, the facial surface is termed the buccal, whereas in anterior teeth it is termed the labial surface.)

Dental decay may involve any one or

all of these five surfaces, and the design and type of the restoration depends upon the extent of destruction. Thus, an occlusal restoration involves only the biting surface, whereas a restoration of the mesial, occlusal, and distal surfaces (MOD) involves three sides of the tooth. Not until dental decay has been removed can the dentist determine the extent of the necessary restoration, which would depend upon the number of surfaces affected; hence the term filling does not indicate the number of surfaces requiring such restoration. Since there are thirty-two permanent teeth with a total of 160 surfaces (32 x 5), and twenty temporary teeth with one hundred surfaces (20 x 5), this makes 260 surfaces which, at one time or another, are potential areas of decay.

TORSION OF TESTIS   When the testis becomes acutely twisted on the spermatic cord, it may become greatly swollen because the blood supply is cut off. This condition is an acute emergency, calling for surgery, but is completely relieved by opening the scrotum and returning the testis to its proper position.

TOXEMIAS OF PREGNANCY   Under the general heading of toxemia are included a whole group of related complications, characteristically occurring during the last few months of pregnancy and disappearing spontaneously after delivery. These diseases have several symptoms in common and vary in severity from relatively benign abnormalities to very serious complications affecting several vital organs and jeopardizing the life of the mother. The cause of toxemia of pregnancy is not known. Accumulations of salt and water often are a part of the toxemic picture, but what causes the retention of salt is unknown. Approximately 10 per cent of all pregnancies are complicated by toxemia, and this, together with hemorrhage and infection, are the three main causes of maternal deaths throughout the world.

Symptoms. The general common denominator of all the symptoms of toxemias of pregnancy are the following abnormalities: hypertension, swelling of the tissues, and presence of proteins in the urine.

Possibly the earliest sign of impending toxemia of pregnancy is excessive weight gain within a short period of time in a patient who is in the last two to three months of pregnancy. This weight gain is mostly in the form of extra water held by salt, infiltrating the tissues and appearing as generalized swelling (edema). The mother presents a "puffy" appearance and the legs and ankles become swollen. Depending on the severity of the condition, her urine will start to show the presence of variable amounts of albumin, and blood pressure may begin rising above normal. Constant headaches follow in more severe cases, and the patient begins to see spots in front of her eyes. The load that the heart has to carry increases suddenly, and the patient may experience shortness of breath.

The worst toxemia of pregnancy, and probably the most serious of all diseases that may complicate pregnancy, is eclampsia. The patient who develops eclampsia may exhibit part or all of the above-mentioned symptoms of preeclampsia, but in addition suddenly goes into convulsions and loses consciousness.

Treatment. Since the cause of toxemias of pregnancy is not known, their appearance cannot be prevented. We are able, however, to keep them under control and avoid serious injuries to the mother and the baby.

Salt-restriction and sometimes salt-free diet will be necessary during the last few months of pregnancy. Diuretic drugs are usually used for excretion of excessive fluids and salts by the kidneys. Antihypertensive and sedative drugs are used to bring the patient's blood pressure down to normal limits. In more severe cases, the patient will have to be put in the hospital for complete bed rest and for frequent analysis of blood and urine, which will help guide the therapy.

The definite treatment of toxemias of pregnancy is accomplished by delivery of the baby. Sometimes the obstetrician may have to terminate the pregnancy, even prematurely, if all other methods fail to produce the desired goal.

TOXIC SHOCK SYNDROME (TSS)   A recently identified condition believed to be caused by a bacteria called staphylococcus aureus. The FDA does not maintain that tampons are the cause of TSS as the disease also occurs among nonusers of tampons.

Symptoms. Sudden fever (usually 102° or more) and vomiting, diarrhea, fainting or near fainting when standing up, dizziness, or a rash that looks like a sunburn.

IF THESE OR OTHER SIGNS OF TSS APPEAR, YOU SHOULD REMOVE THE TAMPON AT ONCE, DISCONTINUE USE, AND SEE YOUR DOCTOR IMMEDIATELY.

There is a risk of TSS to all women using tampons during their menstrual period. TSS is a rare but serious disease that may cause death. The reported risks are higher to women under 30 years of age and teenage girls. The incidence of TSS is estimated to be between 6 and 17 cases of TSS per 100,000 menstruating women and girls per year.

You can avoid any possible risk of getting tampon-associated TSS by not using tampons. You can possibly reduce the risk of getting TSS during your menstrual period by alternating tampon use with sanitary napkin use and by using tampons with the minimum absorbency.

TOXOPLASMOSIS.   A disease varying from the unnoticed to the lethal, now recognized as being very widespread, it is produced by a minute intracellular parasite, the toxoplasma organism. In most instances the disease may be passed off as a mild flu-like infection. Surveys indicate that a third or more of the inhabitants of cities in the United States have had the illness and give positive skin tests. A first episode of toxoplasmosis in the pregnant woman, like rubella, can produce severe brain and retinal damage in the fetus (congenital toxoplasmosis). The disease can be acquired by eating raw beef, and there is evidence that cats may be household carriers.

Treatment. Treatment with sulfa drugs and pyrimethamine (Daraprim®) is of value but does not assure removal of encysted organisms.

TRACHEITIS See Respiratory Tract Infection

TRACHEOTOMY (TRACHEOSTOMY) These terms are applied to the surgical opening of a small aperture in the foreward wall of the windpipe (trachea) through which a tube is inserted to maintain access to air. The procedure is designed to relieve certain types of airway-obstruction, and for many years it was mainly indicated in cases of diphtheric croup. With time, the indications have broadened to incorporate other conditions such as tumors of the upper respiratory tract and, more recently, relief of obstruction in the lower respiratory tract. In the latter case, the operation is obviously not intended to by-pass any point of blockage —the obstruction being on the far side of the tracheal opening—but provides a means to give direct access for cleaning out secretions and for connecting apparatus to produce effective mechanical ventilation (artificial respiration); many different diseases and conditions which threaten or preclude normal breathing may therefore be benefited by temporary or prolonged periods of artificial ventilation through a tracheotomy. Among these are poliomyelitis, chest injuries, extensive burns, tumors, severe respiratory infections, and so forth.

As an emergency procedure, the tracheotomy may be a truly life-saving operation, particularly in children where the complete closure of the larynx may take place in a period of hours. The length of time a tracheotomy is maintained depends on the nature of the underlying disease, and may vary from several days to the occasional case in which it has to be maintained for months, or even indefinitely. Upon removal of the tube and bringing-together of the skin surfaces, the wound will generally close by itself without after-effects.

TRANSPLANTATION Successful transplantation of kidneys is now a routine procedure at many medical centers. Careful matching of donor and recipient and the use of immunosuppressive agents prevent organ rejection. Such kidney transplants may prevent death from uremia or abolish need for frequent dialysis on the artificial kidney. More dramatic but far less successful have been heart transplants. Most recipients experience troublesome complications and eventual rejection of the engrafted heart. Lung transplants have so far been uniformly unsuccessful. Variable results have been reported for pancreas transplants (for diabetes) and thymic and bone marrow transplants for immunologic and hematologic deficiencies. (See also Corneal Transplant.)

TRENCH FOOT Rarely encountered in civilian life, trench foot results from long exposure to cold and moisture of the extremities encased in restricting footgear. Obvious damage to the skin is rarely noted except as a secondary and ominous effect.

Symptoms. Hemorrhage of the small vessels of the skin, ulcers, blisters, and gangrene constitute an extension of the primary condition, in which the damage appears to be to the deep blood vessels and nerves, giving the skin a blanched appearance at first, and then a reddening and swelling. The condition is accompanied by a sensation of "pins and needles" and marked sweating. The sweating may indeed worsen the condition by producing more of the wet-cold local skin environment.

Treatment. Prevention is afforded by the far-sighted wearing of roomy and sturdy footgear in circumstances where this condition can be anticipated. Repeated drying of the feet and gentle massage (under a shirt or outer garment) may seem to be a luxury in military situations conducive to producing trench foot, but they are essential precautions. Treatment consists of bed rest, elevation of the feet, systemic antibiotic remedies, and supportive measures.

TRENCH MOUTH   Trench mouth is an infection of the gums and mouth (occasionally also the throat and tonsil area) caused by a specific bacterium. The infection may be due to poor oral hygiene or exposure to certain poisonous heavy metals such as lead or mercury. Occasionally, chronic vitamin deficiencies or generalized bodily infections will predispose to trench mouth. In unsanitary surroundings it can be rather contagious and may be carried by contaminated food utensils.

Symptoms. The symptoms of trench mouth are a sudden onset of fever, pain on swallowing or talking, bleeding and painful gums, and a foul odor to the breath. If the infection lodges on the tonsils it may resemble diphtheria; here, differentiation is important. The signs of trench mouth are grayish, membrane-covered ulcers on the gums or in the back of the throat. (Other infectious agents can cause similar appearing ulcers so an exact diagnosis is important in initiating proper treatment.)

Treatment. Appropriate antibiotic therapy is uniformly successful in clearing up trench mouth.

TRICHINOSIS   Trichinosis (also called trichiniasis) is a disease caused by a parasite, the roundworm *Trichinella spiralis*. Infection occurs when raw or inadequately cooked pork containing the encysted larvae is eaten. The larvae spread through the body, and those that reach muscle tissue survive.

Symptoms. Many people are believed to have trichinosis and not know it because they have no symptoms. Usually within a week or two after ingestion of poorly cooked pork, there is a bout of fever, severe muscle aches and cramps, and a characteristic swelling of the upper eyelids. Muscles of speech, breathing, swallowing, and chewing are frequently involved. The blood typically shows a high percentage of a reddish-staining white blood cell (eosinophilia). The illness may last for weeks or even a few months. Often it is disabling, but rarely is it fatal or does it produce permanent damage.

Treatment. There is no specific treatment for trichinosis, the physician treating the symptoms. The disease may be prevented by the thorough cooking of all fresh pork. Farmers should not feed raw garbage to hogs for it may contain infected pork wastes.

TRIGEMINAL NERVES   The two trigeminal (or fifth cranial) nerves carry sensory impulses such as pain and temperature from the skin of the face to the brainstem. These nerves also transmit motor responses to the muscles used in chewing.

Neuralgia of the trigeminal nerve results in severe periodic facial pain. This nerve may also be damaged by tumors or infections.

TRIGEMINAL NEURALGIA   Trigeminal neuralgia (tic douloureux) consists of sharp shooting pains in the distribution of one or more branches of the trigeminal (fifth cranial) nerve. It is not associated with any change in sensation in the face. The cause is not known.

488

Symptoms The severe bouts of knife-like pain in the face may be temporarily disabling. Pain may occur in any one or all three divisions of the nerve on one side of the face. The lower portion of the face is more commonly involved than the forehead. A "trigger point" is often present in the area of the pain. Light pressure along the lower lip may set off severe pain extending along the lower jaw on the same side. Similarly, touching the gums, chewing movements, or stimulation of the skin over the cheek or forehead may set off pain. Bouts of pain may occur frequently over a period of weeks or months and then subside, with periods of complete freedom for months. Recurrence is the rule.

Treatment. Although pain-relieving medicines are required in severe cases, it is important to avoid the repeated use of narcotic drugs. Dilantin® Sodium and vitamin B$_{12}$ have been associated with remissions of trigeminal neuralgia. In selected cases, injection of alcohol into the maxillary or mandibular (jaw) divisions of the trigeminal nerve may provide relief of pain. Alcohol injection will, however, result in loss of sensation in the distribution of the injected nerve. In other severe cases direct surgical treatment is indicated.

TUBAL (ECTOPIC) PREGNANCY

This is the most common type of pregnancy outside the womb, also known as ectopic pregnancy. Because the tube is a small and thin-walled structure, the pregnancy cannot be maintained for long (rarely for more than three to four months).

Symptoms. The patient usually misses a period or two and has the usual early symptoms of pregnancy. A few days or weeks later, irregular vaginal bleeding and occasional "crampy" lower abdominal pains begin. (This latter is due to stretching of the thin wall of the tube by the enlarging fetus.) Depending on the site of the pregnancy within the tube, the fetus will even-

tually either be pushed into the abdomen or will rupture the tube. At this time the patient feels a sudden, staggering pain in the lower abdomen, which gradually becomes milder while the patient feels weak and fainty. This is due to internal hemorrhage from the ruptured tube. The patient may collapse if bleeding is severe enough.

Treatment. The patient should be taken to the nearest hospital where an emergency operation can be performed in order to stop the bleeding; blood transfusions are usually necessary. The ruptured tube is removed, and recovery is quite satisfactory once the lost blood has been properly replaced.

TUBAL LIGATION See STERILIZATION

TUBERCLE BACILLUS See TUBERCULOSIS

TUBERCULIN TEST See TUBERCULOSIS

TUBERCULOSIS

Tuberculosis is one of the oldest diseases in recorded history. The earliest medical description called it consumption or phthisis because of its conspicuous feature: wasting-away. The disease is not unique to humans, affecting many animal species as well. No branch of the human race has been known to be immune to it, but the severity or prevalence of tuberculosis varies widely in different communities in relation to multiple factors: genetic (inherited resistance); rate of successive exposure (acquired resistance); changes in the virulence of the bacilli; and socio-economic factors (which affect both the nutritional state and the degree of exposure of individuals to the infected persons spreading the disease). Although great strides have been made in the fight against tuberculosis, it still remains one of the world's greatest killers. Today in the United States, which has one of the lowest mortality rates from tuberculosis, there are at least forty million persons with live tuberculous germs in their bodies. Of these, over two million have actually been ill with the disease.

Despite the impressive accomplishments in the fight against this disease, eradication of tuberculosis is not yet in sight. Furthermore, there have been shifts in the pattern of the disease and its distribution. For instance, formerly tuberculosis was predominantly a disease of young adults with comparatively low incidence in older individuals. As treatment became more effective and diagnosis more adequate, we witnessed an increased incidence of this disease in the elderly. Furthermore, from time to time, significant increase in the number of new cases has been reported in the general population. Whether this represents a true numerical increase or only reflects more intensive case finding and improvement in diagnosis remains to be seen.

The disease is caused by the tubercle bacillus, identified by Koch in 1882. Different strains of the germ affect man or animals preferentially, but crossover is possible. Man is affected by the human or bovine variety, seldom by the avian (bird) form. The bacillus is a rod-shaped organism which is identified by its characteristic staining properties and which grows only in the presence of oxygen. As explained above, the bacillus will have different pathogenic effects (illness potential) according to its variety and the degree of resistance exhibited by the host. As a matter of fact, most first attacks are quickly overcome and the bacilli establish themselves in the body without causing actual damage. Occasionally, when the body defenses are weakened, they become virulent, multiply, and the clinical disease is established. In most cases tuberculosis is directly transmitted from person to person via droplets in the cough. The most common initial site of disease is therefore the lung. Occasionally it may enter the body through contaminated milk from a tuber-culous cow, and the initial site will then be the bowel. Tuberculosis is not a hereditary disease and babies are infected after birth.

In recent years, new strains of tubercle bacilli have been identified. These are generically called anonymous mycobacteria. They differ from the classic Koch bacilli in the biological properties, the nature of the disease they produce in men, and particularly in their apparent resistance to the conventional anti-tuberculous drugs.

Symptoms. The tubercle bacillus may produce disease in almost any organ of the body, and the symptomatology will vary according to the location. Still, tuberculosis of the lungs is by far the most common form and the one from which most of the spread to other organs will originate. Tuberculosis of the lung is an insidious disease. The first attack, also called primary infection, is characterized by a nodular lesion in the lung which tends to heal spontaneously through the formation of a scar and the deposit of layers of calcium. This primary infection, which may attack at any age but preferentially in childhood or adolescence, commonly runs the course of a simple "cold" or "grippe," and usually goes by undetected. Nevertheless, at this time an important phenomenon occurs in the form of an allergic reaction. The organism has been sensitized by the tubercle bacilli, a fact which can be detected by the appearance of a positive tuberculin skin test. Subsequently, although the lesion is cured, it continues to harbor live tubercle bacilli which may, under certain propitious conditions, become reactivated and generate the full-blown disease. Thus the disease may be continuous with the primary infection, or a period of many years may elapse before reappearance.

The symptoms of tuberculosis are insidious and appear only after the anatomical lung lesion has been active for weeks or months. As the bronchopneumonic focus sloughs its way into the bronchial tubes, cough and expectoration make their appearance—first as clear mucus, and later as blood-streaking if ulceration of a small blood vessel has taken place (hemoptysis). Slight toxic symptoms are present, such as moderate evening rise in temperature, easy fatigability, decreased appetite, weight loss, night sweats, vague digestive symptoms, etc.

Unfortunately tuberculosis symptoms can be deceptively inconspicuous. The disease may alternately progress and subside until both lungs are widely involved by successive discharge of the bacilli through the bronchi into hitherto healthy areas. By the same token, the lesion may extend and gain access to the blood circulation and establish itself in the brain covers (meningitis), the bones, kidneys, genitals, etc. The disease is discovered at the time of an exacerbation or through routine examination.

From the above description it becomes obvious that the course of pulmonary tuberculosis for any given individual is unpredictable. The susceptible, weakened patient may show extensive lung cavities (cavern) or tuberculous pneumonia when he first seeks medical attention, while in the less susceptible patient, the disease runs a less stormy course.

The natural defense mechanisms of the body against the tuberculous lesion are manifested by the formation of fibrous (scar) tissue which tends to circumscribe the disease while certain cells called macrophages fight the bacilli. This sort of "cure" is at best a compromise toward arresting the spread of the disease. The bacilli are not killed and may erupt again, and the mutilated tissue—if large enough —will eventually produce either large, suppurating bronchial dilatations (bronchiectasis) or symptoms of respiratory insufficiency manifested by crippling shortness of breath.

The most common complication is an extension of the disease to the contiguous pleura (pleurisy) with the common formation of fluid. The most dreadful complication (particularly in small children) is meningitis because of its difficult diagnosis at an early stage. Otherwise the disease may spread to practically every organ in the body. As previously mentioned, although such localizations usually follow in the wake of an originally pulmonary lesion, tuberculosis in other organs may continue active while the pulmonary lesion has already been arrested.

Absolutely necessary for diagnosis is the presence of the tubercle bacillus. In the course of the disease, the bacillus is usually isolated from the patient's sputum, by examining the pleural fluid, or from the urine or cerebrospinal fluid. In the absence of sputum or because the patient swallows it, an alternate useful procedure is to examine the sucked-out (aspirated) gastric fluid. Occasionally a biopsy (surgical excision) of a small piece of gland tissue or bone marrow may be necessary.

The tuberculin test is a useful diagnostic tool. The purpose of this test is to detect the presence of past or present tuberculin infection. Tuberculin is a material extracted from cultures (growths) of tubercle bacilli and is administered by several ways: (1) as an injection under the skin (Mantoux test); (2) by slightly scratching the skin (scratch test); or (3) by applying an adhesive band (Volmer patch). The result is read after forty-eight hours and is called positive when a little lump and redness develop in the injected area.

A positive result in a tuberculin test only means that the person has been exposed to tuberculosis, and that he harbors some tuberculous lesions; it does not imply that the lesion is presently active. Only in infants and small children is a positive reaction interpreted as actual disease. Many adults will exhibit a positive reaction although most of them were never aware of having had tuberculosis. On the other hand, a negative reaction proves quite conclusively that tubercle bacilli never entered the body. The test has diagnostic value in medical practice, but its greatest usefulness is as a screening tool for determining the prevalence of tuberculous infection in a community, tracing sources of infection, and planning the necessary public-health measures accordingly.

Treatment. The need for treatment is self-evident when the patient has overt symptoms of active disease, but there is a large group of individuals in whom the indications are not so clear-cut. Most of the latter have been brought to notice only by findings during routine chest X-ray, and the present activity of the disease cannot be adequately ascertained. This is a rather common medical dilemma because of the relatively large number of individuals who are infected but in whom the disease has been spontaneously arrested, leaving only a lung scar.

It is obvious that the yield of cure is far superior in new infections with lesions of smaller size, than in the far-advanced. Any treatment for tuberculosis, however, represents a long-term commitment with all its implications and should not be used indiscriminately merely because a suspicious pulmonary lesion has been detected by X-ray. The final decision must rest on a clinical evaluation of the history, physical examination, tuberculin test, repeated examinations of the sputum or gastric aspiration, and especially chest X-rays repeated at regular intervals to detect any changes in the appearance or extent of a lesion.

Treatment is presently based on specific antituberculous drugs, the most important of which are streptomycin, isonicotinic hydrazide (INH), and para-amino salycilic acid (PAS), used most frequently in some combination. The drugs should be administered for prolonged periods of time, until the disease-process has been arrested and the bacilli are no longer recoverable. Sometimes, in advanced cases complete control of the disease is impossible, and the patient must be medicated indefinitely. Recently a new antibiotic, rifampin, has been shown to have marked antituberculous activity, producing negative sputums in cases where other combinations of drugs have failed.

More advanced cases which cannot be resolved by drug treatment are considered for surgical procedures, particularly the selective removal of limited areas of lung tissue (segmentectomy, lobectomy) or sometimes of a whole lung (pneumonectomy). Old surgical procedures such as pneumothorax (collapse of the lung by injection of air) or thoracoplasty (collapse of the lung by removal of several ribs) are much less in use today.

The extraordinary advances in treatment have unfortunately created some new problems, mainly the emergence of drug-resistant strains of bacilli. Tuberculosis is essentially a chronic disease, prone to exacerbations and remissions. Even under the best conditions, when the disease is limited and in an early stage, intensive treatment is necessary for at least several months, followed by several years of antituberculous drug coverage and periodic medical examinations. Since the advent of the "miracle" anti-tuberculous drugs, modern treatment has emphasized the need for early rehabilitation and return to normal activities while continuing active treatment. All this has lured many patients into a false sense of "short cures" with the unfortunate consequence that treatment may not be followed adequately and the disease may relapse. Erratic or insufficient intake of anti-tuberculous drugs carries the serious hazard of allowing the bacilli to become resistant to these drugs. Furthermore, dissemination of such drug-resistant bacilli to other individuals will in turn preclude from the new victim the possibility of being effectively treated by these drugs. Unfortunately, this situation is frequently encountered, forcing the use of new anti-tuberculous drugs, some of which are exceedingly toxic.

The obvious aim in the fight against tuberculosis today is not to discover still newer, more effective drugs, but to prevent the spread of the disease by early detection of new cases which can be effectively treated before they in turn continue to spread the disease. Because of their relative simplicity, in this fight, the most important medical tools are the widespread use of routine chest X-rays and the tuberculin test. These have been successfully tested in the canvassing of entire communities.

In the last twenty years a great controversy has centered about the usefulness of the antituberculous BCG (Bacillus Calmette-Guerin) vaccine. This vaccine is made of an attenuated type of tubercle bacilli which, upon injection into tuberculin-negative persons, transforms them into tuberculin-positive skin reactors. Under such conditions, it is postulated that the individual will develop defenses against future tuberculous infection similar to the relative immunity of individuals who have had a minimal tuberculous infection some time in the past and have thus become tuberculin-positive. The effectiveness of this vaccine is still under discussion, and its use in the United States is limited largely to crowded, poverty-stricken communities with a high incidence of tuberculosis, where other methods of preventing the spread of this disease are not feasible. In such cases, the children in particular should be vaccinated, preferably immediately after birth.

TUMORS   A tumor is any swelling. Thus, a mosquito bite is a tumor; so is inflammation of the parotid gland (mumps). However, the term is generally reserved for a new growth (neoplasm), a proliferation of new cells that may continue to develop but may also become stationary at some point in its growth, or even occcasionally regress. The specific cause of tumors is unknown, although in the case of cancer, more and more attention is being given to viruses as the provocative agents. It is known that even after the precipitating factor (chronic irritation, for example) ceases, the tumor can continue to grow, hinting at an ongoing disorder of cellular multiplication.

A benign tumor is composed of normal or nearly normal cells whose growth is local, well outlined, or encapsulated, and hence, not threatening to life and most always amenable to surgical removal. A malignant tumor or cancer is marked by uncoordinated growth, often without sharp delineation of its borders and able to invade neighboring tissues and spread throughout the body (metastasis). It therefore carries a grave prognosis.

It should be recognized that the term cancer indicates disorders of many causes; physically, chemically, and biologically its meaning is no more specific than "inflammation" or "infection." Therefore, it is almost impossible to generalize about many aspects of neoplastic disease.

Biochemical differences between normal and cancer tissues have been the subject of intensive research but no specific or distinctive alteration has yet been discovered. Even under the microscope a distinction may be difficult to make. For example, cancer of the thyroid gland may be virtually indistinguishable from the thyroid tissue from which it arises.

A malignant tumor that arises from ectodermal or entodermal tissues is a carcinoma. Ectoderm is the outer investing cellular membrane of the body, including any tissue (no matter where it is) that is originally derived from the epiblast of the embryo, (the embryo's outer layer). Entoderm or endoderm, is the cellular lining of the major part of the digestive tract and organs that are derivative outpouchings of the digestive tract. A sarcoma (also a malignant tumor) is born of mesodermal tissue; the mesoderm is cellular tissue of the middle layers of the body.

TUMORS, LUNG   The word tumor is descriptive of many different conditions in which the chief characteristic is the presence of an abnormal mass. The mass may contain any kind of body-tissue, liquid or solid, and may be of different sizes and shapes. Some tumors tend to increase in size, and their nature may be either malignant or benign.

A malignant tumor is usually characterized by increased activity in the form of disordered growth which tends to invade adjacent structures in a destructive fashion: as it develops, it may eventually gain access to the bloodstream and establish "colonies" in other organs (metastases or "daughter-tumors"). A benign tumor usually indicates a mass formed by normal tissue cells which tend to grow locally and are neither destructive nor productive of metastases. Nevertheless, a benign tumor may in fact be of serious importance because of its size or complications.

Tumors of the lung may be of two basic types: benign or malignant. They may originate in any structure within the chest and also, if malignant, may be metastatic—"daughter-tumors" whose parent-tumor started outside the chest. (These latter, malignant tumors most commonly originate in the breasts, prostate, kidney, or digestive system.)

The most common tumor originating in the lung is the bronchogenic carcinoma (cancer starting in a bronchus). This is presently the most prevalent tumor found in males, particularly in the fifty to sixty-five age group. Deaths from this form of cancer have steadily climbed over the past thirty years from 2.5 per 100,000 population in 1930 to 43 per 100,000 in 1960. As with other forms of cancer, little is known about the cause; but present-day statistical studies have produced uncontrovertible evidence that cigarette smoking and other air pollutants are somehow linked to its production.

Symptoms. The symptoms of bronchogenic carcinoma are unfortunately very sparse and non-specific in the early stages of the disease and cannot be relied upon for early diagnosis. Cough is the single most constant symptom. By the time other symptoms appear (such as expectoration, chest pain, temperature, general malaise, weight-loss, or various complications) the disease is usually far advanced locally or has originated metastases within the chest or distantly in the bones, digestive system, or brain. Under such conditions the tumor is incurable. Awareness of any respiratory symptom and/or obtaining routine or early chest X-rays has been demonstrated to be the single most useful procedure for early diagnosis. Physical examination, however careful, will in most cases fail to establish such an early diagnosis. In the majority of cases the unsuspected cancer is diagnosed after a complication (pneumonia, pleurisy, hoarseness) has brought the patient to medical attention.

Diagnosis by chest X-ray is not always simple or easy. Although certain X-ray features of bronchogenic carcinoma are fairly unmistakable, other causes must be considered. Additional diagnostic procedures which are useful are: study of the sputum (which will demonstrate the presence of cancer cells in a significant percentage of cases); addition of specialized radiological techniques (such as bronchography and laminography); direct visual inspection of the bronchi by bronchoscopy (which will also permit the obtaining of a piece of tissue [biopsy] for analysis); biopsy of lymph "glands" (nodes) in the neck; or biopsy of the pleura.

Treatment. The rate of cure for carcinoma of the lung is still disappointingly low because conventional means of therapy are only effective before the tumor has invaded certain areas (metastasized). The percentage of cure—as expressed in terms of five years of survival after treatment—is presently in the neighborhood of 5 to 20 per cent; this, however, has been slowly improving with increased awareness on the part of patients and also because of a more "aggressive" attitude of physicians toward early suspicious lesions. What this means, in fact, is that small early lesions discovered by X-ray, whose nature (after reasonable diagnostic evaluation) has not been adequately clarified, should be considered potentially malignant and treated as such.

Thus, the approach to therapy is essentially surgical, conducted by means of an exploratory chest-opening (thoracotomy). The lesion is closely examined, analyzed on the spot, and if possible removed. If removal is not feasible because of widespread extension, or if there is doubt that the whole tumor has been removed, X-ray irradiation (radiotherapy) is given to the patient after the operation. If the tumor is considered inoperable from the outset, radiotherapy alone is used.

TWINS Twin births occur approximately once in 90 births, triplets once in 8,000, quadruplets once in 750,000. The role of inheritance in the production of twins is not yet very clear.

Twins may be the result of fertilization of one egg (identical twins), or of two separate eggs (fraternal twins). In the second case, the twins may or may not be of the same sex, and will bear no more resemblance to one another than the rest of the children of the same parents. Identical twins, on the other hand, are always of the same sex and resemble one another very closely.

Triplets, quadruplets, and quintuplets, may also be the result of fertilization of one, two, or more eggs, and they may be identical, fraternal, or of assorted variety.

From the obstetrical point of view, a mother who is known to carry twins should have very careful prenatal care, for nutrition should be specially planned to include extra iron and other minerals and vitamins, and she should get more rest than the average pregnant woman. Twin pregnancies usually terminate two to four weeks earlier than single ones, and the babies' weight is proportionately lower. There is also a high incidence of prematurity.

TYPHOID FEVER Typhoid (or enteric) fever is an acute, severe infection caused by the *Salmonella typhosa* with involvement of lymphatic tissue, and characterized by an abnormally slow pulse, high fever, a skin eruption, digestive disorder, and enlargement of the spleen. Improved hygiene and health guards have made the disease rare in North America. Likewise, prevention is easily obtained through vaccination (see below).

Symptoms. The patient first suffers chilliness, headache, loss of appetite, malaise, nosebleed, backache, and possibly diarrhea and/or constipation. If treatment is not instituted, the temperature rises in steplike progression over the next several days, reaches its peak in the third week, and gradually returns to normal in the fourth. The pulse is abnormally slow, and an eruption described as rose spots occurs. The spleen is enlarged and the patient may become delirious and fall into stupor. Sometimes there are sore throat, extreme nausea and vomiting, bronchitis, pneumonia, kidney infection, and even emotional upsets to the point of a frank psychosis.

Complications include intestinal hemorrhage, intestinal perforation, pneumonia, infection and clotting of veins (especially of the lower limbs), mumps, meningitis, inflammatory involvement of the heart, complete or patchy loss of hair, and inflammations of the kidneys, bladder, bones, joints, and gallbladder. Very common are miscarriages in pregnant women.

Treatment. Specific treatment, especially if promptly instituted, will abort the illness and result in prompt and complete recovery. The antibiotic, chloramphenicol, is the agent of choice. Other conditions are treated as outlined under their respective headings. Symptoms are individually cared for, such as analgesics for pain (aspirin, codeine, etc.) and tranquilizers for emotional upsets. Supportive treatment is also prescribed. Prevention and prophylaxis are accomplished by typhoid vaccine inoculations, usually given simultaneously with paratyphoid A and B vaccine. All persons who have come in contact with a typhoid patient or carrier, or those who contemplate travel to foreign countries should be immunized at least two months prior to taking a voyage to allow time for immunity to develop.

ULCER AND ULCERS   An ulcer is an erosion of the surface lining of a tissue, usually accompanied by varying degrees of inflammation. Ulcers may occur in any area and can have various causes. Viral or bacterial infections, burns due to heat or caustic chemicals, peptic ulcers due to increased secretion of pepsin and acid by the stomach are common causes in the digestive tract.

ULCERATIVE COLITIS   This serious chronic disorder of the colon should not be confused with mucous colitis, a relatively benign functional disorder. Ulcerative colitis is characterized by repeated episodes of severe inflammation and ulceration of the large intestine. The exact causes are not well understood, but emotional factors are thought to play a significant role.

Symptoms. Symptoms of ulcerative colitis include abdominal cramping; as many as ten to twenty bowel movements a day; the passage of blood and mucus;

and fever, weight loss, and prostration. The attacks may be mild at first, but with repeated episodes of increasing severity the potential seriousness of the illness becomes evident. The ulceration may become so severe that the stool contains little else but blood. With vigorous treatment the disease may become dormant for long periods of time, only to begin anew. Stools may be relatively normal, depending upon the region of intestine involved. However, between bowel movements there are discharges of blood and pus, and generalized constitutional symptoms of fever, nausea, vomiting, and gradual weight loss are seen. The diagnosis can usually be confirmed by direct examination and X-rays.

Treatment. Conditions such as amoebic dysentery (see diarrhea) must first be ruled out as the treatment is quite dissimilar. The maintenance of adequate nutrition, replacement of blood, control of infection, and a recognition of the emotional aspects of the disease are the foundations of successful therapy. Often the surgical removal of the offending portion of the colon is mandatory.

ULCER DIET   Patients with ulcers of the stomach or duodenum (the first few inches of intestine following the stomach) are usually placed on a bland diet. The principle of the diet is to dilute the acid gastric juice frequently by providing several meals daily of easily digested, palatable, nonirritating foods. Milk is the basic food in a bland ulcer diet; other foods are gradually added as tolerated.

The following types of food neutralize the acid already in the stomach, and are therefore included in an ulcer-diet:

1. Protein foods such as milk and eggs
2. Cream
3. Foods that are soft and smooth (no raw fruits or vegetables)
4. Salt and lemon juice, for seasoning

Meals should be frequent and small in amount so as to take up the acid; three snacks in addition to the regular three meals are usual.

Certain other habits of eating are also recommended:

1. Rest before meals if tired or nervous.
2. Allow plenty of time for meals and eat slowly.
3. Rest fifteen minutes after meals if possible.
4. While on the diet, the bowel functions should be kept normal by using orange juice as a natural laxative. Use the juice of one orange in one glass of warm water before breakfast and, if still constipated, repeat this at the noon meal.

Foods which must definitely be omitted from the diet of the ulcer-patient are:

1. Foods highly seasoned with mustard, pepper, vinegar, or other spices
2. Meat broths, gravies, nuts, pickles, and hot sauces
3. Foods that are ice-cold (ice cream should be partially melted)
4. Coffee, carbonated beverages (cola drinks, soda pop, etc.) and alcohol

A sample ulcer-diet menu follows:

Breakfast:
 Enriched refined cereal with milk and sugar
 Egg
 White bread and butter
 Milk or cocoa
 Strained fruit or juice at meal's end

Lunch:
 Cream soup
 Lean meat
 Potato, rice, or spaghetti
 Bread and butter
 Milk
 Strained fruit juice

Dinner:
 Lean meat, fish, or fowl
 Potato
 2 strained cooked vegetables
 Bread and butter
 Bland dessert (custard)
 Milk

Milk, in one form or another, is often recommended between meals and at bedtime. The physician will modify the general principles described here for the individual patient.

ULNAR NERVE The ulnar nerve supplies many of the muscles which regulate hand-function. It also carries sensory impulses from the little finger and the neighboring portion of the ring finger.

UNCONSCIOUSNESS Abnormal unconsciousness, occurring when a person would ordinarily be in a waking state and from which one can not be aroused by normal stimuli, may be symptomatic of various disorders of the central nervous system which can be diagnosed only by comprehensive medical examination. Loss of consciousness may occur on several levels of severity, ranging from simple transient fainting (syncope), to stupor, from which one can be aroused only with difficulty, to complete unconsciousness or coma, from which the patient can not be aroused at all.

Symptoms. Among the most common causes which should be routinely considered in every case of unconsciousness is circulatory collapse, including fainting, stroke, head injuries, acute alcoholism, poisoning, diabetic shock, and epilepsy. It is very important to secure a case history clarifying the conditions under which loss of consciousness occurred; often the diagnosis can be made from the history alone. Any evidence relating to reasons for loss of consciousness, such as containers suspected of having held alcohol, drugs, or poisons, should be retained for further examination. In cases where collapse has occurred without apparent cause, diabetes should be ruled out first, by means of laboratory tests of urine and blood sugars.

It is particularly important to rule out an expanding lesion such as hemorrhage or tumor within the skull. In many cases of cerebral hemorrhage following head injury, the person loses consciousness for a few minutes immediately after the injury because of cerebral concussion, following which he appears normal for several hours only to lose consciousness again suddenly. This secondary loss of consciousness suggests an expanding hemorrhage and immediate neurologic examination is indicated.

An important diagnostic problem consists in distinguishing organically caused coma from hysterical reactions. In all emotionally unstable young persons and particularly in women, it is common to observe fainting or apparent collapse which is actually a hysterical reaction to acute emotional conflict. (In such cases, application of painful stimuli results in immediate return to consciousness.)

Treatment. Successful treatment of unconsciousness always depends on rapid and successful diagnosis of its causes. Until a physician is obtained, emergency measures should include placing the person flat on his back, loosening tight clothing, checking to see that the nose and throat are clear, treatment of shock by keeping the person warm, and oxygen inhalation where respiratory difficulties are obvious.

"UNDERACTIVE THYROID" (HYPOTHYROIDISM)

In this condition the amount of circulating thyroid hormone is low. In extreme form, it appears as myxedema or, in children, as cretinism. Not many patients, however, are afflicted with this severe form.

Symptoms. Mild cases of hypothyroidism show easy fatigability, dry skin and hair, increase in body weight, decreased tolerance for cold, and increased nervous irritability. The incidence of hypothyroidism is quite high, as has been demonstrated in several studies in which blood iodine measurements have been taken in the general population. It is often present in people with goiter and in patients previously treated for overactive thyroid conditions. Diagnosis is not always easy because the condition can be confused with anemia, underactive pituitary (hypopituitarism), nervous conditions, and general fatigue states. The basal metabolic rate was once the most useful test in diagnosing this condition. In recent years, however, thyroidologists have developed the blood protein-bound iodine (PBI) test and the radioactive iodine-uptake test, as well as a test which measures the relaxation time of the achilles tendon at the heel.

Treatment. Treatment of hypothyroidism is usually quite easy and may be effected with oral adminstration of a variety of thyroid preparations. Patients may have different reactions to these preparations, however, and the physician will often change the type of thyroid medication. Treatment must usually be continued for a long period of time, sometimes indefinitely. Usually the individual thus treated will show remarkable improvement in energy, strength, general vigor, and ability to accomplish his daily activities.

UNDERFEEDING

An infant may receive insufficient food because of poverty, neglect, or community lack of food (as in wartime siege or a widespread transportation strike), and malnutrition may result. Malnutrition may also result from organic conditions such as blockage in the digestive tract (by a tumor, pyloric stenosis, or intestinal obstruction), chronic diarrhea, colitis, liver disease, gastritis, osteoporosis (cystic degeneration of the bones), and tuberculosis. In a child it may be caused by sheer refusal to eat or other emotional or mental conditions.

In the training of an infant, underfeeding may arise when a mother adheres rigidly to a schedule. She may ignore his screams, adamant in her determination not to "spoil" him. The baby may simply be hungry and his diet should be increased (after consultation with the physician). Psychological factors to which varying importance has been attached also color the clinical picture.

UNDERWEIGHT   Below average weight may be normal for an individual, in the absence of pathology, and must be differentiated from "loss of weight." In the healthy person, underweight is actually desirable. In 1962, an investigation involving a million men revealed that a person who was not merely at normal weight but below normal weight had a 79 per cent greater chance of never suffering heart disease of any kind.

Loss of weight may result from starvation, under- or malnutrition, protein deficiency, vitamin deficiency, mineral deficiency, disease processes, and emotional disorders. Once the physician has ascertained the cause of underweight, then he may prescribe the proper treatment. This may include diet—even surgery if tumors, etc. are the cause of the loss of weight.

UNDULANT FEVER (BRUCELLOSIS) Undulant fever is an infectious, febrile disease contracted by humans from animals.

The causative organisms belong to the brucella group. They are found in cattle, hogs, and goats from whose skin, excreta, or milk man contracts the disease.

Symptoms. Within five to twenty-one days after brucella enter the body, the disease begins insidiously (although some cases have been reported as occurring months after exposure to the organism) with influenza-like symptoms. A sudden onset with chills, fever, and extreme weak-

ness sometimes occurs. The spleen is usually enlarged and tender to the touch. Inflammation of the testicles or ovaries may occur. There may be nerve and spinal cord pains, swollen and aching joints, and very rarely, bacterial endocarditis.

A myth has developed over the years that undulant fever is apt to be a long, drawn-out, disabling disorder. To the contrary, it is self-limiting, and, with the advent of antibiotics, the outlook is generally favorable. Relapses and recurrences are not unknown, however.

Treatment. The antibiotics, streptomycin or dihydrostreptomycin, combined with tetracycline comprise the treatment of choice. If the patient appears to be extremely toxic, adrenocortical therapy is employed.

UREMIA   When the kidney is unable to excrete poisons from the body in a normal fashion, these substances—mostly organic acids or nitrogenous substances—collect in the bloodstream and produce characteristic symptoms of uremia. This condition is due to interference with the function of the kidneys, and may be due to disease in the kidney itself, interference with the blood supply of the kidney, or disease and infection in the lower part of the urinary tract.

Symptoms. Symptoms of uremia are usually those of dehydration, clouding of mind, and convulsions.

Treatment. Uremia due to obstruction or renal shutdown is potentially reversible by medical or surgical measures. Chronic uremic states may be managed by dialysis on the artificial kidney or, even better, by a donor kidney. The transplantation of a single healthy kidney can completely reverse all of the disturbances found in uremia.

URETER   The ureter is a muscular tube approximately a foot long which passes from each kidney to the base of the bladder and carries urine to the bladder for storage until its ultimate excretion from the body. Its walls are muscular and are capable of contraction. When the ureter is obstructed, spasm may ensue with resulting severe pain.

URETHRA   This is the tube which carries urine from the bladder to the exterior (via the penis in the male, and to the opening just above the vagina in the female). Lubrication of the tube is accomplished by glands which secrete slippery mucus along its course.

URETHRITIS   Inflammation of the passage from the urinary bladder to the exterior (urethra) is spoken of as urethritis. Since the urethra is short in the female, infection is readily spread from the vagina or the rectum when proper toilet hygiene is not used. The walls of the urethra become inflamed, and passage of urine become difficult and painful. Because in the male the urethra traverses the interior of the penis, it may be the site of infection from gonorrhea or non-specific bacterial organisms acquired during sexual intercourse.

URINARY OBSTRUCTION   Obstruction to the flow of urine may occur in the ureter because of a stone, a blood vessel which passes across the ureter, or a kink in the ureter due to misplacement of the kidney. Usually, however, the term urinary obstruction refers to inability to pass urine through the urethra. In men this is most commonly caused by an enlarged prostate or a stricture of the urethra due to infection. In the days before modern antibiotics, strictures of the urethra were very commonly the result of attacks of gonorrhea.

URINARY-STONE FORMATION Various kinds of stones are found in the urinary tract. Calcium phosphate stones

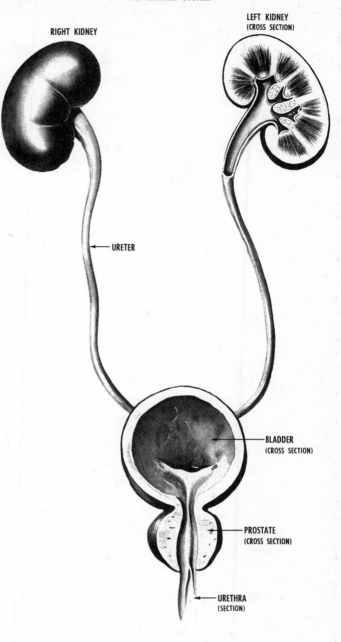

RIGHT KIDNEY

LEFT KIDNEY (CROSS SECTION)

URETER

BLADDER (CROSS SECTION)

PROSTATE (CROSS SECTION)

URETHRA (SECTION)

The organs concerned with containing or secreting urine are the kidneys, ureters, bladder, and urethra. The fluid secreted by the kidneys is stored in the bladder and discharged by the urethra.

are the most common and are formed when there is an excess of calcium in the urine, alkaline or neutral urine favoring deposits of additional calcium phosphate on an already-extant tiny stone. Calcium phosphate stones are usually small and round, of a white or yellow-white color, and show evidence of layering.

The presence of infection in the urinary tract favors the growth of uric-acid stones which form around nuclei or uric acid deposits during the late fetal or early newborn period. These stones are often very soft and crumble easily, accounting for the fact that they are frequently passed from the body in the form of small bits of gravel.

A hereditary condition results in stones made of cystine, a sulphur-containing amino acid.

Urinary stones containing calcium are visible on X-ray films, while uric-acid and cystine stones are not directly visible and may require the use of X-ray opaque (contrast) material given either intravenously or sent directly into the ureters.

URINARY TRACT   The entire system through which urine passes is referred to as the urinary tract. This includes the kidneys, the ureters, the bladder, and the urethra.

URINATION (MICTURITION)   This is the process of expelling urine from the bladder. Voluntary relaxation of the sphincter muscle in the urethra is accompanied by contraction of the detrusor muscle of the bladder, which forces the urine in a stream through the urethra. This process is not ordinarily painful but may become so with the presence of obstructions or constrictions of the urethra.

URINE   The urine is a solution of waste products excreted by the kidneys. Passing from each kidney down the ureter into the bladder, it is expelled by the process of urination (micturition). Urine is usually yellow in color but will be darker or lighter depending on the concentration of dissolved pigments. It usually shows an acid reaction except for a short period after meals or during the presence of urinary infection, at which time it may be alkaline. Normally, urine does not con-

tain either protein or sugar. It may contain a few cells which are washed off in its passage from the kidneys to the bladder and the exterior of the body. There is often a small amount of mucus present. The color of the urine may be affected by the ingestion of various kinds of dyes, and its odor by dietary substances.

A urinalysis is a laboratory investigation of urine. Routine examination reports on the color, turbidity, the acid reaction, specific gravity, the presence or absence of albumin, sugar, ketone elements, pus, or crystals, and a microscopic investigation for casts, blood cells, and epithelial cells. Abnormal findings are followed by special quantitative and qualitative tests.

URINE, RETENTION OF   Urinary retention is an accumulation of urine, with inability to pass it and distention of the bladder. The patient complains of pain, an overwhelming desire to urinate, and frequently attempts to do so without satisfaction. Retention of urine is common in enlargement of the prostate gland, stricture of the urethra (the urinary excretory channel leading from the bladder), prostatic cancer, tabes dorsalis, stone or foreign body in the urethra, dislocation and/or fracture of the spine, inflammatory disease of the spinal cord, tumor of the bladder, in certain emotional states and psychoneurotic conditions. In infants, elongation of the foreskin to the extent that it cannot be pulled back may cause urinary retention. Treatment in this instance is, of course, circumcision.

Treatment. Immediate relief of obstructed urinary flow is catheterization. This consists of the passing of a sterile flexible, very thin tube into the bladder. In extreme bladder distention, all urine is not immediately permitted to escape; otherwise the radical change in intraabdominal pressure, particularly in the aged or those with impaired or weak hearts, may cause unpleasant reactions, often a small amount is permitted to pass every twenty to thirty minutes until the bladder is emptied. If catheterization cannot be done (as in complete urethral block), surgery is the only answer. Treatment of the various basic causes, as listed above, is presented under the respective headings.

UROLOGICAL STONE

A stone anywhere in the urogenital tract is referred to as a urological stone. Such stones may be present in the kidney, ureter, bladder, or urethra.

UTERINE BLEEDING, ABNORMAL

Some forms of abnormal bleeding from the vagina are classified as menorrhagia or metrorrhagia. Menorrhagia is excessive menstruation, either in amount or duration, without intermenstrual bleeding. The extent of bleeding varies but is sometimes profuse enough to produce anemia. Menorrhagia in a teen-ager after onset of menstruation is not uncommon and may be severe and intractable. Metrorrhagia is intermenstrual bleeding. It has numerous causes among which are various kinds of tumors. Women over the age of forty should have a gynecological examination at least every six months.

Many nongynecological conditions may be accompanied by abnormal uterine bleeding. Among these are: certain acute infections, anemia, hemophilia, leukemia, gout, scurvy, malaria, emotional conditions, and diseases of the lungs, heart, and liver.

Gynecological conditions that are marked by irregular and/or abnormal uterine bleeding are abortion, miscarriage, fibroids of the uterus, chronic inflammatory conditions of the uterus, cancer of the uterus, tubal pregnancy (ectopic pregnancy), the menopause, placenta previa (heavy bleeding that may occur during labor), malposition of the uterus, inflammation of the tubes and/or the ovaries, hardening of the arteries, prolapse of the uterus, cervical polyp, and laceration of the uterine cervix.

Less common causes include vaginal ulceration, cervical ulceration, hyperthyroidism, overactivity of the pituitary, alcoholism, cirrhosis of the liver, scurvy, and tuberculosis.

UTERUS, INERTIA OF THE

Occasionally during labor the womb, instead of continuing regular contractions for the completion of labor and delivery, slows down or even stops contracting. Cephalopelvic disproportion or heavy premature sedation may be the cause; on other occasions the cause is unknown. The treatment will depend on the individual case: some patients will require special drugs to stimulate labor, while others will have to be delivered by caesarean section.

UTERUS, RUPTURE OF THE

This is a relatively rare, but very serious, complication in the pregnant woman. It is liable to occur more often in patients who have had previous caesarean sections, whether they are in labor or not. Such patients should report any abnormal sign that comes to their attention to their doctor, such as a sudden sharp abdominal pain, vaginal bleeding, feeling of faintness, etc. Rupture of the pregnant uterus frequently results in the death of the baby and in severe hemorrhage. Immediate surgery, blood transfusions, and the removal of the uterus is often necessary.

UTERUS, SUBINVOLUTION OF THE

This represents the failure of the womb gradually to return to normal size after delivery of the child. It is often accompanied by prolonged vaginal bleeding, and sometimes low-grade fever and backache.

Treatment. Treatment consists of special drugs (oxytocics) that make the uterus contract; quite often, scraping of the womb is also necessary.

UVEA

The middle coat of the eye, the uvea, consists of the iris, ciliary body, and choroid. The iris, the colored portion of the eye visible through the cornea, surrounds a central opening, the pupil, which controls the amount of light entering the eye.

The iris contains two muscles, one for dilating the pupil and the other for making it smaller. Structurally, it is a thin tissue consisting of two layers. The front layer is composed of thin filaments, while the back layer is dark brown. The color of the iris depends upon the number of filaments in the front layer. If many are present, the eye is blue; if fewer, the eye is hazel or green-gray; while if very sparse, the eye is brown.

The size of the pupil is mainly governed by the amount of light entering the eye, but varies first of all with the individual; also with instillation of medicines or medicines taken by mouth; with anger, fear or similar emotions; and with optical defects of the eye.

The ciliary body is continuous with the iris and is located behind it, so that it is not visible from without. This body provides nutrition to the interior of the eye and tends to maintain intraocular pressure. Fine fibers attached to the lens and ciliary body (the zonule) support the lens in position. A muscle in the ciliary body gives rise by contracting and relaxing to changes in shape of the lens, with focusing through the zonular fibers. (Focusing for near objects is known as accommodation.)

The choroid is the blood-vessel layer of the eye and provides nutrition for the portion of the retina adjacent to it. It is continuous with the ciliary body in front and ends at the optic nerve behind. It consists mainly of blood vessels with pigment interspersed between them.

VAGINA (BIRTH CANAL)

This structure, resembling a collapsed tube, serves to connect the vulva with the mouth of the womb. On the average, it is four inches long and is surrounded by strong layers of muscular and connective tissues which allow it to stretch and permit the delivery of a full-term baby, with subsequent return to almost the original dimensions. After repeated childbirth, especially in the white race, the walls of the vagina undergo relaxation and the bladder and rectum may herniate into the birth canal. This can be corrected with plastic surgery of the vagina, almost always combined with sterilization of the patient through tubal ligation or hysterectomy.

VAGINAL DISCHARGE

Discharges from the birth canal (vagina) occur normally in a majority of young girls—even babies. They will frequently be noted on diapers and underpants. During adolescence especially, it may become quite noticeable and yet be entirely normal: there are great differences between individual normal girls. If, however, the discharge becomes sufficiently profuse to be bothersome—especially to the child herself; or if the color turns from grayish to yellow; some attention besides cleanliness may need to be given to it. This is especially true if the discharge is blood-tinged (except where menstruation is expected), if it seems to cause irritation about the orifice (vulvar irritation), or if the condition defies simple cleanliness. In such cases the doctor should be consulted. Adolescence often brings on an increase in a normal discharge of this sort. Except for cleanliness, this too can be disregarded.

Infections, generally mild in nature, are often responsible for the more exaggerated and stubborn types of vaginitis causing discharge. Until recently, gonorrhea (even among more privileged families) was not uncommon as a cause. Nowaday it is rare in children—although more common in teenagers. Its results in children are almost never serious, as they may be in adults. There may be some danger of transmitting the infection to adults or infecting the child's eyes, but this is remote with ordinary cleanliness and if the doctor's instructions are carried out.

Occasionally a vaginal discharge is due to a small object (or tampons or parts of them) inserted by the child and retained in the vagina. This generally causes a discharge with a distinct odor and later some blood. This is not uncommon in children with an exploratory bend.

Treatment. Treatment generally consists in external cleanliness and frequent observation. Occasionally the doctor will need to prescribe antiseptics, either local or general, but unless there is serious resultant irritation of the vulva the situation is seldom, if ever, serious. Foreign bodies must of course be removed.

VAGINITIS   Infection of the vagina may occur at any age, from childhood to postmenopausal years. It is commoner during the reproductive period, and is usually produced by microorganisms such as *Trichomas, Monilia*, gonococcus. In childhood it is often the result of insertion of foreign bodies, or contamination from the rectum through improper wiping. In postmenopausal women it is primarily the result of atrophy of the tissue lining the vagina.

Symptoms. Abnormal whitish, yellowish, greenish, or purulent discharge is the main symptom of infection of the vagina. Burning and itching, and local swelling and soreness are also frequent symptoms of vaginitis.

Treatment. Depending on the cause, treatment will consist of vaginal antibiotic suppositories, oral or injectable drugs, douches, hormonal therapy (if atrophy is present), etc. The results are generally good and only 5 per cent of the cases will present difficulties with treatment.

VAGUS NERVES   The paired vagus (or tenth cranial nerves) control the muscles used in speaking and swallowing. They also carry impulses regulating the function of the heart and of respiration. If the vagus nerve is damaged, the patient will have difficulty in swallowing and his speech will have a nasal quality.

VARICOCELE   The veins along the cord inside the scrotum often become twisted and enlarged. This both looks and feels like a "sack of worms" within the scrotum. The condition in and of itself is painless and not serious; when developing suddenly in adult life, however, it may be an indication of a tumor in the genitourinary tract.

VASCULAR ACCIDENTS   This term refers generally to disease produced by gross circulatory disturbances such as clots or hemorrhages, without overt or identifiable external causation. The term is frequently applied to sudden circulatory events occurring in the central nervous system.

Because of the implied localization to the brain, similar events elsewhere (aorta or other major artery) are referred to as cardiovascular catastrophes. A clot lodged in a lung artery, though a form of vascular accident, would be referred to as a pulmonary embolus.

VAS DEFERENS (SPERMATIC CORD) The vas deferens is a cord-like structure which runs within the scrotum from the testes up to the inguinal region and enters the prostatic urethra at the base of the bladder. It carries sperm, which mature in transit, from the testes to be ejaculated into the urethra through the ejaculatory duct. It is sometimes the site of tuberculosis, which produces a beading of the tubular structure.

VASECTOMY   Cutting of the vas deferens with surgical tying-off of the severed ends is known as vasectomy. It is a common procedure in operations to remove

SEMINAL VESICLES

Relationship of bladder, prostate, and seminal vesicles to vas deferens.

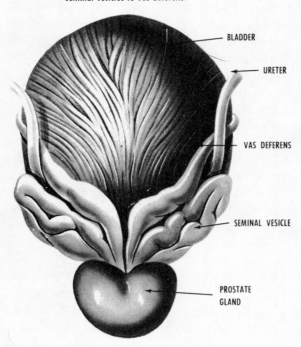

BLADDER

URETER

VAS DEFERENS

SEMINAL VESICLE

PROSTATE GLAND

the prostate gland. This procedure reduces the risk of infection reaching the epididymis and testis; it is also an effective means of producing permanent sterility in the male.

VASOMOTOR (AND ALLERGIC) RHINITIS   See ALLERGIC CORYZA

VASOPRESSIN   Vasopressin (antidiuretic hormone) is secreted by the posterior pituitary gland and is responsible for stimulating contraction of smooth muscle, especially of blood vessels. It also promotes the absorption of water by the kidney tubule, thus producing a urine-reducing (antidiuretic) action. Lack of vasopressin is responsible for a condition known as diabetes insipidus.

VENEREAL DISEASE   Sexually transmitted disease or infection is referred to as venereal disease (VD). Examples include gonorrhea, syphilis, genital herpes, and acquired immunodeficiency syndrome (AIDS). Infestations of pubic lice and scabies (a type of mite) are sometimes included in this category because they too are transmit-

ted during sexual contact. (See AIDS, GONORRHEA, HERPES, and SYPHILIS.)

VERNIX   This is a whitish, cheesy material covering the body of the baby at birth. It does not reappear after having been removed by washing the baby.

VERTIGO (DIZZINESS)   Dizziness involving faintness or lightheadedness should be distinguished from true vertigo, which involves sensations of whirling in space or of seeing the surroundings rotating. A common symptom of vertigo is nystagmus, a rhythmic horizontal or vertical oscillation of the eyeballs which is exaggerated by turning the eyes in different directions. (Many older people experience a transient dizziness on getting out of bed or coming suddenly to an upright position. This is caused by a delay in the body's adjustment of blood pressure to accommodate for a change in posture. It has no particular significance and is relieved simply by moving more slowly, or by resting a moment after standing up, to allow blood pressure to adjust.)

Ordinary dizziness usually involves transient interruption of blood circulation to the brain. True vertigo, in contrast, involves a disturbance of the balancing mechanism of the middle ear.

Treatment. The commonest types of vertigo caused by car and motion sickness are relieved symptomatically by use of Dramamine®. In more complex organic conditions, treatment depends on exact diagnosis and removal of the underlying causes. Ordinary dizziness is far more easily overcome, usually by putting the head between the legs or by lying down until normal blood pressure returns.

VESICLE, SEMINAL   The seminal vesicles lie adjacent to the base of the bladder. They secrete a thick, glairy material, a normal component of the semen; sperm are not stored in them.

VINCENT'S ANGINA, OR INFECTION
See TRENCH MOUTH

VIRAL DISEASES There are a variety of viral diseases that may cause neurosensory hearing loss. Many of them are childhood diseases such as mumps and measles. Hearing loss because of these diseases is not a very common occurrence.

VIRILISM The presence of unwanted hair on the face and body of a girl or woman, together with other features which suggest masculinity, is spoken of as virilism (literally mannishness). It is sometimes difficult to distinguish between excess body hair and true virilism (in which the facial features and body configuration become more definitely male in type).

The development of facial hair and other external evidences of virilism does not in any way change the sex orientation of the individual. Such characteristics are not accompanied by homosexual desires, and do not stimulate homosexual advances. Many women with severe forms of virilism are happily married.

It is not uncommon for physicians to encounter women with minimal amounts of facial and body hair who become quite concerned about being considered homosexual. This concern is often due to a psychological disturbance and is best treated as such. (See ADRENOGENITAL SYNDROME.)

VISION, MEASUREMENT OF The function of the eyes involves several different types of vision.

Central vision is measured by the reading of a chart with different-sized letters, numbers or pictures. The measurement numbers usually used, such as 20/20, 6/6, are not a fraction and do not indicate the percentage of vision present. The first number indicates the distance from the eye to the test-material, in either feet or meters;

the second number indicates the distance at which a normal eye can read the test matter—more accurately, the distance at which the objects subtend a 5 foot angle. "Near tests" are frequently carried out to learn the smallest object or print that can be seen without respect to distance from the eye. In general most attention is given to testing with the best possible correcting lens rather than to vision without lenses.

The most important visual function for moving about is the ability to see to the side (peripheral vision). One may have entirely normal central vision; but if side vision is lost, one is blind for practical purposes. Side vision can be measured accurately by a variety of tests. A rough measurement is made by closing one eye and having someone else signal with fingers from a given side until one can recognize the number of fingers used.

There may be a loss of color vision with loss of central vision, but many individuals are born with a decreased color sense. This loss may be very marked and easily evident by the inability to see color. In others, it may be very slightly depressed and require elaborate testing to demonstrate. There is no treatment for hereditary color blindness.

The ability of the eye to increase in sensitivity in dim illumination is dark-adaptation. Testing is fairly complex and seldom done. Much of the same information may be obtained by testing the electrical response of the nerve network (retina) at the back of the eye.

VISUAL AIDS A number of aids to vision are used, ranging from partially closing the eyes to make the lids act as a pinhole, to looking through a small opening in the closed fingers. (A pinhole admits only parallel rays of light to the eye. These do not have to be bent by the lens or cornea to come to a clear focus at the retina.) A number of pinholes in a piece of paper may also be used.

Spectacles consist of either concave or convex lenses, frequently with different powers at right angles to each other to correct astigmatism. Lenses of additional strength may be fused to them by heat to make bifocals or trifocals.

Spectacles are frequently made of safety glass or plastic, so as not to shatter if struck by a hard object. Plastic lenses have the disadvantage of scratching more easily than glass, but are lighter in weight. Most safety-glass lenses are manufactured by "case-hardening," in which the lens is heated and then cooled suddenly, thus making the outside surface very hard. (This is an industrial, and not a home, technique.) Rarely, safety lenses are made by laminating an unbreakable plastic between two layers of glass, as is done with automobile windshields. Safety glass is provided in ophthalmic or industrial thickness.

A number of different types of lenses are provided for those whose vision is defective with ordinary lenses. The most popular is a magnifying lens held over reading material. An arrangement of lighting so that a bright light is directed on reading material is frequently useful. (Generally the light should be in front of the eyes and strike the reading material at an angle.) Most lenses for improving near vision cause magnification, and the reading material must be held close to the eye. The lens sometimes permits only one or two letters to be seen at a time, and great patience is required to read. Most devices for visual aid are designed only for close work. Rarely, a small collapsible telescope can be used for distance; this is mainly useful in viewing street signs, bus routes, and the like.

Those with legal blindness (vision with correction less than 20/200, or a visual field contracted within a 20 degree radius) are eligible for "talking books" from the Library of Congress (books re-corded on phonograph records, together with a phonograph) and many other aids. (Write to American Foundation for the Blind, 15 West 16 Street, New York 10011, New York, for information.) (See also EYE, ARTIFICIAL.)

VITAMIN A   Vitamin A is an essential fat-soluble vitamin or "accessory food substance." It is involved in vision since it is a part of the purple visual pigment, rhodopsin. It is also needed for the proper maintenance of a very thin layer of cells (the epithelium) which lines or coats certain bodily structures. In the case of vitamin A, the tissues involved are the eyelid and eyeball linings (conjunctiva), the windpipe (trachea), the hair follicles, and the kidneys. Bone growth is also affected by vitamin A levels.

The vitamin is present in such animal food as liver, egg yolk, butter, and cream. It is also derived from many green and yellow vegetables, which contain a plant pigment—carotene—that is converted into the vitamin in the intestinal lining.

Vitamin A deficiency results from a poor diet and inadequate intake. It also follows from failure to absorb the vitamin, as in chronic diarrhea, sprue, certain forms of childhood indigestion (celiac disease) and premature birth, as well as from failure to convert carotene to vitamin A. This last is seen occasionally in diabetes mellitus and advanced liver disease.

Children deficient in vitamin A show retarded growth and, like deficient adults, are susceptible to infections. Night-blindness (nyctalopia), or inability to adjust the eyes to darkened conditions, is the result of inadequate retinal pigment, rhodopsin. A dry, thick roughening of the skin (follicular hyperkeratosis) appears on the arms and legs. In advanced cases, the conjunctiva of the eye is dry and wrinkled, and infections are frequent.

Treatment. The recommended daily

allowance for a healthy adult on a mixed diet (receiving two-thirds of the vitamin as carotene) is 5,000 International Units. In treatment, doses of 10,000 to 50,000 Units a day are used for children and 50,000 to 100,000 Units for adults.

Whereas vitamin A is easily stored and slowly excreted, it follows that repeated large doses may lead to excessive accumulation and "poisoning." A number of instances of abnormal excess of the vitamin in the body have been reported, especially in children. Symptoms of this condition are weight loss, headache, low-grade fever, changes in the bones and hair, anemia, and an enlarged liver. These symptoms usually disappear within one to four weeks after stopping the vitamin.

VITAMIN B$_2$ (RIBOFLAVIN)   Riboflavin is a member of the water-soluble vitamin B complex. It is essential for proper growth and tissue function. Deficiency of this vitamin (ariboflavinosis) results in characteristic oral, skin, and eye lesions. The deficiency may be present when there is an inadequate consumption of milk and other proteins. More often it is found in patients with chronic diarrhea; liver disease; chronic alcoholism; or when, after an operation, infusions are given into the vein for some days without preventive vitamin therapy. Pure riboflavin deficiency rarely occurs. It is more likely to be present with other deficiencies of the vitamin B complex.

In vitamin B$_2$ deficiency, the corners of the mouth may be the site of the first signs of riboflavin deficiency. They may become reddened, and there may be cracks or maceration of the mucosal lining in the angles. These cracks often leave scars in healing. A series of disturbances in the oil-secreting (sebaceous) glands of the skin may also occur, with the following sequence of symptoms: increased oiliness; appearance of yellow, flaky scales—often

in the folds between the nose and the mouth, sometimes behind the ears; and later, plugging-up of sebaceous-gland pores and roughening of the skin. In some cases, the cornea of the eye may develop a prominent network of tiny blood vessels. This may be accompanied by burning, tearing, and itching sensations.

Treatment. General nutritional therapy is essential, and riboflavin may be given by mouth in large doses. In rare instances, it may have to be given by injection. The recommended daily intake for the adult is between 1 and 2 mg. a day. The minimum requirement is less. Riboflavin is widely distributed in foods, but it is destroyed on exposure to light, and considerable loss can occur in such foods as milk.

VITAMIN B$_6$ Actually a group of closely related compounds, vitamin B$_6$ is often designated as pyridoxine. This member of the B complex has a function in the processing (metabolization) of amino acids, the basic components of protein. It also plays other less well-understood roles. Vitamin B$_6$ can relieve a form of neuritis sometimes observed by patients taking isoniazid (a drug for tuberculosis). Another preliminary report suggests that it contributes to the protection against dental caries (cavities) in children. A few cases of anemia in adults respond to large doses if the normal dietary intake is inadequate and a specific high requirement exists. Recent evidence suggests that vitamin B$_6$ may be required in heightened amounts during pregnancy.

The minimum daily requirement has not been firmly established, but the best estimates are that 1 to 2 mg. per day is an adequate amount.

Vitamin B$_6$ is abundant in foods, and a spontaneous dietary deficiency is not likely to occur. However, infants, and perhaps some adults, subsisting on an artificial processed diet not supplemented with vitamins could become deficient. In a few instances of proven vitamin B_6 deficiency, the patients (infants) developed anemia, impaired growth, and convulsions. In experimental deficiency in adults, a type of skin condition (seborrheic dermatitis) developed on the face. In addition, weakness, loss of appetite, a burning tongue, and inflammation around the eyes were noted.

Treatment. For treatment of vitamin B_6 deficiency, large doses of pyridoxine are given by mouth or injection. Ideally, the possibility of vitamin B_6 deficiency can be avoided by giving the vitamin precautionarily in multivitamin preparations—especially to infants, pregnant women, and others who may be eating poorly or whose requirements are higher.

VITAMIN B_{12} This member of the vitamin B complex family is one of the most biologically active substances known. The average daily requirement is only about 1 microgram, one millionth of a gram. It is found in liver, beef, pork, organ-meats, and eggs and milk products, among other sources. Chemically, it is a cobalamin, meaning it contains the element cobalt—the only nutritionally significant compound that does contain it. The usual form used as medication is cyanocobalamin and is derived from microbiologic material—that is, it is produced by certain bacteria when grown under special conditions.

Vitamin B_{12} is necessary for the normal development of red blood cells. If there is a deficiency of this vitamin, the cells do not grow to maturity and the patient becomes anemic. True B_{12} dietary deficiency is extremely rare; certain people, however, lack a substance in their gastric juice called "intrinsic factor" which binds and carries vitamin B_{12} across the intestinal membrane. They therefore cannot absorb the vitamin B_{12} in food. Such patients develop a serious disease known as pernicious anemia, characterized by severe anemia and a progressive deterioration of nerve tracts in the spinal cord, the outcome of which used to be fatal.

Treatment. Some years ago liver (raw or cooked, and later as an injectable extract) was the standard treatment for pernicious anemia. With the discovery of vitamin B_{12}, it became possible to treat the disease with monthly injections of this nontoxic vitamin. The disease is also treated by daily oral administration of vitamin B_{12} plus intrinsic factor obtained from animals. More recently, large oral doses of the vitamin alone have also proved to be effective. So it is that pernicious anemia, a disease of vitamin B_{12} deficiency, is no longer the fatal condition it was a mere generation ago.

VITAMIN B COMPLEX Vitamin B complex is the name given to a number of nutritional factors differing widely in chemical structure, but having in common an essential role in human nutrition. Many of the vitamins in this complex are components of one or more agents which play an important part in the activity of other bodily substances. Included in the group are thiamine (vitamin B_1), riboflavin (vitamin B_2), niacin, pyridoxine (vitamin B_6), and panthothenic acid, together with the "anti-anemia" vitamins, folic acid and vitamin B_{12}. (Choline is also usually included in the B complex.)

Deficiency of B-complex vitamins is a form of malnutrition frequently encountered in medical practice. Many of these vitamins occur in the same foods, and multiple deficiency is therefore observed more often than deficiency of a single substance. Some of the vitamins in this group are closely interrelated, and the clinical signs of deficiency may be similar, whatever the particular vitamin present in inadequate amounts.

If more vitamin B complex is given

than is required, the excess is excreted in the urine; there is therefore no real danger of accumulating too much of it in the body (hypervitaminosis).

Deficiency of vitamin B complex does not necessarily result from inadequate diet alone. Numerous abnormal conditions may bring on, and contribute to, the deficiency. When the metabolic rate is above normal, (as in hyperthyroidism, fever, or leukemia), there is an increase in the requirements for thiamine, riboflavin, and niacin. These vitamins also function in the metabolism of carbohydrate, and the requirement is increased following high carbohydrate consumption.

Vitamin B complex may be poorly absorbed or lost from the body in diarrheal diseases, inflammation of the digestive tract, and certain circulatory disorders. Furthermore, the body may use the vitamins in an abnormal manner in such diseases as diabetes mellitus and cirrhosis of the liver.

The administration of antibiotics by mouth may have an effect on vitamin B complex; in some instances, production of a B vitamin by intestinal bacteria may be impaired by the antibacterial effects of the drug. In other instances the antibiotic may actually reduce vitamin requirements by destroying the bacteria that utilize them.

VITAMIN C   Vitamin C, also known as ascorbic acid, is an essential water-soluble vitamin unrelated to the B complex. Its primary function is to maintain healthy connective tissue such as is found in bone and teeth. Ascorbic acid also has a role in the body's handling of iron and in the functioning of the adrenal gland whose hormones are essential in man's response to stress. For this reason, it is often administered in prolonged stressful situations, as after burns or extensive injury.

Vitamin C deficiency (scurvy) usually occurs in children from failure to supplement the diet with this essential item. All infants need vitamin C during the early months of life; for without it serious illness develops. (In adults, a deficiency may develop from a poorly balanced diet. It may occur in elderly people who live alone, cook their own food without much concern about nutrition, and rarely if ever drink fruit juices.)

The chief dietary source is citrus fruit, orange juice being the most likely source in this country. Other sources are tomato juice, tomatoes, cabbage, and potatoes. The vitamin is rather easily destroyed by cooking (oxidation with exposure to heat and light).

The average daily requirement for normal children is from 30 mg. (infants) to 90 mg. (boys, 13 to 15 years). Adults need about 75 mg. a day (perhaps double this amount in pregnancy). Most well-balanced diets supply this amount. The vitamin is essentially nontoxic, and larger amounts may be given safely if there is reason to think the requirements are high or the diet poor in citrus fruits (grapefruit, lemons, and limes, as well as oranges and tomatoes).

VITAMIN D   Vitamin D is an essential fat-soluble food substance which has its primary effect on the calcium and phosphorus content of body fluids. It is actually a group of closely related substances, chemically resembling cholesterol and certain hormones. A unique feature of vitamin D is its formation in the skin on exposure to sunlight or ultraviolet rays (hence the name sunshine vitamin). The body is therefore only partially dependent on the dietary supply. Deficiency is rarely seen in adults and is becoming uncommon in infants due to the widespread use of dietary supplements and fortified milk(s) in early life. (Milk irradiated with ultraviolet light has an increased vitamin D content.)

Vitamin D increases the absorption of calcium, and possibly phosphorus, from the intestine and helps to maintain the levels of these minerals. A deficiency of the vitamin results in the condition known as rickets. Normal bone and tooth formation requires, however, dissolved in the body-fluids, an adequate supply of calcium and phosphorus as well.

The vitamin is particularly abundant in fat fish, and cod liver oil was for years the main medicinal source. Nowadays vitamin-enriched, irradiated milks and milk products, margarines, etc., permit a reasonable intake which (with exposure to sunlight) meets the vitamin D requirement of many, but not all, children and adults. Many popular vitamin preparations also contain vitamin D.

Treatment. The recommended daily allowance in medical treatment is approximately 400 International Units a day, or about 10 micrograms of crystalline vitamin D_2, known as calciferol. In the darker-skinned races the requirements are about 50 per cent higher because skin pigment interferes with vitamin D production. Premature infants require much larger amounts, often in a water-mixed preparation, because of immature fat absorption.

Massive doses given over long periods of time may lead to toxic reactions such as elevation of serum calcium levels, deposit of calcium in abnormal and unwanted sites, vomiting, and diarrhea. Death may occur from kidney failure. *Note:* The fat-soluble vitamins A and D are the only ones in which the danger of overdosage is a realistic possibility.

VITAMIN E Vitamin E (also known as alpha-tocopherol) is a fat-soluble vitamin which has an essential but still poorly understood role in metabolism. It is widely distributed in foods (especially wheat-germ oil and eggs), so that dietary inadequacy is rare. An uncommon form of anemia in infants has been shown to be specific to vitamin E deficiency. In the experimental animal, vitamin E prolongs the life-span, an effect ascribed to its antioxidant capacity. Hence the older idea that vitamin E was without a role has been abandoned. Nonetheless, many of the claims advanced for its use, as in heart disease and osteoarthritis, have not been substantiated.

VITAMIN K Vitamin K is essential for the formation of prothrombin, a substance necessary for blood coagulation. In vitamin K deficiency, hemorrhage in any tissue or in mucous membranes occurs. Such deficiency, however, is rare unless there is some underlying disturbance. Vitamin K is present in a large variety of foods and is synthesized by bacteria in the intestinal tract. The adult human requirement is easily supplied by the ordinary diet, in addition to the amount produced in the intestines. Natural forms of vitamin K are fat-soluble; deficiencies are therefore observed in conditions in which fat absorption is impaired (jaundice or malabsorption).

In infants whose mothers have not received vitamin K before birth, there is the danger of an inadequate intake in the first ten days of life. Cerebral hemorrhage may be present in such a case. Vitamin K deficiency may be diagnosed by estimating the prothrombin activity of blood.

VITAMINS Most people are aware of the fact that vitamins cannot be manufactured in the body, hence must be included in the diet, and there is, in fact, a tendency to dose children with them too liberally, on the theory that whatever the organism does not need will simply be thrown off, and that an oversupply is safer than an undersupply. This is not accurate: doctors and nutritionists have positive knowledge that here "too much of a good thing" can be harmful. Nevertheless, vitamins may indeed be needed in increasing amounts during periods of rapid growth, during stress, and while convalescing.

Babies especially need to be given vitamins—but only according to the doctor's recommendation—because of their very rapid growth and because they are seldom exposed to the rays of the sun. What is usually prescribed for them is a multivitamin mixture, to be continued through their first year of life; but as soon as the diet becomes reasonably balanced and some meat, fruits or vegetables, as well as grain and dairy products, are consumed almost daily, the vitamin supplement becomes a needless expense and may even be dangerous. In this case, as in so many others, the wise parent will be content to be guided by the advice of the family doctor or pediatrician rather than rely on well-meaning friends or on advertisers.

VITILIGO This disease is characterized by a progressive loss of pigment occurring most often on the face, neck, arms, and the back of the hands, but no portion of the body is exempt from involvement. The lesions appear first as small round or oval alabaster-white spots which grow larger and join with adjacent lesions. When the skin is tanned on exposure to the sun, there appears to be an increase of the pigment at the border of the white lesions. Whether the increase is "real" or whether it is "relative" and due to a larger differential in color (from the border's ability to become tan from the sun) is still an unresolved question. There is no known cause for the disease and there are no significant concomitant symptoms.

Treatment. Before treatment can be started it is necessary to differentiate this disease from several quite similar conditions, namely albinism (congenital loss of the ability to produce pigment, which is not susceptible to treatment), chloasma (partial and irregular hyperpigmentation, in which the paler areas may resemble vitiligo), and pseudoachromia parasitica (or tinea versicolor, a fungous infection causing lesions of both lessened and in-

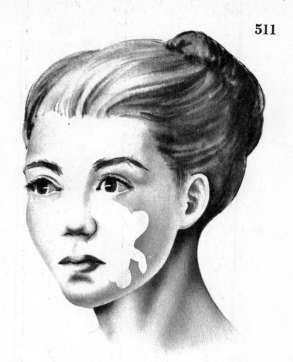

VITILIGO
Vitiligo is an acquired pigmentary disease characterized by irregular, sharply defined, milk-white patches. Except for the loss of pigment, the skin is normal. The condition lasts throughout life.

creased pigmentation). Because spontaneous remission is uncommon, treatment, limited though it is, may afford relief. Among the many and varied kinds of treatment, the recent revival of an ancient remedy, the plant-derived ammoidin which is now synthesized as the psoralenes, has stimulated extensive clinical research of great promise. The psoralenes are worthy of trial, especially in patients with extensive involvment of the skin.

VITREOUS, DISORDERS OF The vitreous is a clear, gel-like structure which fills the eyeball between the lens and the retina. It has very few cells and does not partake actively in any disease process.

Normally the vitreous contains small strands of protein fibers which are opaque and can be seen as dark lines against a bright background such as the blue sky. They are of no significance.

In injury and disease, white or red blood cells may enter the vitreous from adjacent structures. Treatment is directed against the cause.

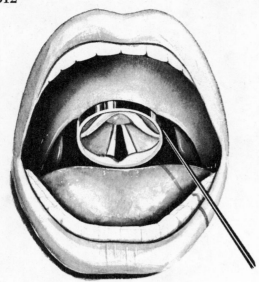

MIRROR-IMAGE OF THE VOCAL CORDS

VOCAL CORDS, PARALYSIS OF THE
Paralysis of one or both vocal cords as the cause of hoarseness is surprisingly common. In about 20 per cent of cases it is not possible to determine the cause.

Symptoms. When one vocal cord is paralyzed there is mild hoarseness at the onset of paralysis, but the larynx compensates and a normal-sounding voice may be the eventual outcome. When both vocal cords (bilateral) are paralyzed and cannot be moved apart from their midline position, the voice usually remains of good quality but the airway is often inadequate under physical stress.

Treatment. The treatment of paralysis is therapy of the causative factors. In addition, in cases of bilateral paralysis, operations are possible which return the vocal cords to a more normal position and thereby enlarge the airway.

VOLUNTARY NERVOUS SYSTEM
Also known as the motor system and the efferent nervous system, this complex consists of the nerve cells and fibers which convey impulses from the central nervous system to the periphery, chiefly the muscles.

VOLVULUS
A volvulus is an obstruction of the intestine due to the twisting or kinking of a segment of the bowel. This not only prevents passage of the intestinal contents but usually shuts off the blood vessels as well. A volvulus most often occurs in the sigmoid portion of the large intestine because of the peculiar anatomic attachments at this point. The most common predisposing cause is the presence of adhesive bands of scar tissue, often as a result of previous abdominal surgery. (Interestingly, a high percentage of volvulus is seen in patients who are vegetarians. It is presumed that this more bulky diet is in some way responsible.)

Twisting may occur in other portions of the large intestine but is rare in the small intestine. Because of the disruption of the blood supply to the involved section, gangrene and perforation of the bowel are common if early surgery is not performed. The symptoms are similar to those in any intestinal obstruction. In occasional instances, the twist will right itself, but surgical treatment is usually necessary.

VOMITING, CYCLIC
Some young children have periodic recurrent vomiting, often accompanied by abdominal pain, migraine headaches, and diarrhea. The nausea and vomiting appear suddenly, last one or two days, then disappear spontaneously.

Among the possible causes of this condition are allergy, glandular disturbance, low blood sugar, faulty fat metabolism, epilepsy, and recurrent infection. It often afflicts children of families with a strong history of migraine headaches.

Treatment. A good thorough medical examination to try to determine the cause is necessary. If allergic in nature, the condition may be cured by removing the suspected food. As the child grows older, the vomiting is less of a problem and headaches become more obvious—usually the severe one-sided types.

VOMITING (EMESIS) IN CHILDREN

Vomiting is the forceful emptying of the stomach via the mouth. It is a sign of a number of conditions, depending on the frequency, amount, color, and projectile force of the attack. The simple "slip-up or wet burp" so often seen in babies is hardly worth considering; the gas bubble in the stomach simply pushes up a little bit of milk.

A baby may lose some or all of a feeding because of injudicious handling or even straining at stool. If a baby vomits some, or what appears to be all, of its feeding, it means the milk is too rich or that the child is sensitive to one of the components of the milk. Simply changing to another type (skimmed) will solve this problem immediately. If within four to six feedings of a new milk the baby is no better—especially if there are cramps, loose stools, and gas—it usually means that the infant has become allergic to cow's-milk and should be tried on goat's-milk or soy-bean milk.

When trying to find the correct food for a baby, the main consideration is weight-gain; if in the first six months the child gains from one to three pounds a month, he is probably getting enough nourishment. If not, a more determined search must be made as to the cause. When stools and urine become scanty because of severe vomiting, and especially if there is a weight loss, skilled care is necessary or the baby may become dehydrated. (See also PYLORIC STENOSIS.)

Most children vomit once or twice when coming down with any illness, but the most common illness which produces vomiting is intestinal flu (viral gastroenteritis): there are great spasms of stomach cramps terminating in forceful emptying of the stomach; this may continue until the dry heaves occur. Usually there is a day of vomiting, with a week of diarrhea following. Urine output may become restricted, but unless it does, the patient may need nothing more by way of care than frequent sips of water, broth, or cola drinks. In any event, milk and heavy, greasy foods are the worst things to be given if there is nausea or vomiting.

Nervous-system disease, especially if there is intracranial pressure (due to concussion, blood clots, tumors, or meningitis), will give rise to vomiting. Vomiting may also occur at the onset of sore throat, kidney infections, or almost any illness: apparently this is the body's way of trying to reject the disease.

A kind of vomiting no longer often seen is "rumination"; this is usually found in a tense home—in the nervous child who seems to derive some sadistic joy from upsetting his mother who has just carefully fed him. He rolls his tongue into his throat, vomits, and then seems content.

VULVA   The vulva surrounds the entrance to the vagina (birth canal) and consists of several structures. On the outside there are two folds of skin (labia majora) and within these two smaller folds (labia minora). At the upper end is the clitoris, and under it, the urethra (opening of the bladder). The hymen separates the vulva from the vagina.

A variety of diseases can involve the structures of the vulva, such as infections, irritations of the labia, and infections or cysts of Bartholin's glands.

VULVA-IRRITATION   Irritations of the outer female genitals are discussed under VAGINITIS; in children and babies these are common in the vulvar area where the child's skin is exceedingly vulnerable. In girls older than babies, the most common cause of redness, soreness, and itching in this area is an irritating or infective vaginal discharge. Indeed, the vulvar condition may often seem to be much the most obstinate and difficult aspect of any of these discharges.

In severe conditions, a child is apt to

scratch or manipulate the vulva locally, causing excoriations (raw lesions) and thus creating a vicious circle. This type of irritation, especially with itching, has been thought to be the occasional cause of beginning autoeroticism; for this reason these irritations, whether mild or severe, must have early and efficient attention. In stubborn cases, sugar in the urine (perhaps from diabetes) should always be suspected for sugar encourages the development of local bacteria and yeast. The urine should always be checked repeatedly.

Numerous skin conditions which also occur elsewhere as well as in older people may be found occasionally in children. Pimples, rashes, or any unusual skin condition should be always called to the attention of a doctor.

The rectal area as well as the genital may be similarly involved, and at the same time.

Treatment. A soothing, cleansing wash with a mild detergent is helpful for frequent and thorough daily washing of the vulvar and rectal areas. These washings must be done, or at least supervised, by the parent, in order to see that they are thorough. The physician will, of course, prescribe and direct the treatment of any disease which may lie behind vulvar irritation, which itself is more a symptom than a disease.

WARTS   This well-known condition, especially common in children, is caused by an identifiable filtrable virus. What is so curious and so baffling about a wart is that even though the condition is that of a tumor mass, it can resist all forms of destructive treatment including irradiation, surgery, and acids, and can regrow in the identical site after seeming total removal and complete healing. Conversely, the most persistent, obdurate, extensive warty masses can disappear overnight for no apparent cause and with no attempt at

treatment. There is considerable evidence indicating the importance of psychic influences in therapy. But the nature of effective psychogenic modality (anger, indifference, acceptance, resentment) is not known.

Treatment. Since the largest number of warts disappear without treatment, it is desirable to treat only those that are easily removable or that are so large as to interfere with function of the affected part. Treatment which may result in permanent damage (scarring, distortion) is almost never indicated because the wart itself is never a threat to life, and because it not only can, but most often does, disappear without treatment. Treatment (aside from patience) varies from the highly technical administration of irradiation (X-ray, grenz ray) and "alteratives," whose function it is to change the immunity to the virus, to the application of local remedies like castor oil, boiled potato, raw onion, silver nitrate, and bi- and trichloracetic acid.

WATER   Like air (oxygen), water is absolutely essential for life. Indeed, one can live for weeks without food but only a few days without water. Water is lost from the body through the kidneys as urine, by which means certain waste products are removed; through the bowel in stools, by which means solid wastes are removed; through the lungs in maintaining the air moist in the respiratory passages; and through the skin (both with and without sweating). Even without sweating, as much as a liter (approximately a little over a quart) is lost every day; with sweating, of course, the amount is considerably higher.

This water must be and is replaced by drinking it in beverages, by whatever water exists in solid foods, and by the small amounts of water produced by the metabolism of foodstuffs. (The words dehydration and overhydration refer to the balance between the amounts of water and of solids in the body.)

About 60 per cent of the total weight of an adult is fluid. Of this total body water, about half is contained within the cells. The remainder is distributed in the blood plasma, in lymph (which circulates between cells), and in other tissues. Dissolved in the body fluids are the electrolytes, such as sodium, potassium, calcium, and magnesium, all of which are essential for normal bodily functions. These electrolytes are very carefully balanced by nature so that precise amounts are present both in and outside the cells. Many serious disturbances associated with disease occur because of abnormalities in the electrolytes.

When water deficiency exists, whether through inadequate intake or excessive loss, the results, in addition to thirst, are concentrated urine and a rise in body temperature; the patient becomes irritable, weak, and tired, his muscles may twitch, and eventually death may result. On the other hand, when there is an excessive amount of fluid, urine volume increases maximally; there may be headache, confusion, nausea, vomiting and muscle cramps.

WATER ON THE BRAIN (HYDROCEPHALY)

Although called water on the brain, this condition is more accurately water (actually cerebrospinal fluid) in the brain. This fluid is found over the surface and within the ventricles of the brain, and is manufactured by certain blood vessels inside these ventricles. Normally, the cerebrospinal fluid travels through small apertures at the base of the brain, circulates over the spinal cord and upper surface of the brain, and is reabsorbed by other blood vessels. If formation of the fluid is more rapid than its removal, or if there is obstruction to the flow of fluid, it will accumulate inside the brain. This accumulation can stretch the ventricles, expand and thin out the brain, and "balloon" both the brain and the thin skull.

Symptoms. In hydrocephalic infants (often before birth) the whole skull and skin will sometimes be stretched to paper thinness, because the soft spots are still open; the face, however, stays relatively normal. Most such infants die in the early weeks or months of life.

Treatment. Once the "skull-stretching" stage has been reached, the brain is irreparably damaged. An occasional patient will, however, be aided by clever neurosurgical techniques which employ tubes to lead the fluid from one area to another where it will be absorbed. Nevertheless the outlook, especially in the advanced cases, is not good.

WET DREAMS   See NOCTURNAL EMISSIONS

WHOOPING COUGH (PERTUSSIS)

Whooping cough, a contagious disease caused by a bacterium, may be mild or severe and may occur at any age—even under one month.

Symptoms. There is a gradual increase of a dry night-cough. At the end of two weeks the cough is very severe and comes in spasms, followed by a "whoop" during inhaling. The patient may vomit, turn blue, develop hemorrhages into the whites of the eyes, become dehydrated, and even interrupt breathing. Typically, this period lasts two weeks and is followed by two weeks of improvement. Altogether, the disease generally lasts six weeks. If the typical whoop is not present, blood counts and cultures are necessary to establish diagnosis. Early "baby shots" are designed to prevent this disease, and while the well-immunized child may still contract the disease, it will be less serious.

Treatment. Steam inhalations, sedative cough syrups, small feedings, oxygen may all be necessary. Antibiotics do not effect a cure; they are, however, necessary if secondary infection develops. There is a serum which is effective in reducing the severity of the spasms, if given early enough in the disease. A doctor should be called in for *all* stubborn chronic coughs.

WISDOM TEETH   These are the permanent third molars, which usually erupt at an age (seventeen to twenty-four years) when individuals may be expected to be reasonably knowledgeable.

WITHDRAWAL (COITUS INTERRUPTUS)   When conception is not desired, the male partner may withdraw the penis during sexual intercourse just before ejaculation. This is a dangerous practice because it often results in failure to reach orgasm, with consequent build-up of tension in either partner or in both. It is likewise risky because it may not as a birth-control measure always be accomplished in time to prevent deposit of sperm in the vagina.

WOMB (UTERUS)   The uterus is located at the bottom of the female pelvis, between the bladder and the rectum, and consists of several layers of strong muscle surrounding the cavity of the womb. In its nonpregnant state, the uterus is the shape and size of a flattened pear, and sits on top of the vagina. Its cavity connects with the vagina through the cervix (neck of the womb) and with the ovaries through the two fallopian tubes. With the onset of puberty, the lining of the cavity of the womb responds to the changing levels of hormones produced by the ovaries and undergoes hypertrophy and eventual shedding; these changes are manifested monthly in the form of menstrual periods. The muscle of the womb has tremendous adaptability and, when pregnancy does occur, hypertrophies and stretches to huge dimensions, still maintaining its ability to contract strongly for expulsion of the baby and the afterbirth (placenta).

A variety of diseases can affect the womb, ranging from infections to tumors, both benign and malignant. Abnormal uterine bleeding may be the result of diseases primarily involving the womb, but more often is the reflection of ovarian problems and abnormal hormone production; the womb is only the final "target organ" through which these latter abnormalities are manifested.

WOMB, CANCER OF THE   About 90 per cent of the cases of cancer of the uterus involve the cervix (neck of the womb); only 10 per cent are of the main body of this organ. Cancer of the body of the womb rarely occurs before menopause, the most common age range being between fifty and sixty-five.

Symptoms. The major symptom of cancer of the body of the womb is bloody discharge, "spotting," or active vaginal bleeding in postmenopausal women. This must be considered as a very dangerous sign and, until proven otherwise, as evidence of cancer of the womb. The diagnosis can be only made by obtaining tissue for biopsy from the inside of the womb, usually by scraping, and examining it microscopically.

Treatment. Treatment will depend on the individual case. As a rule, it consists of radium placed within the womb for two to three days, followed by surgical removal of the womb, both tubes, and the ovaries. The prognosis is quite good if the cancer is detected in its early stages, when confined to the body of the womb.

WORMS   Worms are estimated to inhabit 80 per cent of the intestines of the two-to-ten year olds at one time or another. The most common worm is the pinworm. This white worm is only about three-eighths of an inch long, and is as thick as a piece of thick thread. The adult female comes out of the rectum at night to lay her hundreds of eggs about the anus; this sets up an intense itch, the victim scratches, and gets many eggs on his hands and under the nails. During the day he then transmits these eggs to his toys and clothes, his friends, and of course, to his own mouth. Once the eggs reach the intestines, they hatch and mature, male meets female, the female is fertilized, and the cycle is repeated.

Some children are much more susceptible because they suck their thumbs, pick their noses, or for some reason or other have their hands frequently in contact with their faces. Pinworm-infestation is not caused by eating candy or sitting on cold cement; furthermore, pinworms come from other humans and not from animals (animals have their parasites and we have ours).

Symptoms. Worms will not cause convulsions. The usual symptoms are an itchy anal area, wakefulness at night, stomachaches, and a grouchy disposition. The best method of diagnosing the condition is to inspect the anal region about an hour after the child has retired at night. A strong light is used and the worms may be seen coiling and twisting about, and in a girl even crawling into the vagina, where they may occasionally carry infection, such as vaginitis.

Worm-eggs are microscopic, and can not be seen by the naked eye. For accurate diagnosis it is recommended that the sticky side of transparent adhesive tape be placed against the anal area and then taped to a glass slide; this can then be given to the doctor to be examined under the microscope where the characteristic eggs are seen.

Treatment. Newer and more effective medicines are now on the market to kill pinworms, but physical cleanliness (especially of the hands) is a vital part of the treatment; otherwise the worms will soon

be back. It is also recommended that whole neighborhoods be treated simultaneously, for even if a child is free of worms he will soon get them from his untreated playmates. It is no longer considered a sign of unclean living to be afflicted with worms; it is merely a sign that a child has friends who may have worms.

WRINKLES Degeneration of the connective tissue of the dermis (subcutis) of the skin results in both a loss of elasticity of this tissue and a lessening of the number of connective tissue fibers. Almost always the result of senile changes, the process is irreversible. Relief from the undesired changes in the skin-surface patterns, laxness, folds, etc., can be achieved by reconstructive plastic surgery.

XANTHELASMA Occurring in both sexes between forty and fifty years, although occasionally in younger people, too, this disease is often a manifestation of disturbance of fat (lipid) metabolism or of diabetes. Although sometimes accompanied by fatty tumors elsewhere, xanthelasma usually affects the upper and lower eyelids near, and sometimes extending onto, the nose.

Symptoms. The lesions consist of yellowish or buff-colored, velvety, firm plaques, ranging in size from one-eighth inch to one inch and often joining to form irregularly shaped masses. Occasionally they become large enough to interfere with vision. There are no accompanying subjective symptoms.

Treatment. Because of the high incidence of fat-metabolism disturbance and of diabetes in patients with xanthelasma, examination for the possible existence of these conditions is essential. The lesions can be removed surgically, destroyed by desiccation, or peeled with acids. Recurrence is not uncommon. Marked reduction of fat (plant and animal) intake may cause the lesions to disappear. However, the necessary drastic reduction and attendant monotony and impalatability of diet, may be impractical.

XANTHOMATOSIS Disturbance of fat metabolism resulting in fatty deposits in the skin may occur as a primary, inherited disease (incomplete dominant trait), or may result from the increase of fat in the blood serum from diabetes, nephrosis, pancreatitis, etc. Determining the type of xanthomatosis present in a patient often necessitates extensive observation and investigation.

Symptoms. The lesions consist of yellowish brown tumors or plaques of varying size, usually occurring in groups over the joints, on the buttocks, in the creases of the palms and on the heels, but sometimes scattered elsewhere on the body. They can enlarge and interfere with movement of the hands and feet; and occasionally they can become ulcerated.

Treatment. Drastic reduction of fat in the diet will cause a diminution, and even disappearance, of the lesions. The necessary reduction of fat (both vegetable and animal) intake is difficult to maintain because of the resulting monotony of diet. In cases in which the disease is a secondary result of another condition, treatment of the causative condition in addition to restriction of fat intake is essential. Surgical removal of lesions interfering with function is feasible, especially if recurrence can be avoided by treatment of the causative systemic condition.

XERODERMA PIGMENTOSUM An inherited disease of the skin in which there is an accelerated and persistent reaction to even small exposures to light, with a resultant excessive freckling and aging of the skin.

Symptom. This condition is usually noted soon after the first or second summer of infancy and may first appear as a vague dermatitis accompanied by freckling and by tearing of the eyes. Dryness and wrinkling of the skin of the exposed areas of the face, chest, and upper extremities are followed by the production of warty growths; finally, skin cancers of several types develop in the affected areas. The intolerance of the eyes to light may be severe. Other defects such as deafness and mental deficiency may occur.

Treatment. Rigid avoidance of sunlight is essential in the care of the patient. Protective creams (with ultraviolet-light filters) should be used when even minimal exposure to light is necessary. Removal of warty and malignant growths should be done early to avoid excessive surgery.

YELLOW FEVER Yellow fever is caused by a virus and is seen exclusively in subtropical and tropical climates; it is marked by an acute onset with fever, slow pulse, and, in its severe form, by albumin in the urine, vomiting of blood, jaundice, extreme weakness, and, perhaps, hemorrhage. The virus is brought to man through the bite of the infected *Aedes aegypti* mosquito. There has been no severe outbreak in this country for more than sixty years.

Symptoms. The disease begins suddenly with a relatively high fever that may be preceded by a chill. The pulse becomes slow and the face, gums, and eyes take on a marked redness. There are various digestive manifestations. Within a week to ten days after onset three characteristic indications appear: "black vomit" (blood in the vomitus), albumin in the urine, and jaundice. Nosebleed, signs of hemorrhage in the skin, passage of blood in the stool, and other evidence of bleeding are common. In some countries the prognosis is grave (more than eight out of ten patients dying in an epidemic); in others it is quite good. Prevention by good public hygiene is the best cure. There is no specific drug and treatment consists of good nursing care and supportive care together with treatment aimed at individual symptoms.

First Aid and Emergencies

IRST AID AND EMERGENCY care should be included in the curriculum of every school as a fundamental part of preparation for living. An educated person might reasonably be expected to know how to give mouth-to-mouth resuscitation; he should have some general ideas about the treatment of severe bleeding; and he should know that in moving an accident victim a simple fracture might be made into a compound fracture. The unfortunate thing about emergencies is that they strike with bewildering impact. The very circumstances that call for keeping one's wits together—and for calmly evaluating the situation—may instead produce confusion, even panic. Under these circumstances mistakes are easily made, and one can only hope that they are not irreparable. A knowledge of first aid can reverse this situation; prompt, intelligent action may convert a dangerous, even life-threatening, situation into a controllable one.

First-aid measures are based on the use of common sense. When reading this section, which describes different kinds of emergencies, it is important to understand the why and wherefore of each procedure and the reason or principle governing each action that is taken. It is not possible in this brief space to describe all the variations or combinations of factors that may come together in an emergency. But an understanding of first principles will enable the average person to sort out the fundamental requirements of an emergency and to act correctly.

As an example of basic principle, the first-aid treatment of fracture is to produce immobilization so that the sharp, broken ends of the bones do not move. Any means that provides immobilization—and there are many—may be considered acceptable. The first-aid principle involved in the treatment of bleeding is that direct pressure on a blood vessel will compress it and hence decrease the bleeding. It is only when this does not work that one utilizes the tourniquet principle, based on the fact that placing a constricting material around an extremity and tightening it will compress the artery that goes to the limb. Mouth-to-mouth resuscitation is based on the simple idea that one can force air into a victim's lungs much as one blows up a balloon, and that the elastic recoil of the lungs will expel the air thus pushed in. As for poisons, with some exceptions, first-aid treatment consists of using any of a number of procedures that will produce vomiting, the principle being to get the poison out in the quickest way possible.

ACCIDENT PREVENTION   Not all accidents can be prevented, but analysis of thousands of them indicates that with care and forethought many can be avoided. For example, it is generally agreed that most of the serious cases of childhood poisoning can be prevented if certain precautions are taken. Not all falls are avoidable, but those that occur in a bathtub—because of no rubber mat—most certainly are avoidable. Slippery scatter rugs are a special threat to elderly or feeble individuals and to children, and could well be firmly anchored or removed. The evidence that safety belts can drastically reduce our enormous automobile casualty rate—there are over a million such accidents a year in the United States—cannot be disputed. We are naturally concerned about the food our children eat and the education they get. But are we equally concerned and equally alert when it comes to protecting them against accidents? Accidents are, in fact, the number one threat to the young child's life.

In first aid, major emphasis should be on prevention, and the first and last points stressed in first-aid courses should be the preventability of accidents. Dr. Harry Raybin, of New York City's famous Poison Control Center, has said: "A knowledge of antidotes will not satisfactorily substitute for prudent housekeeping." Here are some safety tips, derived from the sad experiences of others, which you should carefully consider and profit from:

1. When there are small children in the home, be sure to keep medicines where they cannot be reached by creeping, climbing toddlers. Some of the newer medicine chests have safety locks which cannot be opened by the small child. If yours can be opened too easily, you should keep it free of all medicines. This applies especially to aspirin, which is the most common single cause of childhood poisoning. Find a location for medicines which you are sure is inaccessible to the children. A sliding latch placed high on the bathroom door is one solution you might consider.

2. Other common causes of childhood poisoning include bleaches, disinfectants, and cleaning agents which are often kept virtually at floor level in the kitchen. Most detergents are not likely to produce serious poisoning, but bleaches and lyes are major threats. They are best kept under lock and key, or in some inaccessible place.

3. Never leave small children unattended. A minute's negligence can result in tragedy.

4. Many falls in the home can be prevented by using rugs with nonskid backing, by not waxing floors too highly,

and by avoiding rickety step-ladders, or chairs balanced together, for doing repairs. Women are more subject to falls because of fashionable but unsafe shoes. They can avoid many falls by wearing rubber rather than leather soles. Night lights are also an aid in avoiding falls.

5. Children's falls out of windows can be completely prevented by having adequate window-guards.

6. Falls out of bed are always a possibility with the young and the elderly, especially when certain drugs are being taken or when there is fever, confusion, or serious debility. These falls can be prevented by placing chairs against the bed, by side rails, or by similar methods.

7. A small fire extinguisher in the kitchen may be more useful than any other gadget there. It may prevent a grease fire from spreading to wooden cupboards and to curtains.

8. Kerosene, gasoline, benzine, turpentine, and other cleaning fluids are potential poisoning agents as well as fire hazards. Keep them in a safe place and, unless the need for them is frequent, do not keep them at all.

9. Never take a medicine without reading and rereading the label.

10. Do not store cleaning fluids, lye solutions, or any other hazardous substances in soda bottles, wine bottles, or milk containers. Do not trust to your memory to identify chemicals you may have stored away for some vague future use— a moment taken to label them is a worthwhile safety provision.

By their very nature, accidents can occur even to the most careful among us. One should therefore be prepared to cope with many kinds of accidents and emergencies. They can occur in someone else's home, as well as in your own, or on the highway, at the beach, in the woods, or the countryside, at some distance from a medical center or a doctor's office.

Here then, alphabetically arranged, are some of the important aspects of emergency care with which you should be familiar.

ARTIFICIAL RESPIRATION See color insert First Aid and Life Saving, plates F4-F5

BITES Animal and insect bites may be daily events in the lives of some people, and only a small percentage constitute a threat. Obviously, a minor bite from a household pet need hardly cause concern. On the other hand, a child bitten by a stray dog may not only sustain a severe laceration requiring stitches, but the question of rabies inevitably comes up. Every effort must be made to locate the stray animal and have it placed under observation until the question is resolved. Recently, only one or two cases of human rabies per year have been occurring in the United States, but it remains a serious disease and has a high mortality rate. In general, an animal bite may be allowed to bleed at first, for this washes out bacteria, bits of clothing, or other contaminants. The wound may then be washed with soap and water; if bleeding continues, it may be treated as described under BLEEDING.

Most cat bites, like cat scratches, are not likely to be of any consequence. Fever and swelling of nearby lymph glands can occur, often well after the original injury has healed. This is a viral disease known as cat-scratch fever. It is quite rare, however. Bruising without cutting of the skin may occur after some animal bites, such as a horse bite. This is best treated initially by cold water or ice applications which slow down both bleeding or swelling.

BITES AND STINGS (INSECT) Most insect bites fall into the nuisance category. Thus, while mosquito bites in certain parts of the world do transmit such diseases as yellow fever and malaria, the transmission of any disease from mosquito bites in the

United States is rare. In recent years, the public health authorities have been concerned over a few cases of encephalitis which have been traced to viruses carried by the mosquito. Generally, however, all one needs to do is apply some household remedy, such as calamine lotion; and one can dismiss the idea of coming down with an illness from mosquito bites. The bites of certain other insects fall into an entirely separate category, and with these, appropriate medical measures as described under the proper heading should be taken.

BEE STINGS   More deaths occur each year in the United States from bee stings than from the bite of any other insect or animal. This is because certain individuals have allergic or hypersensitive reactions to the sting of bees. Such persons can suffer sudden collapse or respiratory obstruction. Usually, they have shown sensitivity to a bee sting on one or more previous occasions, with reactions such as unusual local swelling, marked weakness, asthmatic breathing, or severe drop in blood pressure. Once an individual has shown some unusual reaction of this kind, special precautions are thereafter necessary. Desensitization, much as one desensitizes for the pollens or against horse serum, should be seriously considered: while this has been shown to have marked protective value, it is still not widely enough employed. In the absence of desensitization, the hypersensitive person should take special precautions to avoid bees and to wear protective clothing and netting if exposure is unavoidable. If such exposure is unavoidable, certain emergency drugs for use after a bee sting may easily be carried on the person. One of these is a tablet (Isuprel®), which can be placed under the tongue; as it is absorbed, it has an adrenalin-like effect. Another remedy is one of the several different types of pocket inhalers used by asthmatics. A few inhalations of this will prevent bronchial spasm.

BITES (SCORPION) (TICKS)   Scorpion bites are not life-threatening, as is widely believed, but the venom of the bite can produce considerable local pain and symptoms of illness. First aid may consist of ice applications. Wood ticks often attach themselves to people passing through certain wooded areas of the United States. They may transmit the disease known as Rocky Mountain spotted fever. In such areas, immunization against the disease is advisable. Ticks that have attached themselves to the skin may be removed by covering them with mineral oil, vaseline, or kerosene, or by touching them with a lighted cigarette. The injured or dead tick is then readily removed.

BITES (SNAKE)   Most snakes are harmless; they are useful scavengers, and they flee from human beings. If by chance they do bite, the bite produces two curved lines or serrations resulting from the indentations of their small, blunt teeth. Poisonous snakes, however, possess fangs, which are specialized hollow, long teeth through which the snake can expel his venom. When a poisonous snake strikes, sharp puncture wounds are produced which appear as two needle-like wounds fairly close together. The injected venom produces severe inflammation with marked swelling, discoloration, and burning pain. The aim of first aid is to limit the absorption of venom, and to draw it out of the wound site.

The following steps should be taken:

1. Place a tourniquet above the puncture wounds and tie tightly enough to make the veins stand out prominently. The tourniquet can be a handkerchief, a belt, twine, or anything else that can adequately encircle the limb, for most snake bites are on the extremities. Too tight a tourniquet will shut off the circulation entirely; this can be recognized by failure of the veins to fill up.

2. With a sharp razor blade, a pocket-

knife, or other sharp object, make an X-shaped cut into each fang mark. Avoid cutting into a vein or any of the cordlike structures under the skin, which are the tendons, and make the cuts approximately one-quarter inch long and one-quarter inch deep. Due to the tourniquet, fairly free oozing of blood should occur.

3. Suck out the venom with a strong sucking effort, spitting out the mixture of blood and venom from time to time. Swallowed venom will not harm you, and there is no absorption of venom from the mouth cavity unless there are sores or open areas in the mouth lining. Keep sucking as continuously as possible until medical attention is obtained. Continue sucking out the venom for at least an hour, and if you get tired have someone else help you.

4. Snake bite kits are available for those who go camping and hiking in areas known to be inhabited by such poisonous snakes as the rattlesnake or the cottonmouth moccasin, the copperhead, and the coral snake. These kits enable you to give first-aid attention promptly. They should be carried along as a routine part of outdoor equipment in such areas.

5. Once the tourniquet is on properly, with veins bulging, do not disturb it, for the venom spreads more quickly when the pressure of the tourniquet is loosened. *Do not* give whiskey or other spirits—these are valueless and, in fact, tend to accelerate the spread of venom.

6. If available, place ice around the bite. It slows the spread of the venom.

BITES (SPIDER)   That the bite of the black widow spider can be dangerous is known to many laymen. This large black spider can be identified by the orange-colored hourglass figure on its abdomen. Its bite produces local pain and swelling, followed by general symptoms which include weakness, muscular cramps, abdominal rigidity, and nausea. Another type of spider bite being reported with increasing

frequency is that of the brown recluse spider. Like the black widow spider, it is found mostly in the southern part of the United States, most of the cases being reported from Texas, Arkansas, and Louisiana. The brown recluse spider gets its name from its pattern of living in dark, secluded locations of man-made dwellings, cellars being a favorite haunt. This spider has to be molested before it bites, and children could be well advised of this fact. It can be identified by its brown color and the violin-shaped figure on its abdomen. Its bite produces a breakdown in the skin, which is sometimes extensive, and it may produce general symptoms such as chills, fever, and anemia.

The bites of either of these two spiders, when on the extremities, may be handled in much the same manner as a snake bite (see BITES (SNAKE)). One can place a tourniquet above the region of the bite and apply ice to the bite itself as a temporary measure. Medical attention is mandatory. The bites of the black widow spider have been treated with antivenins, which are drugs that neutralize venom. Local injection of cortisone-type drugs have been found useful in the treatment of recluse-spider bites.

BLEEDING   The most widely applicable method for the control of bleeding is direct pressure, using a compress. By this is meant the exertion of sufficient pressure on a bleeding area to compress bleeding vessels. For most bleeding, even from fairly large veins, such direct pressure should bring the hemorrhage under control. In most emergency situations, one can use any clean cloth for the compress: a handkerchief, towel, shirt, sheet, or pillowcase folded on itself to make a multi-layered wad. Using either the fingers or the palm of the hand, apply the emergency compress over the bleeding area and exert firm pressure against it. Maintain pressure for ten minutes or so. One may then diminish the pressure, occasionally lifting up part of the compress to judge whether the bleeding has come under control. Pressure can be maintained more or less indefinitely, if necessary. However, if brisk bleeding continues despite firm pressure, particularly if the bleeding comes in good-sized spurts (as may happen when an artery is involved) one should turn to other first-aid measures. The two other are the tourniquet and the pressure point methods.

Tourniquet. A tourniquet is a tightly applied device which encircles a limb and controls the circulation through it. When the pressure exerted by the tourniquet is of sufficient degree, no more blood can flow through the arteries, and the limb is deprived of its circulation. It is this complete cutting off of the blood supply that makes the tourniquet a method to be used only as a last resort, and then only with extreme caution. The overzealous use of a tourniquet for a period of several hours may endanger the entire limb.

A tourniquet is made easily enough by using a handkerchief, strap, belt, suspenders, a strip of cloth, necktie, towel, rubber tubing, or similar material to be tied about the limb. Do not use wire, cord, or anything that will cut the flesh. Place a hard pad or object over the artery so that when the tourniquet is tightened, it will press the pad or object against the artery. Next, a stick or any substitute such as a pencil is placed between the tourniquet and the skin. Twisting the tourniquet one or more times produces an increase in pressure. At first the veins may bulge up, but as the pressure of the tourniquet is increased and the circulation through the artery is cut off, the limb turns white and all visible blood vessels collapse. At this point, bleeding should stop. Continued bleeding indicates that more pressure needs to be applied. Occasionally a stouter tourniquet may be needed to accomplish this.

A tourniquet should never be left in a concealed position where its presence escapes notice. Opinions vary as to how long a tourniquet may be safely allowed to stay on. United States Armed Forces experience indicates that a tourniquet can remain on for several hours without causing damage. However, the wise course is to release it before one hour has passed. One may check after twenty minutes or even less to determine whether bleeding has been controlled. Sometimes, one can use the tourniquet to gain rapid control of bleeding, then switch to the direct pressure method (described above) with considerable success. This also circumvents the drawback of continued use of the tourniquet.

Pressure Point Method. This method can be used for bleeding from a limb and for hemorrhage where a tourniquet is not applicable. (When a tourniquet is to be used, finger pressure should be applied to stem the loss of blood while the tourniquet is being prepared and applied.) The pressure point method is based on the principle that some of the major arteries can be directly compressed to a point where bleeding from one of their branches is either considerably cut down or abolished altogether. The application of pressure should always be between the cut and the heart. There are standard pressure points at which major arteries going to the head and extremities can be readily compressed. You can identify these location on yourself by feeling for your pulse. In fact, it is a good idea to gain some familiarity with their location in this manner. Some of these locations are the following:

1. Brachial. The brachial artery is the major vessel going to the arm. It emerges from the region of the armpit and runs down the inner side of the upper arm. Direct pressure on the inner part of the arm presses the artery against the bone; with sufficient pressure, its pulse can be

abolished. This maneuver will control bleeding from any injury of the arm, forearm, or hand below the level at which pressure is being exerted.

2. Carotid. The carotid arteries are the major vessels supplying the head, including the face and the brain. Ordinarily they can be readily felt on either side of the windpipe, and are compressible against the spinal column below. Pressure on the carotids should be applied only as a last resort, since it may lead to complications attendant on cutting down brain circulation. Prolonged pressure could, in fact, produce paralysis. One may consider intermittent or partial carotid artery pressure (for brief intervals of a minute or so) as a temporary first-aid method, to be followed by direct pressure. In no case should both carotids be compressed simultaneously. For an extensive bleeding wound of the head region where facial and temporal pressures (see below) are not applicable, cautious use of carotid pressure can be of value.

3. Facial. The facial artery, a branch of the carotid, winds over the jawbone, about halfway between the angle of the jaw and chin. Pressure at this point may successfully control bleeding from the face and jaw.

4. Temporal. The temporal artery winds over the bone just in front of the midportion of the attachment of the ear. This is an artery whose pulsations are often visible in older individuals. Pressure on it will control bleeding from the upper part of the head on that side.

5. Femoral. The femoral is a large artery which emerges from the pelvis to nourish the lower extremity. It produces an obvious pulse which can be easily felt in the crease between the thigh and abdomen at about its middle. Pressure here will control bleeding from the thigh, leg, and foot.

Several further pointers to remember about bleeding are:

1. There is no reason why combinations of the above methods cannot be used. Thus, one might combine a compress on the actual wound site with pressure on one of the standard pressure points. Actually, because arterial circulation may form a network (this is known as the collateral circulation), some bleeding can occur from a wound even if the pressure point method is correctly utilized. The bleeding that escapes the pressure point is usually modest, however, and controllable by a local compress to the wound.

2. Another tip to be remembered is that elevation of a limb tends to decrease bleeding and should be routinely employed when possible. Thus, with a bleeding wound of the hand, the first approach might well be to apply a compress with firm pressure to the wound and to elevate the arm as high as possible.

3. Where bleeding is extensive, there is always the possibility of shock. The preferred position for incipient or actual shock is for the victim to lie stretched out flat on his back.

BRUISES See FALLS AND FRACTURES

BURNS Burns are generally described in terms of their extent and their depth. Extent refers to the area of skin involved, and is sometimes stated in percentage. Thus, an extensive burn involving the skin of the arm would be an 8 per cent burn, whereas one involving most of the back would be a 16 per cent burn. A first-degree burn is one that produces reddening of the skin; a second-degree burn produces blister formation; a third degree burn produces injury of tissue at deeper-than-skin level. Extensive third-degree burns may produce shock, and often may require skin grafts to cover the denuded surfaces. Shock may also result from extensive second-degree burns with blistering. Shock results from the rapid loss of fluid, as well as from toxic chemicals pro-

526

duced by the burn. The initial first aid for shock is to stretch the patient out and keep him warm.

Minor Burns. Minor burns involve a limited surface and present no threat of shock or similar reaction. A good first-aid measure for the usual minor burn of the fingers or hand is immediately to dip the hand into ice-cold water. This stops pain almost at once, and tends to cut down the degree of tissue injury. For such burns, a vaseline dressing, which has a protective effect, may be all that is necessary. Annoying blisters of the fingertips may be pricked with a sterile needle and allowed to collapse. The possibility of this leading to infection is quite remote, but one should observe the usual precautions of washing with soap and water and applying a surface disinfectant.

Major Burns. Extensive second- or third-degree burns are major burns. These generally require hospitalization. It is best not to attempt treatment such as cutting away burnt clothing, since this may further aggravate the injury. Also *do not* apply burn ointments or other ointments. An exposed burned area may be covered with the inside portion of a pillow slip or sheet which, as it comes from the laundry, is likely to be relatively free of bacterial contamination. Clothing that adheres to the burned area should not be pulled at, nor should any attempt be made to undress the victim. The patient should be kept covered. If medical aid or removal to a hospital is not possible for some time, and if there is no vomiting, the patient may be given fluids by mouth, since thirst is a common complaint. The fluid might consist of fruit juice to which a sprinkle of salt has been added. "Shock solution" is another fluid that has been advocated. This consists of one teaspoon of salt plus one-half teaspoon of baking soda dissolved in one quart of water.

A chemical burn is produced by the corrosive effect of such agents as lye (caustic soda [Drano®] and similar products), hydrochloric acid (muriatic acid), sulphuric acid, and carbolic acid (phenol). Burns of the skin resulting from phenol, creosote, or carbolic acid should be dabbed or rinsed with alcohol followed up with water. (Alcohol, of course, cannot be used when these substances enter the eye or have been swallowed). Other chemical burns should be promptly washed with water. Burns due to an acid may then be covered with a paste made of bicarbonate of soda, or with vaseline. Chemical burns are usually quite destructive to tissue and hence heal slowly.

CHOKING An error in the complicated swallowing mechanism may result in a lump of food covering the entrance to the air passage or even entering the passage itself. This will produce a breathing obstruction and severe coughing. The coughing itself may dislodge the foreign body. Otherwise, gasping or difficult respiration, together with the classic purplish appearance of the victim, can produce a terrifying sight. Very often the obstructing object can be dislodged by inserting the fingers into the mouth and removing the object. If this fails and the victim is a child, he should be turned upside down and vigorously slapped between the shoulder blades several times. An adult may be positioned over a chair or bed in a head-down position, and similarly slapped between the shoulder blades.

If these simple measures fail and the victim is still in great distress, call the doctor. In the meantime, the more drastic method of inserting one's finger into the back of the throat can be used to dislodge the object. In some cases, where the obstruction is partial and the victim continues to have a purplish color, artificial respiration (see ARTIFICIAL RESPIRATION) should be maintained while rushing the patient to the hospital.

CONVULSIONS The most common form of convulsion is seen in epilepsy. It is sometimes referred to as a fit or a seizure. Often there is a brief warning which the patient may recognize, known as the aura. This is usually followed by his falling to the ground and undergoing a generalized stiffening. Following this, a series of severe and involuntary muscular contractions occur, generally accompanied by grinding movements of the jaws and the appearance of a foamy saliva on the lips. Involuntary emptying of bowels and bladder is usual. The attack lasts for a minute or more, stops abruptly, and is followed by a period of sleep. The victim will have no recollection of what happened.

The aim of first aid is to prevent self-inflicted injury as a result of the powerful, involuntary muscular movements. Biting of the tongue may be severe. In any case, proceed as follows:

1. Insert any handy object between the teeth, such as a wadded handkerchief, the victim's own tie, even a pencil. This will prevent the tongue from being bitten and chewed.

2. Loosen the collar and necktie, and move the patient away from any object that he may strike during the seizure.

3. As soon as the convulsive movements have stopped, turn him on his stomach so his tongue will not fall back into his throat.

In infants and young children, a high fever may produce a seizure. It is important to reduce the body temperature as quickly as possible by an alcohol rub or by wrapping the child in a cool wet sheet. A doctor should be promptly notified. These febrile seizures in children have no relationship to the possible development of epilepsy later in life.

CROUP Croup is produced by an infection involving the larynx and vocal cords, in which a spasm occurs. The spasm may be brought on by a bout of coughing, and most often occurs at night. Croup is generally limited to children with respiratory infections, and is also seen in whooping cough. The usual pattern is for the child to wake at night with a violent attack of coughing followed by obvious difficulty in catching his breath. The attempt to breathe in produces a noisy whooping or crowing sound, and the child turns a dusky red, but normal color is restored as the spasm subsides. This sequence of events may take place night after night. In addition to treating the infection with antibiotics, these measures will be of aid:

1. The child's room should be kept warm and free of drafts.

2. High humidity should be maintained, with one or more vaporizers going all the time. As a routine precautionary measure against possible burns, vaporizers should be placed at a safe distance, with the steam projected toward the head of the bed.

3. Partially covering the crib or the bed with a sheet, as was done in the old-fashioned croup tent, will make a semi-enclosed area which has a high moisture content. Another possibility is to take the patient into the bathroom and run the hot water which will quickly steam up the room. Hot liquids may be of help.

CUTS In contrast to a laceration, which is an irregular tear of the skin, a cut is inflicted by a sharp edge. It often produces a linear opening into the skin. Most cuts are accompanied by bleeding, and if one of the larger vessels is involved, the bleeding may be quite brisk. Control of this is discussed in the entry BLEEDING. Minor cuts generally require no special measures. Cuts received out of doors, as for example when walking barefoot on the ground, may require tetanus antitoxin, a decision which has to be made by the doctor. Sometimes the question arises as to whether or not a cut needs to be stitched. The purpose of stitching is to bring the gaping edges of skin together so as to facilitate healing. Unless this is done, healing is slower and leads to a broad and perhaps unsightly scar. Obviously, then, if the cut is of some length and the skin edges become separated by perhaps one-eighth to one-quarter of an inch or more, then sutures (stitches) will lead to more rapid healing and better cosmetic results as well. Cuts about the face are generally sutured with very fine material, with the stitches closely spaced to secure the least noticeable scar.

ELECTRICAL SHOCK   The usual contact with a 110-volt AC household outlet is not dangerous unless one happens to be wet—in a bathtub or otherwise in full electrical contact with the ground. Most serious injuries are a result of contact with main power lines carrying high currents. Such contact may produce weakness or paralysis, unconsciousness, and a local burn. Under no circumstances should you touch the victim directly, for the current can be conducted to you. Be sure to proceed quickly but calmly. If a switch controlling the line is the fastest thing that can be shut off, do that first. Otherwise push the victim away from the line, or the line away from the victim, always being sure to use a nonconductor such as a long piece of dry wood or cardboard, a dry broom handle, or dry rubber hosing. Dry ropes or dry cloth can also be used. Make sure your hands are dry and you are standing on a dry surface. Pushing the victim off the wire will break the electrical circuit involving the victim. In severe cases, respiration will have usually stopped and artificial respiration may be necessary (see ARTIFICIAL RESPIRATION). In addition, if the pulse is feeble or absent, try pounding the area over the heart several times fairly hard with a clenched fist. Maintain

artificial respiration until medical help arrives.

FAINTING   A sudden, rapid drop in blood pressure with a resulting decrease in circulation to the brain will produce fainting. There may be warning symptoms such as dizziness, lightheadedness, spots before the eyes, sweating, pallor, and a sinking feeling. A simple faint seldom lasts more than a minute. If caught during the stage of early symptoms, fainting may be prevented simply by stretching the victim out on his back. No other measures are usually necessary, although inhaling spirits of ammonia and wiping the face and hands with cold water may be useful. Fainting may be brought on by bad news, or by a disagreeable sight. It occasionally occurs in a physician's office following a needle puncture.

Feeling faint, and fainting, may be secondary to such serious disorders as internal hemorrhage or unusual drop in the blood sugar. A single fainting spell in someone not ordinarily subject to them, should be accounted for, and a doctor consulted. In a known diabetic patient, a faint spell due to low blood sugar is sometimes referred to as a reaction. It may be prevented or counteracted by taking sugar or fruit juice, and it generally indicates that the routine medications being taken by the patient need adjustment.

FALLS AND FRACTURES   The extent of damage sustained when somebody falls can vary from a mild bruise to a major fracture. Sometimes the injury seems disproportionate to the accident; thus, when elderly persons trip inadvertently, the result may be so serious a fracture as a major break involving the thighbone. It is wise to be alert to the possibility of fracture, and it is a basic rule that if such a possibility exists, the victim should be treated as though he had one. It is safer to put on an unnecessary

FIRST AID AND LIFE SAVING

The object of first aid is to give emergency care to people who are injured or ill, to save life, to prevent death, to relieve pain, until such time as professional medical aid arrives.

The United States government publication **First Aid** describes the value of properly administered help in emergencies as follows:

"First aid, rendered correctly, in many instances can restore natural breathing, usually check loss of blood, prevent or moderate shock, protect wounds and burns from infection, immobilize fractures and dislocations, lessen pain, and conserve the patient's strength; and when medical aid can be obtained, his chance of recovery is greatly enhanced.

"The principal objects of first aid are:

(1) Prevention of further injury.
(2) Checking conditions known to be endangering life.
(3) Protecting injuries from infection and complications.
(4) Making the patient as comfortable as possible to conserve his strength.
(5) Transporting the patient to medical assistance, where required, in such a manner as not to complicate the injury or subject him to any more discomfort than is absolutely necessary."

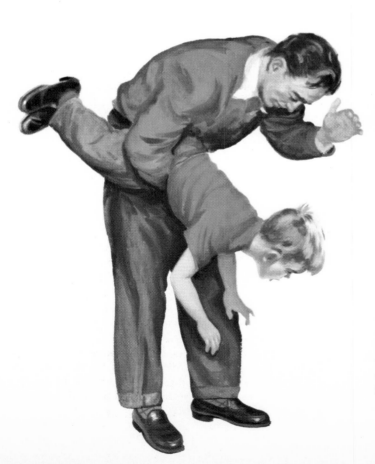

CHOKING (Dislodging Objects From Throat or Mouth)

Very often an obstructing object can be dislodged by inserting the fingers into the child's mouth and removing the object. If this is not successful, turn the child upside down as shown in the illustration. Slap him on the back between the shoulder blades. This may dislodge the obstructing object. Of course, get medical aid immediately if you have not removed the object, and the choking continues.

In the case of a lightweight adult, the same procedure may be followed. If the patient is a large adult, stretch him across a bed face down with the face hanging over the side. Slap the patient on the back between the shoulder blades. In the absence of a bed or table, sit the patient on a chair and bend his head as far downward as possible and slap his back until the object is dislodged.

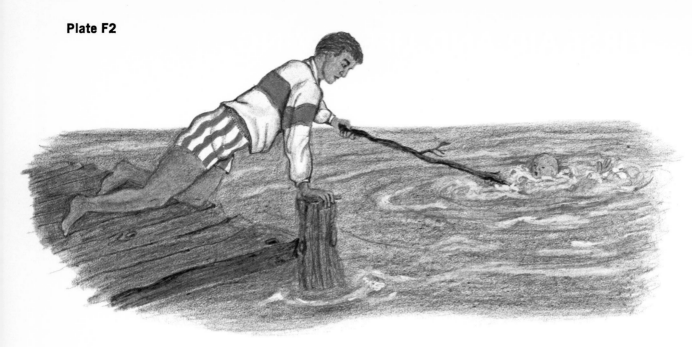

LIFE SAVING — DROWNING

If you cannot swim and the drowning person is near a dock or shore, there are many ways that you can help. The simplest and most effective is to reach out to him with a pole as illustrated. If a line or ring buoy is available, throw it to him. You can also extend your shirt and even tie the shirt and other part of your apparel together to make a longer line. Another way is to grab hold of part of the dock and extend your body to the drowning person; he may be able to grab your feet, and you can then pull him in.

Of course, if you are in a boat, row to the victim and help him grasp part of the boat. If you can pull him into the boat without risking capsizing it, then do so. If you can't safely help him into the boat, then row in with him and if that isn't possible, help him hold on to the boat and keep calling for more help. The American National Red Cross cautions against swimming rescues except by persons trained in life saving.

DROWNING

If there is no way to reach the drowning person by boat or line or other means, and you are a good swimmer and you must swim to him, then the cross-chest carry method of life saving is suggested. Follow this procedure:

Reach over the victim's shoulder and across his chest with your free arm and grasp his side just below the armpit as shown. Hold him so that your hip is directly under the small of his back, and the junction of his chest and head is under your armpit. Swim on your side using the scissors kick and the side arm pull. The side arm pull is executed by pulling the arm outward in a shallow sweep rather than in deep water. The strokes should be short and rapid.

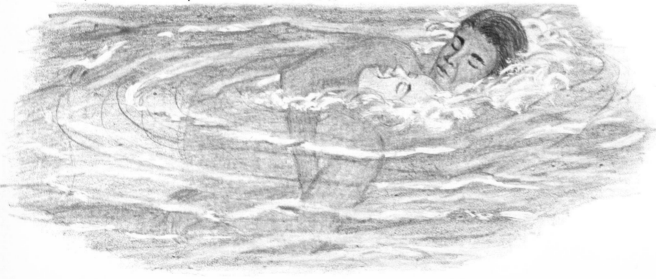

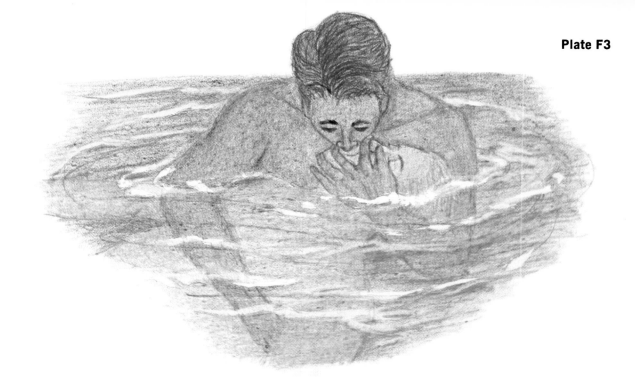

RESCUE BREATHING

The instant you can touch bottom and stand with your own head outside the water, tilt the victim's head back and open his mouth. Place your mouth over his mouth and blow. Make sure to seal his nostrils shut with two of your fingers as shown in the illustration. The first series of breaths should be given as quickly as possible. Continue carrying the victim to shore but blow into his mouth at least once every ten seconds.

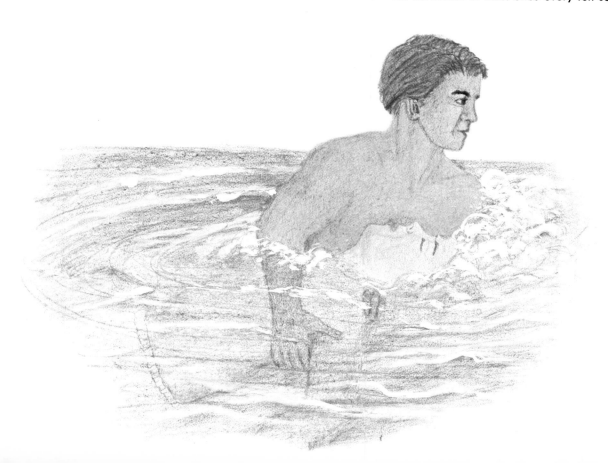

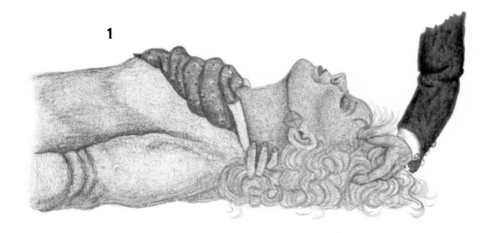

MOUTH - TO - MOUTH RESUSCITATION

Many people are under the mistaken impression that the restoration of breathing is applicable only in cases of drowning. Actually, there are many reasons for loss of breathing besides drowning. These are: choking, electric shock, gas poisoning, overdose of medicines, and many other causes. A knowledge of the four-step method described on these two pages may enable you to save somebody's life. It will only take a few minutes for you to master this knowledge. Once you know it, you will never forget it. It might even be a good idea to practice on someone now so that when an emergency arises, you will actually have some experience with this method.

1. Lay the victim on his back and turn the head to one side and remove with your fingers any foreign objects that may be in the victim's mouth. Now straighten the victim's head as shown in the illustration.

Put one hand under the victim's neck and tilt the head back by holding the head with the other hand.

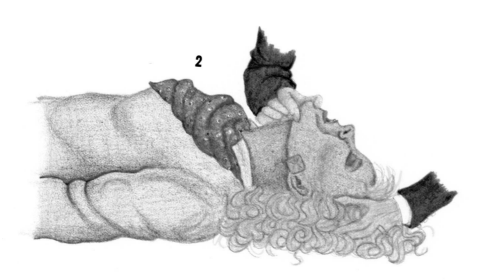

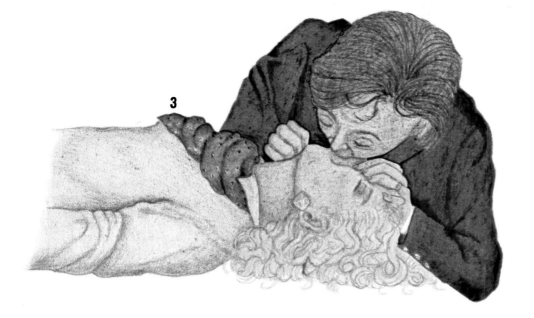

3

2. Pull the chin upward until the head is tilted back fully.

3. Put your mouth tightly over the victim's mouth. Seal the nostrils shut with two fingers of your other hand. Now blow into the victim's mouth in order to make the chest rise.

4. Lift your mouth away from the victim and listen for the sound of returning air. If you don't hear the air, breathe again. If there is still no returning air, then there is a possibility that there is still some obstructing matter in the mouth or throat. Turn the victim's head to the side and attempt to dislodge such obstructing object. Then proceed to breathe into the victim's mouth as before. Always lift your own mouth away each time to permit the escape of air from the victim.

In the case of infants or young children, it is quite possible to obtain an airtight enclosure by covering both nose and mouth of the child with your own mouth. Continue breathing into the victim's mouth — don't give up. For a child, take short breaths, about twenty per minute; for an adult, breathe much more vigorously at the rate of about twelve times a minute. Get professional medical help without delay.

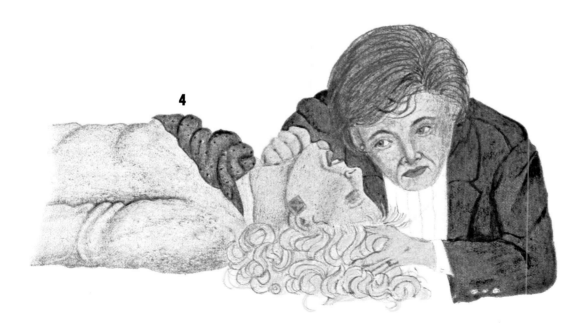

4

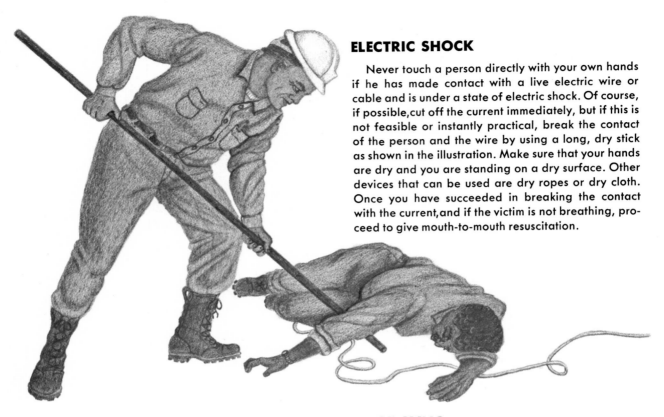

ELECTRIC SHOCK

Never touch a person directly with your own hands if he has made contact with a live electric wire or cable and is under a state of electric shock. Of course, if possible, cut off the current immediately, but if this is not feasible or instantly practical, break the contact of the person and the wire by using a long, dry stick as shown in the illustration. Make sure that your hands are dry and you are standing on a dry surface. Other devices that can be used are dry ropes or dry cloth. Once you have succeeded in breaking the contact with the current, and if the victim is not breathing, proceed to give mouth-to-mouth resuscitation.

TRIANGULAR-BANDAGE SLING

Sometimes it is important to know how to prepare a temporary sling; a very useful one is the triangular bandage sling which is illustrated. It is useful for supporting the arm, elbow, forearm, wrist, hand, or fingers.

Slings may be improvised with any one of objects such as belts, neckties, handkerchiefs and similar materials, but regular bandages are preferable. The illustration shows the triangular bandage sling. Put one end of an open triangular bandage over the shoulder of the injured side and allow the bandage to hang down in front of the chest as shown. Bend the arm at the elbow and bring the injured arm across the chest over the bandage. Now bring the end of the bandage over the shoulder

of the injured side and tie as illustrated. Tuck the other end of the bandage in at the elbow, pinning it with a safety pin. Keep the fingertips exposed to detect the appearance of any interference with blood circulation.

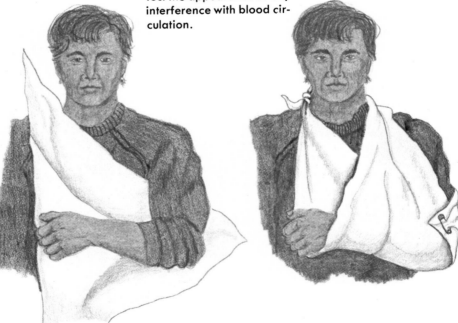

MOVING VICTIM FROM DANGER ZONES

Sometimes it is important to move a victim away from a place of danger such as a fire or automobile accident. This action may even be necessary in the face of the possibility of additional injury but this is the only alternative to saving the victim's life. One quick method of moving the victim to safety is to place him on a blanket as shown and then to pull him away from the danger area. He should be pulled in the direction of the axis of his body, not sideways.

THE THREE-MAN CARRY

Sometimes it is necessary to lift a patient from the floor to carry him either to an ambulance or some other place for emergency medical help. The three-man carry is illustrated below.

In this carrying position two men kneel on one side of the victim and the third carrier faces them as shown. The carriers slide their hands under the victim's back as shown in step 1. The victim is then raised to the carriers' knees and rested on the knees. The carriers then slide their hands farther inwards under the victim and interlock their hands as shown in step

2. Notice that the hands of the carrier on the left are interlocked with the right hand of the front carrier and the left hand of the rear carrier. When the hands are interlocked, all carriers rise and stand erect as shown in step 3 — and carry the victim to the desired location and then lower him by reversing the lifting procedure.

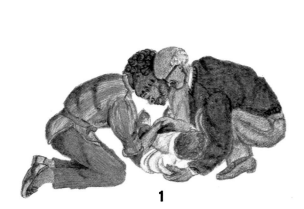

1

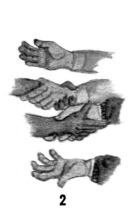

2

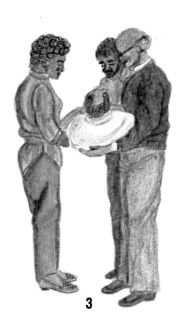

3

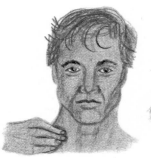
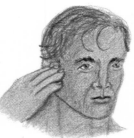
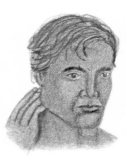

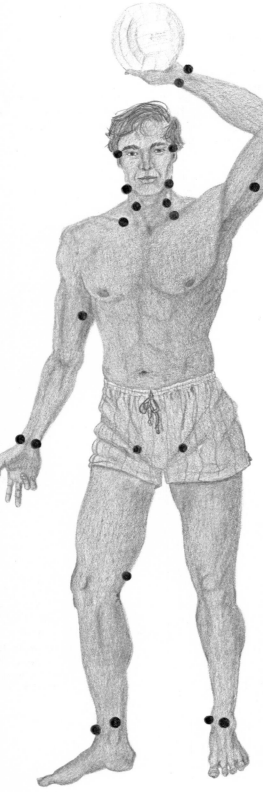

PRESSURE POINTS

Often it is necessary to stop bleeding because of a wound or cut of an artery. Applying pressure at the nearest available pressure point between the heart and the cut may result in stopping or controlling the bleeding. There are actually twenty-two pressure points in the body, eleven on each side. Illustrated on this page are a number of the more important and accessible ones. The principle of the pressure points is somewhat similar to compressing a rubber tube to stop the flow of water through such tube. In some instances finger pressure may be sufficient to stop the bleeding, or it may be the only way to control bleeding. In other cases a tourniquet may be required. When a tourniquet is necessary, finger pressure should be applied first to stem the loss of blood while the tourniquet is being prepared and applied.

Illustrated at the top are various points to apply pressure to stop or control bleeding in shoulder, neck, and head. The application of the pressure should always be between the cut and the heart.

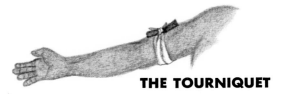

THE TOURNIQUET

The tourniquet can be made from a strap, belt, suspenders, handkerchief, necktie, rubber tubing, towel, or similar material. Do not use wire, cord, or anything that will cut the flesh. Place a hard pad or object over the artery so that when the tourniquet is tightened, it will press the pad or object against the artery. Sometimes a stick is placed through one of the knots as shown in the illustration. This is so that the tourniquet can be twisted and by twisting the stick, extra constricting force can be obtained in order to control the bleeding. Usually after a tourniquet is applied and remains on for several minutes the skin below the tourniquet turns white and then bluish. After the tourniquet is applied, the patient should be rushed to a physician and the physician should be the one to release or remove the tourniquet. United States Armed Forces experience indicates that a tourniquet can remain on for several hours without causing damage. This procedure of permitting the tourniquet to stay on is contrary to the old procedure which required release of the tourniquet after ten minutes and then its reapplication if necessary.

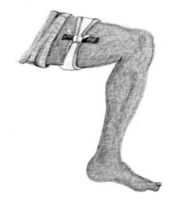

EARLY WARNING SIGNS OF A HEART ATTACK

Many lives might be saved, including your own, if the public learned to recognize early warning signs of a heart attack. A heart attack generally does not occur suddenly; the body gives some warning signs first. Knowing these signs might save your life.

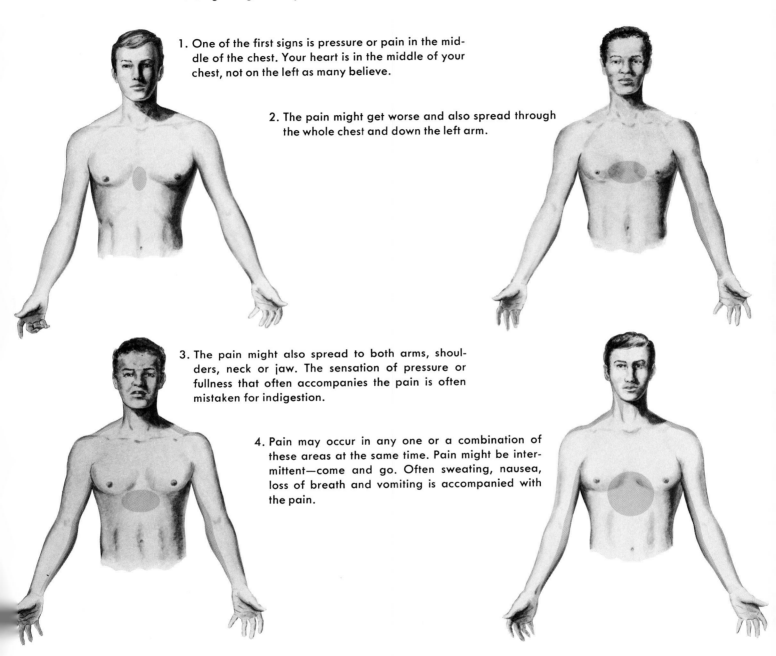

1. One of the first signs is pressure or pain in the middle of the chest. Your heart is in the middle of your chest, not on the left as many believe.

2. The pain might get worse and also spread through the whole chest and down the left arm.

3. The pain might also spread to both arms, shoulders, neck or jaw. The sensation of pressure or fullness that often accompanies the pain is often mistaken for indigestion.

4. Pain may occur in any one or a combination of these areas at the same time. Pain might be intermittent—come and go. Often sweating, nausea, loss of breath and vomiting is accompanied with the pain.

WHAT TO DO IF YOU EXPERIENCE ANY OF THE ABOVE FOUR SIGNS

Call your doctor at once, or if he or any other doctor is not available, immediately go to the nearest hospital emergency room and ask for immediate treatment.

**IN CASE OF AN ACTUAL HEART ATTACK
FIRST AID SHOULD BE ADMINISTERED IMMEDIATELY— SEE PLATE F8D**

NEW LIFE SAVING TECHNIQUE TO HELP VICTIMS OF FOOD CHOKING "THE HEIMLICH MANEUVER"

A victim of food choking, unless helped immediately, will not be able to speak or breathe, usually turns blue, collapses and in most instances dies in about four minutes. Quick help is of the utmost importance. The procedure described below was developed by Dr. Henry Heimlich of the Jewish Hospital, Cincinnati, Ohio.

Place your arms around the victim's waist. Grasp your fist with your other hand. Place it against victim's abdomen above the navel and below the rib cage. Push fist into the abdomen with a quick upward thrust. If the food is not dislodged, repeat the procedure. A doctor should examine the victim after the food is dislodged. The Heimlich Maneuver can be self-administered.

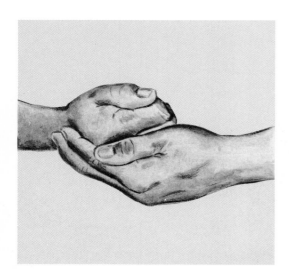

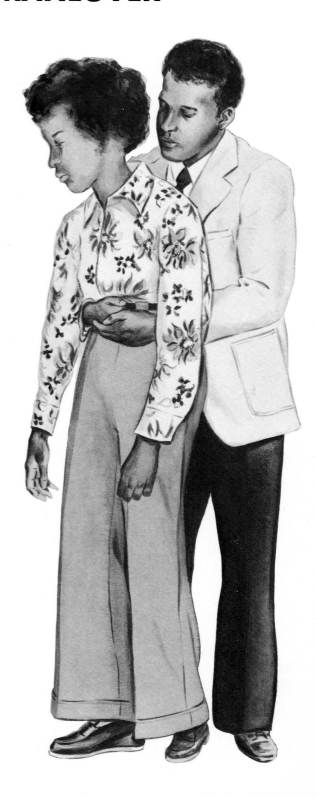

If victim has collapsed and is lying down, kneel astride the victim's hips. Now place one hand on top of the other, as is shown in the picture. Place heel of bottom hand on victim's abdomen above the navel and below the rib cage. Push into the abdomen with a quick upward thrust. If food is not dislodged, repeat the procedure. As soon as the food is dislodged, the victim should be examined by a doctor.

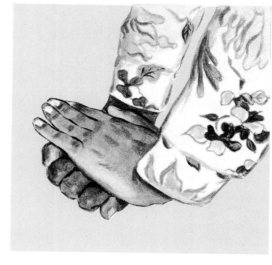

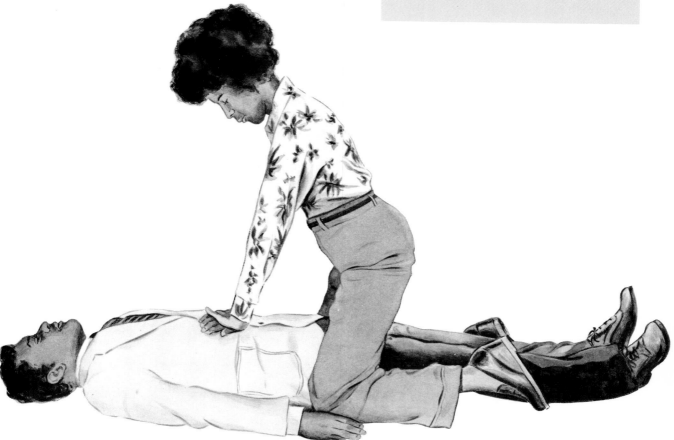

LIFE SAVING TECHNIQUE FOR A HEART ATTACK

CARDIOPULMONARY RESUSCITATION

A heart attack victim may collapse, show no pulse and usually rapidly turns blue from lack of oxygen. The heart may have stopped beating. Often the heart can be restarted by a sharp rap with a clenched fist on the chest area above the heart. However, in most cases, it will be necessary to keep the circulation going and get air into the lungs. The instructions given below were written by Dr. Isadore Rossman, coauthor of *Medical Aid Encyclopedia for the Home* and appeared originally in *Health Digest,* a health newsletter published by *Parents' Magazine.*

This is the procedure called cardiopulmonary resuscitation and is most effective when performed by a two person team; one to compress the heart and another to blow air into the lungs.

1. *Cardiac massage.* Locate the rib margin and follow it to the middle of the body, to the breastbone. At the tip of the breastbone is a flexible, cartilaginous portion which confirms the central location. Three finger breadths above its tip (about 1 ½ inches) is the site for massage. The heel of the one hand is pushed downwards by the other hand. The intent is to depress this part of the lower breastbone by 2 inches, which in turn compresses the heart and ejects some of its blood into the arteries. Pressure is released and reapplied at a rather rapid rate, approximately 60 cycles per minute. Some rescuers count "one thousand and one, one thousand and two, etc.," each count corresponding to one cycle of pressure and release and lasting about one second. There is a pause after the one-thousand-and-five count and then the cycle is repeated.

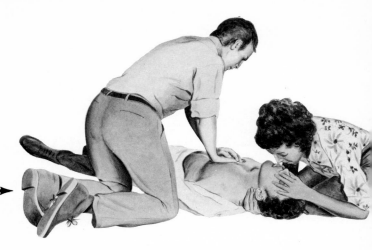

2. *Artificial respiration.* The other rescuer hyperextends the victim's head. (This is the head thrown back position one would assume to look at the top of a skyscraper.) With the thumb in the victim's mouth and the fingers under the chin, the rescuer takes the victim's jaw and brings it forcibly forward. The rescuer takes a deep breath and when the partner's count reaches one thousand and five, blows air into the victim's mouth by tightly sealing his mouth to the victim's. The rescuer should also hold the victim's nose to prevent air loss. There should be an obvious rise in the chest as air is blown into the lungs and a corresponding lowering of the chest as the air is subsequently released. This process (artificial respiration) is repeated once for every five depressions the other rescuer makes on the heart, ideally providing around 12 lung fulls of air every minute.

If only one person is available, he must perform both rescue operations, which is possible but not easy. The steps are the same with the rescuer shifting from pressing on the breastbone to artificial respiration after each fifth count. The maneuver should be kept up until an ambulance crew or medical help arrives. Individuals interested in learning more about cardiopulmonary resuscitation will find that many local communities and Red Cross chapters offer courses in the subject.

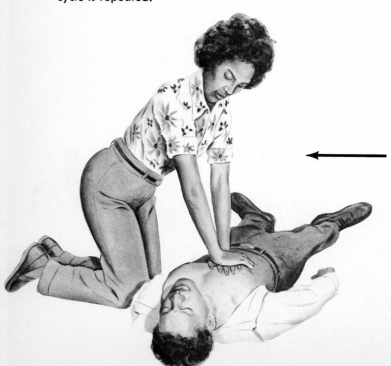

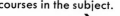

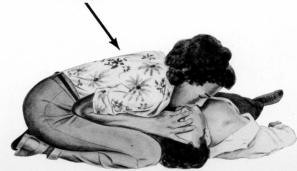

splint than to ignore the possibility of fracture and allow further serious damage to occur. The truth is that even an expert may not always be able to distinguish between a bad sprain and a fracture until an appropriate X-ray film has been taken. However, there are some leads that should alert one in this connection:

1. Obviously, an accident in which the individual has undergone considerable impact, such as falling down a flight of stairs or being knocked down by an auto, makes the probability of fracture high.

2. A fracture will generally produce a deformity, such as an abnormal bulge or a peculiar contour to the surface of an extremity, or a similar obvious change from the usual appearance. One important exception to this rule is skull fracture, which cannot be detected without medical examination.

3. False motion may be produced by attempted movement. What happens is that a muscular contraction acting on the broken bone will produce a type of motion that is obviously abnormal, such as a movement in the middle of the thigh or forearm.

4. A peculiar grating sound may be produced as one lightly runs his hands over the region of the fracture. This is due to the crackling produced by the fragments of bone as they move. It is known as crepitus.

5. Sometimes an obvious shortening of the limb occurs, due to the overriding of the broken bone ends. For example, after a thighbone fracture the entire leg on the affected side may be one or more inches shorter than the other leg.

If any of these findings are present, the victim should be treated for fracture, and special care should be taken not to aggravate the injury while trying to help. A natural impulse when seeing somebody stumble and fall to the ground is to rush over and help him up. It would be wiser first to check for the possibility of fracture.

Otherwise, helping the person to his feet may transform a simple fracture into a compound—that is, one where the bone penetrates the skin and is exposed—or such help may aggravate the injury in other ways, since the broken ends of the bone may produce damage to neighboring structures. Also, one may have to deal with the possibility that the injured person will be unable to bear weight, and may collapse again. Hence, the old first-aid maxim of "splint them where they lie."

One should be particularly careful where the possibility of an injury to the spinal column exists, as for example, after a fall on the back or an accident in which considerable force has been directed against the neck. Here it is always possible that the underlying spinal cord may be damaged, and any aggravation of such injury could produce paralysis.

Once it is clear that no fracture exists and that one is dealing with a bruising injury or contusion, the best first-aid treatment is promptly to chill the affected area. Probably the easiest way to do this is with ice cubes, but if no ice is available, cold compresses may be applied instead. Immediate application of ice serves two purposes: It cuts down bleeding from any vessels that may have been torn, and it diminishes both the local pain and the extent of inflammation and swelling set up by the injury. An ice bag suitably replenished from time to time is a good expedient. For exactly how long this can be continued has never been accurately determined. For severe sprains with evidence indicating a torn vein, the ice bag can be kept on for hours.

At one large Eastern university, the practice in treating athletic injuries, such as a twisted knee, is to strap an ice bag around the injured part by means of an elastic bandage. Fresh ice cubes are added as needed, and this does not interfere with the athlete's attending classes. The ice bag may be kept on not only throughout the day of the injury, but on the following day as well. Bleeding, soreness, and pain have been considerably lessened by this procedure. For smaller injuries, probably a few hours of off-and-on ice applications will do, particularly if it becomes apparent that one is not dealing with extensive bleeding or with torn tissues and ligaments. Sometimes cold or ice applications are recommended for the first day, and thereafter heat—as from a heating pad or hot compresses—may be substituted. The idea here is that the cold will cut down the initial bleeding and swelling, while heat on the following day may aid in resorption of swelling and in increasing local circulation.

Following some falls with torn blood vessels, a large local accumulation of blood with an obvious swelling may occur. This is known as a hematoma. Usually, in addition to the swelling of the hematoma, there is obvious discoloration for some distance beneath the skin as the blood diffuses through the tissues. This process may go on for a period of days so that what initially seemed to be a small black-and-blue spot becomes larger and larger. It also undergoes color changes, turning from the black-and-blue stage to yellowish-brown or a lighter tone. What is happening is that blood in the tissue is acting as a foreign body and may produce local reactions. It can even undergo calcification. The doctor may therefore decide to needle or aspirate a large hematoma in order to evacuate the blood from it. (See also FRACTURES.)

FRACTURES The correct first-aid treatment for a fracture is immobilization, for example, splinting. The basic principle is to run a relatively rigid support, customarily extending down to the adjacent joint, alongside the region of the break. Strapping or tying the support to the limb will help prevent motion of the fracture. Most first-aid stations have padded splints of various sizes available.

In a great many circumstances, however, one has to rely on makeshifts. Such makeshifts may simply be reasonably rigid objects, such as a branch broken off from a tree, a stick, a broom handle, a piece of piping, or even such an odd object as an umbrella. The object can be tied in place with a necktie, strings or rope, torn pieces from a shirt, a man's belt—in short, anything that is handy. Some of the possibilities for dealing with different fractures are to be seen in the illustrations, First Aid And Life Saving, Plates F1-F8. Here is what one can do for specific kinds of common fractures:

Wrist. Fractures of the wrist occur most commonly as a result of a fall on the outstretched hand. The impact may snap the bone of the arm just above the wrist. The deformity that results is sometimes referred to as the silver-fork deformity, since the break results in the hand and wrist presenting a curved elevation somewhat like the curved part of a fork. Technically it is known as a Colles' fracture. The splint should be laid over the upper and lower parts of the wrist. Appropriate ties attaching it to the hand and forearm are made to hold the splint in place. In addition, a sling—or pinning the sleeve to the shirt or coat—will give useful support.

Sometimes, instead of a typical Colles' fracture, a fracture occurs involving one of the small bones of the wrist. It may be hard to distinguish this from a sprain, except by X-ray. Needless to say, this and any other suspected fracture should be routinely X-rayed.

Finger. Crushing injuries in falls may produce a fracture of one of the three little bones that make up the finger. They may be difficult to distinguish from a bruising injury with swelling. A short narrow piece of wood, even a pencil or a portion of a tongue depressor, can be applied with gauze or adhesive strapping as a first-aid measure. Not uncommonly, instead of a fracture there may be a subluxation. In this, the supporting tissues present at each of the individual joints of the finger bones are torn, so that there is a displacement at the joint. It becomes obvious from observation that a portion of the finger is out of alignment. First-aid treatment for this is the same as for a fracture. Ice may be of help in relieving pain.

Forearm and Arm. Fractures of these bones are treated with splints in the usual manner. In addition, a sling or pinning of the sleeve to another part of the clothing will help support the limb. If no splints are available, one should consider any arrangement that will keep the arm or forearm immobilized against the trunk— for example, strapping of the upper arm to the trunk with strips of adhesive tape.

Thigh. Fractures of the thigh are most likely to occur in elderly persons, more often in women than in men, and generally as the result of a fall. Because of the brittleness of the thighbone in the elderly, it may fracture as a result of the impact of falling, most often high up in the region of the hip. A fracture is generally recognized by its pain, shortening of the extremity, and the fact that the leg tends to turn outward, in what is known as external rotation. Splints should be applied to the entire length of the thigh and extend down over the knee.

Knee. Fracture at the knee can occur in the thighbone, just above the knee joint, or may involve one or both of the two bones of the lower leg, below the level of the joint. The latter is sometimes referred to as a bumper fracture, the name deriving from the fact that it is often sustained as a result of the direct impact of an automobile bumper. Fractures in this area will be recognized by the abnormality of contour, and are often compound, meaning that the bone ends protrude through the skin. As with all fractures or suspected fractures, no attempt should be made to help the patient up; he should be splinted where he lies.

Ankle. It is sometimes difficult to distinguish between a bad sprain and an outright fracture of the ankle joint. In both cases there may be a considerable amount of swelling, usually on the outer aspect, just above the ankle joint. If in doubt, treat as a fracture, and do not allow weight-bearing.

Neck and Back. In cases of fracture or suspected fracture of the neck and back, first aid should be directed toward avoiding potential spinal-cord injury. The best procedure may well be to allow the patient to lie where he has fallen, with no attempt to move him until proper medical aid has arrived. If circumstances are such that he must be moved, the basic principle is to avoid any manipulation or motion of the spinal column. Avoid any movement of the back and any rotation of the head. The victim must not be allowed to turn from one side to the other on his own. It takes at least three people properly to move someone with a suspected back injury. One should support the head and neck, a second the trunk, and the third the lower extremities. All the motions should be synchronized in such a way that twisting of the head, the trunk, or the hips is avoided. The basic principle is to keep the patient stiff and immobile. If he has to be transported, it should be on a flat, hard surface such as a door, on which he rests flat on his back. If only a litter or a blanket is available, the patient should be transported in the face-down position.

Skull. Some head injury is an inevitable accompaniment of skull fracture. If the person is knocked out and then recovers consciousness, this is spoken of as a concussion. If someone who has been knocked out comes to, and after a period of consciousness becomes unconscious again, there is a strong suspicion that bleeding within the skull has occurred. There is no specific treatment for a skull fracture, except to transport the patient to a medical institution and not to permit walking.

Rib. Blows and crushing injuries to the chest will often fracture one or more ribs. This will produce severe pain in the affected ribs, made worse with breathing or movement. Sometimes the pain produced by attempting to breathe is so marked that involuntary splinting occurs and the breathing is noticeably shallow. Rarely, a broken fragment of rib may penetrate the lung surface. The pain of a rib fracture is often relieved if the patient lies on the affected side. This will diminish the respiratory motion on that side. If medical aid is not readily available, one may attempt to splint the side with the fractured rib by means of adhesive taping. To do this, the victim is told to breathe out as much as possible. Wide (two to three inch) adhesive tape is run from back to front over the region of the presumed rib fracture. The tape should extend beyond the midline both in back and in front. Two or three such tape strips placed above and below the part of the rib cage involved, will cut down the motion imparted by breathing and will diminish the pain. (See also FALLS AND FRACTURES.)

FROSTBITE Injury to tissues (generally to fingers, toes, nose, or ears) produced by exposure to severe cold is referred to as frostbite. Initially, the affected area looks very white, and is obviously quite cold and stiff to touch. Later, variable amounts of reddening, often accompanied by an increase in pain, may be noted. Severe frostbite lasting many hours may lead to death of the involved tissues, a condition known as gangrene. Such extensive frostbite is seldom seen except in mountain climbers, in persons who are lost in the bitter cold, or in someone who has been injured and remained unconscious out-of-doors during a severe freeze. First-aid treatment of frostbite is to immerse the area in warm water at approximately 105° to 110° F.—in short, to warm up the area as rapidly as possible. In addition, a physician may give anticoagulant drugs or other medications which have been shown to cut down on the extent of cold injury. Rubbing the part with snow is an old procedure which has been completely discarded. It may in fact increase the extent of cold damage.

HEAT EXHAUSTION Heat exhaustion is most common during spells of hot, moist, damp weather. It is sometimes seen among persons gathered into tight crowds who have to stand for prolonged periods. The victim generally complains of faintness, weakness, and dizziness. This is often due to a drop in blood pressure. The skin is moist, but not hot, and the pulse may become weak and rapid. If there has been a good deal of perspiration, there may be further complaints of muscular or abdominal cramps, sometimes associated with nausea and even vomiting. The following steps are useful:

1. Stretch the victim out in a cleared area so that he may benefit from whatever air in motion is available.

2. Give small amounts of cold drinks, such as fruit juices to which a pinch of salt has been added. If there has been excessive perspiration, one might give salt tablets, or a diluted salt solution made by adding a teaspoon of salt to a quart of water.

3. Mild stimulants such as coffee or tea may also be useful.

4. A cold, brisk sponging of the head, face, and arms, and inhaling of spirits of ammonia, stimulate the heart and circulation.

HEAT STROKE During heat stroke the body's temperature-regulating mechanism goes astray. Such a stroke generally comes on after overexposure to the sun, on very hot days, in places such as open fields or beaches. The victim is obviously hot to the touch, and very high temperatures ranging up to 104° or 106° F. are not uncommon. The skin is hot and dry, the pulse full and bounding. The chief complaint is complete weakness.

First aid consists of getting the victim out of the sun and into as cool and as shady a spot as possible. Vigorous measures to lower the body temperature should be taken immediately. These may include pouring cold water over the victim's head and shoulders, or applying ice bags to these areas. Immersion in cool water or rubdowns with alcohol may also be helpful in lowering body temperature. If necessary, the patient can be wrapped in a cold moist sheet and transported to a hospital for further treatment.

NOSEBLEED　　More than 90 per cent of all nosebleeds come from the lower half of the nose and from the nasal septum, the midline structure which divides the nasal pathway into two separate halves. The nasal septum has a very extensive blood supply and is easily damaged when picked at. Its delicacy of structure explains why nosebleeds occur as often as they do. Injury, various kinds of infection, and over-strenuous blowing are the usual causes; very rarely do they result from high blood pressure. This statement also applies to individuals known to have elevated blood pressure but who nevertheless can have nosebleeds for the same reasons as people with normal blood pressure.

Most of the suggested treatments for nosebleed, as, for example, the one that calls for applying ice to the back of the neck, are of little value. The most satisfactory method of controlling it is by direct compression of both nostrils. The nostrils should be firmly grasped with the fingers, exerting an even pressure on the entire fleshy portion of the nose. Maintain the pressure for approximately ten minutes,

then cautiously release to see whether the bleeding has stopped. The clot that forms is easily dislodged, so do not blow the nose or poke about in it for some time after a nosebleed.

When nosebleeds are frequent, cauterization of the septum or similar procedures may occasionally be resorted to by a physician. Nosebleeds that occur behind the fleshy part of the nose may sometimes be severe, and not controllable by the form of compression described here. A possible first-aid measure would be to take a large wad of cotton, sprinkle it with a few drops of nasal decongestant such as neosynephrine nose drops, insert, and then compress the nasal tissue. Severe nosebleeds may require packing by a physician.

POISONING　　Many cases of poisoning occur only because suitable precautions are not taken. Remember that there is nothing a toddler may not sample in his travels around the household, including objects of unpleasant taste and odor. Warning notices, or skull and crossbones identification, will certainly not hold him back. Eternal vigilance is the price not only of liberty, but also of child rearing. The fact that bathrooms come equipped with medicine chests is not necessarily a valid reason for keeping medicines there. With a young child around the house, medicines should be placed under lock and key. See that detergents, bleaches, lye, and acid solutions are completely inaccessible to him. Poisoning precautions should extend to the basement, the attic, the garage, the barn, and the woodshed. Children have been known to swallow insecticides, rodenticides, herbicides, algicides, and fungicides (the so-called "economic poisons") many of which are potentially serious threats.

Here are a few basic facts to keep in mind in relation to chemical poisoning:

1. Milk is a good everyday antidote usually available in every household. It

will neutralize various acids and alkalis, fluorides, and other poisons. Therefore, even if you do not know the exact nature of the poison, or its antidote, you will do well to give milk.

2. With few exceptions, the basic aim of first aid in chemical poisoning is to produce vomiting. Vomiting can be induced by scraping the back of the throat with a spoon or a finger, or by giving an emetic (an agent that produces vomiting), such as ipecac. Other easily made up emetics are a tablespoon of salt or of mustard in a glass of warm water. These can be repeated.

3. The exceptions to the above rule are the corrosives and the carbon tetrachloride, kerosene, and benzine group. The corrosives—agents which produce tissue burns—such as acids and alkalies (lye, Drano®, battery acid) produce whitish changes of the lips and mouth. If any of these has been swallowed, *do not* induce vomiting.

4. Some of the substances swallowed by children are not necessarily poisonous.

However, when in doubt, produce vomiting anyway. In all cases make sure that a doctor or a Poison Control Center is called, and if a doctor cannot get there readily, plan on bringing the victim rapidly to a hospital where the stomach can be washed out if necessary.

5. A universal antidote, active against many different types of poisons, may be purchased at most drug stores. It consists of activated charcoal, tannic acid, and magnesium hydroxide. This will neutralize and absorb various poisons. If available, give a tablespoon of the universal antidote with water or milk. With most poisons, one can induce vomiting after one to two minutes. The alleged household "substitute" for the universal antidote, consisting of burnt toast and tea, is completely worthless. Milk is much better.

6. Always save the container that held the ingested substance. Its label will often specify the exact ingredients and may also give directions for treatment of accidental poisoning. If the victim is brought to a hospital, take the container along.

TABLE OF COMMON POISONS

Poison	Treatment
Acetone. This is found in some nail polish removers and some paint solvents. Small amounts are not dangerous.	Induce vomiting. Give one to two teaspoons of bicarbonate of soda in water.
Acids. Battery acid, sulfuric acid, etc., are corrosive, give off irritating fumes and produce burns about the mouth and lips.	Avoid vomiting. Give milk, repeated doses of milk of magnesia, baking soda, Tums®, or other household remedies for hyperacidity.
Alkalies. Chiefly lye (Drano® and similar products), ammonia, quicklime, produce chemical burns.	Avoid vomiting. Give large amounts of milk, vinegar diluted with water, fruit juices.
Arsenic. Found in some mouse seeds, some ant and rat poisons.	Induce vomiting. Give milk, milk of magnesia, egg white.

Poison	Treatment
Aspirin. (Also found in Anacin®, Empirin®, APC, etc.) Taken in overdoses produces sleepiness, flushing, deep breathing, burning in upper abdomen.	Induce vomiting. Give one to two teaspoons of baking soda in water.
Barbiturates. Phenobarbital, and sleeping pills such as seconal, amytal, nembutal, are poison if taken in overdoses.	Induce vomiting unless the patient is in a coma. Give large amounts of coffee or tea. If comatose, give artificial respiration.
Bleach.	See **Chlorine**
Carbolic Acid (creosote). A corrosive which produces burns on the lips and mouth.	Avoid vomiting. Give large amounts of olive oil, cottonseed oil, or egg whites. Follow with one ounce of Epsom salts in a pint of water.
Chlorine. Found in bleaches.	Give an emetic and produce vomiting. Follow with dilute ammonia water (one teaspoon household ammonia to a glass of water).
Cleaning Fluids: Benzine, kerosene, gasoline, carbon tetrachloride, etc., are poisonous both in liquid form and if inhaled as fumes.	Avoid inducing vomiting unless the cleaning fluid is known to be carbon tetrachloride. Give strong coffee or tea. Artificial respiration as necessary.
Copper. Bordeaux mixture, blue vitriol, found in garden sprays.	Produce vomiting. Give milk or egg whites and repeat vomiting.
DDT. Contained in insect poisons and sprays.	Give one ounce Epsom salts in water and repeat vomiting.
Detergents. Not likely to be dangerous, except those few containing phosphates.	Give milk and induce vomiting.
Digitalis. A common heart medicine, and its derivatives (digoxin, gitalin, digitoxin). Produces weakness, slow pulse, collapse, and delirium.	Within first half-hour, produce vomiting. Otherwise do not do so. Give strong tea.

Poison	Treatment
Fluorides. Found in many ant and mouse poisons. The amount found in children's antidental decay preparations is not likely to be dangerous, even if a whole bottle is taken.	Induce vomiting. Give milk repeatedly.
Iodine. Found usually as tincture of iodine or Lugol's solution.	Give enough of corn starch or flour to induce vomiting; repeat.
Lead. Found in some paints and in white and red lead, may be inhaled in dangerous amounts.	Induce vomiting. Give large amounts of milk.
Narcotics. Demerol, morphine, codeine, paregoric, tincture of opium, all narcotics. Produce drowsiness and coma, markedly constricted eye pupils, depressed breathing.	Give strong tea, or universal antidote (see page 534). Induce vomiting. Give artificial respiration.
Oil of Wintergreen. Produces symptoms similar to aspirin poisoning.	Give one to two teaspoons of baking soda in water. Induce vomiting and repeat.
Phosphorus. An ingredient of some roach and rodent poisons. May fume and has a pungent, garlicky odor.	Avoid vomiting. Give one half to one glass of hydrogen peroxide.
Strychnine. Found in some rodent poisons.	Induce vomiting. Give universal antidote (see page 534), strong tea, or coffee.
Turpentine. Produces burning of mouth and stomach, weakness and shock.	Induce vomiting. Give one to two ounces of Epsom salts in a pint of water.

Over-the-Counter Medications

The rising costs of medical care during recent years has encouraged consumers to treat minor symptoms with the aid of a pharmacist. There are many products on the market to treat everything from the flu to body odor. Minor cuts, abrasions, and burns may be treated with nonprescription ointments, thus saving the patient an expensive visit to the doctor's office. The ability to treat the symptoms of colds, influenza, and viral infections also spares the patient an uncomfortable and often long wait to see the physician. Being able to treat these symptoms is particularly helpful when the patient is a young child or an elderly person. Medicines which relieve the discomfort of arthritis and rheumatism may be purchased without a prescription as well as medicines for diarrhea, constipation and others. Sore throat remedies, ointments for infected cuts, bandages for cuts and sprains are all available at the corner drugstore.

As more drugs enter the over-the-counter market, the consumer may be confused by warnings, dosage schedules, and ingredients. The possibility of dangerous interactions with other drugs, food, and drink demands that the patient proceed cautiously and intelligently. The pharmacist is a valuable resource in the treatment of minor ailments and can explain confusing details regarding medications. This section should answer many questions about nonprescription medications and how to take advantage of them safely.

OTC is short for over the counter, and when we talk about OTC drugs, we mean that vast assortment of medicines you can buy without a doctor's prescription.

Pharmacies and supermarkets have hundreds of thousands of nonprescrip-

538

tion drug items, and we Americans buy them to the tune of $3.5 billion or more each year.

From the antibacterial bar soap with our morning shower to the sleep-aid at bedtime—and everything from a headache remedy to an antacid in between—we use nonprescription medicines to relieve symptoms we feel do not warrant a visit to the doctor.

Over-the-counter (nonprescription) drugs should not be regarded lightly. They are often as powerful and can have the same potential for harmful side effects as their prescription counterparts. The difference between prescription and nonprescription drugs is spelled out in the Food, Drug, and Cosmetic Act, which says that drugs that are habit-forming, toxic, or not safe for use except under a doctor's supervision can be dispensed only on prescription. All other drugs are available over the counter.

Unlike prescription drugs, over-the-counter drugs are not usually intended to *cure* anything. They are used primarily to relieve the symptoms of a particular disease or condition.

THE IMPORTANCE OF LABELS

OTC drug product labels are very different. FDA requires more information and very special information because consumers are pretty much on their own when they use the products. Thus, the label must provide the consumer with adequate information for the safe and effective use of the product. This information is important because OTC drugs are often purchased in supermarkets or convenience stores where there may not be a pharmacist to answer questions.

This is the information that should appear on an OTC drug product label:
• The name and address of the manufacturer, packer or distributor and the lot, control or batch number. This means any distinctive combination of letters, symbols or numbers from which the complete manufacturing history of the drug can be determined.
• The name of the product and what type of drug it is—that is, an antacid, nasal decongestant, pain reliever, antiseptic, or so on.
• A statement of the active ingredients. Consumers should read this list carefully when selecting an OTC drug, not only to

know what they're taking, but also to avoid ingredients to which they may be sensitive.
• Declaration of the presence of the dye Yellow No. 5. Federal regulations require that the presence of this dye be indicated on the labels of all products—foods and cosmetics as well as drugs. People who are allergic to aspirin will also be allergic to this dye and therefore should be especially careful to look for it on product labels.
• The amount of the product in the container—that is, the number of tablets or ounces of liquid, cream or ointment.
• Indications for use—the symptoms or conditions for which the product should be used.
• Directions for use—(sometimes designated "dosage")—explain how much of the drug to take (per dose, time between doses, and maximum number of doses) and when to take it. The directions may also tell how to take or use the product: "Tablet should be chewed," "Take with a glass of water," and so forth. Directions for ointments and creams will explain how often to apply them and how to apply them (thin layer, for example).

• Warnings or cautions—who shouldn't take the drug, when the drug shouldn't be taken, what adverse reactions might develop, and what symptoms signal the need for professional help.

Many OTC medicines should not be used by people when they are using certain other drugs. The label now or in the future will contain a warning to prevent use of the medicine when it could cause a hazardous interaction.

Some information now on labels will be especially helpful to people with special health problems. For example, some labels now contain the sodium content per dose, if it is 5 mg or higher, so people who must limit their intake of salt can be on guard against medicines that have a high salt content.

While OTC drugs may temporarily relieve symptoms, overuse may mask a serious illness. (The indigestion relieved by an antacid may really be caused by an ulcer, for example.) For this reason, the label may warn that the product shouldn't be taken for more than a specific number of days or that it should be discontinued and a doctor consulted if symptoms persist for more than a specific period of time or if certain other symptoms occur.

The labeling of all OTC drug products that are to be taken internally must include the warning "As with any drug, if you are pregnant or nursing a baby, seek the advice of a health professional before using this product."

The most important warning on the OTC drug label is "Keep this and all drugs out of the reach of children."

• Drug interaction precautions—some ingredients in OTC drugs can counteract or interfere with the effectiveness of other drugs. Certain antacids, for example, reduce the effectiveness of the antibiotic tetracycline. Mixing drugs and alcohol is never a good idea, particularly when the drug is one that causes drowsiness.

• Expiration date—the month and year be-

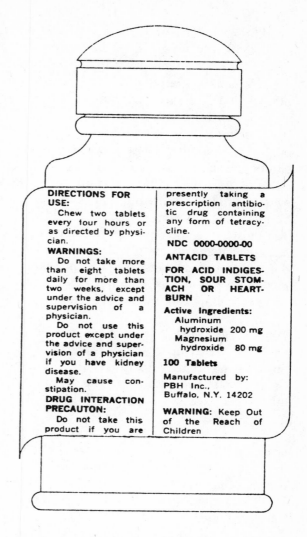

DIRECTIONS FOR USE:
Chew two tablets every four hours or as directed by physician.

WARNINGS:
Do not take more than eight tablets daily for more than two weeks, except under the advice and supervision of a physician.
Do not use this product except under the advice and supervision of a physician if you have kidney disease.
May cause constipation.

DRUG INTERACTION PRECAUTON:
Do not take this product if you are presently taking a prescription antibiotic drug containing any form of tetracycline.

NDC 0000-0000-00

ANTACID TABLETS
FOR ACID INDIGESTION, SOUR STOMACH OR HEARTBURN

Active Ingredients:
Aluminum hydroxide 200 mg
Magnesium hydroxide 80 mg

100 Tablets

Manufactured by:
PBH Inc.,
Buffalo, N.Y. 14202

WARNING: Keep Out of the Reach of Children

yond which the drug will no longer be effective. Not all OTC drug products will have an expiration date, but when it appears, take it seriously. Taking an outdated drug may not provide relief and may be harmful.

CHILDREN AND OTC MEDICINES

To make sure children are protected from accidental use of medicines or other products that could be harmful, the Poison Prevention Packaging Act requires that all such chemicals or drugs be enclosed in safety packaging. When you buy medicines, or other products that pose a potential hazard to children, look for safety packaging. In OTC drugs this means choosing a container with a top designed to be especially difficult for children to open or medicines encased in an individually wrapped package. Also it should be remembered that drug packages are designed especially for keeping the drugs placed in them safe and potent, so you should consult your pharmacist before transferring a drug to a different container or package. Buying safety-packaged drugs can be a tremendous help in preventing accidental injury to children—and perhaps even to careless adults. But don't think that safety packaging alone can protect children. You must remember to keep medicines and all other chemicals out of the reach of children, in locked cabinets, and to avoid taking medicines in front of children, or leading them to believe that medicine is candy.

YOUR PHARMACIST   A pharmacist is naturally relied upon to fill prescriptions, but he can often be just as reliable in answering your questions about the drugs you take. That's one of the responsibilities that goes with the job.

How do you choose your pharmacist? In addition to location, the American Pharmaceutical Association (APhA) suggests these considerations.
• Is the pharmacist accessible, by phone and in person?
• Does the pharmacist offer emergency prescription service?
• Does the pharmacy deliver and can you charge drug purchases?
• Is the pharmacist willing to answer your questions about drugs?
• Does the pharmacist keep patient profiles—that is, records of all drugs the customer buys, including prescription and nonprescription products? Some states require this service. Many people get prescriptions from more than one doctor. Through patient profiles, the pharmacist can be a kind of watchdog, making sure that the patients aren't taking dangerous combinations of drugs.

Having made a choice, how do you get the most out of your pharmacist? First off,

never hesitate to ask a question, even though it may seem insignificant at the time. Patient education—making sure the patient is fully aware of the medicine he is taking—is a major responsibility of the pharmacist.

One thing you will want to verify at the pharmacy is how and when to take your medicine. Often the label on the bottle is not much help. "Take as directed" or "take as needed" is too vague. "Take 4 times a day" isn't much more specific, and "take with meals" could be misleading if your ulcer treatment calls for six small meals a day instead of the standard three. Your pharmacist can advise you on the exact time you should take that medicine in order to get the most benefit from it.

Find out whether your prescription can be refilled. For some drugs your doctor may have indicated you can have one, two, or even more refills. Some drugs that have a potential for abuse are "controlled" under federal law that puts limits on the number of refills.

How to store your medicine is more important than most people realize. Putting a bottle of medicine on the kitchen window ledge may be a handy way to remember to take it, but light may cause it to deteriorate. On the other hand, the bathroom medicine cabinet is misnamed. It is not such a good place to store drugs because of the moisture generated by steam from the bath or shower. Some medicine should be kept cool and dry; some should be refrigerated. Your pharmacist can advise you of the best way to store your medicine to ensure that it doesn't lose its effectiveness.

If you are on a medication schedule that calls for a dose during the day and you have to work, don't put a small supply of tablets in a fancy pill box even though it is more convenient. The tablets may break apart, in which case you may not get the correct dose. Or they could react with the metal the box is made of. Or, in some cases (such as nitroglycerin), they can be absorbed by plastics. Instead, explain your problem to the pharmacist who can put your medication in small containers.

Some people have trouble taking tablets or capsules. If this is a problem for you and you forget to remind your doctor, mention it to your pharmacist. He or she knows whether your medicine comes in a form that's easier to take. Your doctor's permission will be needed to change the prescription. Some tablets can be crushed and easily mixed with food or water; others should not be broken up because they are coated to prevent the drug from being absorbed too rapidly or from irritating the stomach. The pharmacist is the person to ask whether a particular tablet can be crushed and, if so, what liquid can be mixed with it.

OTC drugs of the same type can vary greatly. For instance those preparations lined up on the shelf labeled "cough or cold preparations" will have different ingredients because they are intended to treat different symptoms associated with the common cold. One product may be good for suppressing a cough, while another is intended to help the patient breathe easier. Still another will be for runny noses as well as coughs. Your pharmacist can help you select the appropriate product for your particular symptoms as well as keep you from mixing drugs that have essentially the same ingredients, which could cause an adverse reaction.

Many people might feel uncomfortable discussing the cost of their medication, but this is another area for candor between the pharmacist and the patient, and pharmacists are usually very willing to provide information on the cost of your prescription. For instance, if you must take a diuretic (water pill) daily and you know that you will be taking it for a long time, it would be to your advantage to check with your pharmacist about buying your medicine in large quantities, e.g., a month's supply at a time. On the other hand, there may be reasons why quantity buying is not a good idea. For example, the doctor may want to change the dosage form or prescribe a different drug; or

perhaps you will not need additional drug therapy. Talk it over with the pharmacist.

Then there is the matter of "buying generic." Most states have changed their pharmacy laws to permit or require pharmacists to dispense lower-cost drug products, provided the generic product is equivalent to the product the physician has specified on his prescription. Many drugs are manufactured by only one company and thus do not have generic equivalents. Your pharmacist will know in which cases substitution is possible.

Your pharmacist by law may not diagnose disease or prescribe a prescription medicine, but he may be able to help you. If your pharmacist recommends that you see a doctor, take his advice. If an adverse reaction to an OTC drug—or a prescription drug as well—is serious, consult your physician for advice.

FOOD AND DRUG INTERACTIONS If you're taking a drug, the food you eat could make it work faster or slower or even prevent it from working at all. Eating certain foods while taking certain drugs can be dangerous. And some drugs can affect the way your body uses food.

The extent of interaction between foods and drugs depends on the drug dosage and on the individual's age, size, and specific medical condition. In general, though, the presence of food in the stomach and intestines can influence a drug's effectiveness by slowing down or speeding up the time it takes the medicine to go through the gastrointestinal tract to the site in the body where it is needed.

Food also contains natural and added chemicals that can react with certain drugs in ways that make the drugs virtually useless. Some reactions can be downright dangerous, triggering a medical crisis or, in rare instances, even death.

It is because of these interactions that your doctor tells you to take certain medica-

542

tions on an empty stomach, some just before meals, and some with meals.

More commonly, though, food and beverages interfere with absorption. A classic interaction is the one between tetracycline compounds and dairy products. The calcium in milk, cheese, and yogurt impairs absorption of tetracycline. On the other hand, taking some iron supplements with citrus fruits or juices which contain ascorbic acid enhances absorption of the iron.

In general, it is unwise to take drugs with soda pop or acid fruit or vegetable juices unless you check with your doctor first. These beverages can result in excess acidity that may cause some drugs to dissolve quickly in the stomach instead of the intestines where they can be more readily absorbed into the bloodstream.

Some foods contain active substances which can cause a drug effect or which can interact with a drug to produce an unexpected or counter effect. For example, licorice extracted from natural sources contains a substance which, when consumed regularly in excess amounts, may cause an elevation in blood pressure. Licorice is a favorite ingredient in candy and a flavoring for some pharmaceuticals. Most American manufacturers now use a synthetic flavoring but many imported products still contain licorice from natural sources. Continued regular use of products containing natural licorice extract could aggravate high blood pressure or counteract the effect of medication for high blood pressure.

Excessive consumption of foods high in vitamin K, such as liver and leafy green vegetables, may hinder the effectiveness of anticoagulants. Vitamin K, which promotes clotting of the blood, works in direct opposition to these drugs, which are intended to prevent clotting.

Some foods, such as soybeans, rutabagas, brussels sprouts, turnips, cabbage, and kale, contain substances known as goitrogens which inhibit production of the thyroid hormone and thus can produce goiter. Sci-entists suggest caution in eating these foods when taking thyroid medications.

Perhaps the most hazardous food-drug interaction is the one between monoamine oxidase (MAO) inhibitors, drugs at times prescribed for depression and high blood pressure, and such foods as aged cheese, Chianti wine, and chicken livers. MAO inhibitors can react with these foods and force the blood pressure to dangerous levels, sometimes causing severe headaches, brain hemorrhage, and, in extreme cases, death.

To prevent a possible reaction, anyone taking MAO inhibitor drugs should avoid aged and fermented foods, including pickled herring; fermented sausages, such as salami and pepperoni; sharp or aged cheeses; yogurt and sour cream; beef and chicken livers; broad beans, such as fava beans; canned figs; bananas; avocados; soy sauce; active yeast preparations; beer; Chianti wine, sherry, and other wines in large quantities. MAO inhibitors also are suspected of reacting adversely with cola beverages, coffee, chocolate, and raisins.

Alcohol, which is actually a drug itself, although not regulated as a drug under the Food, Drug, and Cosmetic Act, does not mix well with a wide variety of medications, such as antibiotics; anticoagulants; antidiabetic drugs, including insulin; antihistamines, high blood pressure drugs; MAO inhibitors; and sedatives. Alcohol combined with antihistamines, tranquilizers, or antidepressants causes excessive drowsiness that can be especially hazardous to someone driving a car, operating machinery, or performing some other task that requires mental alertness. A good rule of thumb is to avoid alcoholic beverages when taking any type of prescription or over-the-counter medication.

Just as some foods can affect the way drugs behave in the body, so some drugs can affect the way the body uses food. Drugs may act in various ways to impair proper nutrition: by hastening excretion of certain nutrients, by hindering absorption of nutrients, or by interfering with the body's ability to convert nutrients into usable forms. Nutrient depletion of the body occurs gradually, but for those taking drugs over long periods of time these interactions can lead to deficiencies of certain vitamins and minerals, especially in children, the elderly, those with poor diets, and the chronically ill.

Quite a few drugs—for example, colchicine, oral antidiabetic agents, and the antibiotic neomycin—can impair absorption of vitamin B$_{12}$. But because most Americans have good stores of B$_{12}$ in their livers, it takes prolonged ingestion of these drugs to cause a deficiency.

Long term use of diuretics, or "water pills," to treat such conditions as congestive heart failure, can lead to serious potassium depletion. If the potassium loss is not corrected in heart patients taking digitalis, the heart may become more sensitive to the effects of the drug. People taking diuretics regularly should eat foods which are good sources of potassium. These include tomatoes and tomato juice, oranges and orange juice, dried apricots, cantaloupes, figs, raisins, bananas, prunes, potatoes, sweet potatoes, and winter squash.

Because oral contraceptives are used so widely, their effect on nutrition has been getting increasing attention. The Pill is known to deplete the blood's content of certain vitamins, notably folic acid and vitamin B$_6$, but usually the vitamin depletion is not serious enough to cause overt symptoms. In most healthy women with good diets, these vitamin levels do not go down to a point that is alarming.

Because her requirements for several vitamins may be increased, it is especially important for any woman on The Pill to eat a nutritionally balanced diet.

Drugs readily available without prescription also can lead to nutritional problems. The worst offenders are antacids.

Chronic use of these remedies without a doctor's supervision can cause phosphate depletion, a condition that in its milder form produces muscle weakness and in more severe form leads to a vitamin D deficiency.

Mineral oil, an old-fashioned laxative still widely used by elderly people and in nursing homes, can hinder absorption of vitamin D. One study reported that as little as 20 milliliters (4 teaspoons) of mineral oil twice daily can interfere with absorption of vitamin D, vitamin K, and carotene, a substance the body converts to vitamin A.

What can consumers do to prevent undesirable food-drug interactions? Here are a few suggestions:

• Read the labels on over-the-counter remedies and the package inserts that come with prescription drugs.

• Follow your doctor's orders about when to take drugs and what foods or beverages to avoid while taking medications.

• Don't be afraid to ask how drugs might interact with your favorite edibles, especially if you consume large amounts of certain foods and beverages. While taking drugs, be sure to tell your doctor about any unusual symptoms that follow eating particular foods.

• Eat a nutritionally well-balanced diet from a wide variety of foods. Use of a needed drug, even on a long term basis, is less likely to cause depletion of vitamins and minerals if your overall nutritional status is good.

Drug labeling and informed health professionals can be helpful to you, but your doctor and pharmacist cannot follow you to the dinner table or the snack bar. Remember that warnings about food-drug interactions are only as good as the patient's willingness to heed them.

ASPIRIN: THE GREAT AMERICAN CURE-ALL Americans take over 20 billion aspirin tablets a year. Aspirin is a significant ingredient in many prescription medicines and in a large number of over-the-counter products, such as "cold" and "pain" tablets. Daily consumption of aspirin in this country amounts to more than 20 tons. That makes aspirin America's most widely used drug.

Although "Aspirin" is still a trade name in some European countries, the word has become so widely used that it is treated as a generic name here. You can buy brand-name aspirin such as Bayer or St. Joseph, or tablets simply labeled "aspirin." All aspirin—whether sold under its brand or generic name—must meet the same FDA standards for potency and purity and must be produced under the same manufacturing regulations.

Relatively safe when used properly, aspirin is not harmless. It may injure the stomach, sometimes severely, and may pose special risks for certain groups—including pregnant women, people with bleeding disorders, and those with ulcers. In fact, because of its wide use, aspirin leads over-the-counter drugs as a cause of adverse reactions leading to hospitalization, and is a major cause of childhood poisoning.

It's well known that aspirin lowers fever temperatures rapidly, although it does not affect normal temperatures. During fever, aspirin acts to reset the body's thermostat for normal temperature, and also dissipates the body's excess heat by increasing sweating and blood flow in the skin. However, it may not always be desirable to reduce a fever. A fever is an important symptom of and is helpful in following the course of a disease. It's important to find and treat the cause of a fever, not just the fever itself. When in doubt about whether to use aspirin for fever, consult a doctor.

Using aspirin as a painkiller, or analgesic, does not lead to physical addiction, as may happen with other analgesics. Aspirin is also less toxic than more powerful analgesics. And it's effective. In a 1972 comparison of marketed analgesic drugs, aspirin was superior to all the agents tested, including propoxyphene (brand name Darvon) and codeine, for relieving pain from inoperable cancer.

Aspirin works best on pain of mild to moderate severity, such as muscular aches and pains, backache, toothache, and headache. Any use of aspirin for aches and pains should be for a short period unless otherwise directed by a doctor. In particular, individuals who have frequent tension headaches due to stress should seek counseling instead of relying on chronic use of aspirin.

Aspirin works well for arthritic pain. It also does something even more useful: It can reduce inflammation in joint tissues and surrounding structures. Damage to joints is the most difficult aspect of rheumatoid arthritis to manage, and any drug that reduces inflammation is important, for it can lessen or delay crippling. Aspirin's effectiveness in reducing inflammation also helps in treatment of rheumatic fever.

There are several new anti-inflammatory drugs for treating arthritis, but aspirin is much cheaper, and, for most patients, at least as effective; most physicians still consider it the drug of the first choice for rheumatoid arthritis.

Many over-the-counter cold preparations (Coricidin, for example) contain aspirin. But aspirin has no effect on viruses or bacteria, so it won't cure a cold or the flu, or even shorten its duration. It can only make a cold sufferer more comfortable by reducing fever and relieving headache and muscle ache. However, if this improvement in symptoms tempts the patient to be more active, aspirin could do more harm than good. Gargles containing aspirin have no benefit for a sore throat.

There is some evidence that aspirin and large doses of vitamin C taken together may be more damaging to the stomach than aspirin alone. People with colds who want to take both should try to make sure the stomach is empty of aspirin before taking vitamin C or use enteric-coated aspirin, which doesn't dissolve in the stomach. They should also understand that the excretion of large amounts of vitamin C in the urine can interfere with the excretion of aspirin and raise the levels of aspirin in the blood.

Aspirin interferes with clotting and may help reduce unwanted clots that contribute to heart attacks and strokes. However, there is no clear-cut proof that aspirin reduces cardiac mortality.

Some women believe in using aspirin to treat menstrual cramps. Even though this cramping may be caused by prostaglandins, aspirin hasn't been proved particularly effective for this purpose. Other antiprostaglandin drugs, ibuprofen (brand name Motrin) or mefenamic acid (brand name Ponstel), appear to work better.

Along with discoveries of new uses for aspirin, there is increasing evidence that it can cause side effects which may sometimes be serious. Many are gastrointestinal. Not only can aspirin cause heartburn, dyspepsia, stomach discomfort, nausea, and vomiting, but it can also cause stomach ulcers, erosion of and bleeding from the lining of the stomach, and even gastrointestinal hemorrhage. The more serious of these side effects occur most frequently in patients taking high doses but may occur at low doses in hypersensitive patients. Drinking alcohol can considerably increase aspirin's stomach damage.

Aspirin exposed to air begins to take on moisture and eventually decomposes to salicylic acid and acetic acid, or vinegar. Salicylic acid is even more irritating than aspirin; thus decomposing tablets, which can be detected by their "vinegary" odor, should be discarded.

Aspirin enhances the effects of drugs used to lower the blood sugar, so diabetics should not take aspirin without consulting their physicians. Other interactions can occur between aspirin and prescription drugs; it's a good idea always to check with your doctor or pharmacist before taking aspirin if other medications have been prescribed.

Pregnant women are another group who should avoid aspirin when possible, especially during the last 3 months of pregnancy. Unfortunately, many don't. Recent surveys indicate aspirin is taken during pregnancy more frequently than any other drug, often in large doses. The most serious danger is infant mortality. A study of Australian women showed that the infants of aspirin users had significantly lower birth weights and were more likely to die around the time of birth.

Since prostaglandins are known to initiate uterine contractions, it might be expected that aspirin would delay the onset of labor and prolong its duration, and studies do associate aspirin use with significant increases in postmaturity (birth of an overdeveloped infant), length of time spent in labor, and likelihood of a complicated delivery. Prenatal aspirin use by women is also associated with increased hemorrhaging in both mothers and newborn infants, presumably because of aspirin's effect on clotting. It has also been reported that aspirin taken by the mother can cause constriction of a blood vessel between the heart and lung of the fetus; this can interfere with development of normal blood circulation in the lungs and cause persistent newborn hypertension.

Some people are allergic to aspirin. This allergy can result in varying degrees of reaction to the drug, including minor skin itching, abdominal pain, facial swelling, swelling of the larynx (with symptoms of asphyxiation), falling blood pressure, shock, and death. Even very small amounts of aspirin can have serious effects in people who are sensitive to it, and death may occur within minutes after ingestion unless they get the right medical care quickly.

Aspirin allergy can appear at any time. Absence of such an allergy in the past is no guarantee that the person will not develop a hypersensitivity to aspirin. A first reaction is rarely fatal, but people allergic to aspirin have to make quite an effort to avoid the more than 200 products on the market that contain it.

Aspirin is a remarkably useful drug. When properly used, it can be valuable in the treatment of many conditions, both mild and serious. But every time you take it, it affects a wide variety of biological functions in ways that are only imperfectly understood. Aspirin, like all OTC drugs, shouldn't be used unnecessarily or indiscriminately. It doesn't just have the potential to make sick people healthy; it can also make healthy people sick. As with any drug, use your head before you swallow.

Recommended Aspirin Dosage Schedule for Children

Age in years	Number of children's tablets (80 milligrams or 1.23 grains) than can be taken every 4 hours	Number of standard adult tablets (325 milligrams or 5 grains) that can be taken every 4 hours
Under 2*		
2 to under 4	2 tablets	1/2 tablet
4 to under 6	3 tablets	3/4 tablet
6 to under 9	4 tablets	1 tablet
9 to under 11	5 tablets	1 1/4 tablets
11 to under 12	6 tablets	1 1/2 tablets
12 and over	8 tablets	2 tablets

*Children under 2 should only be given aspirin under the advice and supervision of a physician.

No child should be given aspirin as a pain reliever for more than 5 days, or as a fever-reducer for more than 3 days, except under the advice and supervision of a physician.

ASPIRIN SUBSTITUTE—ACETAMINO-PHEN Acetaminophen is a nonprescription painkiller that does not contain salicylic acid. It is often used as an aspirin substitute. Most people know this drug by such trade names as Datril and Tylenol.

The FDA advisory panel found acetaminophen safe and effective for the relief of minor pain and the reduction of fever. It is not effective for reducing inflammation, however, and should not be used in the treatment of arthritis and rheumatism except under the advice of a physician. While acetaminophen is free of most of the side effects of the salicylates, an overdose can result in serious liver damage. An overdose of acetaminophen does not cause a ringing in the ears or any other warning signal. Severe and possibly fatal liver disease may develop 2-to-4 days after overdose without any early warning sign.

Sexually Transmitted Diseases

The current publicity surrounding the increase of acquired immune deficiency syndrome (AIDS) has focused attention on the wide variety of sexually transmitted diseases and their effects. These diseases occur within many groups, young and old, homosexual and heterosexual. Venereal diseases are caused by various bacteria and viruses and can be contracted only by direct sexual contact. The signs and symptoms usually appear around the genital area. Those afflicted with these diseases may not realize the dangers and permanent consequences. Some sexually transmitted diseases can be cured, others can only be treated. Some cause permanent disability such as sterility. Others may recur without warning. Sexually active people, defined as people who have sex with different individuals, should know how to recognize the early stages of these infections, especially since the more sexually active have the greatest likelihood of contracting an infection. Public health care clinics can provide information in addition to medical tests and treatment.

Pregnant women in particular should know the consequences to mother and child in case either parent has been infected. An estimated 300,000 infants die or suffer birth defects every year because of venereal infections received from their mothers. Women infected with genital herpes are eight times more likely to develop cancer of the cervix. Early diagnosis and treatment can eliminate the severe consequences of these infections. The information in this section describes the more prevalent sexually transmitted diseases, giving an overview of signs, symptoms, side effects and treatment.

WOMEN AND STDs If a pregnant woman has an STD and neglects immediate medical care, her unborn baby can be infected too. An estimated 300,000 infants die or suffer birth defects every year because of STDs they get from their mothers.

In addition, untreated STDs can lead to PID (pelvic inflammatory disease). PID can permanently hinder a woman's ability to have children.

STDs are the leading cause of infertility in the United States. *Chlamydia* and *gonorrhea* are the chief culprits.

Of the women now under 30 years old, at least 100,000 this year will suffer painful permanent damage to their reproductive organs as a consequence of untreated, or inadequately treated, gonorrhea. Many of these women will never be able to bear children.

While scientists have yet to establish a firm link between genital herpes and cancer, women infected with genital herpes are eight times more likely to develop cancer of the cervix as non-infected women. There is similar evidence that chronic trichomonal infection may predispose the cervix to cancer.

Every year in the United States 12,000 to 15,000 pregnant women transmit group B streptococcus to their fetuses. Half of these infected infants die soon after birth; a large percentage of babies who survive suffer brain, sight and hearing damage. Also, many babies die each year as a result of infection with genital herpes transmitted to them at birth by their infected mothers. A few pregnant women with primary genital herpes infection in early pregnancy will suffer miscarriages due to this disease.

Twenty-five percent of all serious infant retardation is caused by congenital cytomegalovirus, a little understood sexually transmissable disease that produces virtually no symptoms in adults who harbor it.

Because of these and other similarly grave consequences, the growing epidemic of venereal disease is of concern. VD is al-most as common as the common cold; but, unlike a cold, it will not go away without treatment, and its aftermath may be lifelong illness and disability or premature death.

Babies born to mothers with untreated STDs can suffer severe health consequences and even death. *Gonorrhea* in the birth canal during delivery can cause eye infections leading to blindness. Because of this all babies born in hospitals are treated promptly with medicated eye drops. Similarly, *chlamydia* and *venereal warts* can cause eye, ear, and potentially fatal lung infections. A woman with active *genital herpes* at the time of delivery can infect her baby. Infants who survive a severe herpes infection usually suffer physical or mental damage. If an unborn child is infected with *syphilis*, it will be born with congenital (present at birth) syphilis. The baby may appear healthy at first, but can later develop a number of consequences of the disease, including a heart defect, bone deformities, or brain damage.

HERPES Herpes is a common viral infection. It causes cold sores or fever blisters (oral herpes), and it also causes genital sores (genital herpes). In the United States, oral herpes affects more than 50 million people, and genital herpes affects about 20 million. Herpes is transmitted by direct skin-to-skin contact. Unlike a flu virus that you can get through the air, herpes is transmitted by direct physical contact with the infected area of another person.

When the virus gets into skin cells, it starts to multiply. As your immune system fights the virus, the skin becomes red and sensitive. Soon after, one or more blisters or bumps appear. The blisters open, and sores that sometimes look like cuts in the skin remain. These heal as new skin tissue forms. During the first outbreak the area is usually painful and may itch, burn or tingle. You may also have swollen glands, headache, muscle aches or fever—similar to flu symptoms. Some people notice itching, or other sensations before they see anything on their skin. These are called "prodromal symptoms," and they warn that virus may be present on the skin. Herpes can be transmitted from the time these first symptoms are noticed until the area is completely healed and the skin looks normal again.

Condoms help to prevent transmission of sexually transmitted diseases (STDs). It is not known how effective they are in preventing transmission of genital herpes. Although laboratory studies have shown that the virus does not pass through condoms, they should not be relied on if you have any symptoms or signs of infection (sores, discharge, painful urination, itching, etc.).

It is important to see the doctor as soon as sores appear and before they begin to heal. A blood test cannot diagnose herpes. Another reason to see a doctor is for treatment. Your doctor knows what medications are available and can talk to you about them. Before using over-the-counter (drug store) medications or home remedies, check with a doctor.

If a woman has ever had genital herpes or if her current (or past) sexual partner has genital herpes, she needs to tell her doctor when she becomes pregnant. Babies can get herpes during delivery if virus is present in the birth canal. Tragically, more than half of the babies who become infected during delivery will die or suffer severe damage.

Babies can also get herpes if they are kissed by someone with a cold sore. A young baby can not fight off infections as easily as an adult can, so serious problems may result. It's important that you do not kiss a baby when you have a cold sore.

Some studies suggest that women with genital herpes may be at greater risk of developing cervical cancer than other women. Since early cell changes can be detected by Pap smears, all women with genital herpes should have regular Pap tests—at least once a year. Early detection and treatment of cervical cancer can prevent serious disease.

Oral and genital herpes can be treated and cared for but, at present, not cured.

Here are some positive things you can do:

- Take good care of your general health—eat well, get enough rest and exercise. Avoid physical and emotional stress as much as possible—don't let yourself get "run down."

- Keep the infected area as clean and dry as possible during an outbreak. This will help your natural healing process.

 Preventing self-spread is simple: do not touch the area during an outbreak. If you do, wash your hands as soon as possible. The herpes virus is easily killed with soap and water.

- Get the information you need so you aren't worrying unnecessarily. Understanding herpes gives you a positive way to deal with your concerns and fears.

CHLAMYDIA Chlamydia (pronounced *kla-mid-e-uh*) are widespread sexually transmitted microorganisms that are causing a national epidemic. An estimated three million Americans get chlamydial infections each year, making it three times more common than gonorrhea and thirty times more common than syphilis. Chlamydia may infect both men and women. It is thought to be a major cause of nongonococcal urethritis (NGU), cervicitis and various pelvic infections (PID).

Tests that give accurate, quick results are now available to diagnose chlamydial infections. These tests can be taken even when there are no symptoms and are not painful.

Chlamydial infections can be treated with several different drugs. Because it is often present with other venereal diseases, such as gonorrhea, your doctor may prescribe a drug that can cure a number of infections at the same time.

NGU NGU stands for nongonococcal urethritis which means an inflammation or infection of the urethra (the tube that carries urine from the bladder) caused by some-

550

thing other than the germ that is responsible for gonorrhea.

NGU is one of the most common forms of sexually transmitted disease (VD). It is estimated that 2.5 million Americans are infected each year. NGU is treated with antibiotics, although not the same drugs used to treat gonorrhea.

PID   Pelvic Inflammatory Disease, also called PID or salpingitis, is the most common serious infection involving a woman's reproductive system. Although PID may be caused by a variety of organisms and conditions, certain sexually transmissible diseases (STD) and the use of an intrauterine device (IUD) for birth control are known to be especially important factors.

If not promptly diagnosed and treated, PID can damage the reproductive system. Scar tissue can form inside the fallopian tubes. This can result in infertility by partially or totally blocking the tubes, thus not allowing the egg to enter the uterus.

Formation of scar tissue can also increase the risk of tubal pregnancy. Tubal pregnancy, which can be life threatening, is the result of a fertilized egg becoming implanted inside the fallopian tube rather than in the uterus.

PID should never be dismissed as insignificant or without consequences. Research has shown that women who have had PID once are at greater risk of developing this condition again. This may further the possibility of infertility and tubal pregnancy.

Diagnosis of PID is based on an in-depth medical and social history, a pelvic examination and laboratory tests. Treatment consists of any number of antibiotics, depending on the cause of the infection. PID can usually be treated on an out-patient basis, although in severe cases hospitalization may be recommended.

(See also GONORRHEA, SYPHILIS, AIDS)

In the treatment of all STDs, physician instructions should be followed carefully and all of the medication must be taken as directed. After treatment, it is important to be rechecked to make sure the infection is completely cured.

Sex partners should be treated for two reasons: 1) to avoid your re-infection and, 2) to prevent them from suffering possible complications.

Avoid sex throughout the time of treatment since, until you're re-tested and proven cured, you might still be infectious.

How can I avoid getting an STD?

☐ Limit your number of sexual partners. Your risk of infection increases with the number of partners you have. If you and your sexual partner have no other partners, and neither of you has VD—neither of you will be exposed. If you have one sexual partner, but that person has other partners, your risk of getting an STD is increased.

☐ Practice and encourage open and honest communication with your partner(s). Remember, some STDs aren't obvious in women. A woman may not know she needs to see a doctor unless her partner tells her she has been exposed to a disease.

☐ Use condoms. If properly used, they provide good (though not perfect) protection. Various foams and creams intended for vaginal use as contraceptives have been found to have some ability to kill VD germs.

☐ If either partner has an STD, *both* partners must be treated in order to avoid re-infection.

☐ If you or your partner have other sexual contacts, you should get regular VD checkups, at least four times a year.

If you need more information about VD, or if you need the name of a private doctor or a public health clinic, call the VD National Hotline, toll-free:

National 1-800-227-8922
In California 1-800-982-5883

PREVALENT SEXUALLY TRANSMITTED DISEASES (STDs)
Developed from American Social Health Association information

DISEASES	SIGNS A WOMAN MAY NOTICE IN HERSELF	SIGNS A WOMAN MAY NOTICE IN A MAN	CONSEQUENCES OF PROLONGED INFECTION	SPECIAL CONSIDERATIONS
GENITAL HERPES	Painful, blister-like, fluid-filled lesion (or cluster of lesions) on, in or around vagina. Often accompanied by swollen glands in groin area.	Same as in women, only on or around penis.	Under study at this time. Genital herpes has been implicated with a form of meningitis and associated with cervical cancer. Consequences to Babies: Damage to internal organs, blindness, retardation, death. Acquired during birth.	Genital Herpes is caused by a virus and cannot be cured. The initial infection will lapse into a latent state with periodic flare-ups often triggered by stress or fatigue. Genital herpes may be passed from an infected pregnant woman to her newborn during birth. A series of tests (cultures) taken from the cervix will help your doctor determine whether a cesarean section is required to protect the baby at time of birth.
GONORRHEA	Pus-like vaginal discharge, vaginal soreness, lower abdominal pain, painful urination.	Pus-like urethral discharge.	Pelvic inflammatory disease (PID)—tubal damage, pelvic adhesions and tubo-ovarian abscesses, tubal pregnancy which can lead to pathological sterility. Consequences to Babies: Eye infection. Acquired during birth.	Even if the original gonococcal infection is cured, PID may predispose the body to repeated episodes of pelvic inflammation caused by a variety of organisms. Untreated gonorrhea and chlamydia are major causes of PID in women. PID can lead to infertility or ectopic (tubal) pregnancy. Symptoms of these two infections are similar, but chlamydia, unlike gonorrhea cannot be cured with penicillin. It requires other antibiotics.

CHLAMYDIA	Symptoms similar to those caused by gonorrhea, but sometimes milder. Symptoms often take weeks or even months to develop.	Discharge from the penis and/or burning when urinating. Burning and itching around the opening of the penis. Symptoms may be present early in the day and go away, but they will come back. Many men will have no noticeable symptoms, or symptoms so mild that they go unnoticed.	For both men and women, a painful infection can develop requiring hospitalization. Can cause permanent damage to the reproductive organs and sterility. For women, the infection can complicate pregnancy resulting in the death of the unborn baby and, occasionally, the mother.	(See Gonorrhea)
Sexually Transmitted NONGONOCOCCAL URETHRITIS (NGU) CERVICITIS	Symptoms similar to those caused by gonorrhea.	Occasionally, heavy pus-like discharge. More frequently, a mild watery discharge.	Pelvic inflammatory disease. (See Gonorrhea) Consequences to Babies: Eye infections and pneumonia in newborn babies if their mothers have NGU.	Like gonococcal PID, non-gonococcal PID could lead to repeated episodes.
SYPHILIS	Rashes appearing almost anywhere on the body, including palms of hands and soles of feet. Chancre (lesion) on or in vagina, anus or mouth. Loss of facial or scalp hair in patches.	Rashes or hair loss in the same pattern as in women. Chancre on or around penis.	Brain or heart damage. Consequences to Babies: An infected pregnant woman may pass syphilis to a developing fetus, which could lead to a variety of birth defects. Blindness, brain damage, heart defect, bone deformities, death. A baby may seem healthy at birth and develop symptoms later in childhood. Acquired in the womb before birth.	Syphilis is particularly dangerous because symptoms will go away by themselves without treatment, but the disease remains in the body and can ultimately cause severe damage and even death. It can remain in the body for years. It can be cured at any time, but damage done cannot be repaired.

Questions and Answers

Some of the most frequent questions heard daily in any doctor's office are discussed in this section. It is hoped that this material will serve to illustrate and clarify the many interesting aspects of medical practice. It should be emphasized, however, that the field of diagnosis is a complicated one, and that no layman should attempt to match any of his symptoms against those in a particular paragraph and conclude that he is necessarily suffering from the specific condition described. Doctors themselves often have difficulty determining which of a great many possible disorders the patient being examined may have. This difficulty belongs under the heading differential diagnosis. To do a differential diagnosis properly may require specialized procedures such as blood counts, X-ray studies, examinations of stones, and the like. Sometimes batteries of tests of this sort may be necessary to evaluate a chest pain or an abdominal pain. Hence, in reading the material which follows, the reader is most definitely urged not to attempt self-diagnosis. Rather, he should consider this section only as a run-down of some of the various disorders that may afflict one of the most complicated of all machines—the human body.

Q. *For years I have been plump around the hips and abdomen. Why do medical men object so strongly to overweight?*
A. Medical objections to obesity have steadily increased in recent years. The average person may look upon his excess weight as something that gives him a bulge around the midriff, necessitates larger clothing sizes, and makes him puff a bit when climbing stairs. A physician regards obesity as a disease which predisposes to many other diseases. Many ailments or conditions which shorten life are associated with excess weight.

Exactly why an overweight person is so much more susceptible to a variety of other illnesses has not been entirely clarified. Sometimes the association is understandable. Thus overweight people are prone to pain and discomfort in their knees and ankles, generally in the form of osteo-arthritis, because of the abnormal load borne by these joints year after year. The correlation between obesity and certain other diseases is less easy to explain but nonetheless real. For example, there is a significantly higher incidence of diabetes among the obese. Reducing the weight of patients with mild diabetes may clear up the diabetic condition. Even if it does not, the weight loss may permit them to get along without taking special drugs for the diabetes.

High blood pressure is likewise more frequent in people who are overweight, and also tends to drop with a curbing of calories and consequent loss in weight. High blood pressure in the obese in turn contributes to the high incidence of such circulatory ailments as heart attacks and strokes. Obese individuals with normal blood pressure are subject to greater degrees of hardening of the arteries than those of normal weight.

It is no secret that treatment of strokes, diabetes, heart attacks, and similar disorders has considerable limitations, and that prevention is preferable to treatment in these disease categories. Hence the emphasis on keeping weight down as a form of prophylaxis against a variety of serious disorders. The influence of weight is dramatically underlined by the fact that, while individuals of normal weight live longer and have fewer illnesses than those who are overweight, the underweight do even better than those of normal weight. All human statistics and even animal experiments indicate that mild undernutrition tends to maintain good health. In short, the thinner the better.

Q. *I avoid cream, butter, ice cream, and fat cuts of meat. Is this advisable?*
A. In recent years a considerable body of data has been accumulated indicating some relationship between the kinds and amounts of fats in the diet and hardening of the arteries.

One important aspect of hardening of the arteries is the deposit of fats in the lining of the blood vessels. As this process goes on the arteries narrow, and eventually the blood may clot in a constricted passage. This is known as thrombosis.

A coronary thrombosis, a clot occurring in one of the arteries of the heart, results in a heart attack. A similar process in one of the blood vessels of the brain may produce a stroke.

More than fifty years ago it was demonstrated that a considerable portion of the fat deposited in the arteries consists of a waxy substance, cholesterol. When large amounts of cholesterol are fed to experimental animals, deposits are found in their arteries too. Because of these findings, the first diets brought forward in relation to hardening of the arteries were low in fats, especially cholesterol.

Cholesterol is found in large amounts in eggs, cream, whole milk, and milk products such as cheese and ice cream. At one time advocates of the dietary approach recomended a reduction of all fats as well as low cholesterol content. This called for such measures as avoiding all fatty foods and trimming all visible meat fat. It was found that the amount of cholesterol in the blood dropped in many subjects when they were shifted from their usual diet to a diet low in cholesterol and in saturated fats.

More recently it has been discovered that reduction of saturated fats (the fats of animal origin, such as those found in meats, butter, and milk) and addition of unsaturated fats (corn oil, safflower oil, and various vegetable oils, coconut oil being the sole exception) produces a further drop in the level of blood cholesterol. In the most recent formulations of the dietary approach to hardening of the arteries, diets have been worked out which are low in saturated fat and contain moderate amounts of unsaturated fats in the form of oils added in cooking and in salads.

Although there has not been sufficient experience with these diets to know what their effect will be in the long run, there is already some evidence that persons who have had heart attacks or other vascular diseases do better if they switch to such diets. The American Heart Association now recommends these diets for heart-attack victims. Other dietary authorities feel that diseases of the heart and blood vessels are so common that everyone could well go on a diet of this kind or at least modify the customary intake of fats to conform to the general guidelines proposed for heart-attack patients.

Given below are some examples of diets which are high in polyunsaturated and low in saturated fats. In general, these diets can be approximated by the approach, recommended by the Bureau of Nutrition of the New York City Department of Health, termed the "prudent diet."

The prudent diet emphasizes fish, lean cuts of meat, and liquid vegetable oils.

The following further suggestions are made:

Fish, Meat, Eggs. Fish and shellfish at least four to five times a week, for any meal. The fat in fish is an excellent source of polyunsaturated fatty acids. Poultry may be taken often; it is low in fat. Veal may be taken frequently; it is a lean meat. Beef, pork, and lamb—not more than three to four times a week, with the serving not to exceed four ounces of cooked meat. Eggs, not more than four a week for adults; four to seven a week for children.

Avoid very fat meats, bacon, sausage, corned beef, pastrami. Select lean cuts of all meats. Trim off all visible fat. Keep portions moderate—four to six ounces before cooking (four ounces after cooking).

Milk and Milk Products. The fat in whole milk is predominantly saturated and is not recommended. Two cups of skim milk daily for adults; two to four cups of milk daily for children—two cups of this milk allowance may be whole milk. More than four cups of milk is not recommended for children, even for adolescents. Use cottage, pot, or farmer cheese often. Avoid butter, cream, ice cream, cream cheese, hard cheeses, and other milk cheeses.

Fats. Vegetable oils should be used for their polyunsaturated fatty acids. To have more of these than saturated fatty acids, use vegetable oils daily. Use 1½ ounce (3 tablespoons) daily in cooking and at the table. Make salad dressings with oil. Substitute oil for other fats in cooking and baking. Butter, ordinary margarine, and other hydrogenated fats must be kept at a minimum.

Q. Everything I eat seems to turn into fat. Why is this so?
A. Undoubtedly you are consuming more calories than you need for your bodily functions and activities. The only way the body can deal with excess calories is to convert them to fat. A switch from high-caloric to low-caloric items might make the difference. Some foods in ordinary portions pack a good deal more in the way of calories than others. When a normal portion of a food is very high in calories, it is referred to as a high-caloric item; when the opposite is true, as a low-caloric item. The difference may easily be illustrated when the choice of desserts facing a dieter is between half a cantaloupe (40 calories) and a three-inch wedge of lemon meringue pie (300 calories). Although a person may become too calorie conscious, a general knowledge of the caloric content of foods can be useful.

For example, the following are desserts fairly high in calories: a brownie, 2 x 2¾ inches, contains 140 calories; a 5-cent chocolate almond bar, 200; a chocolate sundae, 335; an iced cupcake, 250; an ordinary doughnut, 140. In contrast, an apple or an orange has 75 to 100 calories; an average portion of melon, such as honeydew or cantaloupe, perhaps 50 calories; a banana, 75 calories. Not to be disregarded in this connection are the alcoholic beverages, for an 8 ounce glass of beer contains 120 calories, while the usual cocktails, such as martinis or Manhattans, 150 to 175 calories.

Icebox raiders should know that a hamburger on a bun usually represents well over 300 calories; a frankfurter on a roll, 250; a half cup of potato salad with mayonnaise, 200; and 8 to 10 large potato chips, 100. Nuts are high in calories, too, 4 to 5 cashews running to 100, as do 6 pecans. Certain bulky vegetable items, on the other hand, are quite low in calories, including salads with lettuce, tomatoes, and cucumbers, and many of the so-called "5 per cent" vegetables. The 5 per cent vegetables include string beans, wax beans, asparagus, broccoli, Brussels sprouts, and carrots. Ordinary portions will have about 20 to 30 calories. Sometimes with a little effort the number of calories in a food item can be readily decreased. Thus, eating a hamburger made from lean ground round steak, or drinking skim milk instead of whole milk, will cut the calories by half. Dieters are often advised to eat broiled meats and to cut away the visible fat, two methods of getting rid of the highly caloric fat portion.

Similarly, cottage cheese made from skim milk contains fewer calories than pot cheese made from whole milk. The common rather oily cheeses are almost as high in calories as straight butter. Cheeses can be either high- or low-caloric items and have to be identified before they can be classified.

Q. *Are there special programs which will slim me down fast?*
A. These are the programs usually referred to as crash diets or formula diets. Crash diets and special-formula diets are usually too restricted in their range and in their caloric content. They are designed to achieve extremely rapid weight reduction and are sometimes used to start off a long-term reducing program by producing a large initial weight loss. The drastic reduction that can be brought about by a crash program seems to firm up a person's desire to continue reducing, and so, on psychological grounds, the crash diet may be defended. A few examples of crash diets are the following:

1. Grapefruit and cheese diet. Each meal consists of half a grapefruit, one-half to one cup of cottage cheese, and a cup of tea or coffee. One vitamin capsule per day is included.

2. Hard boiled egg diet. This consists of one or two hard-boiled eggs, plus a cup of coffee or tea for each meal, plus one vitamin capsule per day.

3. Milk and banana diet. A glass of skim milk and one banana, with tea or coffee, constitute each meal. One vitamin capsule per day is included.

4. Lettuce-tomato diet. Each meal consists of one-half head of lettuce and one tomato, plus tea or coffee, plus one vitamin capsule per day.

It is obviously possible to select something from each of these groups, alternating them from one meal to another. Crash diets are not medically approved since they are not nutritionally sound. Physicians also feel that the problem of excess weight fundamentally demands a long-term solution of the disproportion between intake of food and actual need, so that short, painful bursts of dieting are not really the answer. However, for someone who wants to lose a few pounds rapidly, such as a woman who wants to be able to get into a special dress for a special occasion, crash diets may have some value.

Formula diets generally consist of flavored skim milk-oil preparations to which vitamins have been added. A representative specimen runs 225 calories per serving so that when taken four times a day, it is a 900-calorie diet, which will certainly induce a loss of weight.

There is very little oral satisfaction in downing a drink of this kind, and a sense of deprivation that users may experience is the absence of chewing satisfaction. Some people cannot tolerate the liquid preparations and have digestive disturbances as a result. One of the secrets of the success of the formula diets is that they permit no leeway. Apart from coffee or tea and sometimes a raw vegetable such as celery or carrot, the dieter has no alternative. He can hardly cheat. From a nutritional point of view, however, the 1,200-calorie diet (see page 617), has the virtue of including the four basic food groups, of not being monotonous, and of affording some eating satisfaction.

The most drastic crash program of all has been the total starvation program, sometimes referred to as the Philadelphia program. It is based on the fact that total starvation produces acidosis, which in turn leads to loss of appetite. The total starvation program was originally recommended for hospitals or other supervised settings. The individual is allowed fluids which include low-caloric, sweetened, carbonated beverages, coffee, and tea. After a day or two of discomfort, the patient on this program may feel unusually well. Of course, considerable weight losses are possible during the starvation periods. Some of the weight loss is due to loss of water from the system which returns after a more normal diet is resumed, even one low in calories. The total starvation program for the treatment of obesity has also been recommended in the form of one- or two-day fasts once or twice a month.

In general, crash diets and starvation programs are last-ditch maneuvers or programs for the desperate. There is no rea-son why a well-balanced, reasonable diet program which will provide satisfactory weight loss week after week cannot be maintained by the average overweight person. Because the overweight problem is chronic and long-term, crash programs which provide only short-term results are bound to fall short of the solution desired.

Q. *Several people have told me my breath is sometimes unpleasant. How can I handle this problem?*

A. A number of different factors may contribute significantly to disagreeable breath. Perhaps the most common is the eating or drinking of certain kinds of foods or liquors. Among some of the items that may cause bad breath are garlic, onions, and various alcoholic beverages. Certain constituents of these substances are excreted through the lung into the air we expire and contribute their odor to the breath. (This is one of the principles behind the drunkometer test for concentration of alcohol in the blood.) Some of these odorous constituents may also be excreted in the saliva and the sweat.

Decaying food particles impacted between the teeth may contribute an odor to the breath. A particle of meat caught between the teeth undergoes a chemical change by bacterial action in the mouth, and as a result can become somewhat odorous. The use of dental floss—a good hygienic idea—often reveals that meat fragments undergo softening and chemical changes which alter their initial odor. The extent to which particles lodge in the teeth varies in different people and depends upon the structure of their teeth. In a normal set of teeth, there are narrow spaces between the teeth at the gum margin. Thus, the dental arrangement which collects food is a normal one.

Various disorders of the nose, throat, and oral cavity, particularly certain kinds of inflammation, may contribute to breath odor. They include various infections of

558

the gums (gingivitis), abscesses, tonsillitis, and others. A condition of the nose and throat known as ozena, which is associated with dryness and crusting, will produce an odor. It may be helped by snuffing up water into the nasal cavity and washing away the crusts.

Various digestive disorders may create an unpleasant breath. Although normally the muscular activity of the digestive tract tends to propel in only one direction—onward from the stomach—there are various conditions in which this movement may be interrupted or reversed to produce regurgitation, burning sensations, unpleasant tastes, and odors. Constipation produces a furry tongue and unpleasant breath. Bad breath may be present in certain fevers and also in some women when they are menstruating.

The treatment of bad breath is, of course, indicated by the cause. He who insists on eating garlic, onions, salami, dill pickles, frankfurters, and similar food may find that his breath produces some social problems. The same may be said for certain kinds of liquors and wines, but reputedly straight gin and vodka do not create breath odor. Good mouth hygiene, including frequent brushing of the teeth and the use of dental floss, may relieve many common forms of bad breath. However, even with due care for all of these factors, there are occasional individuals whose breath will still have a distinct odor. In the absence of any specific cause, the only solution left may be camouflage.

Q. I often have a burning feeling high up in my stomach. What can I do for it?
A. This is probably simple heartburn. Heartburn is a commonly experienced symptom of disordered digestion which is usually described as a burning sensation high in the upper central abdomen. It is sometimes located in the lowest portion of the chest cavity at the tip end of the sternum or breast bone. Heartburn is gen-

erally attributed to irritation of the lining of the gullet (lower esophagus) and stomach wall. In some individuals it regularly follows the eating of certain offending foods for which they have low tolerance. These may include onions, cucumbers, radishes; spicy, smoked, or heavily salted foods; too much coffee or very strong coffee, alcohol, mustard, garlic, chocolate, and certain fried or greasy foods.

It is probable that stomach acids play an important part in this complaint. For example, neutralizing the stomach acids with an alkalinizing agent such as ordinary bicarbonate of soda may give prompt relief of the burning sensation; the common over-the-counter medicinal alkalinizers are also usually helpful. In this respect, heartburn may be compared to the symptoms experienced by peptic ulcer victims, in whom pain is produced by exposure of the ulcerated area to acid stomach fluids. Here, too, neutralization of the stomach acids will relieve the pain. However, heartburn occasionally occurs in individuals who have no acids in their stomach juices, and it may well be that not all heartburn is due to the same cause.

Although heartburn is most often a mild disorder and ordinarily does not signify any grave disease, it may be the chief symptom of an ulcer. Also, in the condition known as hiatus hernia in which a portion of the stomach is above the level of the diaphragm, irritative and even ulcerative states of the pouch or stomach above the diaphragm are often described as heartburn. Some forms of heartburn which are experienced chiefly at night seem to be due to a reflux of acid gastric juices from the stomach up into the lower esophagus. Since the esophagus does not tolerate such exposure to stomach acids, the usual reaction consists of a sort of burning pain. This condition is sometimes referred to as peptic esophagitis. Certainly, if heartburn is not specifically related to a particular food item, and becomes more than just an occasional event, it may require a doctor's checkup to ascertain the cause.

Q. I've been told that I have a "delicate stomach." What sort of foods should I eat?
A. Probably a bland diet may be of value, once it has been ascertained that the specific condition exists. A bland diet is a specially selected dietary program consisting of foods that are relatively easy to digest and that are not likely to be stimulating or irritating to the digestive tract. Spicy, highly seasoned, fried, smoked, marinated, and pickled food items are prohibited. Also eliminated from the bland diet are some so-called "gassy" vegetables, nuts, and fatty cuts of meat. Many people almost automatically put themselves on a bland diet when they have a digestive upset. They may have farina, toast, jam, and tea for breakfast instead of their usual fried eggs, pork sausages, and two cups of strong coffee. Bland diets are recommended after digestive upsets that have included nausea, vomiting, and diarrhea. They are also recommended for certain stages of active ulcer, for functional colitis, for various illnesses in which there is fever and malaise (feeling poorly), and for gallbladder disease.

The following are guidelines for a strict bland diet. The omission of caffeine-containing beverages, such as coffee and tea, is due to their acid-producing characteristics. However, many bland diets permit weak tea or coffee. The diet given on page 620 is based on the Montefiore Hospital, New York, Bland Diet # 3.
General Rules:

1. Meat should be well cooked and tender; it may be baked, boiled, broiled, or roasted.

2. Skins, seeds, nuts, spices, or coconut should be avoided.

3. Fruits or juice should be taken after some food has been eaten or at the end of a meal.

4. Small frequent feedings are better tolerated than large meals.

5. The food should be not only bland, but of moderate temperature.

DAILY FOOD ALLOWANCE:

Milk	3 cups or more
Vegetables	2 portions or more
Fruits	2 portions or more
Cereals, bread, cakes, or starches	6 portions or more
Eggs	1 or more
Meat, fish, or cheese	6 ounces or more
Fats	2 tablespoons or more

Q. Sometimes my stomach swells up, and I have to burp or pass gas. What causes this and how can I take care of it?
A. This appears to be a common form of digestive disturbance often described as bloating and "gaseousness." By bloating most persons mean a distention of the abdomen, often accompanied by sensations of fullness. By gaseousness what is usually meant is either eructations, "burping," or flatulence, the passage of gas rectally. Sometimes all these conditions may occur together, in which case a patient will complain of abdominal swelling, burping, and annoyingly frequent passage of wind. They may also be dissociated from each other and can occur singly. They are all common complaints, and very few individuals have not experienced them at one time or another. However, in some people they occur with far greater frequency and may be a daily event.

When symptoms of this sort appear for the first time in middle or late life, a physician may suspect some organic disease or inflammation in the digestive tract. In fact, he may be impelled to order X-rays or other appropriate studies in order to get at the cause of the underlying difficulty. If, however, the compaints have occurred again and again over the years, it is apparently clear that no new or very

CAUSES OF MINOR DIGESTIVE DISORDERS

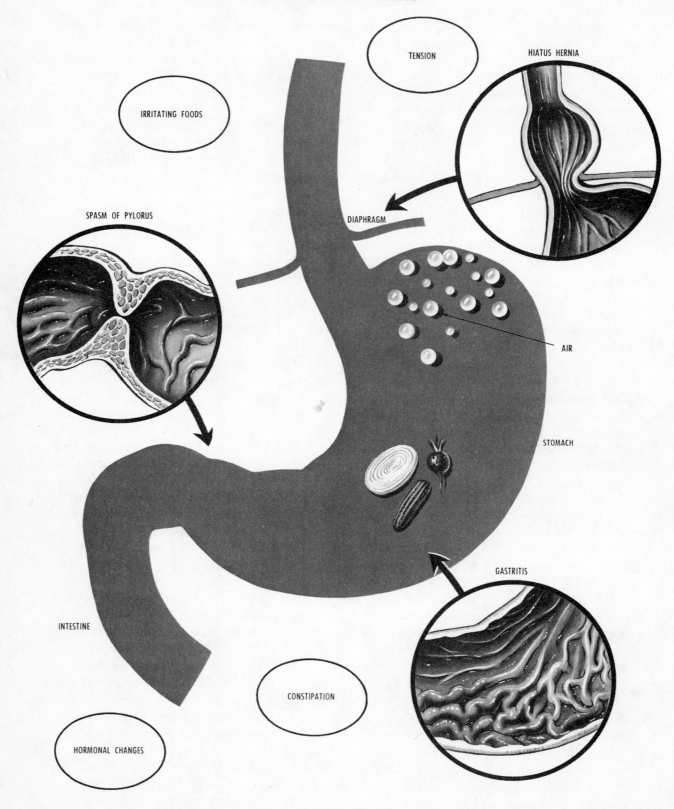

TENSION

HIATUS HERNIA

IRRITATING FOODS

SPASM OF PYLORUS

DIAPHRAGM

AIR

STOMACH

INTESTINE

GASTRITIS

CONSTIPATION

HORMONAL CHANGES

threatening disorder can underlie them.

Certainly these complaints are encountered in persons who otherwise are in excellent health. For a long time it was thought that they were more common in individuals with gallbladder disease, but a recent study indicates that people without any gallbladder difficulties whatever may have these complaints as often as those with chronic disease of the gallbladder. The causes of bloating and gaseousness vary and including the following:

1. Certain mild chronic disorders of the digestive tract may produce these symptoms. Among them are gastritis, a mild inflammation of the stomach lining; hiatus hernia, a protrusion of part of the stomach above the level of the diaphragm; and pylorospasm, a spasm of the muscle between the stomach and the intestine. Any of these disorders can lead to upper abdominal fullness, belching, or related conditions.

2. Anxiety and tension may produce symptoms of this sort. The digestive tract frequently faithfully reflects emotional upsets and changes. Many people know that when they are upset they seem to "fill up" very rapidly, or they become "gassy." When they are nervous, some individuals, with or without being aware of it, make repeated swallowing movements which send air down into the stomach. The swallowed air may produce upper abdominal distention and burpiness.

3. Conditions of this kind are sometimes associated with the hormonal changes in the female cycle. Bloating often occurs at the time of menstruation, and not infrequently heartburn and gaseousness are among the complaints of pregnancy. It is known that the hormonal changes which accompany menstruation and pregnancy can affect the behavior of the digestive tract.

4. Reactions to certain foods, sometimes termed idiosyncrasies, produce these symptoms in many people. Among the common offenders are onions, cucumbers, radishes, cabbage, and smoked or spicy foods. Certain rich or fat foods, including pork, some cuts of beef, large amounts of buttery and creamy substances, chocolate, and fried and greasy foods commonly are also offending items.

5. Constipation, though often without other symptoms, may produce bloating, distention, and gaseousness.

Obviously the treatment of these complaints should be directed to the cause when it is ascertainable. It may mean a process of learning from experience and thereupon avoiding offending foods. The "cast iron stomach" is more of a myth than a reality, and there are few individuals who are not aware that certain foods will give them indigestion accompanied by fullness, bloating, and gas.

In such cases an ounce of prevention is worth a pound of cure. Eating bland and very light foods, particularly when one is nervous or upset, may also be effective. Cutting down on the amount of fats in the diet or, in some cases, on fermentable starchy items may also be useful. When symptoms are frequent, one should go over one's diet and perhaps one's manner of living. This should be done in consultation with a doctor.

For mild or infrequent cases, a physician may prescribe certain drugs. Among them may be an alkalinizer containing familiar neutralizers such as bicarbonate of soda. Perhaps this will "bring up the gas," relieving some of the distention. An antispasmodic—a drug which relaxes the digestive tract—may be of value, as may a sedative or tranquilizer. Some individuals seem to be helped by activated charcoal tablets or by a few drops of peppermint in water. A hot-water bottle or heating pad on the abdomen may give prompt relief. Finally, for persons with chronic or spastic forms of constipation, regularization of bowel habits will possibly alleviate many of these symptoms.

Q. *I regularly experience gnawing pains between meals which are helped by eating. What causes this?*

A. One of the common causes of this type of complaint is the condition termed peptic ulcer. A peptic ulcer is an opening or a small defect in the lining of the digestive tract caused by the action of the digestive juices of the stomach. The peptic ulcer is most commonly found in the upper part of the small intestine, the duodenum. This is ascribed to the fact that during the digestive process this area is sprayed with acid stomach juices. Such ulcers are known as duodenal ulcers. However, ulcers can form within the stomach itself (gastric ulcer) and occasionally in the lowermost portion of the esophagus (esophageal ulcer).

Peptic ulcer is a very common disease. An estimated 10 per cent of the population will, at some time or other, develop an ulcer. For reasons that are unknown, the tendency to peptic ulcer may be chronic in some people who suffer from ulcer symptoms off and on for very long periods of time. Exactly what distinguishes the unlucky few with chronic peptic ulcer formation from other individuals is not known. Peptic ulcer patients often form stomach juice with a higher acid content and in larger amounts than normal individuals, but such excessive acidity is not in itself a cause of ulcer. It is believed that some process in the stomach lining weakens it so that a portion becomes susceptible to acid digestion, and so the ulcer is formed. But what this process in the lining is, remains unknown.

Characteristically, ulcers produce pain that is generally felt somewhere in the upper abdominal region and occasionally in the back. The pain is variously described as burning, gnawing, and like a hunger sensation. Typically, the pain is relieved by eating, drinking milk, or taking an alkalinizing medication. Peptic ulcer pain ordinarily occurs some hours after a meal, is relieved by eating, then recurs several hours later. The characteristic cycle of the ulcer, therefore, is pain . . . eating . . . relief . . . pain . . . eating . . . relief, and so on. Night pain, which arises for the same reason, namely, the accumulation of acid secretion in an empty stomach, occurs frequently. Pain may awaken the patient night after night at approximately the same time. It, too, is relieved by eating or by alkalinizers.

These basic facts about peptic ulcer imply the method of its treatment. Neutralization of acid promotes healing of the ulcer, and milk, milk-and-cream mixtures, and alkalinizers are used for this purpose. The patient may be placed on milk-and-cream mixtures and alkalinizing powders which are the basis of the well-known Sippy treatment. In the early treatment of peptic ulcer, frequent feedings of bland foods, milk, and alkalinizers are prescribed.

Some physicians forbid alcohol, spicy foods, mustard, and fried or greasy foods, but otherwise allow a diet as close to a normal one as possible. Since caffeine seems to stimulate acid formation, coffee may be forbidden entirely or only weak coffee and tea permitted. One program calls for taking something every hour — either food, milk, or an alkalinizing tablet or liquid. If night pain is a problem, the patient may be asked to set the alarm so that he wakes up prior to the expected onset of pain and takes something to eat. Cigarette smoking seems to aggravate peptic ulcer in some individuals, and the incidence of peptic ulcer is higher among smokers than among nonsmokers. Hence patients with peptic ulcer are often advised to stop smoking.

For an unfortunate group of patients, clearing up of a peptic ulcer is not the end of the story. Months or possibly even some years later they may suffer another bout of peptic ulcer. A still more unfortunate few find themselves suffering with peptic ulcer symptoms a good deal of the time. For such intractable and chronic cases of peptic ulcer, and also where bleeding has occurred from an ulcer—especially if it has occurred more than once—surgery is often advocated. There are various surgical procedures in the treatment of ulcer. With one or another of these, it is often possible to promise the victim of a chronic peptic ulcer relief from his longstanding distress.

Q. *I have had severe abdominal pains and have been told my X-ray shows stones. What is going on?*
A. The pains produced by the movement of stones is referred to as colic and occurs in either the bile-fluid system or in the urinary tract. There may be biliary colic or renal colic. These share the reputation of being among the most severe pains produced by any disorders of the human body.

In biliary colic, the pain is generally due to the movement of a stone either down the duct of the gallbladder or down the major bile duct, which runs to the intestine. The patient usually experiences severe pain in the upper abdomen, either in the line of the right nipple or in the central area of the abdomen above the navel, the epigastric region. The pain may double the patient up, and is generally completely incapacitating. It is sometimes felt in the back or in the region of the right shoulder.

Occasionally, there is an onset of steady pain in the region of the gallbladder which mounts in intensity. Waves of intensified pain may then be superimposed on this. The pain may be caused by movement of a stone within the gallbladder, with the communicating channel between it and the bile duct closed off. Or it may be due to the passage of a stone from the gallbladder into the bile duct where it

may either lodge, perhaps producing jaundice, or pass on, with relief of the obstruction.

Renal colic refers to the pain produced by the passage of a stone anywhere in the urinary tract, but generally between the pelvis of the kidney and the bladder. The pain has a severe and knife-like quality. It too may come and go in waves, and when the movement of the stone stops or the stone is passed, the pain may end. The character and location of the pain depend on the location of the stone and its movement. When the stone is high up, perhaps moving from the pelvis of the kidney into the first part of the ureter—the channel which runs from kidney to bladder—pain may be experienced in the flank or in the back, adjacent to the lowest ribs and the spine. As the stone moves outwards and downwards, the pain may be experienced in the side, and radiating down toward the bladder and the genital region. As it moves further along the ureter, it is felt at lower levels, and in males may extend into the scrotum.

Both biliary and renal colic are variable in duration, sometimes lasting only a minute or two, but more often one or more hours unless they are relieved by a potent pain-killing drug. Second and third doses of drugs must often be given before complete relief is possible. The intensity, character, and location of the pain will generally indicate its probable cause to the doctor. In both biliary and renal colic, it is possible to confirm the diagnosis by X-ray studies. Any patient undergoing an attack of renal colic might be well advised to save a urine specimen from the time of the attack. The urine often contains red blood cells, a common accompaniment of the movement of a stone in the urinary tract. A doctor may request a patient to urinate through cheesecloth in the hope that the stone may be preserved; it can then be analyzed chemically and used as a guide for dietary or other treatment.

Q. *Off and on for years I have had loose bowel movements and sometimes pass mucus. What causes this?*

A. If no organic disease is present, this is the condition called colitis. Functional colitis is a disorder of the large bowel that generally results in frequency of bowel movements and irregularity of bowel pattern. Sometimes increased amounts of mucus are passed; occasionally, when there is an impulse to move the bowel, nothing much more than some stained thick mucus may be passed. There may be departures from normal patterns of bowel behavior. Constipation may alternate with mild diarrhea; thus, after two or three days without a movement, there may come a day in which there are three or four fairly active ones. Another pattern is for two or three loose stools to be limited sometimes only to the morning, sometimes scattered throughout the day. This pattern is often related to nervous stress or other tension. See COLITIS

Q. *I often skip a day or two without having a bowel movement. What is responsible?*

A. This is generally referred to as constipation. Constipation is a common problem, yet it is not so common as many people think. To skip a bowel movement for a day is not necessarily a sign of constipation, and there are perfectly normal individuals who have a bowel movement every other day and seem to be in excellent health. On the other hand, one can have a daily bowel movement and still be constipated if by constipation one means the passage of an overly hard, pellety, somewhat smaller than normal stool.

Constipation appearing for the first time in middle age can be serious, especially if it is progressive. Unfortunately, so much functional constipation appears in middle age that X-ray examination of the large intestine and other special procedures may be necessary to determine whether or not it is caused by an organic condition such as a tumor.

In the absence of a disease process in the large intestine, one can make a diagnosis of functional constipation. There are various approaches to the problem:

1. Sometimes constipation is due to inadequate roughage and stimulating foods in the diet. This frequently occurs in individuals who are reducing, and may simply be due to a reduction of food bulk intake. Diminished bulk, or the absence of stimulation produced by such foods as salads, vegetables, and fruits, may result in sluggish action of the colon. One way to correct this, of course, is to add bulk and stimulating foods to the diet.

2. Inadequate intake of water may play a part in some cases of constipation. When fluid intake is inadequate, the colon may abstract more than the usual amount of water from the stool, resulting in a dried-out stool and constipation. This is easily corrected by increasing fluid intake.

3. Other essentially minor dietary manipulations may successfully alleviate mild degrees of constipation. Taking prunes or prune juice, figs, or dates may be of value. Some individuals seem to be helped by drinking a cup of hot water the first thing in the morning.

4. Some cases of constipation result from the pressures of early-morning rush. Often, regularity of bowel habit can be restored by establishing a special time to go to the bathroom every .morning and adhering to it whether or not a strong urge to move the bowels is present.

5. Laxatives may be indicated when constipation persists despite restoration of a balanced diet and routine habits. Laxatives fall into various classes:

(a) Bulk stimulants are substances that mix with the stool and take up water. The increased bulk acts as a mechanical stimulant to evacuation. Extracts of psyllium seed, one commercial preparation of which is known as Metamucil®, are an example of this.

(b) Saline cathartics (a dose of "salts") act by pulling fluid into the bowel and result in an increased watery type of movement.

(c) Direct stimulants are agents that act on the smooth muscle of the intestine, stimulating it to increased activity. Many of them are found in proprietary drugs sold over–the–counter. They include phenolphthalein, cascara, anthraquinone derivatives, and that old standby, castor oil.

(d) In recent years stool softeners, which tend to keep the stool from losing its moisture and thereby its bulk, have been used increasingly. One such agent is known as dioctyl sodium sulfoccinate. It is found in such commercial preparations as Colace®.

On the whole, it is preferable to start with the milder agents, such as the bulk-formers and stool-softeners, rather than those that are essentially laxative, such as the salts. It may not be necessary to take them daily. Sometimes a dose every other day will work. One should use the smallest dose compatible with getting results. For occasional constipation, fast-acting suppositories and prepackaged enemas are available. These can bring relief within minutes.

Q. I can feel several small round growths protruding from the opening after a bowel movement. What are they?
A. Most probably this is the condition termed piles. Piles—known medically as hemorrhoids—are small, dilated veins just within or protruding from the rectal opening. They may be compared to the varicose veins seen on the lower extremities, but they are, of course, much smaller. Internal hemorrhoids are covered by the anal lining and are situated within the canal. External hemorrhoids are covered by skin and can be present individually or as a cluster around the opening. Why some people have difficulty with hemorrhoids and others escape them altogether is not known. Pregnancy, chronic constipation, and several other medical conditions may predispose to their formation. See HEMORRHOIDS

Q. Some days I feel a lack of energy. Can I take vitamin supplements?
A. The widespread promotion and consequent widespread consumption of vitamins has no real relationship to the dietary deficiencies or vitamin needs of most consumers. Many people take vitamins because they believe that this will increase their general health, enable them better to fight off colds and other viral illnesses, or give them more of that vague quality known as "pep." Carefully controlled scientific observations do not support these beliefs.

Divide a large number of individuals, all of them on an adequate diet, into two groups, give one group vitamin supplements and the other sugar pills, and approximately one-third of the persons in each group will claim that they feel better. In other words, the sugar pill works as well as the vitamin pill. The positive effect results from the individual's belief.

It is true that the ill health of individuals suffering from vitamin deficiencies is *corrected* by taking vitamins. But it is not true that the health of individuals not suffering from vitamin deficiencies is *improved* by taking vitamin pills. Neither is it true that large amounts of vitamin C taken at the start of a cold are of any special help. Furthermore, most inflammation of the gums seen in doctors' and dentists' offices is not due to vitamin C deficiency, nor does it respond to increased consumption of vitamin C. Claims that vitamin B improves the circulation to the heart have repeatedly been demonstrated to be untrue.

After a thorough examination of the various claims for various vitamins, the American Medical Association's Council on Nutrition concluded that the average American on the usual balanced diet does not benefit from taking vitamin supplements. The Council recommended that such supplements be taken by women during pregnancy, by individuals on bizarre or restricted diets who persistently refuse to include some important group of foodstuffs, and by certain geriatric patients on poor intakes. Vitamins A and D are recommended for the infant and the growing child. It should be noted, however, that children can be overdosed with these vitamins, and that an overdose of vitamins A or D can produce striking examples of poor health.

It is probable that individuals who dislike vegetables and will eat none of them, as well as strict vegetarians who shun anything resembling meat, may profit from taking a vitamin supplement. But those who think that the consumption of larger and larger amounts of vitamins does more and more good should be warned that there is such a thing as overdosage, that some vitamins produce fermentation and gassiness, and that water-soluble vitamins (such as those of the B complex) cannot be stored in the body—any excess taken in is promptly excreted in the urine.

Another point to remember is that there are still some unknown vitamins and necessary food factors which the manufacturers have been unable to isolate and put into their capsules. Those genuinely interested in securing a balanced vitamin intake must recognize, therefore, that nature puts its vitamins into food and not into pharmacies.

Q. *Since taking birth control pills I've noticed some bloating and swelling of the breasts. What is the pill doing?*
A. The birth control pills work by interfering with the action of the gland regulating the ovary, the pituitary gland. This gland, situated at the base of the brain, controls all the processes going on in the ovary. Pituitary secretions are responsible for the growth of the egg (ovum) and for its release. Taking the birth control pill, which contains hormones similar to those usually produced by the ovary, in effect signals the pituitary gland that enough of these are present in the woman's body. As a result, the pituitary does not produce the hormones that stimulate ovarian activity. The final result is that the ovary does not go through the usual cyclic changes, no egg comes to maturity or is released, and hence the woman remains infertile. However, changes resembling those of the normal cycle do take place in the uterus and the breasts because of the hormones contained in the pills.

If, after taking the pills for three weeks and experiencing these transformations, the pills are stopped, menstruation will ensue. Menstruation occurs whenever the hormone level in the body drops to a significant extent. Whether the hormonal drops occurs normally, or is produced by stopping medication, a menstrual flow will occur.

As a birth control measure, the hormone pill is just about 100 per cent effective, and indeed is considered by most authorities to be the most effective method of contraception presently available. In order to work reliably, however, the pill should be taken daily, as skipping even one day may permit the pituitary to start ovarian stimulation. However, little is known with certainty about all the side-effects of some of these pills.

Q. *Why do I have pain and bloating between periods?*
A. The release of an egg from the ovary (ovulation) is sometimes accompanied by lower-abdominal pain, tenderness, and/or bloating. Sometimes the abdominal pain is severe enough to make it difficult for a

doctor to decide whether a young woman complaining of pain in the lower right abdomen is suffering from appendicitis or is having ovulatory pain. Ovulatory pain or discomfort do not necessarily occur in every menstrual cycle, and many women never experience it.

In others, however, they may occur so regularly that they can be used as a fairly reliable indication of the time of ovulation. Discomfort most often appears between the twelfth and sixteenth days of the usual menstrual cycle, but it can also vary from cycle to cycle.

The discomfort seldom lasts for more than twelve hours, then tends to subside. It is sometimes referred to as *Mittelschmerz*, German for middle pain. Very occasionally it is accompanied by an increased discharge of mucus and occasionally a trace of blood appears with the discharge. Such a pink-stained discharge in midcycle is sometimes referred to as ovulatory bleeding. Again, this may be found in only an occasional cycle. A physician must of course rule out other possibilities that may produce similar symptoms, such as cervical erosions, polyps, and tumors. Women who undergo *Mittelschmerz* may find it of interest (and it may be of use to their physicians) to chart their menstrual cycles on a calendar, and to note the days on which this type of discomfort is experienced. Such information may be of considerable value in family planning.

Q. *What can I do about discomfort during menstruation?*

A. Various degrees of discomfort are often noted, particularly on the first and second days of the menstrual flow. They may consist of backache, a feeling of heaviness in the pelvis due to congestion, a tendency to urinate frequently, and an overall subpar feeling. It is known that a mildly toxic substance may originate in the lining of the uterus during menstruation, some of which is absorbed into the body. This is referred to as menotoxin and undoubtedly contributes to the feeling experienced. Certainly many women do not look their best at this time. They may appear paler than usual, have puffiness under the eyes, and feel headachy. However, the complaints most likely to be disabling are those relating to the rhythmic cramps originating in the menstruating uterus, medically termed dysmenorrhea. Dysmenorrhea is most common on the first and second days.

Painful uterine cramps are more likely to occur during the early reproductive years. With the passage of time, and especially after a pregnancy, dysmenorrhea is greatly diminished or ceases altogether. There seems little reason to doubt that dysmenorrhea arises in the thick muscular wall of the uterus, which is capable of severe contraction. Among the helpful procedures for uterine cramps are the following:

1. A hot-water bottle or heating pad applied to the lower abdomen.

2. Antispasmodic drugs, similar to those used for pains arising in the digestive tract, may also relax the muscle of the uterus and thus cut down the intensity of painful cramps.

3. Various pain-killing drugs are widely employed. They may vary from aspirin alone to combinations of aspirin with an antispasmodic. Sometimes small doses of benzedrine taken along with them appear to reduce the intensity of the pain, and have the further virtue of giving the individual a slight "lift."

4. Occasionally a doctor may find some organic cause contributing to painful uterine cramps. The reason can be an underdeveloped uterus (juvenile uterus) or an abnormally narrow opening of the womb. Hormone injections may be given to build the uterus to mature size, and slight dilatation of the opening is easily done.

Q. *Before my period I feel nervous and snap at everyone. What causes this?*
A. Premenstrual irritability is a common phenomenon which is experienced by some women during every one of their menstrual cycles. It is sometimes of minor degree and passes unnoticed, but it can also be quite marked and produce intense subjective feelings of tension and nervousness. Depression, the "blues," and a tendency to tearfulness may also occur. Not infrequently there are also physical symptoms such as headache, bloating, swelling of the extremities, and tenderness or painful engorgement of the breasts. Usually, with the onset of the menstrual period or by the second day of the flow, symptoms are markedly alleviated. It is generally conceded that most, if not all, of these changes are due to the action of the hormones of the ovary. An important factor is the water retention these hormones produce. The swollen, bloated feeling is due to fluid retention. It is also believed that water retention in the cells of the nervous system may be responsible for premenstrual tension states.

Minor degrees of premenstrual tension are often tolerated without treatment, with the help of the knowledge that the symptoms will pass with the period. For jumpiness and nervousness, mild sedatives or tranquilizers may be prescribed. Where the chief complaint is of feelings of depression, drugs of the dexedrine-benzedrine group may be ordered by the physician. Where water retention seems to be significant (some women gain four to five pounds of fluid in the last week or so of the menstrual cycle), diuretic drugs may be administered. These are drugs which promote the excretion of fluid from the body by way of increased urination.

The diuretics seem to be equally successful in reducing bloat, the swelling of the extremities, and some of the psychic and emotional changes that accompany fluid retention. There are various schedules of administration of the diuretic drugs. They may be given every day or every other day for the last week or ten days of the menstrual cycle, during the phase of increasing fluid retention.

Q. *Some of my menstrual cycles are longer than others. Can I use the rhythm method of birth control?*
A. A knowledge of the "safe period" is the essential approach to the rhythm method of birth control. The rhythm method is the only one permitted by the Catholic Church. It is used extensively by couples who wish to diminish the possibility of pregnancy without using pills or other mechanical techniques.

Calculation of the safe period is based on the following basic considerations:

1. The egg or ovum is released from the ovary only once during a menstrual cycle and remains fertile for only about twenty-four hours after release from the ovary. If a day or so passes, the egg is no longer capable of being fertilized by the sperm.

2. Ovulation does not necessarily occur on the same day in each cycle, and the exact cycle-length varies also. Many women who are sure that they menstruate at twenty-eight day intervals find on charting that the interval may vary from twenty-six to thirty days, or even more widely.

3. Because of fluctuation in cycle length and the day of ovulation, it is necessary to record the dates of menstruation for at least a year in order to calculate the safe period accurately. A cycle always begins with the onset of menstruation, and can conveniently be charted by marking off the dates of menstruation on a calendar.

4. Once the length of the menstrual cycle is known, there are various formulas for calculating the safe period. The following one offers less chance of error than some others: Subtract fifteen days from the shortest recorded cycle and subtract four more—this gives the first day of the

PHYSICAL FITNESS AND REDUCING EXERCISES

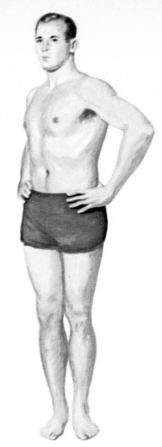

The exercises illustrated in this eight-page full-color insert are useful for general body conditioning and for reducing flabbiness and girth in specific parts of the body. If, for example, the goal is to reduce the size or flabbiness of the hips, spending a few extra minutes each day on the hip exercises will produce the desired results. Success both in body conditioning and weight control will be yours if you spend about thirty minutes a day on the exercises. The United States government publication Adult Physical Fitness, on which some of the exercises in this insert are based, cites a study by the Harvard School of Public Health for the claim that "one-half an hour of proper exercise each day can keep off or take off as much as twenty-six pounds a year."

TRUNK MUSCLES

This exercise is designed to condition and strengthen the trunk muscles. Stand with the feet shoulder-width apart. Turn the trunk to right and bend forward and touch the fingertips to the floor outside that right foot. Return to the starting position by sweeping the trunk and arm upward. Repeat the exercise to the left side. About fifteen repetitions on each side are recommended.

TRUNK AND WAIST

At the start stand erect with hands on waist and hips. Twist the trunk to the right but not the hips and head — they remain to the front. Return to the starting position. Repeat the exercise to the left side. About thirty daily repetitions on each side are suggested.

ABDOMINAL MUSCLES AND SHOULDER GIRDLE

This exercise is designed to strengthen the abdominal muscles and the shoulder girdle. Assume a squatting position with the hands touching the ground inside the knees. Thrust the legs to the rear with toes and heels together. Return to the squatting position and then to the starting position. Repeat about ten times but only if you can do so without strain.

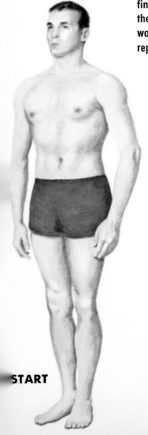

START

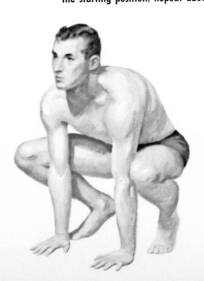

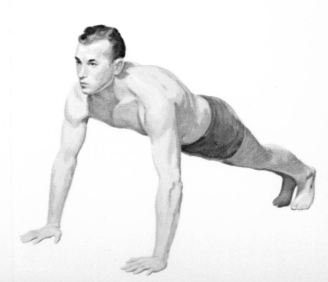

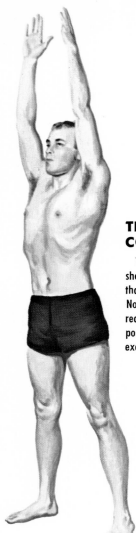

LEG MUSCLES

This exercise builds leg muscles. It is quite strenuous and should be attempted only after considerable conditioning has been achieved. In the starting position, the knees are bent and the feet are set about eight inches apart. One foot is forward toe-to-heel distance. The back is erect. The fingers are joined on top of the head and the elbows are well back.

Now jump into the air, locking the knees and reversing the leg position. The feet come to rest but reversed from the starting position. Repeat up to four times, reversing the starting position from one leg to the other.

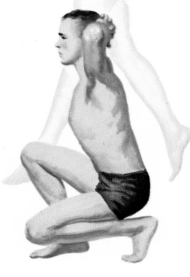

THIGH-TO-SHOULDER CONDITIONING

This is a good exercise for the thigh, abdomen, back and shoulder muscles. In the starting position spread the feet more than shoulder-width apart, arms straight overhead, palms facing. Now bend at the knees and waist, swing the arms down and reach between the legs as far as possible. Return to the starting position with a sharp and quick movement. Repeat, but without exertion or strain.

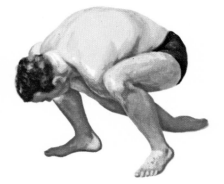

START

START

PUSH UPS—SHOULDER MUSCLES

This exercise will help to build the muscles of the shoulder. To assume the starting position lie on the floor, face down, legs together, hands on floor under shoulders with fingers pointing straight ahead. Now push the body off the floor so that the weight rests on the hands, and the legs and arms are kept straight. Then lower the body until the chest touches the floor. Repeat up to ten times and more if you can do so without strain.

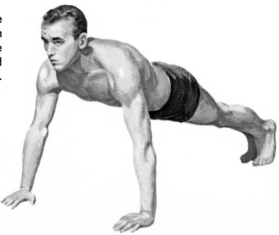

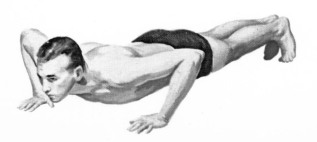

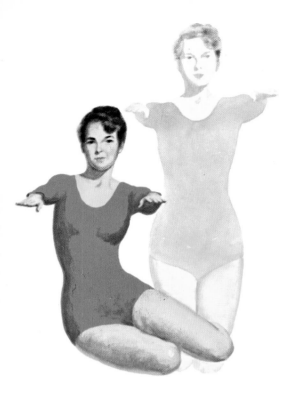

HIPS

This is a good exercise for strengthening the hip muscles and reducing their flabbiness and girth. At the start kneel on the floor with the arms out in front. Now sit down, moving hips to one side as shown. Next, return to the kneeling position and repeat the exercise to the other side.

THIGHS

This exercise, although designed for thigh conditioning, is also effective for the back, neck, and other parts of the body. The exercise should not be attempted until the body has been conditioned by other milder exercises. Lie on the back and place the feet on a chair as in the starting position illustrated. Now raise the hips until the knees, thighs, and trunk are in line. Return to the the starting position. Repeat as often as comfortable without exertion.

ARMS

This exercise is designed to strengthen and condition the arm muscles. Stand in the straddle position (feet spread shoulder-width apart). Take a rubber ball, sponge, or any squeezable object in each hand. Now lean forward and bend the elbows. Next, bring the arms all the way back, at the same time squeezing the objects held in the hands. Repeat a few times until you can do about twenty exercises without exertion.

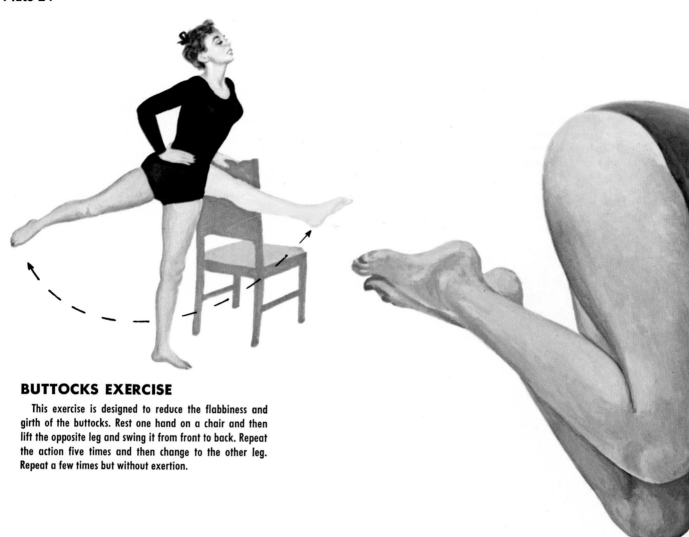

BUTTOCKS EXERCISE

This exercise is designed to reduce the flabbiness and girth of the buttocks. Rest one hand on a chair and then lift the opposite leg and swing it from front to back. Repeat the action five times and then change to the other leg. Repeat a few times but without exertion.

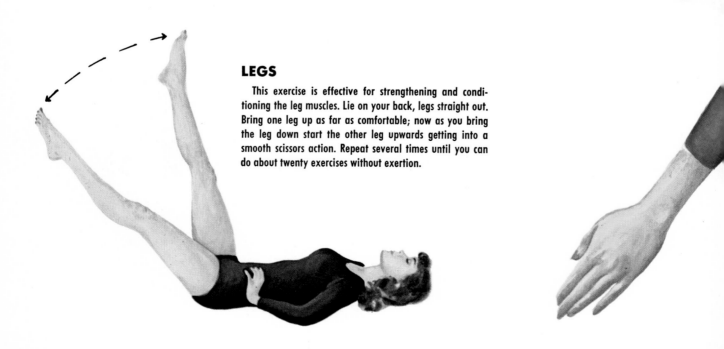

LEGS

This exercise is effective for strengthening and conditioning the leg muscles. Lie on your back, legs straight out. Bring one leg up as far as comfortable; now as you bring the leg down start the other leg upwards getting into a smooth scissors action. Repeat several times until you can do about twenty exercises without exertion.

ABDOMINAL EXERCISE

This abdominal exercise is designed to reduce the flabbiness and girth of the abdomen and to strengthen the abdominal muscles. Stretch out on your back, arms stretched sideways, legs together. Now bend the knees and bring them as close to the chest as possible. Now return the legs to the floor, first to the left side, and then to the right side. Bring the knees back to the chest. On the finish, straighten the legs to the starting position. Repeat several times.

WAIST AND BODY

At the start assume a straddle position (feet about shoulder-length apart). Raise the left arm up, keeping the right arm down. Bend and stretch far to the right with raised left arm following. Return to the starting position. Repeat to the other side.

HEAD AND NECK MUSCLES

This exercise will strengthen the neck muscles and reduce the girth and flabbiness of the chin and neck. The exercise may be done in a standing or in the illustrated sitting position. Hold the back straight and stretch the head as far back as possible. Now turn the head from side to side attempting to make a complete circle. Repeat as many times as you can manage without exertion.

Plate E6

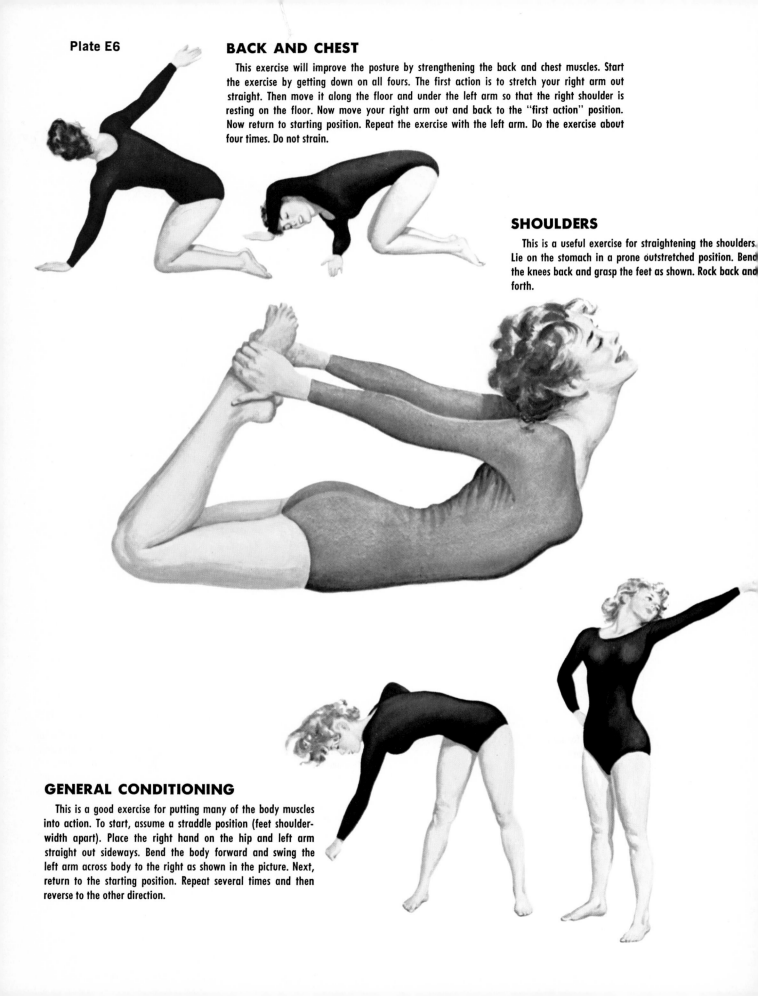

BACK AND CHEST

This exercise will improve the posture by strengthening the back and chest muscles. Start the exercise by getting down on all fours. The first action is to stretch your right arm out straight. Then move it along the floor and under the left arm so that the right shoulder is resting on the floor. Now move your right arm out and back to the "first action" position. Now return to starting position. Repeat the exercise with the left arm. Do the exercise about four times. Do not strain.

SHOULDERS

This is a useful exercise for straightening the shoulders. Lie on the stomach in a prone outstretched position. Bend the knees back and grasp the feet as shown. Rock back and forth.

GENERAL CONDITIONING

This is a good exercise for putting many of the body muscles into action. To start, assume a straddle position (feet shoulder-width apart). Place the right hand on the hip and left arm straight out sideways. Bend the body forward and swing the left arm across body to the right as shown in the picture. Next, return to the starting position. Repeat several times and then reverse to the other direction.

POSTURE

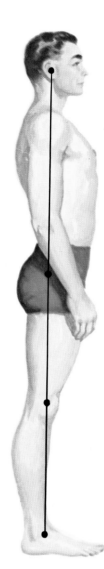

While posture must necessarily vary from person to person due to inheritance and different growth and development characteristics, there is a generally accepted standard followed by physical fitness experts. For example, the United States Army Conditioning Manual describes this standard as follows:

"Good posture is characterized by true vertical aline-ment, in which certain body segments are alined, one above the other, so that they support each other along the line of the pull of gravity."

The publication Adult Physical Fitness, prepared by the President's Council on Physical Fitness, states:

"Good posture acts to avoid cramping of internal organs, permits better circulation, prevents undue tensing of some muscles and undue lengthening of others. It thus contributes to fitness.

"In turn, physical conditioning, by developing muscle tone, helps to make good posture more readily main-tainable — and will help, too, if you have any bad pos-tural habits you need to break.

"For good posture, the centers of gravity of many body parts — feet, legs, hips, trunk, shoulders, and head — must be in a vertical line. As viewed from the side when you are standing, the line should run through ear lobe, tip of shoulder, middle of hips, just back of kneecap, just in front of outer ankle bone."

The posture illustrations and texts shown on these pages are based upon material from these two publications.

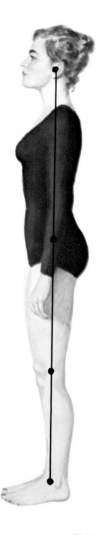

STANDING

The ideal standing position is illustrated by the large figures of the man and the woman on the top left and right. Unfortunately, most people are quite careless about their standing postures and the most common postures with their faults are illustrated below.

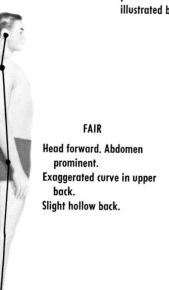

FAIR

Head forward. Abdomen
   prominent.
Exaggerated curve in upper
   back.
Slight hollow back.

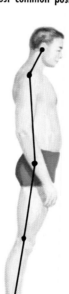

POOR

Relaxed posture.
Head forward.
Abdomen relaxed.
Shoulder blades prominent.
Hollow back.

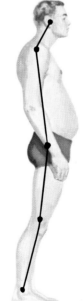

VERY POOR

Head forward badly.
Very exaggerated curve
   upper back.
Abdomen relaxed.
Chest flat — sloping.
Hollow back.

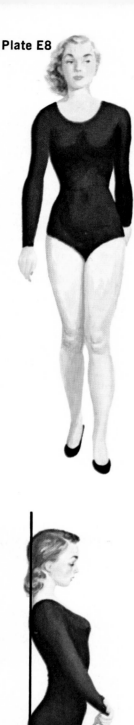

WALK TALL

1. Knees and ankles limber, toes pointed straight ahead. 2. Head and chest high. 3. Swing legs directly forward from hip joints. 4. Push feet off the ground — don't shuffle. 5. Swing shoulders and arms freely and easily.

PLUMB-LINE TEST

Hang a plumb bob or any weight from the top of a mirror as shown. Stand in front of the mirror and position your body so that the string lines up with the lobe of your ear, the tip of the shoulder, the middle of the hip, the middle of the knee, and the front of the ankle bone. Practice keeping this position for a few minutes each day. Soon it will become so natural that you will not have to strain to maintain the position.

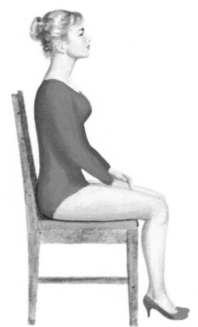

SIT TALL

1. Sit tall and back, with hips touching the back of the chair, feet flat on floor. 2. Chest out, back of neck nearly in line with upper back.

THE BACK-TO-THE-WALL TEST

Stand with your back against the wall. If your figure is as shown on the left illustration (or variations of it), then your posture does not conform to what is considered healthful and physically desirable. To correct this wrong posture, push your back against the wall as shown on the right illustration. Automatically you will stand in a position which more closely conforms to the plumb-line ideal.

WRONG

RIGHT

YOGA EXERCISES FOR HEALTH

Yoga has increasingly become popular in this country as an exercise procedure for achieving and maintaining good physical and mental health. Some of the basic positions are described in the succeeding pages.

THE LOTUS POSTURE

Practitioners of the Lotus Posture claim that it is the ideal position to practice meditation. The Lotus Position should be achieved by stages.

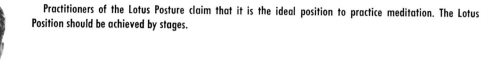

STAGE 1

As demonstrated in the picture, bring the right foot on to the left thigh with the heel touching the root of the left thigh with the sole upturned.

STAGE 2

Bring the other leg over the right leg and thigh so that the heel is close to the root of the thigh. Study the picture carefully, and maintain the position as closely as possible, initially for a brief time. Increase the time as you become more expert at assuming the Lotus Position.

HIP CONTROL

This is a very good exercise to achieve balance. It is also good for controlling the hips.

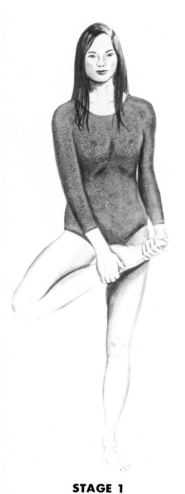

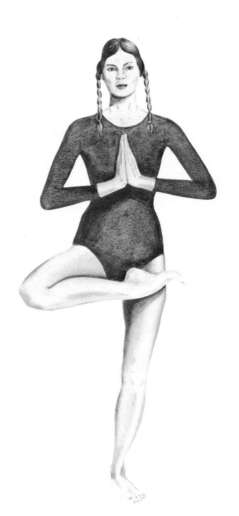

STAGE 1

Place one foot against the opposite thigh, as shown.

STAGE 2

Raise both hands and join the palms together.

STAGE 3

Conclude the position by bringing the palms in front of the chest. Maintain that position for a few seconds and change to the other side.

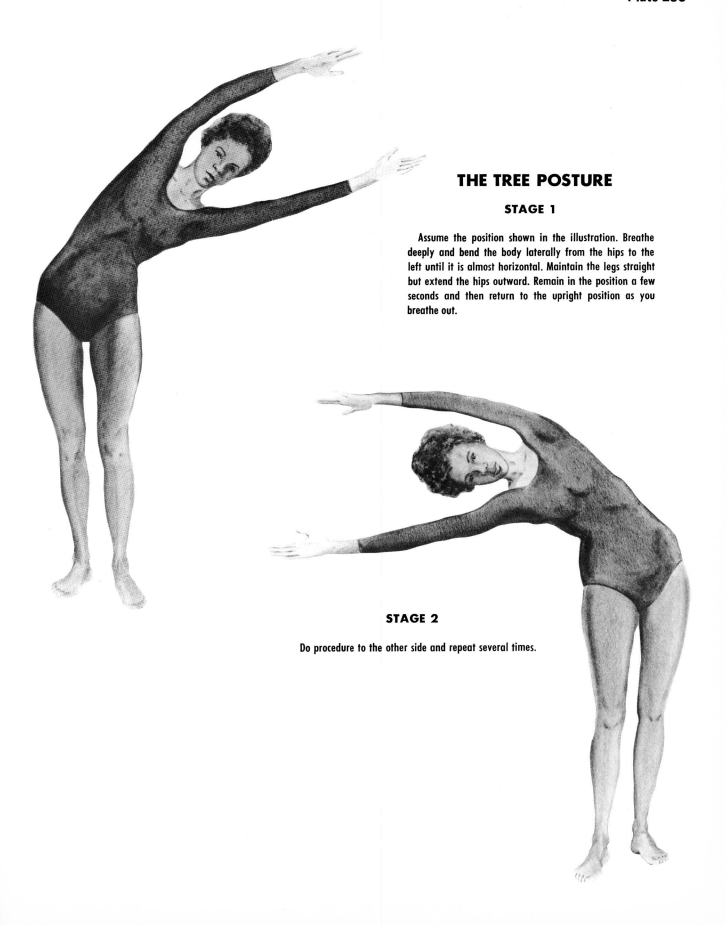

THE TREE POSTURE

STAGE 1

Assume the position shown in the illustration. Breathe deeply and bend the body laterally from the hips to the left until it is almost horizontal. Maintain the legs straight but extend the hips outward. Remain in the position a few seconds and then return to the upright position as you breathe out.

STAGE 2

Do procedure to the other side and repeat several times.

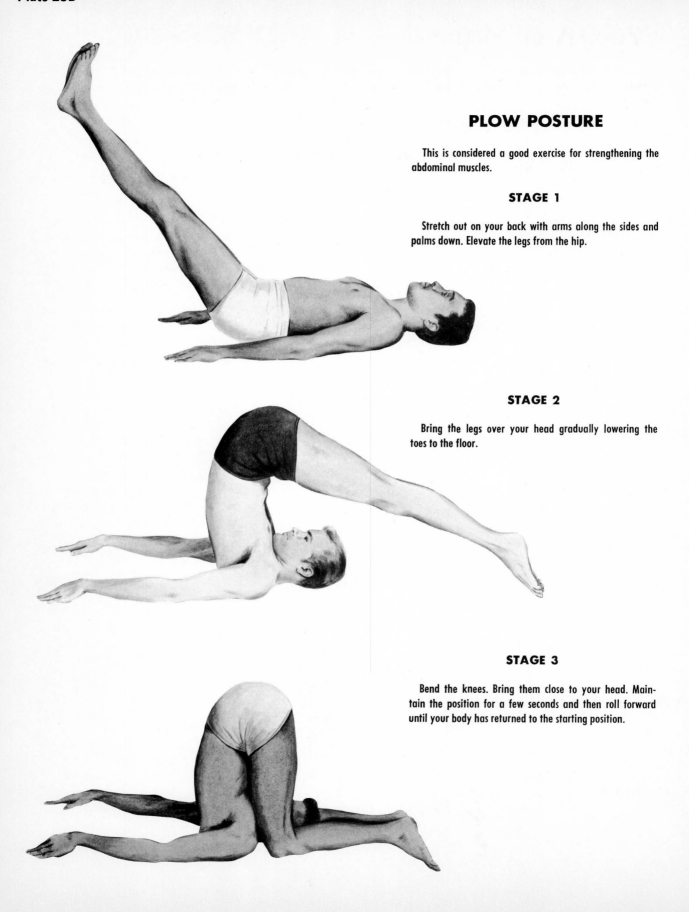

PLOW POSTURE

This is considered a good exercise for strengthening the abdominal muscles.

STAGE 1

Stretch out on your back with arms along the sides and palms down. Elevate the legs from the hip.

STAGE 2

Bring the legs over your head gradually lowering the toes to the floor.

STAGE 3

Bend the knees. Bring them close to your head. Maintain the position for a few seconds and then roll forward until your body has returned to the starting position.

fertile period. Subtract fifteen days from the longest cycle and add four more—this gives the final day of the fertile part of the cycle. For example, suppose that during the preceding year the cycles have varied from twenty-five to thirty days. Subtracting 15 from 25 gives us 10, subtracting 4 more gives us Day 6. Subtracting 15 from 30 gives us 15 and adding 4 more gives us Day 19. Hence Day 6 to Day 19 represents the range of the fertile period. Sexual relations before and after these days would be most unlikely to result in pregnancy.

5. The smaller the variation in the menstrual cycle, the more precisely can the fertile period be calulated and the shorter it is. Thus, if all menstrual cycles during the preceding year have fallen between twenty-seven and twenty-nine days, the calculations give a fertile period from Day 8 to Day 18. On the other hand, if cycles are very irregular, safe period calculations and the rhythm method cannot be used.

Q. I feel waves of heat and perspiration many times a day in recent months. What can I do for this?
A. They are probably menopausal flushes. Flushes, or as they are also sometimes called, "flashes," are transient sensations of warmth experienced by women during the menopause or "change of life." The warm sensation characteristically travels from one part of the body to another—for example, starting in the head and face and moving down to the trunk.

Flushes are often associated with perspiration. Sometimes the waves of perspiration are frequent and annoying, and may be a predominant symptom. The sensation of warmth may be so marked and realistic that the person experiencing it may be impelled to open a window or insist that the furnace is sending up too much heat. Not infrequently the flushes and sweats come on during the night.

It is generally agreed that the flushes are manifestations of a drop in the amount of female hormone in the system. They usually appear at about the time that the menstrual periods become scanty, irregular, or are skipped altogether. They are likely to vary considerably from day to day, and are aggravated by nervous tension, fatigue, or fluctuations in the weather. Waves of warmth and similar sensations, experienced by a woman who is still menstruating regularly, need not necessarily be regarded as a sign of oncoming menopause.

The flushes may come and go in erratic manner for months and even years. Following an initial period during which they are mild and occasional, they may increase in intensity. Then, after a period of months or even years, they slowly begin to decrease, both in number and intensity. Occasional flushes may be experienced even years after the menopause.

Where the flushes are marked, and considerable discomfort and annoyance are repeatedly experienced, a physician may prescribe moderate amounts of female hormone. These are usually taken in decreasing amounts over a period of time. Their purpose is to give enough female hormone to tide a woman over the acute period of hormone withdrawal. By gradually decreasing the amounts taken, the period of withdrawal is less abrupt, and there are fewer symptoms. The hormone can be given orally or by injection, both methods being of equal efficacy.

Q. I have noticed some red tingeing to the semen. What causes this?
A. This is generally due to the presence of some blood in the semen. Men are occasionally disturbed to notice a pink or bloody tinge to the ejaculated semen. There is a great deal of circulatory congestion in the genital region during sexual stimulation, and this is the usual background for some slight bleeding that may

occur in the male reproductive system at the time. Most commonly, it is an isolated event which happens once or twice and may not be seen again for a long time.

Very rarely, it occurs frequently. A doctor will check for various possible contributory causes, including considerable prostatic enlargement, possible chronic inflammatory disease in the prostate or seminal vesicles, or other potentially aggravating or causative factors. Very often no specific cause can be determined in the more usual types of investigation. The man who sees some blood in the semen should not be unduly alarmed, although he should of course take the precaution of reporting to a doctor.

Q. *I have slight irritation around the vaginal area. Sometimes moist secretions go with it. What is this?*
A. This is probably due to mild inflammation of the vagina, called vaginitis. There is usually vaginal discharge with this. However, not all vaginal discharges are signs of disease. In some women, there is sufficient hormonal stimulus to secretion at certain times in the menstrual cycle to produce a slight mucous discharge. This may occur around the middle of the cycle, and is not infrequent just prior to the onset of menstrual flow. In such cases, there may be enough secretion to stain the underclothing, but there will be little or no accompanying itching or other irritation. Perhaps the most common cause of vaginal discharge is a very common organism known as the trichomonas. This produces a slightly greenish, frothy discharge accompanied, when marked, by some redness of the external genital parts. See Vaginitis

Q. *I have had chills, fever, and aching in both flanks. What can be the cause of this?*
A. This is most probably a urinary tract infection, known as pyelitis, which involves the kidneys. Pyelitis refers to an infection in the central collecting portion of the kidney, into which the urine flows. This central collecting portion has a distinctive white irregular lining, and narrows into the ureter, the duct that runs from the kidney to the bladder. Although pyelitis is an old and well entrenched term, it is doubtful that a pure form of pyelitis ever exists. In all instances there is associated inflammation of the kidney itself, so that a more descriptive term is pyelonephritis, indcating a mixed infection both of the pelvis of the kidney and of the kidney substance itself.

Acute pyelonephritis is generally easy to recognize. There are chills and fever, pain in the flank, turbid urine, and such general symptoms as weakness, headache, and malaise. There are also chronic forms of pyelonephritis, in which careful search reveals the continuous existence of excessive bacteria in the urine, perhaps with such other evidence of infection as casts and white blood cells in excess. Occasionally there is also bleeding, which quite often accompanies infection of the urinary tract.

However, only in recent years has the existence of very stealthy and quiet forms of chronic pyelonephritis been recognized. Careful studies have shown that very low-grade persistent infections may be present in the kidneys for months or years without producing significant symptoms. They may lead to such eventual difficulties as impaired function and high blood pressure.

It is not always clear how the kidney becomes infected. Bacteria in the blood stream undoubtedly may be filtered out through the kidney and set up an infection in that organ. It is also likely that in many instances the infection reaches the kidney from the bladder below. It is common for a woman who first has symptoms of bladder inflammation, such as frequent urination and a sense of inability to empty the bladder completely, subsequently to suffer chills and fever and other symptoms indicating that the infection has spread up into the kidney. In young children, particularly girls, it has been demonstrated that there may be a reflux of urine from the bladder up the ureter and into the kidney because of inadequacy of the valve-like arrangement between bladder and ureter. Whenever there is obstruction of the free flow of urine from the bladder, infection appears in the bladder urine first, then often ascends into the kidney. This is true whether it occurs in a child with a congenital obstruction of the bladder opening, or in an elderly male with obstruction due to an enlarged prostate.

Prevention of chronic pyelonephritis can be accomplished only by recognition and full treatment of cases of acute pyelitis or pyelonephritis. It is very easy to bring an acute urinary-tract infection under apparent control within a few days. Appropriate antibiotics or other medication quickly bring the fever down to normal, and many of the symptoms disappear. However, in order to eradicate the lingering traces of infection within the kidney itself, experience has shown that the drugs should be continued for a longer period —perhaps even weeks—after the original symptoms have subsided. Otherwise the door may be opened to a chronic kidney infection.

It may also be necessary to investigate the reasons for recurrent attacks of acute pyelitis. Repeated attacks may be due to a complication of some kind, such as a stone or some structural change producing partial obstruction; this may vary from a stricture or narrowing of a portion of the urinary channel to pressure on it externally from an enlarged prostate. Recurrent pyelitis can be avoided only if such a predisposing condition is corrected. If, as occasionally happens, it cannot be corrected, a doctor may decide to place a patient on medication designed to prevent infection on an almost indefinite basis.

A great many medications are available for the treatment of both acute and chronic pyelonephritis. They include various antibiotics and various sulfa drugs. In practice, the problem is not starting treatment with the appropriate drug; rather the question is how long to continue treatment before there can be assurance that the infection in the kidney is completely eradicated.

Q. *I have to urinate frequently. What causes this?*
A. In women, the most common cause of frequent urination is cystitis, an inflammation involving the bladder. The channel between the bladder and the exterior of the urethra is very short in women—less than one inch long—and it is not difficult for an infection to work its way up the urethral passage into the bladder. Inflammation of the bladder produces a group of symptoms, often including the following: a frequent desire to void, pain or burning on urination, and a sensation of fullness in the bladder even after voiding. The desire to urinate may be felt at intervals of only a few minutes, and only a few drops may be passed with each voiding. With severe cystitis, there may even be some bleeding with urination, more frequently at the end of urination. Cystitis is generally treated by giving an antibiotic or other medication to clear the bacterial infection.

In men, the most common cause of frequent urination is enlargement of the prostate gland, an accessory sex gland located just at the base of the bladder. Enlargement of the prostate occurs in a considerable number of men as they grow older. The enlarged prostate may impede the passage of urine from the bladder, producing such symptoms as weakness of the stream, difficulty in starting (hesitancy), dribbling, difficulty in ending the stream, and the feeling that complete emptying is impossible. The bladder does not in fact normally empty entirely with the act of urination. A certain amount of urine is left behind; this is called residual urine. The residual urine normally does not exceed one ounce, but in some men with enlarged prostates from four to twelve ounces may remain. A doctor can determine the amount by passing a catheter, a hollow tube, into the bladder after urination and draining it.

Not infrequently, bladder infection occurs in the presence of retention of urine, and the symptoms of cystitis that the male then experiences are much like those noted above for the female. Mild enlargement of the prostate requires no treatment. It simply results in higher urinative frequency with perhaps a need for getting up one or more times at night. More advanced enlargement, producing severe symptoms, may require surgery.

Other causes of frequent urination are numerous. Nervousness often gives rise to repeated desire to void. Sometimes exposure to cold, or wading in cold water, produces a contraction of the bladder and a need for voiding. Certain substances in the diet may stimulate or irritate the bladder and produce a desire to void. There are also substances called diuretics which promote the passage of urine. They result in passing larger amounts of urine more frequently than usual. Among common substances that may have diuretic effect are coffee, tea, alcohol, and a variety of drugs used in the treatment of certain conditions of the heart and of blood pressure. In diabetes, the spillover of sugar into the urine is associated with an increased amount of fluid passing through the kidneys and bladder; consequently, one of the early symptoms of diabetes is frequent urination.

Other causes may be noted. Tumors and stones in the bladder may lead to a desire to urinate often. In some women, swelling of the uterus or womb at the time of menstruation may lead to pressure on the bladder and result in frequent urination. Other structures pressing on the bladder may do likewise. Finally, various kinds of inflammation and scarring in the bladder may produce contraction with a need for frequent urination because of the loss of normal bladder capacity.

Q. *Over recent years, I have had frequency of urination, difficulty in starting urination, and dribbling. What causes this?*

A. In a man past fifty the most likely cause of this is enlargement of the prostate gland. There are all degrees of enlargement of the prostate occurring in aging men. Even in the complete absence of symptoms, routine examination may reveal a considerable enlargement of the prostate. This is so because considerable enlargement can occur without obstruction of the bladder. On the other hand, a prostate which is not much larger than normal may result in considerable obstruction. In general, however, there is a proportionate relationship between the amount of prostate enlargement and the degree of obstruction associated with it. Obviously, if extensive enlargement produces no particular symptoms, no problem exists and the man can consider himself lucky.

The early symptoms due to obstructive enlargement of the prostate usually consist of frequency of urination and weakness of the stream. Frequency of urination may increase from three or four times daily to six or eight times. Instead of urinating once at night, a man may find himself getting up two or three times. This state of affairs may level off and persist unchanged for months and years. However, if obstruction progresses, the frequency usually increases until the need for voiding may be felt as often as hourly throughout the day, with a further increase in nocturia, the passing of urine during the night. Difficulty in starting the stream, weakness of the stream, and a prolonged dribbling conclusion rather than a sharply cut off end to urination are characteristic.

Infection and complete obstruction often follow. Whenever there is obstruction of the urinary tract, a condition favorable to infection exists. It is therefore not uncommon for a urinary tract infection to occur at some point in the development of prostatic enlargement with obstruction. This generally takes the form of cystitis, with the usual symptoms of a need for voiding, painful urination, frequency of urination, and a constant sense of incomplete evacuation. These may be followed by the symptoms of an ascending urinary tract infection, which include chills, fever, and other signs. An equally threatening and more dramatic event is the sudden onset of complete obstruction. After months or years during which difficulty in voiding and other signs of enlargement have been experienced, there may be a fairly abrupt onset of total obstruction. The patient finds himself unable to urinate despite an increasing accumulation of bladder urine and consequently pain.

Certain measures may be salutary in these circumstances. The application of a warm, moist towel to the genitals, a warm bath to induce relaxation, or the application of an ice-cold compress to the pubic region may stimulate the desire and the capacity to void. If none of these maneuvers works, catheterization may have to be resorted to. This consists of the passage of a hollow tube into the bladder to permit the urine to drain. The catheter may be kept in for a considerable period of time—catheter drainage—since it is likely that it will be necessary to drain the urine again within a few hours.

Although a man may successfully "live with" moderate symptoms due to enlargement of the prostate, repeated episodes of infection, or complete obstruction, indicate the need for surgical intervention. Individual urologists favor various surgical approaches to the enlarged prostate. In addition to removal of portions of the obstructing prostate by an instrument passed into the urinary channel itself (transurethral resection), several direct operative approaches to the prostate gland are used. One involves an abdominal operation and a one- or two-stage removal of the prostate gland. Another (the perineal prostatectomy) avoids the abdominal approach by operating in the region between the anus and scrotum, the perineum.

Each of the various surgical approaches has its merits and drawbacks and involves the pros and cons of many technical considerations. Suffice it to say that relief of obstruction can be definitely promised.

Q. I have been passing a reddish urine. What is the cause of this symptom?
A. This is most likely due to the presence of blood in the urine, a condition referred to as hematuria. There are many causes but a few are far more common than all the others combined. Congestion, infection, stones, and tumors are among the leading causes. Among the most common conditions in which hematuria occurs are the following:

1. Bladder infection (cystitis). Perhaps the most common cause of hematuria is that associated with infections of the bladder, most often seen in women. In addition to such "bladder symptoms" as frequent desire to void, and pain in the bladder region with feelings of fullness not relieved by urinating, some bleeding may occur. The bleeding sometimes takes the form of a terminal hematuria, the passage of a small amount of blood after passing the urine. In men, similar bleeding associated with a bladder infection can occur. With the clearing of the infection, the bleeding promptly ceases.

2. Congestion, especially prostatic. Congestion, especially when there is prostate enlargement, may lead to some bleed-

ing. It is likely to be made worse by alcohol and sexual stimulation and intercourse.

3. Stones. Stones at various levels of the urinary tract may produce bleeding. Stones can occur at any level, from the pelvis of the kidney to the ureter, the bladder, and even the urethra, the channel between the bladder and the outside. The movement of a stone often produces severe pain, known as renal colic, and there is frequently associated bleeding into the urine. When the possibility that there is a stone in the urinary tract is being considered, it is important that the patient save the urine to be examined for blood cells.

4. Tumors. Various kinds of tumors of the bladder and of the kidney may produce enough bleeding to color the urine.

5. Other disease. A variety of other conditions may produce bleeding into the urine. Among them are acute nephritis, blood disorders, even including infectious mononucleosis, circulatory disorders involving the kidney blood supply, overdosage of anticoagulant drugs, damage to the kidney due to direct blows or other causes.

Finding the specific cause for hematuria may be easy—for example, when cystitis is present—or very complicated, when one of the less common causes is operating. Then the investigation may require various technical procedures for visualizing the kidney and its passages, procedures which are generally performed by a specialist known as a urologist.

Q. *I have recently noticed a yellow tinge to my skin and eyeballs. What is this?*
A. This is probably the condition known as jaundice. It is due to the accumulation of bile pigments in the blood and tissues, and the degree of yellow staining roughly parallels the degree of accumulation of bile substances. One of the chief constituents of bile, bilirubin, is formed by the breaking down of red blood cells, a process that goes on continuously in the body. Massive sudden destruction of red blood cells (as in hemolytic anemia) may produce so much bilirubin that the capacity of the liver to handle it is temporarily overwhelmed. Transient jaundice will result. In ordinary circumstances the bilirubin is passed into the bloodstream, brought to the liver, and excreted by it into the bile. Two common mechanisms which may interfere with the process, and therefore produce jaundice, are injury to the liver resulting in impairment of its function, and obstruction of the bile ducts, reducing the volume of fluid they can carry.

Damage to the liver may be caused by a variety of agents, including drugs and heavy and prolonged alcoholism; but perhaps most commonly occurs as a result of the inflammation produced by the virus of hepatitis. Hepatitis can exist without jaundice, in which case it may then go undetected. Jaundice, however, is such a striking finding that it always demands a diagnostic explanation. In viral hepatitis, liver cells may be so greatly damaged that they are unable to function adequately, and usually enough bilirubin accumulates in the bloodstream to produce obvious jaundice. The urine turns dark because of the overflow of bile into it. In many cases of hepatitis, the jaundice intensifies for one or more weeks, and severe degrees of it may be encountered. In the average case, the recovery process sets in after some weeks; the liver cells begin to return to normal functioning and the jaundice slowly subsides.

In healthy persons, there is a continuous secretion of bile by the liver cells into a system of fine canals which increase in size until finally they empty into a pencil-size canal known as the common bile duct. Obstruction of the flow of bile through this duct leads to a backing up of the bile, and a reversal of the normal process occurs: The accumulation produces a dilation of all the ducts, and there is a reverse flow of bile into the bloodstream. Because of the continued production of bilirubin and the continued inability of the liver to excrete it, increasing bilirubin accumulation and jaundice occur as a result of obstruction of the bile duct. Among the common causes of such obstruction are a stone or a tumor pressing on the duct. Obstruction can result from inflammation and swelling, leading to a narrowing of the duct.

It is not always easy to tell which of the various possible causes are producing the jaundice. Certain tests tend to draw a line between hepatitis and obstructive jaundice. Sometimes a needle biopsy of the liver is indicated. Examination of tissue under the microscope may lead to a diagnosis. It may sometimes seem quite probable that a stone is the cause—for example when there is a history of gallstones—and although an exact diagnosis cannot be reached by testing, it may be considered wise to operate in order to relieve the jaundice produced by the presumed stone.

Although X-raying the upper digestive tract may occasionally suggest the possibility of a tumor, operation may again be necessary to arrive at a final conclusion. In recent years, with new and potent drugs coming into use, some of which occasionally lead to jaundice, the problem of distinguishing among the various causes of jaundice has become somewhat complicated. Serial tests and prolonged observations may be necessary before a sound opinion can be reached.

Q. *I have been told several times now that I have anemia. Why do I get it?*
A. Anemia is a deficiency of red blood cells. The red cells are formed in the bone marrow, and the process can be retarded in any of a number of ways, with anemia as a result. By far the most common form of anemia is iron-deficiency anemia. This results from a lack of iron, which is an essential building block in the formation of hemoglobin, the basic constituent of the red blood cell. Iron deficiency can cause a reduction in the number of red blood cells. Individual cells may be smaller and more irregular than normal and contain less than their normal amount of hemoglobin. Insufficient iron in the diet may be an important factor. Even in infancy, iron-deficiency anemia can occur when the child is maintained on milk alone for a year or more. Similarly, at puberty, the combination of an inadequate diet and a rapidly growing organism may result in a form of anemia, which once was known as the green sickness—chlorosis.

Occasionally, women in whom menstrual blood loss is excessive suffer from iron-deficiency anemia. In other forms of bleeding in which iron is lost, such as bleeding from an ulcer, prolonged nosebleeds, or bleeding from hemorrhoids, iron-deficiency anemia may result. The treatment of iron-deficiency anemia is relatively simple and consists of the administration of iron in a number of ways. The body will quickly utilize any iron furnished under these circumstances, and the correction of anemia takes place quite promptly.

Other forms of anemia not involving the iron mechanism may also occur, although they are less common. Absence of certain essential elements in the diet or in the body may interfere with the proper maturation of blood cells in the bone marrow. One well-known form of this condition is known as pernicious anemia. In this disease, the system fails properly to assimilate vitamin B_{12} from the diet, and severe anemia may result. The condition is rapidly correctable by direct administration of vitamin B_{12}. A somewhat similar form of anemia due to metabolic difficulties with another substance, folic acid, is occasionally seen in pregnant women and in persons suffering from certain nutritional disorders, or in association with disorders of assimilation in the intestinal tract.

Various disorders of the bone marrow may lead to anemia, sometimes quite severe. The activity of the bone marrow may be inhibited by a number of known factors, and also probably by some unknown ones, so that its cells are reduced in number—a condition known as aplastic anemia. In leukemia and similar disorders, there seems to be an overproduction of white blood cells together with a severe reduction in the number of red blood cells, so that anemia may be the most prominent feature. There are some disorders in which there is a rapid destruction of red blood cells, or hemolytic anemia. Inhibition of bone marrow activity accompanied by anemia is found in uremia. All of these causes of anemia are relatively uncommon, but of course require consideration for accurate diagnosis and treatment. This may mean referral to a hematologist, a physician who specializes in blood disorders.

Q. *I seem to lack pep. Could this be a glandular trouble?*

A. The chief gland regulating the rate at which the body functions is the thyroid gland. The thyroid gland is held responsible for many of the difficulties about which people commonly complain. Thyroid underactivity is blamed for the tendency to put on weight easily, for proneness to fatigue, for lack of "pep," for sluggishness and inertia, and for subpar feelings. The truth is that these complaints are seldom due to underactivity of the thyroid. Most overweight, whatever its real basis, is not specifically related to inadequate amounts of thyroid secretion. Overweight is generally due to a combination of sedentary living and an overhealthy desire for foods, particularly for carbohydrates. Tiredness, fatigue, and inertia—

the common complaints of many people —are seldom due to a single cause; they are seldom traceable to the thyroid.

True underfunctioning of the thyroid is referred to as hypothyroidism. Most commonly seen in middle-aged women, it usually comes on very gradually. Surprisingly, many hypothyroid persons are not overweight; rather, they appear puffy. This puffiness may be noted in the skin generally, but is most marked around the eyes. The condition is referred to as myxedema.

One of the characteristic findings of hypothyroidism is excessive dryness of the skin. The skin looks and feels dry. There is a striking absence of both oils and sweat. In severe cases the skin may have a leathery appearance. The best body site to observe this is not on the hands and forearms—which in many housewives are often dry due to excessive exposure to soaps and detergents—but on the skin of the trunk. The scalp and hair also tend to dryness. Hair loss and thinning of the eyebrows are other common complaints. The pitch of the voice commonly drops to the point of marked huskiness.

There are various degrees of hypothyroidism, but in the advanced stages everything appears to be slowed down—thinking and speaking appear slowed, the appetite seems less than normal, the bowels are sluggish, and there is a lack of drive and energy. Menstrual periods often go awry, the periods being prolonged and the menstrual cycle itself being shortened. Chronic headache is sometimes a major problem, and so are occasional nervousness, irritability, and depression. Considerable derangement of brain functioning may occur in advanced stages, and there is little doubt that some people who are considered mentally ill may be unrecognized hypothyroids.

Diagnosis of hypothyroidism includes special blood tests, basal metabolism tests, or uptake of radioactive iodine by the gland. In borderline cases, a "therapeutic test" with thyroid may be undertaken. This is simply administration of thyroid in gradually increasing doses while the patient's reaction is being observed. Hypothyroid persons are very sensitive to even small doses of thyroid, and will generally show a prompt response: there will be clearing of the puffiness, while the skin becomes more moist and more supple, the pulse rate speeds up, and general stimulation is discernible. On the other hand, individuals whose thyroids are reasonably normal—whatever their other symptoms of fatigue or weight gain may be—do not possess the same unique sensitivity to administered thyroid. Hence, little improvement of consequence will occur if they take thyroid.

Q. I am high-strung and thin. Can this be a glandular problem?

A. The only gland that could contribute to this is the thyroid when it becomes overactive, a condition called hyperthyroidism. In hyperthyroidism, an excessive amount of thyroid hormone is secreted. The condition is a good deal more common in women than in men. It is frequently precipitated by psychic stress such as death, a separation, or an accident in the family. It may come on during or after pregnancy, and it has been known to occur in several members of a family, as for example, a mother and a daughter. In young women the condition is sometimes referred to as Graves' disease. There may be an obvious swelling in the thyroid region (the thyroid is located in the lower part of the neck to either side of the windpipe) along with a rapid heartbeat, a forceful pulse, excessive perspiration, and, not infrequently, a bulging appearance of the eyes.

Hyperthyroid women usually complain of heat sensations, nervousness, and crying spells. They may manifest restlessness, jitteriness, sleeplessness, and similar signs of overstimulation. There may be various abnormalities of the menstrual cycle, including scanty periods or disappearance of the periods. Marked weight losses can occur as well as a variable amount of overactivity of the bowels, including frank diarrhea. Milder cases may go unrecognized and may even seem to abate for a while, but then a recurrence of symptoms is likely.

In the older age group, hyperthyroidism may be milder and harder to recognize. All degrees of an overstimulated state between the normal and the obviously hyperthyroid may be found. Hence mild degrees of hyperthyroidism may exist for years, manifested only by a rapid pulse, palpitations of the heart, a tendency to excessive perspiration, feelings of warmth, or various symptoms likely to be attributed to "nervousness."

There is now a choice of treatment for hyperthyroidism. In addition to surgery, in which a large portion of the thyroid gland is removed, drugs are available that will cut down thyroid hyperactivity. In certain individuals, partial destruction of the thyroid by radioactive iodine may be employed. Some of the complaints of rapid heart rate are improved by the class of drugs derived from the Indian snake root, the Rauwolfia drugs, now frequently employed in the treatment of high blood pressure. Of course, most nervous states in women are not due to excessive thyroid activity. On the other hand, no woman should be characterized as being "just plain nervous" unless the possibility of thyroid overactivity has been investigated.

Q. What can be done for swelling of the legs?

A. Swelling of the legs is known medically as edema. When advanced it is often referred to as dropsy by the layman. The condition generally results from an accumulation of fluid in the skin, and is due to various factors. Probably the most common of them has to do with simple mechanics and is brought on by gravity. When a person has settled down in a chair, with legs hanging down, or has stood for a long time, a noticeable degree of swelling may develop in his feet or ankles. This happens to many perfectly normal individuals, particularly on a hot day.

Another factor related to edema is any difficulty, new or old, a person may have with the veins and the circulation through them. An aftereffect of a clot in one of the larger leg veins may be a tendency to troublesome swelling of that extremity. The usual factors that aggravate this condition are a dependent position of the legs, inactivity, hot moist weather, and increased amounts of salt in the diet. Swelling often occurs in association with varicose veins, since in a varicose vein the return blood flow from the legs is impaired. Other factors that augment pressure within the veins may also predispose to swelling. Thus, clots of the large veins of the pelvis into which the leg veins drain, or pressure upon these veins from nearby organs, may sometimes result in leg swelling.

The condition known as congestive heart-failure is followed by a rise in pressure in the veins, and congestion can occur in various parts of the body. Frequently this results in leg swelling. Sometimes the puffiness may be marked.

In addition to cardiac causes, certain diseases of the kidney may underlie leg swelling, particularly conditions in which albumin is lost in the urine. When loss of albumin in the urine occurs for any length of time, body tissues puff up, and this may be most marked in the legs. It should be kept in mind, however, that such relatively trivial things as altered circulation in the veins are responsible for swelling of the legs most of the time, and that the heart and kidneys are most usually in no way involved.

There are various ways of dealing with troublesome leg swelling. Obviously, if disorders of the heart and kidney are involved, a physician will direct treatment specifically toward these organs. If the swelling is due to local circulatory disorders, as mentioned above, the patient will be advised to keep the affected leg in an elevated position as much as possible to diminish the force of gravity. The use of elastic stockings may also be advised, and the patient will be told to curtail the salt content of his diet. Finally, diuretic drugs may be prescribed. By pulling salt and water out of the kidneys, these drugs may rapidly diminish the degree of swelling of the legs.

Q. *I sometimes have a lightheaded feeling and things seem to swim about. What is responsible for this condition?*
A. This is generally referred to as dizziness, and dizziness is very variable. It can vary from a mild sensation of lightheadedness or giddiness (which is not truly dizziness) to what is medically known as true vertigo, in which objects around the patient seem to be in motion; this sensation is often accompanied by nausea. At the risk of a slightly inaccurate stretching of the term to include all of these sensations, the following may be considered as important causes:

1. Mild sensations of lightheadedness or giddiness may be due to insufficient sleep, to a hangover from alcohol or drugs, and sometimes to a psychosomatic disturbance resulting from depression or emotional stress.

2. Some viral illnesses attack the labyrinth—the semicircular canals of the internal ear which regulate equilibrium. This disturbance is called labyrinthitis and may produce severe symptoms of dizziness, nausea, and vomiting. The slightest attempt to get up or even a movement of the head may produce a marked increase in all these disagreeable sensations.

3. Ménière's disease affects the labyrinth, and comes and goes in irregular fashion. It is usually found in individuals

past middle age, most often men, and is frequently associated with a diminished sense of hearing on the affected side. The attacks often come without warning and produce intense dizziness and vomiting. These attacks may last from minutes to hours, during which time the patient is quite prostrated. Ménière's disease is considered to be a primary disturbance of the semicircular canals. The symptoms may be precipitated by an excessive distention with accumulated fluid. Occasionally, they may be brought about by stressful situations. Other neurological disturbances can lead to such symptoms as head noises and dizziness.

4. Finally, dizziness may be secondary to disturbances such as very low blood pressure, hemorrhage, or severe anemia. This is sometimes observed when patients who are taking drugs for high blood pressure experience a sudden drop in blood pressure, as may occasionally happen when the person remains standing for any length of time. The reverse of this is also seen: high blood pressure by itself may produce moderately severe sensations of dizziness. Bouts of dizziness are also seen in elderly persons and may be associated with circulatory changes to the brain.

The treatment of dizziness will depend upon the particular cause. If due to anemia, the anemia will have to be corrected; if due to high blood pressure, judicious lowering of the blood pressure may be helpful; and if due to the effect of drugs, changes in the drug program may be necessary. Acute attacks of dizziness such as seen in Ménière's disease do not usually last long, and it is often difficult to tell whether any drug has been of help or whether the attack has not in fact passed spontaneously. Where the disturbance seems to be in the semicircular canals, as with some viral illnesses, the drugs that have been developed for the treatment of motion sickness (seasickness) are often quite useful. Among these are

Dramamine®, Bonamine®, and Marezine®. These drugs seem to break up the "seasick" feeling and may markedly diminish nausea and the tendency to vomit.

The physican will prescribe the appropriate dosage of the drug. If it cannot be taken by mouth, injectable and suppository forms are available. In the case of some individuals who have frequent attacks of labyrinthitis, moderate doses may be taken for fairly long periods of time. Various forms of vitamin therapy are employed in the treatment of Ménière's disease, and may produce a diminution in the frequency and severity of the attacks.

Q. *I have headaches and sometimes dizziness. Several members of my family have had elevated blood pressure. What can I do?*
A. High blood pressure frequently exists without producing any symptoms. The diagnosis can only be made by having the blood pressure measured in the doctor's office. If your symptom is due to elevated blood pressure, here are some facts you should know:

High blood pressure is a common disease. It affects about 20 per cent of the population; it seems to run in families; and it is found to an increasing degree in the older age groups. The old definition of normal blood pressure as consisting of 100 plus the age implied a recognition of the aging factor. Actually, there are many exceptions to this, and the saying has relatively little significance. It seems quite clear that elevated blood pressure contributes materially to the aging of the heart and the blood vessels. Thus hardening of the arteries, heart attacks, and strokes have an increased incidence among people with elevated blood pressure, as compared to those with normal blood pressure.

Treatment for high blood pressure was unsatisfactory for many years. It consisted of difficult programs such as rigid salt restriction, or special dietary programs such as the rice diet. The problem of treatment has been greatly eased in recent years by a variety of new drugs. Indeed, the physician may now choose from a range of medications, some of which are for mild cases, others for the more severe ones. Depending upon the patient's reaction to the drugs and to the degree of elevation of blood pressure, a combination can be worked out for controlling the pressure, usually with gratifying results. First, however, it must be established that none of the less common causes of high blood pressure are present. Among these are certain tumors of the adrenal gland and various kidney disorders. On the other hand, most cases of high blood pressure are known as essential hypertension; that is, no specific disease of an organ seems to underlie the elevated pressure.

Q. *I often have dull aching in the fore-head, which is sometimes throbbing. What could be responsible for this?*
A. These sensations in the head are classified as headaches. There are literally dozens of factors that may produce headache, some uncommon, others so common as to be almost everyday occurrences. A very incomplete list of some common causes of headache includes the following: tension, inadequate sleep, oversleeping, colds and other respiratory illnesses such as grippe and flu, menstruation, elevated blood pressure, sinus infections, eye strain, constipation, missing of meals, overindulgence in tobacco or in alcohol, and a variety of illnesses in which fever is also a symptom. Other far less common causes of headache include brain tumors, infections within the brain or its coverings, marked anemia, lead and certain other forms of poisoning, hemorrhages and clots within the arteries of the brain (strokes), uremia, severe hemorrhage, and sunstroke.

Some headaches have a throbbing quality, with the throbs synchronous with the pulse, and are sometimes referred to as vascular headaches. One well-known type of vascular headache is migraine, which has a hereditary component, since it seems to run in some families. Typically, it produces a throbbing headache on one side of the head, generally followed, before it runs its course, by nausea and often by vomiting. In some allergic persons eating certain kinds of foods may precipitate a headache.

Many apparently healthy persons have an occasional headache which cannot readily be accounted for. However, many people learn to identify the various likely causes of their own headaches. An alcoholic hangover on Sunday following a Saturday night drinking bout, or an emotional upset, or staying up very late looking at television all regularly lead to headaches in some people. However, the cause-and-effect relationship may not operate all of the time. Thus it is well known that some patients with elevated blood pressure have headaches when their pressure is high; but since the levels of the blood pressure vary, sometimes headache may be experienced when the blood pressure is in the lower range, and not when it is higher.

Q. *What can I do for pains in the head?*
A. It is commonly desirable to determine the cause of the headache as the first step in treatment. If the ache is due to some organic disease, the doctor will attempt to define the disease and institute appropriate treatment. This may mean taking medication to reduce the blood pressure, perhaps giving up smoking, or perhaps changing dietary habits so that the blood sugar does not drop too low. One may suspect that a definite disease process is producing headache if the headaches are frequent or chronic and if this is a new occurrence; if their location is different from previous headaches; if they do not follow the pattern of headaches in the

past; or if they are resistant to the usual simple measures.

In order to determine the cause of headaches, a physician may have to make extensive examinations. In addition to determining the level of the blood pressure and studying the chemistry of the blood, a skull X-ray, a study of brain-wave patterns (electroencephalogram) and, perhaps, careful examination of the eyes and of the nervous system may all be necessary. A migraine headache may be spotted by the existence of a family history of it, a tendency to recurrence under certain circumstances such as undue stress, excessively hard work, or perhaps menstruation, and also because the headache pursues a progressive course involving throbbing, visual disturbances, nausea, and vomiting. Certain drugs are now available for the treatment of migraine, and even for its prevention.

It must be conceded that in more than 80 per cent of the cases an organic cause for headache may not be found. Sometimes talking things over with a doctor or psychiatrist may relieve some of the stresses that form a background to migraine and other tension headaches.

However, most headaches are simple headaches and not a sign of an underlying threatening or severe disease process. Most people take a couple of aspirins for them and try to do the best they can. Occasionally, stronger medications, such as combinations of aspirin with codeine or other pain killers, may be required. Some patients find that an ice bag applied to the head may give considerable relief. For some of the headaches that arise in the back of the neck and are due to stiffening of muscles or to an arthritic involvement of the upper portion of the spine, heat is useful. They may be further helped by following up with some massage.

Sometimes tension-producing experiences may lead to repeated headaches, and the best answer may be a change in environment, as for example, a switch to another job if a person cannot develop a less intense attitude toward the stresses and strains of his life. Sedatives or tranquilizers, sometimes combined with muscle relaxants, may be useful drugs in the treatment of headache due to nervous tension. Finally, when eyestrain or sun glare are the causes, appropriate glasses or smoked lenses may clear up the headaches.

Q. *I have such trouble falling asleep at night. I also wake up frequently during the night and find it difficult to get back to sleep. What can I do?*
A. Difficulties in falling asleep or in staying asleep are common symptoms of nervous tension. Insecurity and anxiety frequently contribute to insomnia. The student worried about a major final exam, the executive harried over a difficult decision he must make, the mother worried over her child's illness, or the husband and father about losing his job—all these may have sleep difficulties. The difficulty may take various forms. It may consist of an inability to fall asleep reasonably quickly, or of a light and uneasy slumber with many awakenings during the night. Sometimes it may take the form of early-morning insomnia in which the person falls asleep much as usual, but wakens several hours ahead of schedule.

Whatever form it takes, a sleep difficulty can be very trying and can lead to intense feelings of wretchedness and tiredness. Its widespread existence no doubt accounts for the many popular remedies against it. In addition to counting sheep —which apparently no one ever does— recommendations have included: a warm tub bath, a glass of warm milk prior to retiring, a nightcap such as beer or some other alcoholic beverage, strict avoidance of coffee and similar stimulants, reading or looking at television until the eyes get tired and the lids droop, and taking a walk before retiring. Another suggestion is to disregard the problem of sleepless-ness altogether, that is, to stay up and just hope that sooner or later normal sleepiness and the sleep pattern will be restored. But this seldom works.

There is no doubt that insomnia may be due to sedentary patterns of living. Many sedentary people living in cities have no physical activity, and when bed-time arrives, the lack of normal physical fatigue may contribute to difficulty in sleeping. Also, many persons are exposed to various kinds of nervous stimulation throughout the day and find themselves in an overstimulated state at bedtime, un-able to relax and fall asleep. Thus, many businessmen find that they are unable to stop thinking of their business problems when they go to bed.

Sometimes an appropriate change in one's pattern of life may be necessary be-fore relief from bouts of insomnia can be achieved. A program of increased physical activity may be of value to some. A shift to a less tension-producing job may be helpful. Certainly, when insomnia is fre-quent, reexamination of one's pattern of life and stresses, perhaps in consultation with a physician or psychotherapist, may be worthwhile.

Ours has been described as a sleep-ing-pill age. Widespread use of pills to induce sleep is perhaps more of a reflec-tion on the kind of world in which we live than on the many sleepless persons in it. Sleeping pills are not recommended as an initial solution to sleeplessness, but it may also be a mistake stubbornly to refuse any kind of medication when insomnia is pro-ducing great fatigue and difficulty in con-centration and in work. A great many medications are available, other than the typical sleeping pill, which may be of help in solving the problem. Mild sedatives and tranquilizers and some of the antihista-mines (these are not sleeping pills but are drugs used for allergies, and often pro-duce mild drowsiness) will often help

without producing hangovers or other un-toward effects. If a sleeping medication is necessary, the dose and the type should be suited to the person taking it, and the mildest one that works will be the best. Temporary recourse to a sedative to se-cure sleep may be extremely worthwhile during periods of great stress. One need not be afraid of becoming "addicted" to the drug. Generally, as the stress subsides and the tension diminishes, the capacity to sleep is restored.

Q. *Should I make a point of doing exer-cises?*
A. The contribution to health that ex-ercise makes has been appreciated more and more in recent years. For example, some important studies have revealed that in persons who are physically active throughout their lifetime heart attacks seem to be less frequent, are more apt to occur later in life, if at all, and are less likely to be fatal. For this reason the pru-dent person might well consider some pro-gram of regular exercise. There are other values to regular exercising. These include the following:

1. Some evidence exists that the ten-dency to grow fat may in large measure be due to a disproportion between output of energy, as represented by work and exercise, and intake of calories, as dictated by one's appetite. This has been demon-strated even with animals. Experiments have shown that when an animal is not allowed to exercise, it may grow fat, whereas when the animal is allowed per-haps an hour or so of exercise per day, it will maintain an even weight. Although at one time the value of exercise was downgraded in programs for reducing for overweight, there has been an increasing tendency to advocate moderate exercise, at least some walking daily, as part of the total program of keeping weight under control.

2. Most doctors now agree that exer-

cise tends to improve the performance and capability of the heart and lungs in the face of unexpected or strenuous effort. This is due to its toning or conditioning effect. Many aspects of this are not well understood, although it is known that the trained athlete's heart can pump much larger amounts of blood with greater ease than the heart of the former athlete who has lost his conditioning.

3. In the absence of exercise, muscles do not merely remain what they were; they tend to shrink and lose their power. Flabbiness of the muscles may contribute to various kinds of stresses and strains which are not experienced by the physically well-conditioned person. One example is the low backache. This is more likely to occur in sedentary persons with poor musculature than in active ones with well-developed muscles. Indeed, there is a growing belief that for certain kinds of low backache, the best long-term answer may be a program of exercises.

4. Exercise has a tonic and stimulating effect on the organism. Sedentary persons who constantly feel tired find that when they exercise, the tiredness disappears and they feel invigorated. They may also find that they have more "pep" and an improved sense of well-being.

The exercise problem is growing as the white-collar population increases, as labor-saving machinery is more widely adopted, and as cars and readily available public transportation lead to less walking. Housework and similar tasks are not the equivalent of exercise—there is considerable difference between standing in the kitchen washing dishes and taking a bracing walk out of doors.

Various booklets and articles dealing with exercises have been available in recent years. Two well-known ones are those published by the United States government and by the Royal Canadian Air Force. Both describe a system of progressively graded exercises which, when followed by a sedentary person whose muscles have had very little use for many years, will produce muscle-toning and conditioning without the risk of harmful over-exertion at the beginning. In the absence of graded exercises, walking for a mile or more per day has much to recommend it. Some exercises for low backache (see page 595) are also good as toning-up exercises, and can be performed routinely by anyone in his own bedroom.

Q. *Since I turned sixty, I have noticed that my hearing seems poorer. What can I do for this?*
A. The hearing mechanism involves:

1. The external auditory canal, which runs from the opening in the outer ear to the eardrum

2. A series of small bones in the middle ear

3. The cochlea, or the hearing organ itself, in which sound impulses are changed into nerve impulses

4. The auditory nerve, which conducts the nerve impulses to the brain

Disease processes at any point on this path can interfere with hearing. A plug of wax in the external canal, a bony engulfment of little bones in the middle ear by otosclerosis, or damage to the cochlea and auditory nerve are among the many conditions that can cause hearing impairment.

The diminished hearing that occurs in the elderly primarily involves the hearing organ and the auditory nerve. The exact cause of senescent hearing loss is unknown but may be regarded as a deteriorative process perhaps comparable to cataracts in the eyes. The diminished acuity of hearing is sometimes called presbyacusis (presby- meaning old and -acusis, hearing). Hearing loss attributable to aging comes on very gradually and, in fact, some hearing loss may be demonstrable fairly early in life. Thus there are very few persons past the age of thirty who can hear the high-pitched squeak of the bat. Hearing loss severe enough to interfere with ordinary conversation is not likely to occur before the age of fifty or sixty, but thereafter tends to be somewhat progressive.

The loss is greater in the higher frequencies, so that a person may understand such words as "one" and "mother" better than higher pitched words such as "six" and "sister." A certain amount of "figuring out" goes on with a person who is hard-of-hearing. Sometimes he guesses wrong, with confusion and embarrassment for those concerned.

There seems to be no reliable treatment for presbyacusis. Large doses of vitamin B complex occasionally help. The most practical solution is a hearing aid. A doctor should prescribe the type of hearing aid needed. As long as the auditory nerve functions reasonably well, the hearing aid will help the elderly in ordinary social situations. When the auditory nerve is too badly damaged, however, even a hearing aid may not be of any help. The thoughtfulness and consideration of persons who deal with the afflicted person on a continuing basis are also of value.

Q. *Since reaching the age of seventy, I have noticed increasing dimness of vision. What could be doing this?*

A. This is most likely due to cataract formation, a not uncommon condition in the eyes of the elderly.

As light passes through the eyeball it is focused on the retina at the back of the eye by a clear crystalline structure called the lens. Any opacity in the lens is referred to as a cataract. Some cataracts are present at birth (congenital cataracts); others are caused by injury (traumatic cataracts). By far the most frequent type is the one that appears in old age. Such cataracts are at first small, produce no significant impairment of vision, and often

the person who has one is unaware of its existence. A small cataract produces no visual problem. However, any of a number of factors may cause a small cataract to progress slowly. It may become large enough to be clearly visible as a whitish area within the pupil.

Certain metabolic disorders, such as diabetes, thyroid disease, or disorders of the parathyroids (the glands regulating the calcium content of the body), may predispose to cataract formation. However, cataracts often occur in aged or aging persons who are apparently in sound general health.

There is no treatment for cataracts other than surgical removal when they reach a certain point of maturation ("ripe" cataracts). Until that point is reached, changes in prescriptions for glasses, good illumination, and magnifying devices may be helpful. Cataracts tend to appear in both eyes, but their rate of development is generally unequal, and only one cataract at a time will be operated upon. Surgery consists of removal of the lens, a procedure that is performed without difficulty or complication thousands of times each day. To make up for the loss of the lens, compensating glasses must be worn. With such glasses, excellent restoration of vision can be expected to follow cataract removal.

Q. *I have frequent colds. What can I do for this?*

A. The fact that solutions for the common cold are less than satisfactory is indicated by the numerous remedies and programs advocated. Colds vary, are undoubtedly caused by different viruses, and are far more severe in some epidemics than in others. These variations undoubtedly contribute to the belief in certain "cures" which people claim to have experienced.

Actually, shortening of the duration of the cold or lessening of symptoms after taking medication "X" may be due to the fact that the attacking virus is less vicious than usual, or that one's resistance and capacity to shake off the cold may be somewhat higher than previously, rather than to any value in medication "X" itself. Nevertheless, once medication "X" seems to have worked, its "beneficiaries" persist in taking it whenever they have a cold, however improbable it is that "X" could have any effect.

At the first sign of a cold, many people dose themselves with whisky. Others take a laxative. Nothing that we know about the tissue reactions to colds, or about the effect of agents like alcohol or laxatives on the body as a whole, or the body's resistance and defense mechanisms, indicates that either procedure can be of any value.

But even the skeptic will admit that there are some useful procedures and drugs:

1. Cutting down on one's work and activities, even to the point of loafing in bed for a day or so, may reduce the intensity of the symptoms and the feeling of wretchedness, and certainly may lower the fever (not generally high in most colds).

2. Aspirin is likely to offer some relief for the headaches or vague muscular aches that accompany respiratory illnesses.

3. In recent years there has been a boom in the use of drugs such as the antihistamines and other decongestant agents known as the sympathomimetic amines, very often in combination. These appear to decrease congestion and the amount of nasal secretion formed, results not to be shrugged off.

When nasal congestion is intolerable, the sparing use of nose drops may unblock the nasal passages sufficiently to permit a reasonably free nasal breathing. Infants with nasal congestion may experience a great deal of difficulty and be most uncomfortable when attempting to nurse. This results from an inability to take in air because of the stoppage of the nasal passages and the presence of the bottle or breast in the mouth. Sparing use of nose drops may make the baby a good deal more comfortable.

There has been considerable argument back and forth as to whether antibiotics or other germ-killing drugs should be used for the treatment of simple colds. The concensus, concurred in United States government statements, is that antibiotics are of no help in the therapy of the simple cold. In addition, quite a few studies, mostly based upon college students and similar groups, have indicated that the course of the cold is the same whether or not antibiotics are also given.

For the overwhelming majority of people the simple cold is a nuisance disease, not a threat. For the cough itself, there are innumerable preparations sold over-the-counter at any drug store. Among the classic cold and cough remedies are such familiar ones as elixir of terpinhydrate (ETH) and codeine, syrup of wild cherry, and syrup of coccilana. When the cough is more severe, the doctor may prescribe medications containing codeine and codeine-like drugs which have a cough-suppressant effect.

Expectorants which increase the amount of phlegm are common ingredients of cough syrups and mixtures. Sucking on cough drops is often of some help for a harassing cough, and so is the inhalation of steam and the maintenance of humidity in the sickroom by vaporizers. Finally, it may be noted that avoidance of colds is always better than treating them. While most people feel that there is no escape, here are several facts to be kept in mind:

1. The common cold is a contagious disease, hence one should avoid undue exposure to individuals with colds who are coughing and sneezing.

2. There is a resistance factor to colds. For many individuals, excessive fatigue seems to be a predisposing cause and should be avoided. The fatigue may be

physical or emotional. Since it may be a long time before we have immunization against colds, it is wise to study the pattern which precedes the development of one's own colds and learn from such experiences.

Q. I have a definite pain in the throat when I try to swallow. What can I do for this?

A. This is usually due to inflammation of the pharynx, producing pharyngitis or sore throat. It is of some importance to establish the type of sore throat that is causing the pain. For example, sore throats due to the streptococcus (strep throat) usually produce a beefy red throat with some white exudation. It is important that the patient with a strep infection be treated with penicillin or some other antibiotic. Statistically, however, the most frequent causes of sore throat are the various viral respiratory illnesses. Whatever the other symptoms they may give rise to in the nose, sinuses, or bronchial tubes, they are very likely to produce a sore throat as well. Since there are no specific drugs for viruses, treatment should be directed toward allaying the discomfort and other symptoms they produce. Among treatments which have proved to be of value are the following:

1. Heat, or alternatively, cold may relieve discomfort. Heat may be applied by means of a heating pad wrapped around the neck, or possibly an infrared lamp or ordinary light bulb directed toward the same area. (Precautions, of course, should be taken against possible burns.) Occasionally, when heat is not helpful and when congestion, swelling, and difficulty in swallowing persist, cold may be effective. Chips of ice may be slowly sucked and swallowed. Here the cold has a numbing effect. It tends to cut down congestion and so may help diminish the inflammation and swelling that goes with the infection.

2. Various types of gargles have been prescribed at one time or another. One consists of a teaspoon of salt in a glass of hot water. The addition of ten to fifteen drops of tincture of iodine to a glass of hot salt water sometimes seems to increase effectiveness, but precautions must be taken not to swallow this gargle; its use therefore cannot be recommended for small children. Still another gargle consists of one or two aspirin tablets crushed in a glass of hot water.

3. Pain-killing drugs ranging from aspirin to stronger compounds such as Darvon® and codeine or its derivatives may be necessary to relieve more painful sore throats.

4. Lozenges containing a local anesthetic are sometimes used to relieve the discomfort of a sore throat. There are a few individuals, however, who have local allergic reactions to these anesthetics. Unless you are quite sure that you will not have this type of reaction, the anesthetic lozenges are best avoided.

5. With certain kinds of infection, where swallowing is very painful, cortisone-type drugs are occasionally used under a doctor's guidance.

6. Some of the liniments, rubs, and ointments used for sore muscles, which work by producing local heat (rubefacients), may occasionally be helpful with sore throats. Care must be taken, however, not to allow the fumes which some of these give off to get into the nostrils and eyes.

7. If warmth seems to be helpful, it may be wise to wear a scarf around the neck not only outdoors but indoors as well. Hot drinks such as tea may also have a soothing effect. For children, milk as warm as they can tolerate it may be used.

Q. I develop nasal stuffiness in the early fall of each year which lasts for weeks. What causes this?

A. This is probably a form of hay fever.

At least five million Americans suffer from hay fever, an allergic disease affecting the lining of the nose. The sensitivity generally is to pollens and hence is more likely to be noted around June (grasses) and August (ragweed). Depending on climatic conditions and the pollen count, the victim may have a variable amount of nasal stuffiness, sneezing, a watery nasal discharge, itching of the eyes, and tearing. One of the earliest fundamental treatments for this condition was to give increasing doses of pollen extracts, which bring about a sort of increased resistance or tolerance for the pollens. This process of desensitization is still fundamentally sound. When successful, it may effect a complete cure. Desensitization is particularly desirable if there is accompanying asthma, an allergic condition involving the bronchial tubes. For mild cases and as a supplementary aid, the antihistamine drugs have proved very useful. These are combined with sympathomimetic amines (neosynephrine, ephedrine, and isopropylaterenol, an adrenalin-like substance), which are often efficacious in diminishing nasal congestion, thereby permitting a reasonable degree of free breathing through the nose.

In addition, the sparing use of nose drops may be of value when the nasal blockage seems intolerable. For severe degrees of nasal blockage, drugs of the cortisone group may be helpful; their use in any but small doses over brief periods of time, however, is not usually recommended. One of the consequences of this form of nasal allergy is the formation of polyps—pale, grapelike growths within the nasal cavity. The polyps by themselves may be, if not entirely, at any rate significantly responsible for nasal blockage. They are not likely to respond to medication and may have to be removed, a minor surgical procedure which may be performed at a doctor's office.

A somewhat similar condition involving nasal obstruction, increased secretion, and even the formation of polyps may be found in individuals who have not been previously allergic. This condition may appear for the first time in adult life—unlike hay fever, which is likely to be manifested in the child or the teenager.

Probably some of the cases that occur in middle life represent unusual allergies. Others have been classified under the term vasomotor rhinitis. This is thought to be an irritable and overreactive state in the nasal lining and not a true allergy. Middle-aged individuals with vasomotor rhinitis may notice more nasal difficulty when they are tense, after they have been drinking, or when they undergo temperature and humidity changes. They complain of being unduly disturbed by various kinds of dust, smoke, and fumes. The treatment for this condition is similar to that advocated for hay fever, but injections are unnecessary since the condition is not a reaction to an offending external agent such as a pollen. Generally, antihistamines are of value, the amount taken depending upon the extent of the disability and the doctor's prescription.

Q. I get aching in the cheek bones and over the eyes, especially with colds. What causes this symptom?
A. This is doubtless due to involvement of the sinuses. The sinuses are cavities within the bones of the face, and communicate with the nasal cavity. They are lined by a mucus-secreting layer of cells, just like the nasal lining; they behave in general as the nasal lining does with respect to infections, allergic responses, dust, and other substances. Between the sinus and the nasal cavity is a small opening called the ostium. It is this anatomical construction that is likely to create difficulty since, if enough swelling of the lining occurs to close off the ostium, swelling and accumulated secretions within the sinus may cause increasing pain.

One or another set of sinuses may take

part in this process: the maxillary sinuses, which are in the cheek bones just below the eyes; the frontal sinuses, located in the bones just above the eyes; or the ethmoid sinuses, located in the nasal bones between the eyes. When this occurs, a painful headache may be noted. In addition, severe infection may be accompanied by fever.

When there is fever, antibiotics or other germ-killing drugs are generally prescribed. Antihistamines and nose drops may be of value in unblocking the openings of the sinuses to permit drainage. Once drainage has been established, pain is likely to diminish. Heat is often soothing, and can be given in the form of hot wet compresses or a heating pad applied to the face. Special narrow heating pads designed for use in sinusitis are available. Aspirin and other pain-killing drugs may also make a useful contribution.

Sinusitis may be intermittent, occurring several times during the winter, and not at all at other times of the year. However, for chronic sinusitis, surgical methods are sometimes employed. For the very common kind of chronic sinusitis in the maxillary sinuses, a useful procedure can be to establish a new opening between the sinus and the nasal cavity to provide free drainage. The procedure may be compared to opening up a boil, for once the pus is discharged, relief of the pain, swelling, and inflammation generally occurs.

Since the introduction of antibiotics, severe sinusitis and chronic sinusitis have markedly diminished. Before trying surgical methods for severe forms of chronic sinusitis, these drugs or antihistamines, as well as similar medications, are generally tried first; they frequently produce satisfactory results. Another procedure that can be performed at the doctor's office is to puncture the sinus. It can then be irrigated or washed out. This treatment is designed to relieve the infection and with it the discomfort. Sometimes, several such treatments may lead to a marked improvement.

Q. *Why do I sometimes feel mucus in the back of my throat?*
A. This is probably due to the condition sometimes referred to as postnasal drip. Postnasal drip refers to the dripping into the upper back part of the throat of mucus from the nasal cavity. It is a condition that occurs regularly with most colds and similar respiratory illnesses. A postnasal drip that is associated with a viral respiratory illness normally ceases as the illness abates. Where there is chronic infection of the nose and sinuses, however, postnasal drip may be present much of the time. Obviously, the treatment of such a condition would be directed toward clearing up the infection, as described in the discussion of sinusitis (page 587). Chronic irritation, in which cigarette smoking may be the leading offender, can also be responsible for postnasal drip.

Q. *I have cough with phlegm for long periods of time. How can I clear this up?*
A. A cough of long duration is generally an indication of an irritation either in the larynx and trachea (the vocal cords and windpipe), or the bronchial tubes themselves.

It should always be possible to account for a chronic cough. A cough should not be allowed to go on indefinitely without being brought under close scrutiny and the reasons for it ascertained. There are dozens of possible causes for chronic cough, but in actual practice a few of the more common ones far exceed the others in incidence.

Perhaps the most common of all is chronic bronchitis, which is an infection of the bronchial tubes usually due to bacterial infection. Normally, because of good self-cleansing mechanisms, the bronchial tubes are virtually free of bacteria. If bacterial infection gains a foothold and lasts for any length of time, increased secretions (phlegm) and chronic cough may be the body's answer to the infection. Both of these are mechanisms for getting rid of the invading bacteria. The phlegm formed under these circumstances may have a yellow tinge and a thickened consistency.

Chronic bronchitis seems to be on the increase and may predispose to emphysema, another lung condition in which the sacs of the lung are overdistended and shortness of breath is experienced. It should not be disregarded, and efforts should be made to treat it rather than to put up with it. The single most important contributing factor to chronic bronchitis is undoubtedly cigarette smoking, and it is idle to treat chronic bronchitis if the victim continues to smoke.

However, chronic bronchitis does exist in nonsmokers. Not infrequently it is secondary to an infection of the sinuses, with a chronic postnasal drip, and the condition is referred to as sinobronchitis. Antibiotics and germ-killing drugs are often useful in the treatment of sinobronchitis. Occasionally, special treatment may be necessary for the sinusitis before the bronchitis clears up.

Some cases of chronic bronchitis seem to follow the acute bronchitis set up by certain respiratory infections. Here again, antibiotics may be administered for a period of time. When large amounts of phlegm are produced, postural drainage is indicated. This involves the placement of the body into various positions, generally with the head lower than the waist. This facilitates the outward flow of the phlegm. By lying first on one side, then on the other, gravity may aid in bringing the phlegm from the smaller bronchial tubes out toward the larger ones. From there, the phlegm can easily be brought up by less strenuous coughing. Often the chronic cough itself will improve as a result of postural drainage. Inhalations of steam, sometimes mixed with other agents, and the use of various expectorant mixtures,

may also be helpful.

No one should attempt self-diagnosis of a cough. Coughs may arise from such serious conditions as pulmonary tuberculosis and tumors of the lung. Also, they may occur in association with mild degrees of asthma, inflammation due to fungous and other organisms, not to mention certain forms of heart disease, emboli (or clots) in the lung, and other possibilities too numerous to mention here. Coughs, phlegm, and chest pains should never be lightly dismissed. All too frequently they are attributed to cigarette smoking and to other banal causes, with the result that serious underlying conditions are allowed to proceed undiagnosed and untreated. Anyone with a chronic cough who brings up phlegm or has frequent chest pains should avoid self-help measures and should instead seek professional advice at once.

Q. Why do I often feel "all out of breath"?
A. A variety of heart, circulatory, and lung conditions may contribute to shortness of breath. We must remember, however, that shortness of breath can be experienced without any serious underlying disease. Sedentary persons, unaccustomed to physical effort, may experience shortness of breath when called on to exert themselves physically, even if the effort is nothing more than climbing a low hill or a few flights of stairs. The fact that this condition is due to a lack of conditioning, and is reversible, is indicated by the observation that performance improves following suitably graded exercises. Persons who are moderately or markedly overweight often complain of shortness of breath on exertion. Contributing factors here include not only the dead weight of the fat, but also the fact that the heavy deposits of fat on the chest and abdomen mechanically interfere with breathing.

Smokers often complain of shortness

of breath. This is due to obstructive bronchiolitis, an inflammation of the lining of the tubes, with accumulation of mucus. This leads to partial clogging of the smaller bronchial tubes. Fortunately, this is usually cleared when smoking is discontinued, so that several weeks afterward, the ex-smoker may find himself able to perform without shortness of breath, tasks that were formerly very trying. All of the factors just mentioned—lack of training, obesity, and cigarette smoking—are reversible.

Other conditions of the lung that impair ventilation and produce shortness of breath may not be so successfully reversed. This is true of certain kinds of chronic inflammation, for example, when there has been a good deal of scarring (fibrosis) which interferes with the ability of the lungs to expand and contract. Sometimes extensive scarring interferes with the exchange of oxygen around the innumerable small blood vessels of the lung, thus setting up a mechanical barrier to oxygenation.

A condition that seems to be on the increase, known as emphysema, may also contribute to shortness of breath. A form of this is seen in many aging people. The more severe grades of emphysema are a consequence of chronic bronchitis and are seen especially in persons who have smoked for long periods. The basic trouble in emphysema is that the little air-containing sacs of the lungs are overdistended and have lost their elasticity. Hence they do not properly expand with inspiration and contract with expiration, and the total flow of air in and out of the lungs is considerably decreased.

In addition to lung factors, heart factors are also involved. Often, as people get older, the capacity of the heart to handle the increased demands produced by exercise diminishes. Hence shortness of breath is experienced as one attempts to run for a bus or train, climb several flights of stairs, shovel snow, or perform any other physical effort that taxes the heart muscle. The ability to face up to an unexpected or unusual demand on the heart's pumping function is sometimes referred to as the myocardial reserve (myocardium being equivalent to heart muscle). Various illnesses, past and present, may diminish the myocardial reserve. A heart attack that knocks out a portion of the heart muscle can do this; so can hardening of the coronary arteries that nourish the heart. Damage to the heart valves produced by rheumatic heart disease may lead to a considerable decrease of this reserve, as can various forms of congenital heart disease and such glandular disturbances as thyroid disease.

A variety of heart troubles may lead to congestive heart-failure. This is a condition produced when the heart's pumping function is inadequate, so that congestion in the lungs, the liver, or the lower extremities becomes apparent, and is manifested by accumulation of fluid in these sites. Pulmonary congestion or fluid in the lungs may be greatly improved by various prescribed programs. These may include instituting the use of such drugs as digitalis and the diuretic drugs, which pull water out of the body. These drugs may clear up pulmonary congestion and lead to marked relief from shortness of breath. Rest alone leads to temporary relief but the shortness of breath returns with exertion or other special effort. The patient may even experience spasm of the bronchial tubes with wheezing, quite like that seen in asthma. Obviously, shortness of breath is only a symptom, one that can arise in a variety of situations. The determination of the precise cause or causes will require examination by a physician.

Q. *I sometimes develop wheezing and feel short of breath. What is the cause of this?*

A. One probable cause is a form of asthma.

In asthma, the chief difficulty is due to an intense spasm of the bronchial tubes. When this is marked, the victim finds it difficult to breathe. Also, expiration, which is normally a passive process requiring no effort, becomes difficult and energy-consuming. In a severe case, the victim seems to gasp for air, and is obviously laboring hard to perform the act of breathing.

Most cases of asthma are due to some allergic reaction, most commonly to pollens, but occasionally to various other items including foods and drugs. If the reaction is to pollens, the discomfort is experienced at particular seasons. Desensitization is brought about by giving injections of the pollen extract. This may gradually build up the body's capacity to tolerate the offending agents and thereby result in cure. Often, however, there may be a multiplicity of substances to which the asthmatic patient is allergic. For these patients, desensitization may be a complicated and protracted process. Whatever the offending agent, drugs of various kinds may be necessary to relax the bronchial spasm. These drugs are known as bronchodilators. They include such agents as ephedrine, aminophylline, and certain related synthetic drugs. These are the drugs commonly found in various asthma remedies and may be given in pills or, occasionally, in suppositories, or in enema form. For very severe cases of asthma, steroid drugs (cortisone derivatives) may be helpful in tiding over a severe episode. Pocket inhalators, small enough to be carried around, are available. A few whiffs of these inhalators may give prompt relief in an asthma attack.

Asthmatoid bronchitis is a somewhat similar condition in which there is also bronchial spasm. This condition tends to appear in middle or later life, although occasionally it is found in some individuals in association with respiratory illnesses at any age. Patients with this condition do not have a history of allergic reactions to pollens, and their bronchospastic disorders are not limited to a particular season of the year. Instead, they seem to develop asthma in association with a bronchial infection—bronchitis—hence the term asthmatoid bronchitis.

Since it is often difficult to clear up bronchitis, the asthmatic tendency manifested by wheezing, coughing, and shortness of breath—particularly on exertion—may be present a considerable part of the year. Many of the drugs used for the treatment of asthma will help with asthmatoid bronchitis. Often combinations of drugs have to be used to achieve maximum control. In addition, since there is an infectious component to asthmatoid bronchitis, antibiotics may be prescribed. Antibiotics may be particularly useful when a person who is subject to asthmatoid bronchitis starts coming down with a cold or similar respiratory illness.

Antibiotics are seldom of value in the treatment of uncomplicated allergic asthma, except when the individual develops a superimposed infection, not infrequently a bronchopneumonia.

Mild forms of asthmatoid bronchitis frequently escape detection. They have all the qualities of a chest cold with cough, but may be more drawn out than usual. A wheeze and a long siege of a choking, hacking cough may well connote asthmatoid bronchitis.

Q. *How can I break the cigarette habit?*
A. Smokers are sometimes surprised to find that giving up cigarettes is far less of a struggle than they had supposed. This includes, to begin with, persons who have stopped smoking for several days during a bout with a cold, persons who light a cigarette and can forget it so that it burns itself out, and persons who, in places of employment that forbid smoking, manage to go for a substantial number of hours without lighting a cigarette. Unfortunately for the majority of individuals, a true

habituation or addiction does seem to exist, so that for them to stop smoking does in fact produce tension and disagreeable symptoms. In addition to their preoccupation with the idea of smoking, some people feel definitely under par during the withdrawal period, and they may experience trouble in concentrating on their work.

Other symptoms are a tendency to constipation during the first few days, some difficulty in falling asleep, marked feelings of hunger, and sensations of warmth in the extremities together with a noticeable slowing of the pulse rate. Withdrawal symptoms are most marked during the first few days, then tend to taper off over the next two weeks. Those abandoning the habit, however, should be advised that, from time to time during the early weeks following cessation of smoking, an intense though brief craving for smoking may reappear and must be firmly denied.

There is no doubt that considerable firmness or self-discipline is necessary for most hardened cigarette smokers who wish to give up the habit. A person seriously interested may wish to consult a doctor who will be in a position to prescribe mild stimulants, sedatives, or alternatives and substitutes that may partially compensate for the tobacco craving. Some people, those who feel truly wretched during the first few days, may be helped by drugs of the dexedrene-benzedrene group, while those who feel nervous may profit by small doses of sedatives. A drug of variable efficacy known as lobeline, which is distantly related to nicotine, has been used on and off for the past fifty years to help relieve the symptoms. When an individual who wishes to stop makes a compact with another smoker, the knowledge that someone else is faced with the same problems is a barrier to falling back into the habit and a help in fighting temptation.

A cigarette smoker who stops should be good to himself and should seek other satisfactions. Since he often has an increased appetite, he should eat, suck on candy and mints, and be prepared to gain a few pounds—a temporary indulgence well worth the price. Women who hesitate to stop smoking due to a fear of gaining weight should be advised that a modest weight gain is no health hazard and that the increase can be reversed once the non-smoking status has been achieved.

It is important for those giving up the smoking habit to realize that not only will they escape such statistical possibilities as lung cancer and heart attack, but that within a few weeks various kinds of pleasant improvements may be noted. Usually the wind is markedly improved, and shortness of breath disappears. The "cigarette cough" vanishes as the chronic bronchitis which afflicts most smokers generally clears. There is sometimes an enormous improvement in the sense of taste and smell, and the flavor of food seems to be doubled or tripled. In addition, many ex-smokers notice that their pep increases, and that sometimes sexual drives and capacities improve. The latter may represent an overall improvement in performance and health brought about by the discontinuance of smoking.

Q. *I seem to cough less on filter cigarettes. May I continue with them?*

A. There is no evidence that present-day filters will necessarily change the picture, as no one knows whether the particular agent responsible for some of these illnesses is held back or passes through the filters. The risk of such conditions as lung cancer seems to be markedly lower in pipe smokers and cigar smokers, perhaps in large measure because they do not customarily inhale the smoke.

The special committee set up by the Surgeon General of the United States, which reported its findings early in 1964, simply corroborated the conclusions reached by many other investigations made both here and abroad over the preceding ten to twenty years. As early as 1938, it was demonstrated that heavy smokers live on an average four years less than nonsmokers. The American Cancer Society studies have repeatedly shown that the chances of developing lung cancer are multiplied a hundredfold when one compares the incidence of lung cancer in heavy smokers as against nonsmokers.

Even more perturbing was the American Cancer Society's finding that the incidence of coronary thrombosis (heart attacks) was definitely higher in heavy smokers than in nonsmokers. In addition, in 1962, the same group published studies indicating that chronic bronchitis and emphysema, a condition which produces shortness of breath and which is most difficult to treat, was almost exclusively a disease of cigarette smokers, and so was cancer of the larynx (voice box), as well as cancer of the mouth and tongue.

The risk inherent in cigarette smoking is significant at the ten-cigarette-per-day level. The risk moves markedly upwards as the amount of cigarette smoking increases. For example, a man of sixty, smoking two packs per day, has one chance in ten of dying of lung cancer alone, not to mention the other smoking-related illnesses to which he may succumb.

All investigations point to the dramatic but inescapable fact that cigarette smoking is by far the most important single preventable agent contributing to illness and death on the American health scene today. It becomes the clear responsibility of every individual, therefore, with even a modest regard for the health of his own body, to desist from cigarette smoking.

Q. Why do I often have dull pains in the lower back?
A. Most chronic backaches arise in the musculoskeletal system, in this case the spinal column, the pelvis, and their associated muscles and ligaments. Various kinds of pulls, stresses, and strains on these structures will produce backaches. They are most commonly felt in the region of the lower back, the "small of the back," and will sometimes be more pronounced on one side than on the other. Back pains in this area may have a constant dull aching quality. Changes in posture or in the physical demands made on the low-back structure will have an effect on the pain. Such changes may be taken as a good indication that the ache does arise in the musculoskeletal system.

Quite often, sitting in certain positions, driving, or standing in one spot may make the backache worse. Bending so that the body goes into a partial stooping position may relieve the backache, as may supporting some of the body's weight on the outstretched hands. A backache which occurs mostly upon arising in the morning raises the possibility that a sagging mattress may be responsible. Backache of a similar quality may be experienced in the upper part of the back by individuals who have a curvature of the spinal column in this region. Here again special stress, which results in the ache, is being placed on muscles and ligaments.

Laymen tend to assume that aching in a particular region signifies some disorder in an organ nearby. Thus they assume incorrectly that an ache in the low back is due to something wrong with the underlying kidneys; or that, when it occurs higher up, it is due to pleurisy. But ninety-nine times out of a hundred the pain is in the muscle walls and ligaments rather than in a diseased organ underneath. This is not to deny that disease in the kidney is occasionally felt in the low back, or that a uterus which is tipped back (retroverted uterus) may produce a chronic low backache.

In addition, a physician will keep in mind other possible causes for backache, since various diseases of the mus-

594

culoskeletal apparatus may be present. Such disorders include osteoarthritis; another form of arthritis known as spondylitis; osteoporosis, a condition in which the vertebrae become weak because of their loss of protein and calcium; herniated discs; tumors; neuritis or inflammation of nerves; and other rare possibilities.

Q. *What should I do for frequent nagging aching in the back?*
A. If, after an examination by the doctor, it becomes clear that this is the usual postural type of chronic low backache, it should nevertheless be treated as a definitely individual problem. However, experience indicates that these backaches often have common features and that certain common approaches may be of value.

1. A mild low backache may occasionally intensify rapidly after a sudden stress or pull on the back. In severe cases, the victim may be unable to straighten up, and every movement of the back may be agonizing. Sometimes chronic low backaches are ushered in by an acute, severe one. Generally, it is best that the individual get off his feet and go to bed. In bed, a slightly bent position of the back is usually the most comfortable. This can be achieved by elevating the knees and the lower extremities on several pillows, perhaps also raising the mattress at the head of the bed. Pain-killers, varying from aspirin to stronger combinations, may be necessary. A heating pad placed on the lower back is often helpful. During this stage, a tight support such as a sacroiliac belt or a girdle may be of value.

2. The victim of low backache should pay special attention to his bed and mattress. As mentioned earlier, if the backache is worse on arising in the morning, it is often found that a sagging mattress is to blame. A mattress should be quite firm and should provide good support under the hips and low back. A mattress that is too soft or has too much "give" may

be firmed by inserting boards between the mattress and spring. Sometimes placing newspapers, books, or a pillow under the center of the mattress helps give additional support in this region.

3. Similar attention should be paid to seating. Pillows placed so as to support the small of the back may enable one to drive a car or work at a desk without getting backache.

4. Supports for the back, such as sacroiliac belts, are often helpful. Women sometimes find that wearing a tight girdle is useful. A pad exerting moderate pressure against the small of the back will be of further value.

5. Stresses and pulls on the back should be avoided. When one stoops to pick up a heavy object, this should be done by bending the knees, never by bending with the knees held stiffly. To keep the knees straight while lifting places all the strain on the low back.

6. The best sitting posture for people with low backache is one which keeps the back slightly rounded. This is best achieved by insuring that the knees are at a higher level than the hips. Thus a good chair for someone with low backache would slope downward from front to back. Another helpful arrangement is to have the feet elevated on a low hassock or stool.

7. Finally, back-strengthening exercises should be seriously considered.

Q. *What sort of exercises are useful for chronic low backaches?*
A. Because low backaches may be a source of discomfort for months or years, and because they often suddenly give rise to episodes of aggravated or disabling pain, there have been increasing efforts to work out long-range solutions to the low-back problem.

In a few instances this may be easy, for example the disappearance of the low backache when the victim shifts from a sagging to a firm mattress. Not uncommonly, however, low backaches may persist, coming and going but never quite gone.

For many sufferers, exercises designed to strengthen the muscles of the low back may afford the best permanent relief. These not only strengthen the supporting muscles of the back, but are also sometimes intended to correct a tendency of the hollow in the small of the back to increase. Many authorities agree that the key to low backaches is a structural weakness in the lumbosacral region, or hollow, on which the weight of the trunk falls. Increasing strength in this region may therefore be of fundamental importance in dealing with low backache.

It has been clearly shown that daily exercise will cure, or significantly help, some low backaches. When, because of inertia or for other reasons, exercise is discontinued, the backache returns. Among the exercises that have been advocated are the following:

1. Lying on the back, raise each leg alternately ten to fifteen times. Then repeat with both legs. The legs need not be returned to the resting position, and it is in fact preferable that they be lowered to from six to twelve inches above bed or floor level, from where the exercise is repeated.

2. "Kissing the knees." While lying on the right side in the straight position, bring the left leg toward the chin, bending the knee. Repeat on the opposite side. While lying on the back, draw the legs upward, bending them at the knees. At the same time bend the trunk forward as far as it can go. With some practice it should be possible to bring the knees up to the face, first on one side, then on the other. This exercise should also be repeated ten to fifteen times.

3. Knees-over-head exercise. In this exercise, the extended legs are brought up over the head as far back as they will go, then returned to a position in which the legs are six to ten inches off the floor. This can be repeated several times.

4. The familiar touch-the-toe exercise should be modified. The knees should be kept slightly bent rather than rigidly straight. It is not necessary to touch the toes, nor should the back be completely straightened in the return sweep of the exercise.

5. Squats. From a slightly stooped position, with knees slightly bent and arms hanging downward between the lower extremities, bend the knees until the knuckles touch the floor. Then straighten up to the partially erect position, and repeat.

These exercises should be started cautiously by sedentary individuals, and are best not done at all when the backache is acute. The number of repetitions can be slowly increased. If there is any increase in backache, the number of exercises may have to be decreased, and a physician should be consulted. The general aim of these exercises is to strengthen the back muscles, but in none of them should the hollow of the back be accentuated. This is the reason for not completely straightening out in some of them, and also the reason why the emphasis is placed on such others, as "kissing the knees," which have a tendency to straighten out the hollow. In addition, the back may be strengthened by exercises such as bowling, swimming, golfing, and pulling of weights.

Q. I have noticed in recent years some thickening around my finger joints. What causes this?
A. The thickening of the finger joints which appears in some people in their forties is a form of the disease called osteoarthritis. The thickening is due to an increased formation of bone around the joint. The condition is sometimes called Heberden's node. It seems to be more common in women, may run in some families, and may show some progression, but

sometimes long periods will pass without any apparent further thickening. Very few people reach their sixties and seventies without some degree of osteoarthritis of the fingers. Occasionally, it may produce angulation so that the fingertip appears to be slightly crooked.

Mild degrees of this disorder may produce no discomfort. At times stiffness and slight aching in a joint may be noted. This may be more marked on arising in the morning, and may improve soon after a person gets up and starts using the hand. The condition is seen in sedentary individuals as well as those who work with their hands, so that work is not a primary cause. Women who are proud of their grooming and appearance will, of course, find the condition a little more annoying than those who are more philosophic about their appearance.

Unfortunately, nothing is known about the cause of this disease or how to alter its course. When pain or stiffness are present, soaking the hands in hot water usually limbers up the fingers and alleviates pain. Aspirin or similar drugs may be taken to decrease the ache. If exposure to cold seems to increase the discomfort, gloves should be worn. In most individuals, the condition is more of a nuisance than a disease process. It has no special relation to osteoarthritis elsewhere in the body, has nothing to do with rheumatoid arthritis, a far more crippling disorder, and is perfectly compatible with excellent health.

Q. *Why do I have pains and difficulty in turning my head?*
A. This is sometimes referred to as a stiff neck and is usually due to a painful spasm in one of the major muscles at the back of the neck. The spasm produces pain, often increased by attempts to move the head about. Such movement generally is restricted to one side. The spasm may make the affected muscle appear to stand

out more than the corresponding one on the opposite side of the neck. Stiff necks produce all degrees of incapacity, from slight discomfort to a severely painful spasm of the neck muscles which makes any motion impossible. Most such conditions are set up by a stress or unusual strain on the neck. Occasionally people wake up with such a stiff neck because the neck has been in an awkward position during sleep.

Occasionally, a stiff neck may occur after a twisting motion of the neck, just as a severe backache can result from an innocent maneuver such as reaching down to pick up a shoe. This is due to a slippage between the connections of the spinal vertebrae, setting up a reflex spasm in the muscles producing pain and then immobilization. Exposure to a cold wind or draft sometimes results in a stiff neck. It is thought that the cold produces some temporary change in the muscle, leading to the stiffness and pain. A variety of other neck pains are somewhat similar to the stiff neck. Arthritis in the neck area, degeneration of the discs between the vertebrae, pressures on the nerves where they exit through the vertebrae, and changes in the alignment of the vertebrae of the neck may all lead to uncomfortable and painful sensations in the neck region. These too are often aggravated on attempted motion.

Many of these conditions are treated by traction, in essence a stretching of the neck produced by a collar and weights. The collar is slung around the head and jaw and is connected to a rope passed over a pulley. The opposite side of the pulley is weighted, and produces a degree of tension that can be regulated and varied by a physician. The neck is stretched by this device for periods of five to fifteen minutes per day. Traction may relieve pain considerably. Aspirin and other pain-killers are often useful in treatment. Also effective is massage

Q. *My daughter has a breaking out of the face for some days before her period. What is this?*

A. This is probably acne (pimples) which is almost an inevitable part of every adolescent's development. Its appearance during adolescence is due to the fact that acne is related to sex hormones stimulation of the oil glands of the skin. Acne is a good deal more common in boys than in girls, but is found in both sexes. As a matter of fact, both male (androgen) and female (estrogen) sexual hormones are found in each sex. In girls, the flare-up of acne that occurs just prior to the menstrual period is related to the altered hormonal secretions at that time. Fortunately, in the great majority of adolescents acne is mild. It may consist of occasional crops of pimples on the face, forehead, or back which vary in number, and perhaps form whiteheads, but which leave little or no scarring. When the acne has run its course, as it generally does by the age of twenty, little in the way of significant skin blemishes can usually be noted. See ACNE

Q. *What can I do for excessive perspiration?*

A. Excessive perspiration is an accompaniment of some diseases, such as overactivity of the thyroid, and episodes of excessive sweating are complained of by some women during the menopause. But many persons have this affliction without any obvious link with disease or organic condition. Hyperhidrosis, the medical term for it, is most often confined to a specific part of the body. A not uncommon complaint is excessive perspiration from the palms of the hands. It occurs in moderate degree when people are nervous or tense, as the result of adjusting to a new business or social situation, or when they are experiencing anxiety or fear. Occasionally, excessive perspiration from the hands seems unrelated to the emotions, and may reach the point of dripping. Excessive perspiration is also complained of in the armpits and on the feet.

There are, of course, innumerable antiperspirants for use in the armpits. Most of them contain an aluminum salt which inhibits the activity of the sweat glands. They generally also incorporate agents to reduce the odor of the sweat. Some seem to be a little more effective than others, and some individuals have to apply them more than once a day. Generally, however, washing the underarm region daily with an antibacterial soap such as Phisohex® or Dial®, and then using the antiperspirant, gives adequate relief. Even with antiperspirants, some women find dress shields necessary to protect their clothing. Similar measures will generally help excessive perspiration of the feet. Wearing sandals or open-toed shoes and porous cotton stockings, rather than synthetics, is of further help.

Excessive perspiration may sometimes be partially but not completely controlled. In the unusual cases in which the excessive perspiration reaches the point of large-scale dripping and is not controlled by the usual measures, surgical procedures may be effective. One of these is the severing of the sympathetic nerves which control the particular area. When they are cut, marked dryness in that part of the skin to which the nerves go will occur. The operation is by no means a minor one, however, and should be considered only when the degree of hyperhidrosis warrants it. More recently, sweat glands have been removed to control excessive sweating from the armpits. The operation is simpler than cutting the nerve supply and, while it has not been used extensively, early reports on the operative results seem quite encouraging.

Q. *How much exposure to sun should I give my skin?*

A. In general, sun exposure and sun tanning are of medical value for only a limited number of people. Where there is excessive oiliness of the skin and acne formation, tanning the skin may have therapeutic value. However, many individuals, particularly sun-worshipers who toast themselves on the beach for prolonged periods, are only injuring their skin. The tanning reaction is the skin's and the body's attempt to protect against further injury.

Excessive exposure to the sun has been demonstrated to age the skin. Loss of elasticity and tone, and thinning and atrophy of the subcutaneous tissue (the tissue just under the skin) are all aging changes which are hastened by excessive, prolonged, or repeated exposure to sunlight. Thus, although a tan is prized as a sign of good health and, admittedly, gives that healthy outdoors look, overindulgence should be viewed with considerable restraint. This is not to say that getting an occasional sunburn, or developing a tan during a summer vacation, is not all right. It is frequent and prolonged exposure to the sun that should be avoided.

A further factor to be considered is the fact that large doses of sunlight over long periods of time increase the rate of formation of skin cancers. Cancer of the skin is known to be more prevalent in people who work out of doors, with constant exposure to the elements, as do farmers and sailors. While slight tanning and exposure to the sun may be defended from the cosmetic point of view, and even, perhaps, from the medical point of view as giving rise to vitamin D formation, like all other desirable activities they should be indulged in with restraint.

Q. Sometimes I feel as though I "itched all over." Yet when I look, I can't see anything wrong with my skin at the place that itches. What can be the reason for this?
A. Many individuals suffering from nerv-

ous stress experience itchiness of the scalp or other parts of the body. The itching is essentially transient, and need not call for special measures. Some persons complain of itching as they lie in bed before falling asleep. They experience prickling, itching sensations in different parts of the body which respond to scratching; after a time, the sensations diminish, and the person falls asleep.

Other forms of nervous itching can be quite chronic, sometimes very stubborn, and present a variety of skin changes. Some patients undergoing particularly stressful periods experience diffuse itching sensations which are relieved by scratching. The scratching may produce a welt-like or reddish elevation of the skin, a condition technically called dermographism— literally, skinwriting. Sometimes, however, there is a full-fledged skin eruption, which is very often symmetrical in shape. The eruption may be on both elbows, or on the backs of both knees, or it may be on various other parts of the body, such as the neck. The skin in these regions becomes reddened or purplish, appears slightly thickened, and the normal linear skin markings are somewhat more prominent than usual. Itching may be so intense as to lead to repeated scratching even to the point of drawing blood.

Q. What can be done for cracking and itching between the toes?
A. The most common cause for these complaints is the condition termed athlete's foot. Athlete's foot is the popular term for a skin disease of the feet produced by a fungus organism. (A fungus organism differs somewhat from bacteria, one of the important distinctions being a greater hardiness and resistance to treatment.) See ATHLETE'S FOOT

Q. I have slight itching and flakiness of the scalp. What can be done for this?
A. This is most often due to the disorder

popularly termed dandruff. A wide range of scalp disorders, from light flakiness to extensive reddened and weeping, crusted patches, may be referred to as dandruff, or more properly as seborrheic dermatitis. Mild cases, which produce a little flakiness on one's collar, need not cause concern. Sometimes, particularly when the hair is not shampooed for a period, some itching may be noted. With any form of seborrhea, it is advisable not to let the hair grow too long, nor to use oily or greasy lotions and dressings. Thick hair and greasy lotions prevent proper aeration of the scalp and consequently promote dandruff. When considerable flaking, itching, and redness occur, a crew cut or a very short haircut may be advisable. See SEBORRHEIC DERMATITIS

Q. *On waking up this morning, my father couldn't move his left arm and leg. What is happening?*

A. The most common cause for this is a stroke. In a stroke, a certain number of brain cells are damaged. The damage may occur because of a thrombosis or clot in the artery which supplies blood to these cells or, less commonly, a cerebral hemorrhage due to a leakage of blood from the blood vessel. Often the physician cannot be sure which has happened, and the event is referred to generally as a cerebral vascular accident, or CVA. A CVA can occur in any part of the brain, and multiple CVA's occur in which small groups of brain cells are damaged, sometimes with surprisingly little functional evidence of impairment. However, most people think of stroke-caused brain damage in terms of the control of voluntary motion. The brain cells involved are sometimes referred to as the motor cells, and are the ones that enable a person to move his arms or legs, speak, swallow, and smile, or perform other facial movements at will.

The motor cells which control each half of the body are located in the op-posite half of the brain, that is, damage in the left side of the brain will produce paralysis on the right side of the body, and vice versa. There is but one speech center in the brain, the center that controls the complicated movements and acquired information that go into the process of talking. In right-handed persons, this center is located in the left half of the brain, in left-handed individuals, it is on the right side. As a result, impairment or loss of speech, known as aphasia, will not occur if a right-handed individual suffers a stroke affecting the left side of his body.

The extent of loss of function that occurs with a stroke varies from slight weakness affecting a limb, with or without speech difficulty, to full paralysis in which the entire affected half of the body appears to be knocked out. The latter condition is referred to as a hemiplegia. In the early stages of a hemiplegia the victim may be completely unable to move either the arm or the leg. Fortunately, however, it is generally found after the passage of some days that a degree of voluntary motion is coming back. Most often voluntary control returns first to the lower extremity, in which some motion can be achieved, even though requiring considerable effort.

As a rule, so long as some motion is evident it is safe to predict that the victim will be able to walk after a period of rehabilitation. The degree to which control returns to the upper extremity is variable. Because of the complexity of human hand motion, and also because a very large number of motor cells are involved in controlling the arm, hand, and fingers, impairment of hand and finger motion is generally more apparent and also more distressing than loss of function in the leg. Particularly, of course, if the dominant side (the right side in a right-handed individual, and vice versa) is affected, difficulties and tribulations will be more marked. Characteristically, finely coordinated finger motions such as those involved in writing, picking up objects, or other everyday motions may be lost or severely impaired.

Various degrees of functional restoration usually take place during the days and weeks immediately following a stroke. This slow healing process may go on for months, at a rate that varies considerably from one person to another. Therefore, one cannot be certain of the permanent damage caused by a stroke for several months. Improvement may continue for as long as a year. Rehabilitation therapy is of great value following a stroke. If the stroke victim can raise his foot even slightly off the bed, the outlook for his eventually walking is quite good. However, before he walks again, a considerable program of effort, exercise, and persistence on his part and that of those caring for him may be necessary. Generally, the affected limb is quite stiff (the technical term for this is spasticity) and control over the spastic extremity is at first slow, weak, and distressingly inadequate. With practice, however, more and more control over the damaged extremity ordinarily returns.

The situation of the stroke victim can be likened to that experienced by the infant when he first attempts to walk. Before he can gain the necessary control and mastery of his muscles, many weeks of trying and of practice are necessary. The person who has suffered a stroke must go through a somewhat similar process of re-education before he can walk again. A brace is of great help in this process. The brace may be a long one, which runs from the hip down to the foot, or a short one starting below the knee. Braces are designed to stabilize the spastic extremity. With the aid of a brace, and perhaps with the help of canes, the use of a "walker," and manual support from an attendant, the patient eventually learns to walk again. Not uncommonly, his rehabilitation progresses from the use of a long leg brace to a short one, and he may even be able to discard all bracing after a period of time. As a rule, however, a cane or other support is useful in stabilizing the individual who has had a stroke.

The outlook for the hand and fingers is often less certain. It is not uncommon to see excellent restoration of function in the lower extremity, with only poor or partial restoration of function in the corresponding upper extremity. Again, only the passage of time, and earnest rehabilitation efforts, will enable one to judge what the residual disability is going to be.

The rehabilitation programs of the past twenty years have clearly shown that the outlook following a stroke is better than had previously been believed possible. Many a stroke patient who once would have been consigned to a wheelchair or bed for life can be made independent again in the activities of daily living, so that he is able to dress himself, feed himself, and take care of his bodily needs. The attainment of this level of competence, however, ordinarily requires the aid of certain specialists. The physiatrist is a doctor who specializes in rehabilitation. The physical therapist (physiotherapist) is a person trained in giving and supervising remedial and restorative exercises.

Q. *Some days I notice a forceful thumping in the left chest. What causes this?*
A. This is probably what many laymen refer to as palpitations. Most individuals look upon palpitations in terms of heart consciousness; they are aware of the beating of the heart, which is described as beating with greater force than usual. Often they describe a longer pause than usual between beats, or a series of rapid beats followed by a pause. The sequence of one or more strong beats followed by a slight pause is sometimes indicated on an electrocardiogram, or ECG. Not uncommonly, this condition is produced by a premature beat, one which comes a little ahead of schedule, followed by a com-

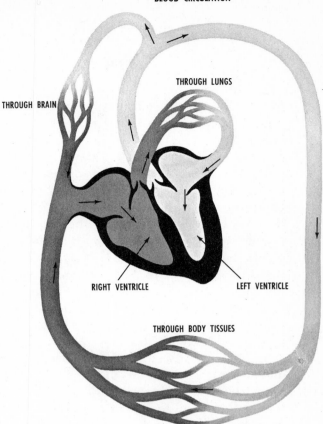

THROUGH BRAIN

THROUGH LUNGS

RIGHT VENTRICLE

LEFT VENTRICLE

THROUGH BODY TISSUES

pensatory pause, a rest interval which is longer than usual. Other variations in the heart rate and beat may contribute to the sensation described as palpitation. This may be noted at irregular intervals during the day, sometimes in "bursts." At other times palpitations recur in fairly regular fashion, every minute or two.

In general, palpitations are not a sign of heart disease. They can occur in persons whose heart, blood pressure, and general status are perfectly normal. However surprising or upsetting the sensation may be, there is usually no legitimate cause for worry. Palpitations may sometimes occur as a result of known causes which can be identified. Among these are fatigue and stress, too much smoking, or too much coffee or other stimulants. Palpitations often occur after a period of illness and in convalescence, or following abdominal distention or other digestive upsets. Overindulgence in tobacco, particularly cigarette smoking, may regularly produce skipped beats and other transient disorders, and can be regarded as a warning to cut down or even cut out smoking.

Q. *I notice large bluish veins over the upper leg, especially after standing. What causes this?*

A. This is probably the condition termed varicose veins. The chief difficulty in varicose veins is that the usual flow of blood through them is reversed. Instead of conducting blood upward toward the heart, the varicose vein often carries it in a reversed direction. The blood is finally siphoned off into the deep veins, and through them it is carried back on up to the heart. Varicose veins have a hereditary aspect, for the condition is sometimes seen in several members of a family.

Mild degrees are not a cause for concern. Women, however, often regard varicose veins as objectionable enough to demand treatment. Elastic stockings, by compressing the varicose veins, may afford

relief of pain and diminish the swelling of the legs associated with the varicosities. Very small varicose veins are sometimes injected with a sclerosing solution. This is a chemical agent that is injected into a segment of the vein. It produces inflammation and scarring, so that the vein is transformed into a scarred, little vessel.

Often, when the varicose vein is large and extensive, a stripping operation is performed. The segment of the vein is tied off at its upper portion, and through a series of small incisions the entire length of the varicose vein (it may extend from the groin down to the calf) is removed. The operation, of course, offers a total cure by virtue of total removal.

Q. *Why does my child throw himself on the floor and then kicks and screams?*
A. These are doubtless temper tantrums. Temper tantrums may take various forms and be most disturbing to parents. One is breath-holding, in which the child may hold his breath long enough so that he turns purple. More often, the temper tan-

trums consist of outbursts of stamping, kicking, and crying, with the child seemingly out of control and responding poorly to attempts to admonish or soothe him. Temper tantrums are by no means rare in children.

There are phases in the development of the child during which bouts of negativism are quite common. It is as though the child has sensed that he is an independent human being and is flaunting this fact by saying "no" to all requests, and by indulging in tantrums. Very often, the child is quite unresponsive to persuasion or discipline during the tantrum. One may have to stand by and wait for the tempest to blow itself out. Sometimes the child can be picked firmly off the floor, taken to his own room, and placed on his own bed. One may appropriately sit by the bedside and await the end of the tantrum. Some children will respond to a quiet talking-to, but with others this may be of no value.

Occasionally temper tantrums and breath-holding are used as weapons to frighten or blackmail parents into certain kinds of indulgences. Here firmness and consistency are necessary. Once the child learns that the maneuver will not work, and once this fact is increasingly driven home to him, the episodes may end. Sometimes temper tantrums represent an outlet for a sense of dissatisfaction and discontent that has developed within the child. The rivalry with a new baby, jealousy of the attention being given to another child in the family, a feeling of neglect, and the desire to gain attention may be contributing factors. Frequent and prolonged or persistent use of the temper tantrum by the child should lead the thoughtful parent searching for causes and for ways and means of dealing with the problem to consultation with a specialist.

Q. I often have spells of jumpiness and irritability. What causes this?
A. Symptoms of this sort are grouped into the category referred to as nervous tensions. By nervous tension most people mean a whole range of subjective sensations, including feeling of inner turmoil, jitters, and irritability. In some individuals the tension is manifested by a feeling of uneasiness, an anticipation that things may go badly. It may be associated with a sinking sensation in the abdomen, sometimes described as "butterflies in the stomach." This sensation, technically known as anxiety, is a fundamental aspect of nervous tension. Therefore, the fundamental question to be asked when someone describes such symptoms is: "What is the cause of the anxiety?"

In this age of physical violence, ranging from threats of worldwide atomic war to assassinations of presidents and all sorts of local acts of violence, many people experience tension caused by anxiety over the possibility of physical damage to themselves and their families. Many of us harbor anxieties generated by concern over the opinions of those about us, that is, fear of their disapproval or criticism. Sometimes our fears may be related to figures in authority, such as a parent, a boss, or a teacher. These examples show that sometimes the cause of tensions can be pinpointed fairly precisely while at other times, in the course of focusing on it and evaluating it, it may be seen by the patient as quite unjustified. Some reduction in anxiety and tension may then occur. What happens in psychotherapy is a prolonged investigation into the causes and origins of anxiety, and it is well established that this process does in fact free many people, to a considerable extent, from many of their nervous tensions.

The reality of many tensions is undeniable, and they may be experienced by many people. For immediate relief, medications are available which will allay the feelings of tension. Originally called sedatives, of which phenobarbital was a well-known early example, more recent drugs are referred to as tranquilizers. The presumed advantage of the tranquilizer is that it diminishes anxiety with relatively little effect on intellectual performance, so that feelings of sleepiness and difficulty in concentration need not be marked. The drugs meprobamate (Miltown®, Equanil®) and Librium® are some of the better-known tranquilizers that have been developed in recent years. Their advantage over old-fashioned phenobarbital is still being debated. Another group of drugs known as the phenothiazine drugs are sometimes referred to as major tranquilizers. They are prescribed for very disturbed states and have been effective in the control of various forms of psychosis, a major mental disturbance.

However, many people find ways and means of reducing their nervous tension without taking drugs. A warm bath or shower, a walk or some other physical activity, various kinds of diversion, all may have a tension-reducing effect. Certainly many people become overweight because they find that eating has a relaxing value for them. Anyone who experiences feelings of nervous tension frequently or repetitively should discuss this with a physician much as he would a fever or any other symptom, with the reasonable expectation that the doctor will be equally ready to treat emotional or psychic complaints.

Q. *My grandfather is getting on and is forgetful and sometimes seems silly. What causes this?*
A. This is most likely the condition referred to as senility. With the markedly increased life span of the United States population in recent decades, more and more elderly individuals are showing an impairment of brain activity. There seems to be little question that most of this is due to a progressive hardening of the arteries that lead to the brain. The result is a progressive enfeeblement of brain function. It starts off at first with signs of increased forgetfulness, wavering attention, difficulty in concentration, poor judgment in business and social dealings, negativism and irritability, and poor temper control. This sort of impairment can be somewhat trying on family and friends, but if it progresses no further than this, little difficulty in relations with the aging person is likely to occur.

In some individuals, however, further symptoms begin to appear. These include increased confusion, especially at night; insomnia, with a tendency to reverse the day-night cycle, so that the individual is up at night and drowses during the day; tendencies to wander and perhaps to level unjust accusations at other members of the household. Obviously, senility to this degree is difficult to live with; it also presents safety factors, since the individual may absentmindedly turn on the gas jet and not light it, or, wandering off, may get lost.

Sometimess, a "total-push" program involving good nutrition, supplementary vitamins, pleasant stimulation, and encouragement to participate in activities at some level, may bring improvement. When it does not, and when the care of such a patient becomes very trying to the members of the family—as it often does because of the round-the-clock care that may be involved—custodial placement may be advised. This generally means a nursing home, where custodial nursing care and supervision are available. This solution is often difficult for families to face, and sometimes it is only a last resort when patience and strength have been exhausted.

Helpful
Public Agencies

SEVERAL YEARS AGO, A physician from the United States was visiting a hospital in Central Africa. He was shown a patient suffering from severe beriberi, a case so far advanced that it went beyond any textbook description of the disease.

Afterwards, discussing the case with his guest, the resident senior physician made a significant comment. "In your country you could never even see such a case because society would not permit any illness to progress to this stage." This remark seems to characterize the spirit in which are organized so many of the community facilities that make aid freely available to our people. True, a wide range of difference exists from community to community as to the number and kind of agencies operating there; but even in the smaller town and rural area some, at least, are to be found.

A word should first be said about the role of the family doctor, whose steadfast work has long sustained and protected us and our families. The doctor's efforts are largely in the realm of clinical services for the sick, and he also makes himself available for preventive measures as well as for medical counseling. The public agencies, on the other hand, deal to a lesser extent with illness, concentrating most of their work on prevention, education, and in some instances on research.

The advent of Medicare and Medicaid (the former a Federal financing of health services for those over age 65, the latter a state-administered financing for the medically indigent) is indication of governmental interest in the delivery of health services. Also, recent legislation leading to a massive Federally sponsored attack on the cancer problem emphasizes the governmental potential.

Governmental and Nongovernmental Agencies

In this country, health services are provided through local public health departments that are organized on a county, city, or in some instances a township basis. In certain areas, several such different units may combine to form a single district health unit. The main objectives of the public health agency are the prevention of disease and the promotion of health. This is accomplished largely through improved environmental sanitation, control of communicable diseases, public-health education, and various services to the individual which will be described later. Ultimate responsibility is vested in a state health department or a state board of health, whose function it is to institute standards for health work, to provide expert technical consultation, and to give material as well as professional assistance to localities.

On the Federal level, the principal health agency is the Department of Health and Human Services. Another agency within this department is the Children's Bureau, which deals with health problems of children, as well as with social matters, child labor questions, and other concerns relating to children.

Additional governmental—tax-supported—agencies, although primarily concerned with other functions, are also instrumental in protecting and promoting the health of the public. National, state, and local levels of government often have agencies, such as departments of agriculture, education, fire, labor, mental hygiene, police, and social welfare, which are involved in public health.

Nongovernmental agencies active in health work are so numerous that they cannot possibly all be listed by name, except in relation to specific programs. However, citing a few of the categories will doubtless bring to mind the particular facilities with which the individual citizen may be familiar. A number of the national health societies and associations have state and local chapters, and it is largely through these that their programs are implemented. Identification in a telephone directory may follow a pattern like this: the local branch of the National Diabetes Association may be listed as the Manhattan County Diabetes Association. Church and fraternal associations, service clubs, farm and home groups, youth organizations, and many other groups perform important health services in many various kinds of communities. An upsurge in the construction of community hospitals is making patient care facilities accessible to many more people than was the case only a few years ago.

This brief summary of the kinds of health services made potentially available to us on a community basis serves only to suggest the list of circumstances under which persons may seek assistance as they need it. Not all apply to any one community. But there is definite value in the individual citizen's being aware of what does exist beyond his own area, so that he may better realize what might be required by way of added facilities in his locality as well.

Accidents and Emergencies

In the case of most accidents, particularly those involving motor vehicles, the most effective agency is the police department, be it state or municipal, or else the county sheriff's office. Not only do they respond quickly to calls for assistance, but they also possess certain equipment which enables them to deal with emergencies. In those types of emergencies where respirators may be needed, the assistance of the fire department is most valuable.

An important public service has for many years been rendered by the American Red Cross and its many state and local chapters in offering, among other valuable services, first-aid instruction. The training thus provided is of incalculable value, and it is urged that everyone take the course particularly those persons likely to be confronted by emergencies where no medical aid is readily available. A word of commendation should also be directed to the Boy Scouts of America (and the counterpart organizations for girls) who have given so many young people an understanding of the nature of accidents, of how to avoid them, and what to do in the face of an emergency.

In many communities, Poison Control centers have been established. These centers, which respond to telephone calls twenty-four hours a day, maintain up-to-date information on commercial and industrial products, particularly those which are potentially dangerous, and can offer prompt suggestions as to antidotes. Householders and persons who handle chemicals should therefore routinely take the following precautions: (1) determine where the nearest such center is located (generally listed in the telephone directory as Poison Control Center) and post its telephone number in a prominent place; (2) in case of accident, be prepared to name the products involved and to write down the suggestions they are given for antidotes and other emergency treatment.

A word might be added regarding the work of the Red Cross, Civilian Defense Organizations, National Guard, and other agencies in disaster relief. Considerable planning has resulted in a promptness with which people and materials may be brought together when community emergencies arise.

Communicable Diseases

In this era of rapid travel epidemics tend to be more widespread than before, and health departments continue with the control of communicable diseases as their major activity. Especially effective against most of these diseases has been control of various channels of transmission.

This includes purification of water supplies, sanitary disposal of sewage, pasteurization of milk, restriction of disease carriers, control of insect and animal sources of infection, examination and education of food handlers, and similar measures, all of which are assigned by law to the health department. It is clear that the prevailing principle in this work is prevention.

Equally characteristic of the principle of preventive medicine is the attempt to increase immunity against certain diseases through the use of vaccines in various forms. In this activity, the family physician plays a leading role, although in many communities the public health department supplements his work by promoting wider use of immunizations and by conducting mass campaigns on specific occasions.

Valuable contributions have been made to our knowledge of communicable diseases and their prevention by research work carried on in many areas. For many years, support for such work had been forthcoming from agencies which relied on public contributions; now, however, governmental sources of funds for research work are proportionately increasing. This is all to the good, for the more we learn about means of prevention of disease, the sooner will the public reap the resulting benefits.

Some communicable diseases have long been singled out for special attention by public health departments, among them the venereal diseases, tuberculosis, and leprosy. Since the potential public hazards they represented were considerable, lasting over a period of time, governmental agencies took full responsibility for control and care of the infected individuals. For example, a promiscuous person affected with a venereal disease could be detained by court order until such time as he or she was rendered noninfectious. Governmental action went even further in the case of tuberculosis, when state, as well as many county and municipal sanatoriums were built for the dual purpose of providing proper treatment for the tuberculous patient and of keeping him "out of circulation" until he was no longer a threat to others. Although leprosy is not a widespread disease in this country, the Federal government maintains a leprosarium in Carville, Louisiana. Its purposes are in a general sense similar to those of tuberculosis sanatoriums.

In the realm of voluntary health agencies dealing with communicable diseases, the National Tuberculosis Association, and its local chapters, is among the oldest and best known to the general public. Others are the National Foundation, whose work was popularized by the late President Franklin D. Roosevelt, and the American Social Health Association, whose concern is with the venereal diseases. These voluntary agencies, and others like them, through public contributions support widespread educational campaigns, research programs, and in some instances direct community services.

Prenatal and Infant Care

Public health departments have, for many years, been interested in maternal and infant health. Causes of illness and death among mothers and children have been carefully studied, and preventive measures developed. In general, early and regular medical supervision has been the principle under which prenatal and infant programs have operated.

Health departments have long urged the expectant mother to visit her physician early in pregnancy, and over the years this has become an accepted pattern. In those communities where appreciable numbers of persons were without a physician, or where for some reason such services were not readily available, public health departments have established prenatal clinics, sometimes in cooperation with hospitals. Actual home delivery care services have also been developed in certain areas, although this is not so necessary because of

the existence of hospitals in most areas.

The public health nurse has been a valuable aid in promoting early prenatal care and regular baby supervision. As a member of the health department staff, she visits homes and makes contact with parents, in order to teach the value of medical attention during these two crucial periods. She works closely with the physicians in the community, as well as with the personnel of the health department or hospital clinic, and interprets the doctor's instructions to the patient or parent. Particularly important are demonstrations of baby care, food preparation, bathing, and other similar instructions. The community-wide immunization program has, of course, been part of infant care.

In many parts of the country, especially areas remote from medical centers and specialists, the tracking down, identification, treatment, and rehabilitation of handicapped children have occupied the attention of state and local health departments, as well as of Crippled Children's societies and others. The public health nurse has been responsible for finding many such children and bringing them to medical attention, either to the physicians in the community itself or to one of the itinerant clinics established by the health department. The expenditure of public funds in such an instance is more than justified by an attempt insofar as possible to remove whatever physical barriers might otherwise prevent an individual from becoming self-supporting, as well as on humanitarian grounds.

School Health Services

Health services for school children, extending even into secondary schools and colleges, are now an accepted part of our way of life. Teachers and other school personnel are expected to refer children to the school nurse whenever any suspicion of ill health is aroused. Further investigation of the child's condition is then carried on by the school physician, with referral for care to the family doctor.

In addition, routine physical examinations are performed on each child at certain stages of his school career, with the same purpose in mind, namely to discover previously unknown defects. One important responsibility of the parent is to follow through the recommendations of the school nurse and physician so that some advantageous results may be achieved; otherwise the child will merely continue to suffer from a condition that will constantly be "re-discovered" without his benefiting from the efforts expended in his behalf.

The physician and nurse are assisted by a school dentist, who examines all school children at regular intervals and refers them for dental care when needed. In some communities, certain treatment procedures are undertaken by the school dentist, but in most instances referrals are made to the family dentist. Dental hygienists also work with school children in screening them for the examination by the dentist and in performing prophylactic procedures.

Special tests, such as those for hearing and vision, are performed by teachers trained to make such tests or, in larger areas, by special personnel in these fields. The use of modern equipment provides considerably more information about a child than was possible even a few years ago, and in those instances where indicated referral is made to the school physician. In some communities, treatment facilities have been developed by Parent-Teacher Associations (the PTA) and by some of the service clubs.

Medical and Hospital Care

While medical care is traditionally provided by the private physician, in some communities public facilities have been established for certain population groups. Particularly in the larger centers, those persons who are unable to pay for physicians' services are now able to obtain care through free or low-cost clinics. Also, eligible for public care is the veteran with a service-connected disability. In addition, military personnel and their dependents have had medical care made available to them. Now the plight of persons over sixty-five years of age is being recognized by government agencies, and assistance is being developed for them.

The insurance principle has become a popular means of providing medical care for individuals as well as for groups. Most numerous are the health plans sponsored by labor unions and other employee groups, whereby payment is made into a fund which then reimburses the patient or physician, or both, at the time of illness. Some groups maintain their own full-time medical facilities and staff, paid out of the funds collected from members and employers.

In addition to medical care in times of illness, provision is made in many places to protect the life and health of workers, especially in the hazardous trades. Industrial plants employ physicians, nurses, engineers, and others to examine employees, detect ill effects (depending on the nature of the work), provide emergency care, and maintain safe and healthful working conditions.

The construction of a large number of hospitals in the last decade has made facilities for in-patient care available to many more persons than ever before. Simultaneously, the growth of local and national hospitalization plans has provided increased opportunities for people to take advantage of modern scientific developments. In fact, hospital bed utilization has swelled to such an extent that other, less expensive, community facilities are being established in many places. One of the most useful devices is the nursing home, where patients who are convalescing or who need long-term care may enjoy the facilities they require without paying for the more costly hospital stay. Another approach to reducing prolonged hospitalization has been the home care program. Here visiting nurses assist relatives in providing adequate care by teaching what a patient's requirements may be and how to meet them. Back in his own home, with trained persons employed to assist him, the patient usually finds himself recovering rapidly—granted his condition permits early discharge from the hospital. Some persons, on the advice of their physicians, undertake home care rather than hospitalization or nursing home treatment throughout the illness.

The Visiting Nurse Association, through its local branches, has long been a valuable adjunct to the private physician, hospital, and nursing home in providing home services in case of illness.

Mental Health Agencies

Care of the mentally ill in institutions designed for that purpose has long been a public community responsibility, usually under a branch of the state government. With the development of better general understanding of the nature of mental illness, active treatment of these patients both in and out of hospital has been growing in importance. Community mental health clinics have been organized, sometimes under the sponsorship of the public health agency, and preventive as well as therapeutic measures are being used. The term preventive, it should be noted, is not used here in the same sense when applied to a communicable disease, since specific agents are not available for immunization. However, the availability of clinical facilities where a trained, sympathetic professional worker can discuss personal problems has in many instances aided in preventing further emotional distress or disturbance. This facility may generally be located as the "Mental Health Clinic," or through inquiry of the health department.

One of the most valuable public services made possible by such clinics is the creation of a "suicide squad," with pro-

visions for twenty-four-hour emergency duty. Trained health workers usually combine forces with social workers, clergy, and other volunteers in responding to calls when impending suicide attempts are suspected. The goal of such a squad is to keep the patient from carrying out his threat until he can be safely placed under psychiatric care.

Some communities have established programs to combat alcoholism, generally in the Mental Health Clinic, whether under the aegis of public health departments, nongovernmental agencies, or both. Alcoholism may be variously considered as a physical affliction, a psychological illness, a social disease, a moral weakness, or any combination of these; and therefore in any community only a multiple attack on the problem offers reasonable hope of success. While professional help, as obtained in clinics, is important in effecting treatment for this condition, many sufferers have achieved gratifying results through adherence to programs like those of Alcoholics Anonymous. This is a fellowship of men and women who group together for the purpose of remaining sober and helping each other attain sobriety.

An ever-growing problem in many communities is that of narcotic addiction. While this too is a social problem, its features are largely medical, and patients require adequate medical supervision to "cure" the habit. In some places, mental hygiene clinics have their own narcotic sections, elsewhere separate treatment facilities are provided within the hospital or health department framework. The United States Public Health Service maintains a hospital for treatment of addicts and for research in Lexington, Kentucky. In addition, many state mental hospitals accept this type of patient. Police cooperation is of course necessary in dealing with the law-breaking aspects of narcotics.

Special Health Problems

A unique phenomenon of our society

is the existence of a large number of associations devoted to individual diseases or separate organs. The National Tuberculosis Association, mentioned earlier, is an example of the former type; the American Heart Association, of the latter. A few others include the American Cancer Society, the Arthritis and Rheumatism Foundation, the Guide Dog Foundation for the Blind, the National Amputation Foundation, the National Association for Mental Health, and the Parkinson's Disease Foundation. These are listed only because they exemplify the wide range of interests represented, and not because they are larger or more important than others which have been omitted. Certainly a comprehensive list of the voluntary health agencies would be beyond the scope of this chapter. However, a coordinating agency known as the National Health Council, located at 1790 Broadway, New York 19, N.Y., can provide information about the existence of associations devoted to any particular health problem.

Most of the voluntary health agencies are national in scope, with some of them maintaining international relationships with similar groups in other countries and with the World Health Organization. Their support is through financial contributions by the public, the funds being used for research, public education, and direct service programs in many localities. Some of these agencies operate only nationally, while others have state and local branches (located as described earlier). A great proportion of the actual tasks is done by interested volunteers under the direction of a relatively small staff of professional workers. Collaboration with governmental health agencies (federal, state, and local) is a principle to which these voluntary groups adhere.

In some communities, a valuable aid to physicians, educators, and social workers is a Guidebook to Social and Health Agencies. Here are listed the various facilities to which persons with special problems may be referred, together with a description of the services offered.

In recent years, health departments have recognized a growing need for providing special health problem facilities, and have thus established services for cancer detection, diabetes testing, chronic disease programs, nutrition clinics, and others. For those conditions for which a readily performed test is available, mass surveys are often conducted by health departments. Multiphasic screening involves two or more tests performed on a population group during a single operation. Where positive or suspected results are obtained, patients are referred to their own physicians for follow-up.

Educational Materials

Health departments and local branches of the national voluntary health agencies are prepared to distribute literature on many pertinent health subjects. In some instances, these agencies are able to provide lecturers, motion pictures, film strips, and other education programs and materials. Information regarding television and other scripts is also available from the national association or from the local branch (which may be identified and located as described earlier).

Many young people are interested in career opportunities in one of the health professions, such as medicine, dentistry, nursing, veterinary medicine, nutrition, health education, and a host of others. The local health agency is of course a valuable source of information, especially with regard to the functions performed by various persons in health work. However, supplementary to a personal visit to the health department or a voluntary health agency, a person may obtain further information from the national association dealing with the profession of his interest.

Appendix

CALORIES USED TO PERFORM CERTAIN ACTIVITIES
CALORIE VALUES IN COMMON FOODS
FAST FOODS CALORIE CHART
SAMPLE DIETS
RECOMMENDED DAILY DIETARY ALLOWANCES

CALORIES USED TO PERFORM CERTAIN ACTIVITIES*

Type of activity	Calories per hour
Sedentary activities, such as: Reading; writing; eating; watching television or movies; listening to the radio; sewing; playing cards; and typing, miscellaneous officework, and other activities done while sitting that require little or no arm movement.	80 to 100.
Light activities, such as: Preparing and cooking food; doing dishes; dusting; handwashing small articles of clothing; ironing; walking slowly; personal care; miscellaneous officework and other activities done while standing that require some arm movement; and rapid typing and other activities done while sitting that are more strenuous.	110 to 160.
Moderate activities, such as: Making beds; mopping and scrubbing; sweeping; light polishing and waxing; laundering by machine; light gardening and carpentry work; walking moderately fast; other activities done while standing that require moderate arm movement; and activities done while sitting that require more vigorous arm movement.	170 to 240.
Vigorous activities, such as: Heavy scrubbing and waxing; handwashing large articles of clothing; hanging out clothes; stripping beds; other heavy work; walking fast; bowling; golfing; and gardening.	250 to 350.
Strenuous activities, such as: Swimming; playing tennis; running; bicycling; dancing; skiing; and playing football.	350 and more.

CALORIE VALUES IN COMMON FOODS*

MILK, CHEESE, AND ICE CREAM

		Number of Calories
Fluid milk:		
Whole	1 cup or glass	165
Skim (fresh or nonfat dry reconstituted).	1 cup or glass	90
Buttermilk	1 cup or glass	90
Evaporated, (undiluted) ..	½ cup	170
Condensed, sweetened (undiluted).	½ cup	490
Half-and-half (milk and cream.	1 cup	330
Cream, light	1 tablespoon	20
Cream, heavy whipping	1 tablespoon	35
Yoghurt (made from partially skimmed milk).	1 tablespoon	55
	1 cup	120
Cheese:		
American, Cheddar-type ...	1 ounce	115
	1-inch cube (3/5 ounce) .	70
	½ cup, grated (2 ounces)	225
Process American, Cheddar-type.	1 ounce	105
Blue-mold (or Roquefort-type).	1 ounce	105
Cottage, not creamed	2 tablespoons (1 ounce).	25
Cottage, creamed	2 tablespoons (1 ounce).	30
Cream	2 tablespoons (1 ounce).	105
Parmesan, dry, grated	2 tablespoons (1/3 ounce)	40
Swiss	1 ounce	105
Milk beverages:		
Cocoa (all milk)	1 cup	235
Chocolate-flavored milk drink.	1 cup	190
Malted milk	1 cup	280
Chocolate milkshake	One 12-ounce container .	520
Ice cream, plain	1 container (3½ fluid ounces	130
Ice milk	½ cup (4 fluid ounces) ..	140
Ice cream soda, chocolate	1 large glass	455

MEAT, POULTRY, FISH, EGGS, DRY BEANS AND PEAS, NUTS

Meat, cooked, without bone:
Beef:
Pot roast or braised:

MEAT, POULTRY, FISH, EGGS, DRY BEANS AND PEAS, NUTS—Continued

		Number of Calories
Lean and fat	3 ounces (1 thick or 2 thin slices, 4 by 2½ inches).	245
Lean only	2½ ounces (1 thick or 2 thin slices, 4 by 2 inches).	140
Oven roast:		
Cut having relatively large proportion of fat to lean:		
Lean and fat	3 ounces (1 thick or 2 thin slices, 4 by 2½ inches).	390
Lean only	2 ounces (1 thick or 2 thin slices, 4 by 1½ inches).	120
Cut having relatively low proportion of fat to lean:		
Lean and fat	3 ounces (1 thick or 2 thin slices, 4 by 2½ inches).	220
Lean only	2½ ounces (1 thick or 2 thin slices, 4 by 2 inches).	130
Steak, broiled:		
Lean and fat	3 ounces (1 piece, 4 by 2½ inches by ½ inch).	330
Lean only	2 ounces (1 piece, 4 by 1½ inches by ½ inch).	115
Hamburger patty:		
Regular ground beef ..	3-ounce patty (about 4 patties per pound of raw meat).	245
Lean ground round ...	3-ounce patty (about 4 patties per pound of raw meat).	185
Corned beef, canned	3 ounces (1 piece, 4 by 2½ inches by ½ inch).	180
Corned beef hash, canned	3 ounces (scant half cup)	120
Dried beef, chipped	2 ounces (about ½ cup).	115
Meat loaf	2 ounces (1 piece, 4 by 2½ inches by ½ inch).	115
Beef and vegetable stew..	½ cup	90
Beef potpie, baked	1 pie, 4¼ inch diameter, about 8 ounces before baking.	460
Chile con carne, canned:		

*Food and Your Weight Bulletin No. 74 U.S. Department of Agriculture.

CALORIE VALUES IN COMMON FOODS

MEAT, POULTRY, FISH, EGGS, DRY BEANS AND PEAS, NUTS—Continued		Number of Calories
Without beans	½ cup	255
With beans	½ cup	170
Veal:		
Cutlet, broiled, meat only..	3 ounces (1 piece, 4 by 2½ inches by ½ inch).	185
Lamb:		
Chop (about 2½ chops to a pound, as purchased):		
Lean and fat	4 ounces	405
Lean only	2-3/5 ounces	140
Roast, leg:		
Lean and fat	3 ounces (1 thick or 2 thin slices, 3½ by 3 inches).	235
Lean only	2½ ounces (1 thick or 2 thin slices, 3½ by 2½ inches).	130
Pork:		
Fresh:		
Chop (about 3 chops to a pound, as purchased):		
Lean and fat	2½ ounces	260
Lean only	2 ounces	130
Roast, loin:		
Lean and fat	3 ounces (1 thick or 2 thin slices, 4 by 2½ inches.	310
Lean only	2-2/5 ounces (1 thick or 2 thin slices, 3 by 2½ inches).	175
Cured: Ham:		
Lean and fat	3 ounces (1 thick or 2 thin slices, 4 by 2 inches).	290
Lean only	2-1/5 ounces (1 thick or 2 thin slices, 3½ by 2 inches).	125
Bacon, broiled or fried	2 very thin slices	95
Sausage and variety and luncheon meats:		
Bologna sausage	2 ounces (2 very thin slices, 4 inches in diameter).	170
Liver sausage (liverwurst)	2 ounces (4 very thin slices, 3 inches in diameter).	175
Vienna sausage, canned..	2 ounces (4 to 5 sausages)	135
Pork sausage, bulk	2 ounces (1 patty, 2 inches in diameter), (4 to 5 patties per pound, raw).	170
Liver, beef, fried (includes fat for frying).	2 ounces (1 thick piece, 3 by 2½ inches).	120
Heart, beef, braised, trimmed of fat.	3 ounces (1 thick piece, 4 by 2½ inches).	160
Tongue, beef, boiled	3 ounces (1 thick slice, 4 by 2½ inches).	205
Frankfurter	1 frankfurter	155
Boiled ham (luncheon meat).	2 ounces (2 very thin slices, 3½ by 3½ inches).	170
Spiced ham, canned	2 ounces (2 thin slices, 3 by 2½ inches).	165
Poultry, cooked, without bone:		
Chicken:		
Broiled	3 ounces, about ¼ of a small broiler).	185
Fried	½ breast, 2-4/5 ounces	215
	1 leg (thigh and drumstick), 3 ounces.	245
Canned	3½ ounces (½ cup)	190
Poultry pie (with potatoes, peas, and gravy).	1 small pie, 4¼ inches in diameter (about 8 ounces before cooking).	485
Fish and shellfish:		
Bluefish, baked	3 ounces (1 piece, 3½ by 2 inches by ½ inch).	135
Clams, shelled:		
Raw, meat only	3 ounces (about 4 medium clams).	70
Canned, clams and juice	3 ounces (1 scant half cup, 3 medium clams and juice.)	45
Crab meat, canned or cooked	3 ounces, ½ cup	90
Fish sticks, breaded, cooked, frozen (including breading and fat for frying).	4 ounces (5 fish sticks)	200
Haddock, fried (including fat for frying).	3 ounces (1 fillet, 4 by 2½ inches by ½ inch).	135
Mackerel:		
Broiled	3 ounces (1 piece, 4 by 3 inches by ½ inch).	200
Canned	3 ounces, solids and liquid (about 3/5 cup).	155
Ocean perch, fried (includ-	3 ounces (1 piece, 4 by	

MEAT, POULTRY, FISH, EGGS, DRY BEANS AND PEAS, NUTS—Continued		Number of Calories
ing egg, breadcrumbs, and fat for frying).	2½ inches by ½ inch).	195
Oysters, shucked: Raw meat only.	½ cup (6 to 10 medium-size oysters, selects).	80
Salmon:		
Broiled or baked	4 ounces (1 steak, 4½ by 2½ inches by ½ inch).	205
Canned (pink)	3 ounces, solids and liquid, about 3/5 cup.	120
Sardines, canned in oil	3 ounces, drained solids (5 to 7 medium sardines).	180
Shrimp, canned, meat only.	3 ounces (about 17 medium shrimp).	110
Tunafish, canned in oil, meat only.	3 ounces (about 2/5 cup)	170
Eggs:		
Fried (including fat for frying).	1 large egg	100
Hard or soft cooked, "boiled"	1 large egg	80
Scrambled or omelet including milk and fat for cooking).	1 large egg	110
Poached	1 large egg	80
Dry beans and peas:		
Red kidney beans, canned or cooked.	½ cup, solids and liquid..	115
Lima, cooked	½ cup, solids and liquid..	130
Baked beans, with tomato or molasses:		
With pork	½ cup	165
Without pork	½ cup	160
Nuts:		
Almonds, shelled	2 tablespoons (about 13 to 15 almonds).	105
Brazil nuts, shelled, broken pieces.	2 tablespoons	115
Cashew nuts, roasted	2 tablespoons (about 4 to 5 nuts).	95
Coconut:		
Fresh, shredded meat	2 tablespoons	40
Dried, shredded, sweetened.	2 tablespoons	45
Peanuts, roasted, shelled	2 tablespoons	105
Peanut butter	1 tablespoon	90
Pecans, shelled halves	2 tablespoons (about 12 to 14 halves).	90
Walnuts, shelled:		
Black or native, chopped	2 tablespoons	100
English or Persian, halves	2 tablespoons (about 7 to 12 halves).	80

VEGETABLES AND FRUITS

Vegetables:		
Asparagus, cooked or canned	6 medium spears or ½ cup cut spears.	20
Beans:		
Lima, green, cooked or canned.	½ cup	75
Snap, green, wax or yellow, cooked or canned.	½ cup	15
Beets, cooked or canned	½ cup, diced	35
Beet greens, cooked	½ cup	20
Broccoli, cooked	½ cup flower stalks	20
Brussels sprouts, cooked	½ cup	30
Cabbage:		
Raw	½ cup, shredded	10
	1 wedge, 3½ by 4½ inches	25
Coleslaw (with salad dressing).	½ cup	50
Cooked	½ cup	20
Carrots:		
Raw	1 carrot, 5½ inches by 1 inch in diameter, or 25 thin slices.	20
	½ cup, grated	20
Cooked	½ cup, diced	20
Cauliflower, cooked	½ cup flower buds	15
Celery, raw	2 large stalks, 8 inches long, or 3 small stalks, 5 inches long.	10
Chard, cooked	½ cup leaves	25
	½ cup leaves and stalks.	15
Collards, cooked	½ cup	40
Corn:		
On cob, cooked	1 ear, 5 inches long	65
Kernels, cooked or canned	½ cup	85
Cress, garden, cooked	½ cup	35
Cucumbers, raw, pared	6 slices, ⅛ inch thick, center section.	5
Kale, cooked	½ cup	20
Kohlrabi, cooked	½ cup	25

CALORIE VALUES IN COMMON FOODS

VEGETABLES AND FRUITS—Continued		Number of Calories
Lettuce, raw	2 large or 4 small leaves	5
Mushrooms, canned	½ cup	15
Mustard greens, cooked	½ cup	15
Okra, cooked	4 pods, 3 inches long, ⅝ inch in diameter.	15
Onions:		
Young, green, raw	6 small, without tops	25
Mature:		
Raw	1 onion, 2½ inches in diameter.	50
	1 tablespoon, chopped	5
Cooked	½ cup	40
Parsnips, cooked	½ cup	50
Peas, green:		
Cooked or canned	½ cup	60
Peppers, green:		
Raw or cooked	1 medium	15
Potatoes:		
Baked or broiled	1 medium, 2½ inches in diameter (5 ounces raw).	90
Chips (including fat for frying).	10 medium, 2 inches in diameter.	110
French-fried (including fat for frying):		
Ready-to-eat	10 pieces, 2 inches by ½ inch by ½ inch.	155
Frozen, ready to be heated for serving.	10 pieces, 2 inches by ½ inch by ½ inch.	95
Hash-browned	½ cup	235
Mashed:		
Milk added	½ cup	70
Milk and fat added	½ cup	115
Pan-fried, beginning with raw potatoes.	½ cup	240
Radishes, raw	4 small	10
Sauerkraut, canned	½ cup	15
Spinach, cooked or canned	½ cup	20
Squash:		
Summer, cooked	½ cup	20
Winter, baked, mashed	½ cup	50
Sweetpotatoes:		
Baked in jacket	1 medium, 5 by 2 inches (6 ounces raw).	155
Canned, vacuum or solid pack.	½ cup	120
Tomatoes:		
Raw	1 medium, 2 by 2½ inches (about ⅓ pound).	30
Cooked or canned	½ cup	25
Tomato juice, canned	½ cup	25
Turnips, cooked	½ cup	20
Turnip greens, cooked	½ cup	20
Fruits:		
Apples, raw	1 medium, 2½ inches in diameter (about ⅓ pound).	70
Applejuice, fresh or canned	½ cup	60
Applesauce:		
Sweetened	½ cup	90
Unsweetened	½ cup	50
Apricots:		
Raw	3 (about 12 to a pound, as purchased).	55
Canned:		
Water packed	½ cup, halves and liquid	45
Heavy sirup pack	½ cup, halves and sirup	110
Dried, cooked, unsweetened.	½ cup, fruit and juice	120
Frozen, sweetened	½ cup	125
Avocados:		
California varieties	½ of a 10-ounce avocado (3⅓ by 4¼ inches).	185
Florida varieties	½ of a 13-ounce avocado (4 by 3 inches).	160
Bananas, raw	1 medium (6 by 1½ inches, about ⅓ pound).	85
Berries:		
Blackberries, raw	½ cup	40
Blueberries, raw	½ cup	45
Raspberries:		
Fresh, red, raw	½ cup	35
Frozen, red, sweetened	½ cup	120
Fresh, black, raw	½ cup	40
Strawberries:		
Fresh, raw	½ cup	30
Frozen, sweetened	½ cup	120
Cantaloup, raw	½ melon, 5 inches in diameter.	40
Cherries:		
Raw (sour, sweet, and hybrid).	½ cup	30
Canned (red, sour, pitted)	½ cup	55
Cranberry sauce, cooked or canned, sweetened.	1 tablespoon	30

VEGETABLES AND FRUITS—Continued		Number of Calories
Cranberry juice cocktail, canned.	½ cup	70
Dates, "fresh" and dried, pitted, cut.	½ cup	250
Figs:		
Raw	3 small (1½ inches in diameter, about ¼ pound)	90
Canned, heavy sirup	½ cup	110
Dried	1 large (2 inches by 1 inch).	60
Fruit cocktail, canned in heavy sirup.	½ cup	100
Grapefruit:		
Raw:		
White	½ medium (4¼ inches in diameter, No. 64's).	50
	½ cup sections	40
Pink or red	½ medium (4¼ inches in diameter, No. 64's).	55
Canned:		
Water pack	½ cup	35
Sirup pack	½ cup	80
Grapefruit juice:		
Raw	½ cup	50
Canned:		
Unsweetened	½ cup	50
Sweetened	½ cup	65
Frozen concentrate, diluted, ready to serve:		
Unsweetened	½ cup	50
Sweetened	½ cup	55
Grapes, raw:		
American type (including Concord, Delaware, Niagara, and Scuppernong), slip skin.	1 bunch (3½ by 3 inches; about 3½ ounces)	45
	½ cup, with skins and seeds	35
European type (including Malaga, Muscat, Thompson seedless, and Flame Tokay), adherent skin.	½ cup	50
Grapejuice, bottled	½ cup	75
Honeydew melon, raw	1 wedge, 2 by 7 inches	50
Lemon juice, raw or canned	½ cup	30
	1 tablespoon	5
Lemonade, frozen concentrate, sweetened, diluted, ready to serve.	½ cup	55
Orange, raw	1 orange, 3 inches in diameter.	70
Orange juice:		
Raw	½ cup	60
Canned, unsweetened	½ cup	60
Frozen concentrate, diluted, ready to serve.	½ cup	55
Peaches:		
Raw	1 medium, 2 inches in diameter (about ¼ pound).	35
	½ cup, sliced	30
Canned:		
Water packed	½ cup	40
Heavy sirup pack	½ cup	100
Dried, cooked, unsweetened.	½ cup (5 to 6 halves and 3 tablespoons sirup).	110
Frozen, sweetened	½ cup	105
Pears:		
Raw	1 pear, 3 by 2½ inches in diameter.	100
Canned in heavy sirup	½ cup	100
Pineapple:		
Raw	½ cup, diced	35
Canned in heavy sirup:		
Crushed	½ cup	100
Sliced	2 small or 1 large slice and 2 tablespoons juice.	95
Pineapple juice, canned	½ cup	60
Plums:		
Raw	1 plum, 2 inches in diameter (about 2 ounces).	30
Canned, sirup pack	½ cup	90
Prunes, dried, cooked:		
Unsweetened	½ cup (8 to 9 prunes and 2 tablespoons liquid).	150
Sweetened	½ cup (8 to 9 prunes and 2 tablespoons liquid).	260
Prune juice, canned	½ cup	85
Raisins, dried	½ cup	230
Rhubarb, cooked, sweetened	½ cup	190
Tangerine, raw	1 medium, 2½ inches in diameter, (about ¼ pound).	40
Tangerine juice, canned	½ cup	50
Watermelon, raw	1 wedge, 4 by 8 inches long (about 2 pounds, including rind).	120

CALORIE VALUES IN COMMON FOODS

BREADS AND CEREALS

		Number of Calories
Bread:		
Cracked wheat	1 slice, ½ inch thick ...	60
Raisin	1 slice, ½ inch thick ...	60
Rye	1 slice, ½ inch thick ...	55
White	1 slice, ½ inch thick ...	60
Whole Wheat	1 slice, ½ inch thick ...	55
Other baked goods:		
Baking powder biscuit	1 biscuit, 2½ inches in diameter.	130
Crackers:		
Graham	4 small or 2 medium	55
Saltines	2 crackers, 2 inches square	35
Soda	2 crackers, 2½ inches square, or 10 oyster crackers.	45
Doughnuts (cake type) ...	1 doughnut	135
Muffins:		
Plain	1 muffin, 2¾ inches in diameter.	135
Bran	1 muffin, 2¾ inches in diameter.	125
Corn	1 muffin, 2¾ inches in diameter.	155
Pancakes (griddle cakes):		
Wheat(home recipe) ..	1 cake, 4 inches in diameter.	60
Buckwheat (with buckwheat pancake mix).	1 cake, 4 inches in diameter.	45
Pizza (cheese)	5½-inch sector, ⅛ of a 14-inch pie.	180
Pretzels	5 small sticks	20
Rolls:		
Plain, pan	1 roll (16 ounces per dozen)	115
Hard, round	1 roll (22 ounces per dozen).	160
Sweet, pan	1 roll (18 ounces per dozen).	135
Rye wafers	2 wafers, 1⅞ by 3½ inches	45
Waffles	1 waffle, 4½ by 5½ inches by ½ inch.	240
Cakes, cookies, pies. (See Desserts).		
Cereals and other grain products:		
Bran flakes (40-percent bran)	1 ounce (about 4/5 cup)	85
Corn, puffed, presweetened	1 ounce (about 1 cup)..	110
Corn and soy shreds	1 ounce (about 4/5 cup)	100
Corn flakes	1 ounce (about 1-1/3 cups)	110
Corn grits, degermed, cooked	¾ cup	90
Farina, cooked	¾ cup	80
Macaroni, cooked	¾ cup	115
Macaroni and cheese	½ cup	240
Noodles, cooked	¾ cup	150
Oat cereal (mixture mainly oat flour).	1 ounce (about 1⅛ cups)	115
Oatmeal or rolled oats, cooked.	¾ cup	110
Rice, cooked	¾ cup	150
Rice flakes	1 cup (about 1 ounce)	115
Rice, puffed	1 cup (about ½ ounce).	55
Spaghetti, cooked	¾ cup	115
Spaghetti with meat sauce..	¾ cup	215
Spaghetti in tomato sauce, with cheese.	¾ cup	160
Wheat, puffed	1 ounce (about 2⅛ cups)	100
Wheet, puffed, presweetened	1 ounce (about 2⅛ cups)	105
Wheat, rolled, cooked	¾ cup	130
Wheat, shredded, plain (long, round, or bite-size).	1 ounce (1 large biscuit or about ½ cup bite-size).	100
Wheat flakes	1 ounce (about ¾ cup)..	100
Wheat flours:		
Whole wheat	¾ cup, stirred	300
All-purpose (or family) flour.	¾ cup, sifted	300
Wheat germ	¾ cup, stirred	185

FATS, OILS AND RELATED PRODUCTS

Butter or margarine	1 tablespoon	100
	1 pat or square (64 per pound).	50
Cooking fat:		
Vegetable	1 tablespoon	110
Lard	1 tablespoon	135
Salad or cooking oils	1 tablespoon	125
Salad dressings:		
French	1 tablespoon	60
Blue cheese, French	1 tablespoon	90
Home-cooked, boiled	1 tablespoon	30
Low-calorie	1 tablespoon	15
Mayonnaise	1 tablespoon	110

FATS, OILS AND RELATED PRODUCTS—Continued

		Number of Calories
Salad dressing, commercial, plain (mayonnaise type).	1 tablespoon	60
Thousand Island	1 tablespoon	75

SUGARS, SWEETS AND RELATED PRODUCTS

Candy:		
Caramels	1 ounce (3 medium caramels).	120
Chocolate creams	1 ounce (2 to 3 pieces, 35 to a pound).	110
Chocolate, milk, sweetened .	1-ounce bar	145
Chocolate, milk, sweetened, with almonds.	1-ounce bar	150
Chocolate mints	1 ounce (1 to 2 mints, 20 to a pound).	110
Fudge, milk chocolate, plain	1 ounce (1 piece, 1 to 1½ inches square).	115
Gumdrops	1 ounce (about 2½ large or 20 small).	95
Hard candy	1 ounce (3 to 4 candy balls, ¾ inch in diameter).	110
Jellybeans	1 ounce (10 beans)	65
Marshmallows	1 ounce (3 to 4 marshmallows, 60 to a pound).	90
Peanut brittle	1 ounce (1½ pieces, 2½ by 1¼ inches by ⅜ inch).	125
Sirup, honey, molasses:		
Chocolate sirup	1 tablespoon	40
Honey, strained or extracted	1 tablespoon	60
Molasses, cane, light	1 tablespoon	50
Sirup, table blends	1 tablespoon	55
Jelly	1 tablespoon	50
Jam, marmalade, preserves ...	1 tablespoon	55
Sugar: White, granulated, or brown.	1 teaspoon	15

SOUPS

Bean	1 cup	190
Beef	1 cup	100
Bouillon, broth, and consomme	1 cup	10
Chicken	1 cup	75
Clam chowder	1 cup	85
Cream soup (asparagus, celery, or mushroom).	1 cup	200
Noodle, rice, or barley	1 cup	115
Oyster stew	1 cup (3 to 4 oysters) ...	200
Tomato	1 cup	90
Vegetable	1 cup	80

DESSERTS

Apple betty	½ cup	175
Cakes:		
Angelcake	2-inch sector (1/12 of 8-inch round cake).	110
Butter cakes:		
Plain, without icing	1 piece, 3 by 2 by 1½ inches.	180
	1 cupcake, 2¾ inches in diameter.	130
Plain, with icing	2-inch sector (1/16 of 10-inch round layer cake).	320
	1 cupcake, 2¾ inches in diameter.	160
Chocolate, with fudge icing.	2-inch sector (1/16 of 10-inch round layer cake).	420
Fruitcake, dark	1 piece, 2 by 2 inches by ½ inch.	105
Gingerbread	1 piece, 2 by 2 inches by ½ inch.	180
Pound cake	1 slice, 2¾ by 3 inches by ⅝ inch.	130
Sponge cake	2-inch sector (1/12 of 8-inch round cake).	115
Cookies, plain and assorted ..	1 cooky, 3 inches in diameter.	110
Cornstarch pudding	½ cup	140
Custard, baked	½ cup	140
Fig bars, small	1 fig bar	55
Fruit ice	½ cup	75
Gelatin dessert, plain, ready-to-serve.	½ cup	80
Ice cream, plain	1 container (3½ fluid ounces).	130
Ice milk	½ cup (4 fluid ounces)..	140

CALORIE VALUES IN COMMON FOODS

DESSERTS—Continued		Number of Calories
Pies:		
Apple	4-inch sector (1/7 of 9-inch pie).	330
Cherry	4-inch sector (1/7 of 9-inch pie).	340
Custard	4-inch sector (1/7 of 9-inch pie).	265
Lemon meringue	4-inch sector (1/7 of 9-inch pie).	300
Mince	4-inch sector (1/7 of 9-inch pie).	340
Pumpkin	4-inch sector (1/7 of 9-inch pie).	265
Prune whip	½ cup	100
Rennet dessert pudding, ready-to-serve.	½ cup	125
Sherbet	½ cup	120

BEVERAGES

Carbonated beverages:		
Ginger ale	8-ounce glass	80
Kola type	8-ounce glass	105
"Low-calorie" type beverage (with artificial sweetener).	8-ounce glass	10
Postum	1 cup	5
Coffee or tea		0
Alcoholic beverages:		
Beer, 4 percent alcohol	8-ounce glass	115
Whisky, gin, rum:		
100-proof	1 jigger (1½ ounces)	125
90-proof	1 jigger (1½ ounces)	110
86-proof	1 jigger (1½ ounces)	105
80-proof	1 jigger (1½ ounces)	100
70-proof	1 jigger (1½ ounces)	85

BEVERAGES—Continued		Number of Calories
Wines:		
Table wines (such as Chablis, claret, Rhine wine, and sauterne).	1 wine glass (about 3 ounces).	70-90
Sweet or dessert wines (such as muscatel, port, sherry, and Tokay).	1 wine glass (about 3 ounces).	120-160

MISCELLANEOUS

Bouillon cubes	2 cubes, small	5
Olives:		
Green	6 "Extra large" or 3 "Jumbo" size.	30
Ripe	6 "Extra large" or 3 "Jumbo" size.	40
Pickles, cucumber:		
Dill	1 large, 1¾ inches in diameter by 4 inches long.	15
Sweet	1 pickle, ¾ inch in diameter by 2¾ inches long.	20
Mixed, chopped	1 tablespoon	15
Popcorn, popped (with 1 teaspoon added fat).	1 cup	90
Relishes and sauces:		
Chili sauce	1 tablespoon	15
Tomato catsup	1 tablespoon	15
Gravy	2 tablespoons	35
White sauce, medium (1 cup milk, 2 tablespoons fat, and 2 tablespoons flour.)	½ cup	215
Cheese sauce (medium white sauce with 2 tablespoons cheese per cup).	½ cup	250

FAST FOODS CALORIE CHART

Items	Calories	Items	Calories	Items	Calories
KENTUCKY FRIED CHICKEN		Bellbeefer	243	Onion Rings	
Original Recipe Chicken		Burrito Supreme	387	Regular	266
Wing	136			Large	331
Drumstick	117	**JACK IN THE BOX**		French Fries	
Keel	235	Hamburger	263	Regular	209
Rib	199	Cheeseburger	310	Large	359
Thigh	257	Hamburger Deluxe	260	Chocolate Shake	337
Extra Crispy Chicken		Cheeseburger Deluxe	314	Vanilla Shake	336
Wing	201	Bonus Jack®	461		
Drumstick	155	Jumbo Jack®	551	**WENDY'S OLD**	
Keel	297	with cheese	628	**FASHIONED**	
Rib	286	Regular Taco	189	**HAMBURGERS**	
Thigh	343	Super Taco	285	Hamburgers	
		Jack Burrito®	448	Single	472
McDONALD'S		Moby Jack®	455	Double	669
Egg McMuffin	352	Jack Steak®	428	Triple	853
Hot cakes with butter		Breakfast Jack®	301	Single w/cheese	577
& syrup	472	French Fries	270	Double w/cheese	797
Scrambled eggs	162	Onion Rings	351	Triple w/cheese	1,036
Hash browns	130	Lemon Turnover	446	Chili	229
Pork sausage	184	Apple Turnover	411	French Fries	327
English Muffin with butter	186			Frosty	391
Hamburger	257	**BURGER KING®**			
Cheeseburger	306	Hamburger	293	**ARBY'S®**	
Quarter Pounder	418	with cheese	347	Sandwich	
Quarter Pounder with cheese	518	Doublemeat	413	Roast Beef	350
Big Mac	541	with cheese	519	Beef 'n' Cheese	450
		WHOPPER	631	Super Roast Beef	620
TACO BELL		with cheese	740	Junior Roast Beef	220
Taco	159	WHOPPER		Swiss King	660
Pintos 'n' cheese	231	Doublemeat	843	Ham 'n' Cheese	380
Tostada	206	with cheese	951	Turkey	410
Bean Burrito	345	WHOPPER Jr.	369	Turkey Deluxe	510
Enchirito	391	with cheese	424	Club	560
Beefy Tostada	291	Apple Pie	250	Cole Slaw	83
				French Fries	211
				Apple Turnover	300

SAMPLE DIETS
FIRST DAY

LOW CALORIE — 1,200 Calories   **NORMAL — 3,000 Calories**

BREAKFAST

Low Calorie		Normal	
Grapefruit	½ medium.	Grapefruit	½ medium.
Wheat flakes	1 ounce.	Wheat flakes	1 ounce.
Skim milk	1½ cups.	Banana	1 medium.
Coffee (black), if desired.		Whole milk	1½ cups.
		Toast, enriched	2 slices.
		Butter or margarine	1½ teaspoons.
		Coffee	1 cup.
		Cream	1 tablespoon.
		Sugar	1 teaspoon.

LUNCH

Low Calorie		Normal	
Chef's salad:		Chef's salad:	
Julienne chicken	1 ounce.	Julienne chicken	2 ounces.
Cheddar cheese	½ ounce.	Cheddar cheese	1 ounce.
Hard-cooked egg	½ egg.	Hard-cooked egg	½ egg.
Tomato	1 large.	Tomato	1 large.
Cucumber	6 slices.	Cucumber	6 slices.
Endive	½ ounce.	Endive	½ ounce.
Lettuce	⅛ head.	Lettuce	⅛ head.
French dressing	2 tablespoons.	French dressing	2 tablespoons.
Rye wafers	4 wafers.	Rye wafers	4 wafers.
Skim milk	1 cup.	Gingerbread	2-inch square piece.
		Lemon sauce	¼ cup.
		Whole milk	1 cup.

DINNER

Low Calorie		Normal	
Beef pot roast	3 ounces.	Beef pot roast	3 ounces.
Mashed potatoes	⅓ cup.	Gravy	¼ cup.
Green peas	½ cup.	Mashed potatoes	⅔ cup.
Whole-wheat bread	1 slice.	Green peas, buttered	½ cup.
Butter or margarine	½ teaspoon.	Rolls, enriched	2 small.
Fruit cup:		Butter or margarine	1 teaspoon.
Orange	½ small.	Fruit cup:	
Apple	½ small.	Orange	½ small.
Banana	½ medium.	Apple	½ small.
		Banana	½ medium.
		Plain cooky	1 medium.

BETWEEN-MEAL SNACK

Sandwich:	
Enriched bread	2 slices.
Beef pot roast	2 ounces.
Mayonnaise	2 teaspoons.
Lettuce	1 large leaf.
Whole milk	1 cup.

SAMPLE DIETS

SECOND DAY

LOW CALORIE — 1,200 Calories   **NORMAL — 3,000 Calories**

BREAKFAST

Orange juice	½ cup.	Orange juice	½ cup.
Soft-cooked egg	1 egg.	Soft-cooked egg	1 egg.
Whole-wheat toast	1 slice.	Bacon	2 strips.
Butter or margarine	1 teaspoon.	Whole-wheat toast	2 slices.
Skim milk	1 cup.	Butter or margarine	2 teaspoons.
Coffee (black), if desired.		Whole milk	1 cup.
		Coffee	1 cup.
		Cream	1 tablespoon.
		Sugar	1 teaspoon.

LUNCH

Sandwich:		Tomato soup	1 cup.
Enriched bread	2 slices.	Sandwich:	
Boiled ham	1½ ounces.	Enriched bread	3 slices.
Mayonnaise	2 teaspoons.	Boiled ham	3 ounces.
Mustard		Mayonnaise	2½ teaspoons.
Lettuce	1 large leaf.	Mustard	
Celery	1 small stalk.	Lettuce	2 large leaves.
Radishes	4 radishes.	Celery	1 small stalk.
Dill pickle	½ large.	Radishes	4 radishes.
Skim milk	1 cup.	Dill pickle	½ large.
		Apple	1 medium.
		Whole milk	1 cup.

DINNER

Roast lamb	3 ounces.	Roast lamb	4 ounces.
Rice, converted	½ cup.	Rice, converted	⅔ cup.
Spinach	¾ cup.	Spinach, buttered	⅔ cup.
Lemon	¼ medium.	Lemon	¼ medium.
Salad:		Salad:	
Peaches, canned	1 half peach.	Peaches, canned	2 halves.
Cottage cheese	⅓ cup.	Cottage cheese	⅓ cup.
Lettuce	1 large leaf.	Lettuce	1 large leaf.
		Rolls, enriched	2 small.
		Butter or margarine	1 teaspoon.
		Plain cake, iced	2-inch piece layer cake.

BETWEEN-MEAL SNACK

Apple	1 medium.	Soda crackers	4 crackers.
		Peanut butter	2 tablespoons.
		Whole milk	1 cup.

SAMPLE DIETS

THIRD DAY

LOW CALORIE — 1,200 Calories   **NORMAL — 3,000 Calories**

BREAKFAST

Tomato juice . . . .   ½ cup.   Tomato juice . . . .   ½ cup.
French toast: French toast:
  Enriched bread . . . . . .   1 slice.   Enriched bread . . . . . .   2 slices.
  Egg . . . .   ½ egg.   Egg . . . .   ½ egg.
  Milk   Milk
Butter or margarine . . . .   1 teaspoon.   Butter or margarine . . . .   1½ teaspoons.
Jelly . . . .   1½ teaspoons.   Sirup . . . .   4 tablespoons.
Skim milk . . . .   1 cup.   Whole milk . . . .   1 cup.
Coffee (black), if desired.   Coffee . . . .   1 cup.
                                                      Cream . . . .   1 tablespoon.
                                                      Sugar . . . .   1 teaspoon.

LUNCH

Tunafish salad: Tunafish salad:
  Tunafish . . . .   2 ounces.   Tunafish . . . .   3 ounces.
  Hard-cooked egg . . . .   ½ egg.   Hard-cooked egg . . . .   ½ egg.
  Celery . . . .   1 small stalk.   Celery . . . .   1 small stalk.
  Lemon juice . . . .   1 teaspoon.   Lemon juice . . . .   1 teaspoon.
  Salad dressing . . . . . .   1½ tablespoons.   Salad dressing . . . .   2½ tablespoons.
  Lettuce . . . .   1 large leaf.   Lettuce . . . .   1 large leaf.
Whole-wheat bread . . . .   2 slices.   Whole-wheat bread . . . .   2 slices.
Butter or margarine . . . .   1 teaspoon.   Butter or margarine . . . .   1 teaspoon.
Carrot sticks . . . .   ½ carrot.   Carrot sticks . . . .   ½ carrot.
Skim milk . . . .   1 cup.   Grapes . . . .   1 large bunch.
                                                    Whole milk . . . .   1 cup.

DINNER

Beef liver . . . .   3 ounces.   Beef liver . . . .   4 ounces.
Green snap beans . . . . . .   ⅔ cup.   Bacon . . . .   2 strips.
Shredded cabbage . . . . .   ⅔ cup.   Mashed potatoes . . . .   ⅔ cup.
  with vinegar   Green snap beans,   ⅔ cup.
  dressing.   buttered.
Roll, enriched . . . .   1 small.   Coleslaw . . . .   ⅔ cup.
Butter or margarine . . . .   ½ teaspoon.   Rolls, enriched . . . .   2 small.
Grapes . . . .   1 small bunch.   Butter or margarine . . . .   1 teaspoon.
                                                    Cherry pie . . . .   4-inch piece.

BETWEEN-MEAL SNACK

Orange . . . .   1 medium.   Orange . . . .   1 medium.
                                                    Iced cupcake . . . .   1 medium.
                                                    Whole milk . . . .   1 cup.

BLAND DIET

FOOD CLASS	FOODS ALLOWED	FOODS TO AVOID
Milk	Reconstituted or Fresh Whole—Skim or Evaporated Milk Buttermilk Yogurt Sweet or Sour Cream Bland Cream Soups Flavored Milks Ice Cream Milk Desserts Ex: Junket—Custard	Very Cold Milk Drinks
Vegetables	CANNED or COOKED WITHOUT HARD SKINS— SEEDS or FIBERS— Asparagus Celery Juice Mushrooms—Spinach Tomato Juice or Puree (not Tomato Paste, Sauce or Catsup) String or Wax Beans Beets—Carrots Pumpkin—Peas Winter Squash Uncooked, Tender Lettuce	HARD SKINS, SEEDS or FIBERS Raw Vegetables or Salads Celery—Brussel Sprouts—Broccoli Cabbage—Cauliflower Corn—Cucumbers Eggplant—Kale Garlic—Okra—Onions Peppers—Radishes Rutabagas—Turnips Summer Squash Zucchini Fresh or Unstrained Tomatoes Dried Lentils
Fruits	COOKED or CANNED WITHOUT SKINS or SEEDS— Apple—Apricots Canned Fruit— Cocktail Cherries Peaches—Pears and Skinned Purple Plums 1 Fresh Ripe Banana JUICES: Grapefruit Orange—Lemon for flavor Peach-Pear-Apricot Apple—Prune Pineapple Clear Fruit Jellies	HARD SKINS, SEEDS or FIBERS— Raw—Dried Fruits Apples—Berries Cherries—Dates Figs—Grapes Raisins—Mangos Grapefruit—Orange Tangerine—Peaches Pears—Plums (Prunes) Pineapple—Melon Jams Conserves Marmalades
Eggs	Poached Soft Cooked Eggnog Soft Scrambled Baked Omelet	Fried Egg or Fried Omelet
Meats	Well Cooked and Tender—Lean Beef—Lamb—Liver Sweetbreads Brains-Lungs, etc. Veal	Less Tender— Patty or Fried Meats, Spices or Gravies Pork Canned Meats and Sausages
Poultry	White or Dark Meat of Chicken or Turkey	Duck or Goose
Fish or	Canned—Unspiced Fish—Salmon and Tuna Fish Fresh Fish Flounder—Cod, etc.	Spiced—Pickled or Smoked Fish Sardines— Anchovies, etc.

FOOD CLASS	FOODS ALLOWED	FOODS TO AVOID
Cheese	Cream—Cottage Farmer or Riccotta Mild Processed American Cheese Muenster or Swiss Small amounts of Cheddar Cheese for flavor	Vegetable, Spice, or Nuts in American Cheese Cottage or Cream Cheese Limburger—Blue Sharp Cheese
Bread or Cereals or	Enriched White Bread—Crackers Biscuits Melba Toast Zwieback Strained Oatmeal or Pettijohns Farina—White Rice—Pearled Barley—All Dry Cereal—without Bran Wheatena or Ralston Strained Oatmeal	Whole Grain Breads or Cereals Seeded Bread Whole Oatmeal or Pettijohns Kasha—Brown Rice—Bran Corn Flakes
Starches and Substitutes	Skinless White Potatoes or Yams Spaghetti Macaroni Noodles or Rice	Fried Noodles Popcorn Skins—Sweet Potatoes Fried Potatoes Potato Chips
Desserts	Cookies or Plain Cakes Yeast Cakes Meringue Eclairs Simple Puddings Jello—Custard Junket Plain Ice Cream— Sherbets Fruit Puree—Whips Sugar—Honey Molasses Corn—Maple or Fruit Syrups Clear Jellies	Rich—Spiced or Fruited Cakes Pies—Doughnuts or Rich Pastries Nuts—Fruit or Cocoanut Jams—Conserves Preserves Marmalades
Fats	NOT FOR FRYING Butter—Margarine Sweet or Sour Cream Mayonnaise	Fried Foods of any kind Meat Suet or Drippings—(Bacon) Peanut or other Nut Butters
Miscellaneous	Salt Sugar Lemon Juice Small amounts of Papricka or Cinnamon—Vanilla Coffee—Tea—Cocoa or Substitutes if permitted by Doctor Cream Soups made with allowed Vegetables or Cereals	Carbonated Beverages Beer—Liquors Most Canned Soups Highly Seasoned Soups or Bouillon Herbs—Spices Condiments Chocolate Nuts or Cocoanuts

Food and Nutrition Board, National Academy of Sciences—National Research Council**
Recommended daily dietary allowances[1]

Designed for the maintenance of good nutrition of practically all healthy persons in the U.S.A.
(Allowances are intended for persons normally active in a temperate climate)

Age[2] Years	Weight kg. (lbs.)	Height cm. (in.)	Calories[3]	Protein Gm.	Calcium Gm.	Iron mg.	Vitamin A I.U.	Thiamine mg.	Riboflavin mg.	Equiv.[4] Niacin mg.	Ascorbic Acid mg.	Vitamin D I.U.
Men												
18–35	70 (154)	175 (69)	2,900	70	0.8	10	5,000*	1.2	1.7	19	70	...
35–55	70 (154)	175 (69)	2,600	70	0.8	10	5,000	1.0	1.6	17	70	...
55–75	70 (154)	175 (69)	2,200	70	0.8	10	5,000	0.9	1.3	15	70	...
Women												
18–35	58 (128)	163 (64)	2,100	58	0.8	15	5,000	0.8	1.3	14	70	...
35–55	58 (128)	163 (64)	1,900	58	0.8	15	5,000	0.8	1.2	13	70	...
55–75	58 (128)	163 (64)	1,600	58	0.8	10	5,000	0.8	1.2	13	70	...
Pregnant (2nd & 3rd trimester)			+200	+20	+0.5	+5	+1,000	+0.2	+0.3	+3	+30	400
Lactating			+1,000	+40	+0.5	+5	+3,000	+0.4	+0.6	+7	+30	400
Infants[5]												
0–1	8 (18)		kg. x 115 ±15	kg. x 2.5 ±0.5	0.7 kg. x 1.0		1,500	0.4	0.6	6	30	400
Children												
1–3	13 (29)	87 (34)	1,300	32	0.8	8	2,000	0.5	0.8	9	40	400
3–6	18 (40)	107 (42)	1,600	40	0.8	10	2,500	0.6	1.0	11	50	400
6–9	24 (53)	124 (49)	2,100	52	0.8	12	3,500	0.8	1.3	14	60	400
Boys												
9–12	33 (72)	140 (55)	2,400	60	1.1	15	4,500	1.0	1.4	16	70	400
12–15	45 (98)	156 (61)	3,000	75	1.4	15	5,000	1.2	1.8	20	80	400
15–18	61 (134)	172 (68)	3,400	85	1.4	15	5,000	1.4	2.0	22	80	400
Girls												
9–12	33 (72)	140 (55)	2,200	55	1.1	15	4,500	0.9	1.3	15	80	400
12–15	47 (103)	158 (62)	2,500	62	1.3	15	5,000	1.0	1.5	17	80	400
15–18	53 (117)	163 (64)	2,300	58	1.3	15	5,000	0.9	1.3	15	70	400

[1] The allowance levels are intended to cover individual variations among most normal persons as they live in the United States under usual environmental stresses. The recommended allowances can be attained with a variety of common foods, providing other nutrients for which human requirements have been less well defined.

[2] Entries on lines for age range 18–35 year represent the 25-year age. All other entries represent allowances for the midpoint of the specified age periods, i.e., line for children 1–3 is for age 2 years (24 months); 3–6 is for age 4½ (54 months), etc.

[3] Table shows calorie adjustments for weight and age.

[4] Niacin equivalents include dietary sources of the preformed vitamin and the precursor, tryptophan. 60 mg. tryptophan represents 1 mg. niacin.

[5] The calorie and protein allowances per kg. for infants are considered to decrease progressively from birth. Allowances for calcium, thiamine, riboflavin, and niacin increase proportionately with calories to the maximum values shown.

* 1,000 I.U. from preformed vitamin A and 4,000 I.U. from beta-carotene.

**Reprinted by permission, revised

Index of Black-and-White
Anatomical and Medical Illustrations

Index

Cross references without numbers refer to the Index.

Murray, Dr. Henry A.; see Thematic apperception test, 476

Muscle
 contractions; see Tension symptoms, 475-76
 disease; see Infantile paralysis (poliomyelitis), 307; Muscular dystrophy, 359; Myasthenia gravis, 359-60
 flabbiness; see Exercises
 spasticity, 459
 sphincter, 460
 tics, 480

Muscular and Skeletal systems, (Plates D1-D8) following page 160
 anatomy of a bone, Plate D5
 articulation of bone at a joint, Plate D8
 control of the muscles, Plate D3
 femero-pelvic joint, cross section, Plate D8
 femur, posterior view, Plate D5
 growth of a bone, Plate D7
 head and neck of femur, cross section, Plate D5
 muscle action, Plate D4
 muscle bundle, cross section, Plate D2
 muscles, Plate D1
 newborn femur, cross section, Plate D6
 shaft, cross section, Plate D5
 skeleton in adult, Plate D7
 skeleton in infancy, Plate D6

Muscular dystrophy, 359
Mushroom poisoning, 359
Myasthenia gravis, 359-60
Mycobacterium balnei; see Swimming pool granuloma, 469
Mycosis fungoides, 360
Myopia (nearsightedness), 362
Myxedema, 360; see also "Underactive Thyroid" (hypothyroidism), 497

Nail-biting, 360
Nail polish remover; see Table of common poisons, 534-36
Nails; see Fingernails; Skin, function and structure; Toenail
Narcoanalysis, 360-61
Narcolepsy, 361
Narcotics, 180-86, 199-201
 addiction, 183-86
 cough-controlling, 193
 as pain-lesseners, 201
 see also Table of common poisons, 534-36
Nasal polyps, 361
Nasopharynx, 361
National Amputation Foundation, 610
National Association for Mental Health; see Special health problems, 609-10
National Diabetes Association, 605
National Foundation; see Communicable diseases, 606-7
National Guard; see Accidents and emergencies, 605-6
National Health Council; see Special health problems, 609-10
National Hospital for Speech Disorders; see Stuttering and stammering, 466-67
National Tuberculosis Association; see Communicable diseases, 606-7; Special health problems, 609-10
Nausea and vomiting, 361-62
 in pregnancy; see Morning sickness, 356-57

treatment; see Bland diet, 559, 620
 see also Vomiting, cyclic, 512; Vomiting (emesis) in children, 512-13
Navel (umbilicus), 362
 cord, umbilical, 140-41
Nearsightedness (myopia), 362
Neck
 fracture, see Fractures, 530-32
 stiff; see Head pain, 596; Lockjaw, 335; Meningitis, 350
 see also Throat
Nembutal; see Table of common poisons, 534-36
Neoplasm; see Cancer, 91; Tumors
Nephritis, 362-63; see also Dropsy, 180
Nephrolithiasis, 363
Nephron, 363
Nephrosis; see Nephrotic syndrome and nephrosis, 363
Nephrotic syndrome and nephrosis, 363
Nerve cell (neuron), 363
 sensory, 445
Nerve disorders
 causalgia, 108-9
 general paresis, 382
 neuralgia, 365
 neuritis, 365-66
 shingles (herpes zoster), 446-47
Nerve fibers, 363-64
Nerves
 cell (neuron), 363, 445
 cranial, 144-45; see also Spinal accessory nerves, 460
 facial, 236
 facial and acoustic; see Acoustic neuroma, 17
 fibers, 363-64
 glossopharyngeal, 267
 hypoglossal, 300
 median, 347
 optic, 374
 peripheral, 390-91
 phrenic, 396
 radial, 423
 sciatic, 441
 sensory cells, 445
 spinal accessory, 460
 trigeminal, 487
 ulnar, 496
 vagus, 503
 see also Nerve disorders; Spinal cord, 460-61; Synapse, 469-70
"Nervous breakdown," 364
"Nervousness," 364
 anxiety and fear, 44-45
 Graves' disease, 269-70
 high-strung and thin, 577
 jumpiness and irritability, 602-3
 "nervous breakdown," 364
 premenstrual syndrome, 409, 568
 tension symptoms, 475-76
 see also Tension
Nervous system, 364-65
 autonomic, 63
 central, 109-10
 voluntary, 512
 see also Nerve disorders, Nerves
Nervous system, (Plates H1-H8) following page 288
 anatomy of central nervous system, Plate H3

brain, cross section, Plate H3
contact with internal organs, Plate H7
contact with muscles, Plate H6
flexor withdrawal, Plate H8
major nerves, Plate H1
motor cell, Plate H4
neuron—location and anatomy, Plate H4
parts of nervous system, Plate H2
reflex activities of spinal cord, Plate H8
relationship between central, peripheral, and autonomic systems, Plate H3
sensation—contact with environment, Plate H5
sensory cell, Plate H4
spinal cord, cross section, Plate H3
stretch reflex, Plate H8
Neuralgia, 365
 trigeminal, 487-88
Neurasthenia; see Neurosis, 366-67
Neuritis, 365
Neurodermatitis; see Eczema, 213
Neurologist, 366
Neuron (nerve cell), 363, 445
Neurosis, 366-67
 alcohol and alcoholism, 23-25
 anxiety and fear, 44-45
 claustrophobia, 120-21
 compulsions, 127
 conduct disorders, 128
 conflict, mental, 129
 conversion reaction, 139
 depression, 167-68
 electra complex, 214
 emotions in allergy, 217-18
 excoriations, 367-68
 guilt, 270-71
 hypochondriasis, 299-300
 hysteria, 139, 462
 insecurity, 310-11
 insomnia, 311-12
 mental illness, 353
 obsessions, 372
 Oedipus complex, 373-74
 overprotection, psychological, 378
 paranoid states, 381-82
 personal social behavior, 393
 phobia, 395-96
 promiscuity, 411
 regression, 425
 repression, 425-26
 self-consciousness, 444
 sociopathic reactions, 457-58
 "split personality," 462
 stuttering and stammering, 466-67
 tension symptoms, 475-76
 see also Psychoneurosis; Psychoses
Neurotic excoriations, 367-68
Neutralizing agents; see Alkalinizing agents
Nevus flammeus (port-wine stain), 406-7
Nevus, spider; see Spider nevus, 460
Newborn
 acne, 16
 jaundice, 323
 Rh factor and Rh sensitization, 433-34
 see also Babies; Children; Infants
NGU, 549-50
Nicotine; see Drugs, 200; Smoking, 456-57
Niemann-Pick's disease; see Splenic disorders 461-63
Night blindness (nyctalopia), 368

prolapse of, 411
Rectus muscle, 425
Red Cross, American, 605-6
Reflex arc, 425
Regression, 425; *see also* Infantilism, 307-8; Schizophrenia, 440-41
Rehabilitation, 425
Renal colic, 563-64
Repression, 425-26
Reproduction; *see* Ovulation, 380
Reproduction and fetal development, (Plates J1-J8) following page 352
comparative sizes in embryos, Plate J6
estrogen stage, Plate J2
external appearance of embryo, Plate J6
female reproductive organs, Plate J1
implantation, Plate J4
lunar months, Plate J7
menstrual cycle, Plate J2
ovulation, Plate J2
period of fetus, Plate J7
pregnancy (first week), Plate J3
pregnancy (second month), Plate J6
pregnancy (second week), Plate J4
pregnancy (third and fourth weeks), Plate J5
progesterone stage, Plate J2
Reserpine; *see* Blood pressure, high, drugs for, 192-93; Tranquilizers, 203
Residue diet, low-, 336-37
Respiration (breathing), 426-27
Respiratory and digestive systems, (Plates A1-A8) following page 64
alveoli (in cross section), Plate A3
bronchial tree, Plate A2
chemistry of digestion, Plates A6, A7
digestive system, Plate A4
empty stomach, Plate A8
expiration, Plate A2
food in the intestines, Plate A8
food in the stomach, Plate A8
function of bronchial tree, Plate A2
inspiration, Plate A2
mechanics of digestion, Plate A4
nervous control of digestion, Plate A8
respiratory movements, Plate A2
Respiratory disorders
bronchiectasis, 83-84
bronchitis, 84-85
bronchopneumonia, 85-86
infection, 427-29
Respiratory system; *see* Respiration (breathing), 426-27
Respiratory tract infection, 427-29
Restoration, 429
Retina, 429
blood vessel changes in, 429
closure of central artery, 429
closure of central vein, 429-30
detachment, 430
disorders, 430
hemorrhage, 430
macular disease, 430
oxygen damage (retrolental fibroplasia), 430
pigmented degeneration (retinitis pigmentosa), 431
Retinoblastoma; *see* Eye, tumors of the, 235-36
RH antigen, 433-34
Rheumatic fever, 431

Rheumatic heart disease, 431-32
Rheumatism and arthritis, 432-33
American Rheumatism Association, 432
Arthritis and Rheumatism Foundation, 610
Rh factor and Rh sensitization, 433-34
Rhinitis
allergic coryza, 26
atrophic, 60
hyperplastic, 298
nasal polyps, 361
sicca, 434
Rhinoplasty, 434
Rhythm method, 138
irregular menstrual cycles, 568-69
Rib
fracture, 532
Riboflavin, 507
Rickets, 434-35
Rickettsia, quintana; *see* Trench foot, 486
Riedel's struma; *see* Thyroiditis, 479-80
Ringworm of the scalp, 435
Rivalry among children, 448
Roach poison, 536
Rocky Mountain spotted fever, 522
Rodent poison, 534, 536
Role-playing, 435
Root-canal treatment, 435-36
Rorschach test, 436
Rosacea, 436
Roseola, 436-37
Rough marsh elder; *see* Ragweed pollen, 423
Roundworm
drugs for; *see* Intestinal parasitic disease drugs, 197-98
trichinosis, 487
Rubella (German measles), 437
Rumination; *see* vomiting (emesis) in children, 512-13
Rupture
uterus, 501
see also Hernia

Sabin vaccine; *see* Infantile paralysis (poliomyelitis), 307
"Safe period"; *see* Rhythm method, 138
Safety belts; *see* Accident prevention, 520-21
Safety, sickroom; *see* Sickroom equipment, 548-51
Safety tips; *see* Accident prevention, 520-21
St. Anthony's Fire; *see* Erysipelas, 225-26
St. Vitus' dance (Sydenham's chorea), 437
Saline laxatives; *see* Laxatives, 198-99
Saliva, 437-38
Salivary glands, 438; *see also* Parotid glands, 383
Salk vaccine; *see* Infantile paralysis (poliomyelitis), 307
Salmonella typhosa; see Typhoid fever, 494-95
Salpingitis, 438-39
Salt; *see* Sodium
Salt diet, low-, 337-38
Sample diets; *see* Appendix, 617-19
Sarcoma; *see* Tumors, 492-93; Types of cancer, 93-94
Sarcoptes scabiei; see Scabies, 439
Scabies, 439
Scalp

caput succedaneum (swollen scalp, infant), 104
itching and flakiness, 598-99
ringworm, 435
seborrheic dermatitis (dandruff), 443-44
Scalp, ringworm of the, 435
Scarlatina; *see* Scarlet fever, 439
Scarlet fever, 439
Scars, 439-40
Schizophrenia, 440-41
School health services, 607-8
Sciatica; see Low-back pain, 335-36; Slipped disk, 455
Sciatic nerve, 441
Sclera, inflammation of; *see* Scleritis, 441-42
Scleritis, 441-42
Scleroderma, diffuse systemic, 442
Scleroderma, localized (morphea), 442-43
Scleroma, 443
Sclerosis; *see* Multiple sclerosis, 357-58
Scoliosis, 443
Scorpion; *see* Bites (scorpion) (ticks), 522
Scratching; *see* Neurotic excoriations, 367-68
Scratch test; *see* Allergies, diagnosis of, 30-31
Scrotum, 443
varicocele, 503
Scurvy, 443
Seasonal allergies, 443
Sebaceous (oil) glands; *see* Skin, function and structure, 449-52
seborrheic dermatitis, 443-44
Seborrheic dermatitis, 443-44
Seborrheic keratosis, 324
Seconal; *see* Table of common poisons, 534-36
Sedatives, 183, 201
Segmentectomy; *see* Thoracotomy, 477; Tuberculosis, 488-92
Seizures; *see* Convulsions
febrile, first aid for; *see* Convulsions, 527
Self-concept, 444
Self-consciousness, 444
Selfishness; *see* Sibling rivalry, 448
Self psychologies; *see* Self-concept, 444
Semen; *see* Sperm (atozoa) reddish, 569-70
Seminal vesicle; *see* Vesicle, seminal, 504
Senescence and senility, 444-45
forgetfulness and silliness, 603
Senile keratosis, 324
Senility; *see* Senescence and senility
Senses, *see* Sensory nerve cell (neuron), 445
Sensory nerve cell (neuron), 445
Septic sore throat; *see* Pharyngitis, streptococcal, 394-95
Septum, nasal; *see* Nosebleed, 533
Serum sickness; *see* Drug allergy, 186-87
Seven danger signals (cancer), 94
Sex determination of fetus, 36
Sex instruction and sex-organ concern, 445-46
Sex inversion; *see* Homosexuality, 293-94
Sex-organ concern and sex instruction, 445-46
Sexual act, 446
Sexual Behavior in the Human Female, 325
Sexual Behavior in the Human Male, 325
Sexual development
adrenogenital syndrome, 21-22
breast, the immature female, 81
eunuchoidism, 227-28
fixation, developmental, 241
Freud, Sigmund, 247-48

Rescue Breathing

1. Clear the airway.

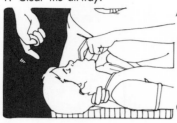

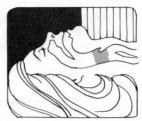

A. Hold the victim's mouth open with one hand using your thumb to depress the tongue . . .

B. Make a **Hook** with the **pointer finger** of your other hand, and in a gentle sweeping motion reach into the victim's throat and feel for a swallowed foreign object which may be blocking the air passage.

C. If **you need to,** reach all the way down to the voice box (larynx) and if there is a foreign object **remove** it.

2. Give mouth to mouth rescue breathing.

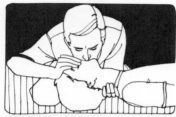

A. Put your hand on the victim's forehead, pinching the nose shut with your fingers, while holding the forehead back.

B. Your other hand is under the victim's neck **supporting and lifting up** slightly to maintain an **open airway.**

C. **Take a deep breath.** Open your mouth wide. Place it over the victim's mouth. **Blow air** into the victim until you see his or her chest rise . . .

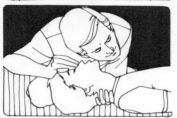

D. **Remove your mouth from the victim's.** Turn your head to the side and watch the chest for a falling movement while you **listen for air escaping** from the victim's mouth as he or she exhales.

E. If you **hear air escaping** and see the chest **fall** you know that rescue breathing is working. **Continue until help arrives.**

F. **Repeat** the cycle every **5 seconds. 12 breaths per minute.**

3. Mouth-to-mouth rescue breathing for a small child.

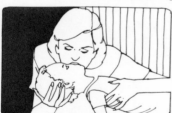

A. Be careful tilting a small child's head back to clear the airway. It **cannot tilt as far back** as an adult's.

B. Cover the child's **mouth and nose** with your mouth.

C. **Blow air in** with less pressure than for an adult. Give **small puffs.** A child needs less.

D. **Feel the chest inflate** as you blow . . .

E. **Listen** for exhales.

F. **Repeat** once **every 3 seconds. 20 breaths per minute.**

Note: It may take several hours to revive someone. Keep up **rescue breathing** until help arrives to relieve you. Remember you are doing the breathing for the victim. If you stop—in about 5 minutes—he or she could be dead!

Unconscious Person

Be careful approaching an unconscious person. **He or she may be in contact with electrical current. If that is the case, turn off the** electricity before you touch the victim.

There are hundreds of other possible causes of unconsciousness, but **the first thing you must check for is breathing.**

1. **Try to awaken the person:** Shake the victim's shoulder vigorously. Shout: "Are you all right?"

2. **If there is no response check for signs of breathing.**

   A. Be sure the victim is lying flat on his or her back. If you have to roll the victim over, move his or her entire body at one time.

   B. Loosen tight clothing around the neck and chest.

3. **Open the airway:**

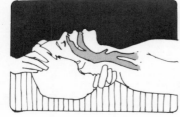

A. Lift up the neck **gently** with one hand.

B. Push down and back on the forehead with the other hand.

C. Place your ear close to the victim's mouth. **Listen for breath sounds.** Watch his or her chest and stomach for movement.

D. If there is any question in your mind, or if breathing is so faint that you are unsure . . . assume the worst!

E. **Give rescue breathing immediately.** Have someone else summon professional help.